# Clinical Approach and Management Strategies of Medical Ailments in Women
## Oorja—The Power of Her

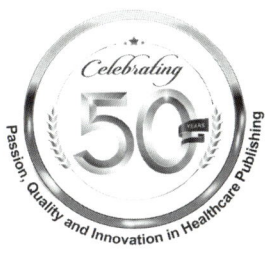

# Clinical Approach and Management Strategies of Medical Ailments in Women
## Oorja—The Power of Her

**Chief Editor**

**Shibba Takkar Chhabra** MBBS MD (Medicine) DM (Cardiology) FACC
Professor
Department of Cardiology
Dayanand Medical College and Hospital
Unit Hero DMC Heart Institute
Ludhiana, Punjab, India

**Co-Editors**

**Aastha Takkar Kapila** MBBS MD (Medicine) DM (Neurology)
Assistant Professor
Department of Neurology
Postgraduate Institute of Medical Education and Research
Chandigarh, India

**Anubha Rathi** MD
Consultant
The Cornea Institute
LV Prasad Eye Institute (LVPEI)
Hyderabad, Telangana, India

**Forewords**

Prem K Gupta
Daljit Singh
Gurpreet S Wander
Sandeep Puri

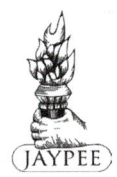

JAYPEE

**JAYPEE BROTHERS MEDICAL PUBLISHERS**
The Health Sciences Publisher
New Delhi | London

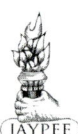 **Jaypee Brothers Medical Publishers (P) Ltd**

**Headquarters**
Jaypee Brothers Medical Publishers (P) Ltd
4838/24, Ansari Road, Daryaganj
New Delhi 110 002, India
Phone: +91-11-43574357
Fax: +91-11-43574314
Email: jaypee@jaypeebrothers.com

**Overseas Offices**
J.P. Medical Ltd
83 Victoria Street, London
SW1H 0HW (UK)
Phone: +44 20 3170 8910
Fax: +44 (0)20 3008 6180
Email: info@jpmedpub.com

Website: www.jaypeebrothers.com
Website: www.jaypeedigital.com

© 2020, Jaypee Brothers Medical Publishers

The views and opinions expressed in this book are solely those of the original contributor(s)/author(s) and do not necessarily represent those of editor(s) of the book.

All rights reserved. No part of this publication may be reproduced, stored or transmitted in any form or by any means, electronic, mechanical, photocopying, recording or otherwise, without the prior permission in writing of the publishers.

All brand names and product names used in this book are trade names, service marks, trademarks or registered trademarks of their respective owners. The publisher is not associated with any product or vendor mentioned in this book.

Medical knowledge and practice change constantly. This book is designed to provide accurate, authoritative information about the subject matter in question. However, readers are advised to check the most current information available on procedures included and check information from the manufacturer of each product to be administered, to verify the recommended dose, formula, method and duration of administration, adverse effects and contraindications. It is the responsibility of the practitioner to take all appropriate safety precautions. Neither the publisher nor the author(s)/editor(s) assume any liability for any injury and/or damage to persons or property arising from or related to use of material in this book.

This book is sold on the understanding that the publisher is not engaged in providing professional medical services. If such advice or services are required, the services of a competent medical professional should be sought.

Every effort has been made where necessary to contact holders of copyright to obtain permission to reproduce copyright material. If any have been inadvertently overlooked, the publisher will be pleased to make the necessary arrangements at the first opportunity. The **CD/DVD-ROM** (if any) provided in the sealed envelope with this book is complimentary and free of cost. **Not meant for sale.**

Inquiries for bulk sales may be solicited at: jaypee@jaypeebrothers.com

*Clinical Approach and Management Strategies of Medical Ailments in Women:*
*Oorja—The Power of Her* / Shibba Takkar Chhabra, Aastha Takkar Kapila, Anubha Rathi

*First Edition*: **2020**

ISBN: 978-93-89776-86-7

*Printed at: Sterling Graphics Pvt. Ltd. India.*

## *Dedication*

From the daughter to her father
"Who raised her, enabled her, and gave her the vision"

From the daughter to her mother
"Who gave her birth, inspired her and nurtured with strength"

From the wife to her husband
"Who was her armor, her strength, her confidence,
her belief and shield through everything"

From the disciple to the mentor
"Who trained, carved and polished her into a physician"

From the mother to her child
"Who is her angel and her world"

— **Shibba Takkar Chhabra**

# CONTRIBUTORS

## Chief Editor

**Shibba Takkar Chhabra** MBBS MD (Medicine) DM (Cardiology) FACC
Professor
Department of Cardiology
Dayanand Medical College and Hospital
Unit Hero DMC Heart Institute
Ludhiana, Punjab, India

## Co-Editors

**Aastha Takkar Kapila** MBBS MD (Medicine) DM (Neurology)
Assistant Professor
Department of Neurology
Postgraduate Institute of Medical Education and Research
Chandigarh, India

**Anubha Rathi** MD
Consultant
The Cornea Institute
LV Prasad Eye Institute (LVPEI)
Hyderabad, Telangana, India

## Section Editors

| | | |
|---|---|---|
| **Cardiology** | **Shibba Takkar Chhabra** MBBS MD (Medicine) DM (Cardiology) FACC<br>Professor<br>Department of Cardiology<br>Dayanand Medical College and Hospital<br>Unit Hero DMC Heart Institute<br>Ludhiana, Punjab, India | **Gurbhej Singh** MBBS MD (Medicine) DM (Cardiology)<br>Assistant Professor<br>Department of Cardiology<br>Dayanand Medical College and Hospital<br>Unit Hero DMC Heart Institute<br>Ludhiana, Punjab, India |
| **Endocrinology** | **Gagan Priya** MBBS MD (Medicine) DM (Endocrinology)<br>Senior Consultant<br>Department of Endocrinology<br>Fortis Hospital<br>Mohali, Punjab, India | |
| **Rheumatology** | **Mohanjeet Kaur** MBBS MD (Medicine) FICP FIACM<br>Senior Consultant Physician<br>Department of Medicine<br>Shree Raghunath Hospital<br>Ludhiana, Punjab, India | **Vikas Gupta** MBBS MD (Medicine) DM (Rheumatology)<br>Assistant Professor<br>Department of Medicine<br>Dayanand Medical College and Hospital<br>Ludhiana, Punjab, India |

| | | |
|---|---|---|
| **Neurology** | **Monika Singla** MBBS MD (Medicine) DM (Neurology)<br>Associate Professor<br>Department of Neurology<br>Dayanand Medical College and Hospital<br>Ludhiana, Punjab, India | **Aastha Takkar Kapila** MBBS MD (Medicine) DM (Neurology)<br>Assistant Professor<br>Department of Neurology<br>Postgraduate Institute of Medical Education and Research<br>Chandigarh, India |
| **Gastro-enterology** | **Vandana Midha** MBBS MD (Medicine)<br>Professor<br>Department of Medicine<br>Dayanand Medical College and Hospital<br>Ludhiana, Punjab, India | |
| **Oncology** | **Shibba Takkar Chhabra** MBBS MD (Medicine) DM (Cardiology) FACC<br>Professor<br>Department of Cardiology<br>Dayanand Medical College and Hospital<br>Unit Hero DMC Heart Institute<br>Ludhiana, Punjab, India | **Mohanjeet Kaur** MBBS MD (Medicine) FICP FIACM<br>Senior Consultant Physician<br>Department of Medicine<br>Shree Raghunath Hospital<br>Ludhiana, Punjab, India |
| **Nephrology** | **Simran Kaur** MBBS MD (Medicine) DM (Nephrology)<br>Assistant Professor<br>Department of Nephrology<br>Dayanand Medical College and Hospital<br>Ludhiana, Punjab, India | **Suman Sethi** MBBS MD (Medicine) DM (Nephrology)<br>Assistant Professor<br>Department of Nephrology<br>Dayanand Medical College and Hospital<br>Ludhiana, Punjab, India |
| **Pulmonology** | **Shibba Takkar Chhabra** MBBS MD (Medicine) DM (Cardiology) FACC<br>Professor<br>Department of Cardiology<br>Dayanand Medical College and Hospital<br>Unit Hero DMC Heart Institute<br>Ludhiana, Punjab, India | **Akashdeep Singh** MBBS MD (Medicine) DM (Pulmonology)<br>Professor<br>Department of Pulmonology<br>Dayanand Medical College and Hospital<br>Ludhiana, Punjab, India |
| **Infectious Disease** | **Mohanjeet Kaur** MBBS MD (Medicine) FICP FIACM<br>Senior Consultant Physician<br>Department of Medicine<br>Shree Raghunath Hospital<br>Ludhiana, Punjab, India | |
| **Miscellaneous** | **Anubha Rathi** MD<br>Consultant<br>The Cornea Institute<br>LV Prasad Eye Institute (LVPEI)<br>Hyderabad, Telangana, India | |

# Contributing Authors

**Aastha Takkar Kapila** MBBS MD (Medicine) DM (Neurology)
Assistant Professor
Department of Neurology
Postgraduate Institute of Medical Education and Research
Chandigarh, India

**Aditi Jha** MD
Assistant Professor
Department of Dermatology
Adesh Medical College and Hospital
Haryana, India

**Amit Lakhani** MS (Orthopedic)
Professor
Maharishi Markandeshwar Medical College and Hospital, Kumarhatti-Solan
Himachal Pradesh, India

**Anita Saxena** MD DM FACC FAMS
Professor
Department of Cardiology
All India Institute of Medical Sciences
New Delhi, India

**Ankia Coetzee** MBChB MMed (Internal Medicine) FCP (Internal Medicine) Cert Endo and Metabolism (South Africa) MPhil (Endo)
Department of Internal Medicine
Division of Endocrinology
Stellenbosch University
Faculty of Health Sciences
Tygerberg Hospital
Cape Town, South Africa

**Anubha Rathi** MD
Consultant
The Cornea Institute
LV Prasad Eye Institute (LVPEI)
Hyderabad, Telangana, India

**Anu Gupta** MBBS MD (Medicine) DM (Neurology)
Assistant Professor
Department of Neurology
All India Institute of Medical Sciences (AIIMS)
New Delhi, India

**Anuja Patil** MD DM (Neurology)
Consultant Neurology
Department of Neurology
KIMS Hospital
Secunderabad, Telangana, India

**Arati Dave Lalchandani** MD DM (Cardiology) FCSI FAPVIS
Principal and Dean
GSVM Medical College
Kanpur, Uttar Pradesh, India

**Arundhati Dasgupta** MD DM
Consultant Endocrinologist
Department of Endocrinology
Rudraksh Superspeciality Care
Siliguri, West Bengal, India

**Asha Kishore** MD DM
Director
Sree Chitra Tirunal Institute for Medical Sciences and Technology
(An Institute of National Importance
Department of Science and Technology,
Government of India)
Thiruvananthapuram, Kerala, India

**Asha Moorthy** MD DM FCCP FICP FIACM FIMSA FICC
Senior Consultant Cardiologist
Department of Cardiology
SRM Institutes for Medical Science
Chennai, Tamil Nadu, India

**Basant** MBBS MD (Medicine) DM (Cardiology)
Assistant Professor
Department of Cardiology, Postgraduate Institute of Medical Education and Research
Chandigarh, India

**Battu Chaithanya** DNB (Respiratory Diseases) DTCD
Consultant Transplant Pulmonologist
Department of Pulmonology
Apollo Hospital, Jubilee Hills
Hyderabad, Telangana, India

**Belinda George** DM (Endocrinology)
Associate Professor
Department of Endocrinology
St John's Medical College Hospital
Bengaluru, Karnataka, India

**Benzeeta Pinto** MD DM
Assistant Professor
Department of Clinical Immunology and Rheumatology
St John's National Academy of Health Sciences
Bengaluru, Karnataka, India

**Bhumika Sharma** MS DNB
Consultant, Department of ENT
Indus Superspeciality Hospital
Mohali, Punjab, India

**Chandan Kumar Kedarisetty** MBBS
MD (Medicine) DM (Gastroenterology)
Assistant Professor
Department of Hepatology
Sri Ramachandra Institute of
Higher Education and Research
Chennai, Tamil Nadu, India

**Davinder Paul** MD DM
Assistant Professor
Department of Oncology
Dayanand Medical College and Hospital
Ludhiana, Punjab, India

**Debasish Mishra** MD DM
Senior Resident
Rheumatology Wing
Department of Internal Medicine
Postgraduate Institute of Medical Education
and Research
Chandigarh, India

**Dina Shreshtha** MD DM
Consultant
Department of Endocrinology
Norvic International Hospital and Medical
College
Kathmandu, Nepal

**Divya Arora** MBBS
PG Student Periodontics
Maharishi Markandeshwar College of
Dental Science and Research
Mullana, Ambala, Haryana, India

**Divya Seshadri** MD
Consultant
Department of Dermatology
Changi General Hospital
Singapore

**Elenjickal Elias John** MBBS MD (Medicine)
DM (Nephrology) FRACP
Assistant Professor
Department of Nephrology
Christian Medical College
Vellore, Tamil Nadu, India

**Ena Sharma** MDS
Associate Professor
Department of Periodontics and
Oral Implantology
Maharishi Markandeshwar College of
Dental and Research
Mullana, Ambala, Haryana, India

**Faria Afsana** MD DM
Assistant Professor
Department of Endocrinology
BIRDEM
Dhaka, Bangladesh

**Gagan Priya** MBBS MD (Medicine)
DM (Endocrinology)
Senior Consultant
Department of Endocrinology
Fortis Hospital
Mohali, Punjab, India

**Harbir Kaur Rao** MBBS MD (Medicine)
Professor and Head
Department of General Medicine
Maharishi Markandeshwar (Deemed to be
University)
Mullana, Ambala, Haryana, India

**Harmeet Kaur** MBBS DFM PGDMCH
Resident
Department of Obstetrics and Gynecology
Dayanand Medical College and Hospital
Ludhiana, Punjab, India

**Harmeet Riyait** MD (Medicine) DM (Nephrology)
(IPGMER Kolkata)
Formerly Consultant Nephrologist at
Sacred Heart Hospital, Jalandhar
Presently Consultant Nephrologist
Department of Nephrology
Tamanna Kidney Care
Joshi Hospital
Jalandhar, Punjab, India

**Hetan C Shah** MD DNB (Cardiology) FACC
FESC FSCAI
Associate Professor of Cardiology
Department of Cardiology
GSMC and KEM Hospital
Mumbai, Maharashtra, India

# Contributors

**IB Vijayalakshmi** Professor Emeritus MD DM DSc FICC FIAMS FIAE FCSI FICP FAMS FISH FRCP (London)
Professor of Pediatric Cardiology
Department of Cardiology
Super Specialty Hospital
Bangalore Medical College and Research Institute, (PMSSY)
Bengaluru, Karnataka, India

**Jain T Kallarakkal** MD FRCP DM
Senior Interventional Cardiologist
Department of Cardiology
St Mary's Hospital
Thodupuzha, Kerala, India

**Jasmine Das** MD (Medicine) DNB (Nephrology)
Associate Professor
Department of Nephrology
Christian Medical College and Hospital
Ludhiana, Punjab, India

**Jaya Gosh** MD DM
Professor
Department of Medical Oncology
Tata Memorial Center
Mumbai, Maharashtra, India

**Jayanthi Venkataraman** MBBS MD (Medicine) DM (Gastroenterology)
Professor
Department of Hepatology
Sri Ramachandra Institute of Higher Education and Research
Chennai, Tamil Nadu, India

**Jayasri Helen Gali** MD (Pulmonology)
Professor
Department of Pulmonary Medicine
Apollo Medical College and Research Center
Jubilee Hills
Hyderabad, Telangana

**Jeji Pukhraj** MBBS
Resident, Department of Medicine
Maharishi Markandeshwar Institute of Medical Sciences and Research
Mullana, Ambala, Haryana, India

**Jyoti Jindal** MD (Medicine)
Assistant Professor of Medicine
Department of Medicine
Dayanand Medical College and Hospital
Ludhiana, Punjab, India

**Jyotsana** MD DM FACC FESC FICC
Chief Editor of IJCDW
Secretary of WINCARS
Professor of Cardiology
Department of Cardiology
Nizam's Institute of Medical Sciences
Hyderabad, Telangana, India

**Krishna Prasad** MD
Senior Resident
Department of Cardiology
Postgraduate Institute of Medical Education and Research
Chandigarh, India

**Kusum Thakur** MD PGDMCH PGDHHM
Senior Consultant
Department of Transfusion Medicine
Maharishi Markandeshwar Institute of Medical Sciences and Research
Mullana, Ambala, Haryana, India

**Lalitha Nimani** MBBS MD (Medicine) DM (Cardiology)
Associate Professor
Department of Cardiology
Nizam's Institute of Medical Sciences
Hyderabad, Telangana, India

**Lipi Uppal** MBBS MD (Medicine) DM (Cardiology)
Senior Resident
Department of Cardiology
Postgraduate Institute of Medical Education and Research
Chandigarh, India

**Lt Col Julie Sachdeva** MD (Medicine) DM (Neurology)
Lieutenant Colonel, Department of Neurology
Classified Specialist (Medicine and Neurology)
Command Hospital (Western Command)
Panchkula, Haryana, India

**Madhushmita Mahapatra** MBBS
Junior Resident
Department of Ophthalmology
Dayanand Medical College and Hospital
Ludhiana, Punjab, India

**Manpreet Kaur** MD
Assistant Professor
Department of Ophthalmology
All India Institute of Medical Sciences (AIIMS)
New Delhi, India

**Mary John** MD FACP FICP
Professor
Department of Medicine
Christian Medical College and Hospital
Ludhiana, Punjab, India

**Mayank Jain** MBBS MD (Medicine)
DM (Gastroenterology)
Consultant Gastroenterologist and Hepatologist
Arihant Hospital and Research Centre
Indore, Madhya Pradesh, India

**Mohanjeet Kaur** MBBS MD (Medicine) FICP FIACM
Senior Consultant Physician
Department of Medicine
Shree Raghunath Hospital
Ludhiana, Punjab, India

**Monika Singla** MBBS MD (Medicine)
DM (Neurology)
Associate Professor
Department of Neurology
Dayanand Medical College and Hospital
Ludhiana, Punjab, India

**MV Padma Srivastava** MD DM
FRCP (Edinburgh) FAMS FNASc FIAN
Professor and Head
Department of Neurology
Chief Neurosciences Center
All India Institute of Medical Sciences
New Delhi, India

**Namrata Sharma** MD DNB MNAMS
Professor
Department of Ophthalmology
All India Institute of Medical Sciences (AIIMS)
New Delhi, India

**Naveen Kumar** MBBS MD (Medicine)
DM (Cardiology)
Assistant Professor
Department of Cardiology
Nizam's Institute of Medical Sciences
Hyderabad, Telangana, India

**Navkiran Mahajan** MD
Professor
Department of Psychiatry
Dayanand Medical College and Hospital
Ludhiana, Punjab, India

**Neelam Dahiya** MD DM (Cardiology)
Assistant Professor
Department of Cardiology
Postgraduate Institute of Medical Education and Research
Changigarh, India

**Neha Berry** MD DM (PGIMER)
Consultant
Department of Gastroenterology
BLK Hospital
New Delhi, India

**Neha Chauhan** MBBS MS (ENT) DNB
Consultant ENT
Department of ENT
Ivy Hospital
Mohali, Punjab, India

**Nidhi Bhim Sain** MD DNB
Specialist Grade I Cardiology
Department of Cardiology
ESIC - PGIMSR and Model Hospital
New Delhi, India

**Nitin Sethi** MS Mch (Plastic Surgery)
Additional Director
Department of Plastic and Cosmetic Surgery
Fortis Hospital
Ludhiana, Punjab, India

**Nupoor Acharya** MD (General Medicine)
DM (Clinical Immunology and Rheumatology)
Junior Consultant
Department of Rheumatology
Pushpawati Singhania Research Institute
New Delhi, India

**Parul Verma** MD
Associate Professor
Department of Dermatology
Venereology and Leprosy King George's Medical University
Lucknow, Uttar Pradesh, India

**Pooja Tandon** MD
Associate Professor
Department of Gynecology
Dayanand Medical College and Hospital
Ludhiana, Punjab, India

## Contributors

**Poonam Malhotra** MD DNB MNAMS
Professor
Department of Cardiac Anesthesia
Cardio Thoracic Center
All India Institute of Medical Sciences
New Delhi, India

**Praneet Wander** MD
Gastroenterology Fellow
Department of Gastroenterology
Donald and Barbara Zucker School of
Medicine at Hofstra/Northwell
North Shore Long Island Jewish Hospital
New York, United States

**Puneet A Pooni** MD
Pediatrics Professor and Head of Pediatrics
Department of Pediatrics
Dayanand Medical College and Hospital
Ludhiana, Punjab, India

**Rahul Purbey** MBBS
Post Graduate, Junior Resident
Department of General Medicine
Mullana, Ambala, Haryana, India

**Rajesh Matta** MD DM (Cardiology)
Senior Cardiology Register
Department of Cardiology
GSMC and KEM Hospital
Mumbai, Maharashtra, India

**Rajinder Singh Gupta** MD (Medicine)
Professor
Department of General Medicine
Mullana, Ambala, Haryana, India

**Rajiv Gupta** MS MCh
Professor and Head
Department of Cardiovascular and Surgery
Dayanand Medical College
Ludhiana, Punjab, India

**Ramya Janardana** MD
Associate Professor
Clinical Immunology and Rheumatology
St John's Medical College
Bengaluru, Karnataka, India

**Roopali Khanna** MD DM
Associate Professor
Department of Cardiology
Sanjay Gandhi Postgraduate Institute of
Medical Sciences
Lucknow, Uttar Pradesh, India

**Roopa Rajan** MD DM (Neurology)
PDF (Movement Disorders)
Consultant Neurologist and
Movement Disorders Specialist
Assistant Professor, Department of Neurology
All India Institute of Medical Sciences
New Delhi, India

**Ruchita Shah** MD
Associate Professor, Department of Psychiatry
Postgraduate Institute of Medical Education
and Research
Chandigarh, India

**Rupinder Kaur** MD
Assistant Professor
Department of Emergency Medicine
Dayanand Medical College and Hospital
Ludhiana, Punjab, India

**Sana Yumnam Devi** MBBS MD (Medicine)
Senior Resident
Department of Psychiatry, Postgraduate
Institute of Medical Education and Research
Chandigarh, India

**Sandeep Kaur** MD (Medicine)
Senior Resident, Department of Medicine
Dayanand Medical College and Hospital
Ludhiana, Punjab, India

**Santosh Varughese** MBBS MD (Medicine)
DM (Nephrology) FRACP
Professor
Department of Nephrology
Christian Medical College
Vellore, Tamil Nadu, India

**Sarah Nadeem** MD FACE
Assistant Professor
Department of Endocrinology
Aga Khan University
Stadium Road, Karachi, Pakistan

**Savita Jain** MD (Internal Medicine)
DNB (Endocrinology)
Consultant
Department of Endocrinology, DEEP Hospital
Ludhiana, Punjab, India

**Savita Kapila** MBBS MD (Medicine)
Professor, Department of Medicine
Maharishi Markandeshwar Institute of
Medical Research
Mullana, Ambala, Haryana, India

**Senthil Kumar** MP MS FRCS
Professor
Hepatopancreatic Biliary Surgery and
Liver Transplant, Sri Ramachandra Institute of
Higher Education and Research
Chennai, Tamil Nadu, India

**Shashank S Telang** DNB
Resident Cardiology
Department of Cardiology
Apollo Health City
Hyderabad, Telangana, India

**Shibba Takkar Chhabra** MBBS MD (Medicine)
DM (Cardiology) FACC
Professor
Department of Cardiology
Dayanand Medical College and Hospital
Unit Hero DMC Heart Institute
Ludhiana, Punjab, India

**Shivani Mehta** MBBS
Junior Resident
Department of Cardiology
Dayanand Medical college and Hospital City
Ludhiana, Punjab, India

**Shobna Bhatia** MBBS MD (Medicine)
DNB (Gastroenterology)
Professor
Consultant Gastroenterologist
Department of Gastroenterology and
HepatoBiliary Sciences
Sir HN Reliance Foundation Hospital
Mumbai, Maharashtra, India

**Shruti Kakkar** MD
Fellowship in Comprehensive Hemato-Oncology
Assistant Professor
Department of Pediatrics
Dayanand Medical College and Hospital
Ludhiana, Punjab, India

**Shubra Mishra** MBBS MD (Internal Medicine)
Senior Resident
Department of Gestroenterology
Postgraduate Institute of Medical Education
and Research
Chandigarh, India

**Simran Kaur** MBBS MD (Medicine)
DM (Nephrology)
Assistant Professor of Nephrology
Department of Nephrology
Dayanand Medical College and Hospital
Ludhiana, Punjab, India

**Sita Jayalakshmi** MD DM (Neurology)
Consultant Neurology
Department of Neurology, KIMS Hospital
Secunderabad, Telangana, India

**Somashiela Murthy** MS
Consultant and Head of Services (HoS)
Cornea and Anterior Segment Services
Department of Ophthalmology
LV Prasad Eye Institute (LVPEI)
Hyderabad, Telangana, India

**Sridhar Sundaram** MBBS MD (Medicine)
DM (Gastroenterology)
Assistant Professor
Department of Gastroenterology
Seth GS Medical College and KEM Hospital
Mumbai, Maharashtra, India

**Suceena Alexander** MD DM (Nephrology)
FASN
Professor, Department of Nephrology
Christian Medical College
Vellore, Tamil Nadu, India

**Sucharita Ray** MD DM PDF (Stroke and
Cerebrovascular Diseases)
Assistant Professor
Department of Neurology
Postgraduate Institute of Medical Education
and Research
Chandigarh, India

**Sujata Bhatti** MD (Pediatrics)
ICU Consultant, Department of Pediatrics
Satguru Partap Singh Hospitals
Ludhiana, Punjab, India

**Sulena** DM (Neurology)
Associate Professor
Department of Neurology
Government Medical College and Hospital
Faridkot, Punjab, India

**Suman Puri** MD
Professor
Department of Obstetrics and Gynecology
Dayanand Medical College and Hospital
Ludhiana, Punjab, India

**Suman Sethi** MBBS MD (Medicine)
DM (Nephrology)
Assistant Professor
Department of Nephrology
Dayanand Medical College and Hospital
Ludhiana, Punjab, India

**Supriya Arora** MS
Consultant
Department of Ophthalmology
Princess Margaret Hospital
Nassau, Bahamas

**Supriya Sharma** DNB
Fellow, Cornea and Anterior Segment Services
Department of Ophthalmology
LV Prasad Eye Institute (LVPEI)
Hyderabad, Telangana, India

**Swapna Shanbhag** MS
Consultant
Department of Ophthalmology
LV Prasad Eye Institute (LVPEI)
Hyderabad, Telangana, India

**Tamarai Selvan** MBBS MD (Medicine)
DM (Gastroenterology)
Assistant Professor
Department of Hepatology
Sri Ramachandra Institute of
Higher Education and Research
Chennai, Tamil Nadu, India

**Tejal Lathia** MD DM (Endocrinology)
Consultant
Department of Endocrinology
Fortis and Apollo Hospitals
Navi Mumbai, Mahashtra

**Than Than Aye** MMedSc DTM&H (London)
MRCP (UK) DMedSc FRCP (Edinburgh, London)
Professor Emeritus
Department of Endocrinology
University of Medicine 2
Yangon, Myanmar

**Tripti Deb** MD DNB (Cardiology)
Fellow in Interventional Cardiology (France)
Senior Consultant and Interventional
Cardiologist
Department of Cardiology
Apollo Health City
Hyderabad, Telangana, India

**Usha Dutta** MBBS (AIIMS) MD (AIIMS)
DM (Gastroenterology) AIIMS MSc HRM (McMaster University)
Fellow American College of Gastroenterology
Clinical Fellow Storr Liver Unit
University of Sydney Clinical
Fellow, McMaster University Professor
Department of Gastroenterology
Postgraduate Institute of Medical Education
and Research
Chandigarh, India

**Vaishali Deshmukh** MBBS MD (Medicine)
DM (Endocrinology)
Consultant and Head
Department of Endocrinology
Deenanath Mangeshkar Hospital and
Research Centre
Deshmukh Clinic and Research Centre
Pune, Maharashtra, India

**Vandana Midha** MBBS MD (Medicine)
Professor
Department of Medicine
Dayanand Medical College and Hospital
Ludhiana, Punjab, India

**Vikas Makkar** MBBS MD (Medicine)
DM (Nephrology)
Professor and Head
Department of Nephrology
Dayanand Medical College and Hospital
Ludhiana, Punjab, India

**Vinita Mani Daniel** MBBS MD (Medicine)
DM (Neurology)
Assistant Professor
Department of Neurology
Sanjay Gandhi Postgraduate Institute of
Medical Science
Lucknow, Uttar Pradesh, India

# FOREWORD

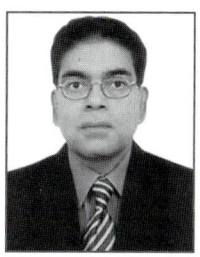

**Prem K Gupta**
Secretary
Managing Society
Dayanand Medical College and Hospital
Ludhiana, Punjab, India

It gives me a great pleasure to see that the women medical fraternity of Dayanand Medical College and Hospital, Ludhiana is working toward the cause of a woman's health in society. I am all the more pleased that they have attempted to compile the medical literature in communion with their lady physician colleagues across the globe. I congratulate Dr Shibba Takkar Chhabra and wish her all the best in her endeavor which will benefit not only the medical profession but have socialistic implications by improving the health of women who lay the foundation of a healthy society.

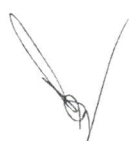

**Prem K Gupta**

# FOREWORD

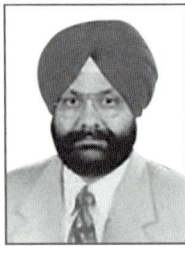

**Daljit Singh**
Vice Chancellor
Sri Guru Ram Das University of Health Sciences, Amritsar
Ex Principal, Dayanand Medical College and Hospital
Ludhiana, Punjab, India

In my years of journey through the medical profession I have seen an amazing progress in the way women have excelled not only in academics but have also proven their skills as astute physicians and surgeons. However, there still persists a lag as regards gender representation in major trials and other aspects of medical literature. It gives me immense pleasure to know that this book being compiled by Female Physicians and Superspecialists across the globe attempts to address this pertinent issue. The effort appears to be innovative and one of its kind. I congratulate Dr Shibba Takkar Chhabra for the endeavor and hope the book stands true to its title "Oorja".....i.e., the epitome of power..... May the empowered women keep working to improvise the health of women who are backbone of a healthy society.

Wishing Team "Oorja" all the best!

**Daljit Singh**

# FOREWORD

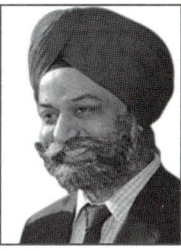

**Gurpreet S Wander**
Vice Principal
Professor and HOD Cardiology
Chief Cardiologist Cum Coordinator
Dayanand Medical College and Hospital
Hero DMC Heart Institute
Ludhiana, Punjab, India

Medical literature since times immemorial has been gender neutral with implications of most studies and trials being imposed on the fair sex even though it is under represented in data collection. I am glad that the lady physicians of Dayanand Medical College and Hospital have collaborated with their colleagues and attempted to address the issue by compiling the literature pertaining to women's medical ailments in the form of book. Besides accumulating the relevant women-oriented scientific text in one go for the reader, this book sensitizes the medical fraternity to manage their female patients with aggression and care they deserve.

I congratulate the Team "Oorja", especially Dr Shibba, my dear student, for beautifully coming out with this unique and innovative project and hope that they build it up further in years to come.

**Gurpreet S Wander**

# FOREWORD

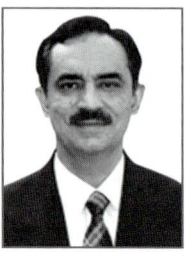

**Sandeep Puri**
Principal
Professor of Medicine
Dayanand Medical College and Hospital
Ludhiana, Punjab, India

Presenting a textbook on a common yet complex agenda which addresses the health issues of the female gender is indeed very laudable.

Gender disparities in delivery of healthcare to the women and their feeble representation in medical literature is a known phenomenon. It gives me immense pleasure to know that the Lady Physicians are now joining hands to gather, accumulate and fortify data on medical ailments in women. I am sure that this endeavor shall instigate the doctors in medicine to manage their female patients in a transformed manner. Given their differences—anatomical, hormonal, and environmental, women do deserve an approach different than men. The insightful suggestions compiled in this book will surely benefit the Women's health.

My compliments to Team "Oorja" for their efforts in this direction and I am confident that this spark that they have ignited shall illuminate and stimulate all of us for the cause.
My Best Wishes!

**Sandeep Puri**

# PREFACE

यत्र नार्यस्तु पूज्यन्ते रमन्ते तत्र देवता: ।

Meaning: "Where Women are honored, divinity blossoms there"

Women are the caregivers of the society. The hand that rocks the cradle not only molds the current generation but pedigrees in the future as well. The discussion on gender equality has been going on since eons. The novel concept of gender "equity" sounds more promising as compared to "equality". A man and a woman are as similar as yin and yang and as diverse as well. Most of the health-related literature till date has been gender neutral with most studies essentially matching for the gender during case recruitment. This trend is changing off late with more focus on gender-based research and outlining different treatment strategies for men and women. With these facts in mind, this book has been compiled to address the various issues pertaining to Women's health and well-being. Across a volume of 52 chapters, it covers all the major organ systems of a woman's body including cardiology, neurology, endocrinology, gastroenterology, nephrology, rheumatology, psychiatry, ophthalmology, infectious disease, etc. It goes on to discuss the various clinical methods and management strategies of medical ailments in women.

The title of the book "*The Oorja*" (*Clinical Approach and Management Strategies of Medical Ailments in Women Oorja—The Power of Her*) speaks of the empowered women, the women physicians in our club who jointly have made an endeavor to highlight the medical ailments in this gender. A healthy woman is the foundation of a healthy family, a healthy society, a healthy nation, and a healthy universe. This book is a unique effort to tap the so far less read and studied aspect of medical science "**The Woman**". The First edition looks ahead in future to pile up even more literature and scientific work with its socialistic implications in years to come.

Gender bias in terms of women presenting late to clinic with their symptoms or not being able to reach at all, is also addressed in the pages to come. For several decades, men have ruled the household court and have taken the liberty to decide for a woman too even when it caters to her health. Public health strategies specifically targeted for women to bring them up and speak for their well-being are the need of the hour.

The medical profession in itself is not untouched by the gender bias. One can actually count the number of women on fingertips in most medical meetings or groups world over. It is even more disappointing to see that most of the patients in remote areas do not look up to a female doctor and almost always consider her to be potentially less competent than her male counterparts.

But all is not gray in the world. With education, comes change. With education, knowledge and strength, we women can pave the way forward for our future generations to follow. Let every woman be heard. Let us be their ears.

*"Here's to strong women. May we know them. May we be them. May we raise them."*
— Anonymous

**Shibba Takkar Chhabra**
**Aastha Takkar Kapila**
**Anubha Rathi**

# ACKNOWLEDGMENTS

My parents, Rita and Ved Parkash Takkar; Rama and Ramesh Chhabra; my heart beats, Ritesh and Vidyut; my mentor, Professor Gurpreet S Wander. I also acknowledge the untiring efforts of my coeditors, Dr Aastha and Dr Anubha and all the section editors who have made "Oorja" possible. Also thanks to Mr Raja Gupta and Mr Satinder Pal Singh who worked day and night for this project. Extremely grateful to the patients who have taught us. Above all, I thank almighty, the supreme power who has guided us throughout.

**Shibba Takkar Chhabra**

I am ever indebted to my pillars of strength, my parents Rita and VP Takkar; Savita and Abhilash Kapila, and my lifelines Amit and Aadita for their endless love and motivation. I am grateful to my mentor Professor Vivek Lal who has been my guiding spirit.

**Aastha Takkar Kapila**

My parents JS Rathi, Mithlesh Rathi, Dr VP Takkar, and Dr Rita Takkar, my brother Aman, husband Brijesh, and son Arjun. Special thanks to Dr Shibba Takkar Chhabra for being the backbone of this book.

**Anubha Rathi**

We would also like to thank Mr Jitendar P Vij, Mr Mani, Dr Richa Saxena and Dr Nidhi Sood for their brilliant efforts in bringing out the book.

# CONTENTS

## Section 1: Cardiology
### Shibba Takkar Chhabra, Gurbhej Singh

1. Role of Women in Development of Cardiology in India — 3
   *IB Vijayalakshmi*

2. Cardiovascular Risk Assessment and Primary Prevention Strategies in Women — 13
   *Jyotsana, Naveen Kumar, Lalitha Nimani*

3. IHD in Women: Epidemiology, Presentation, Diagnosis and Management Strategies — 31
   *Shibba Takkar Chhabra, Jyoti Jindal, Pooja Tandon*

4. Women with Heart Failure: Etiopathogenesis, Clinical Presentation, Diagnostic, and Management Strategies — 38
   *Neelam Dahiya, Lipi Uppal, Krishna Prasad, Basant*

5. Coronary Intervention in Women: How is it Different? — 49
   *Hetan C Shah, Rajesh Matta*

6. Structural Heart Disease in Women: Age-based Presentation, Medical, and Interventional Strategies — 56
   *Tripti Deb, Shashank S Telang, Sandeep Kaur, Rajiv Gupta*

7. A to Z of Rheumatic Heart Disease in Women — 63
   *Arati Dave Lalchandani*

8. Congenital Heart Disease: Pertinent Issues in the Fair Sex — 69
   *Anita Saxena, Nidhi Bhim Sain*

9. Pregnancy and The Heart — 78
   *Asha Moorthy, Jain T Kallarakkal*

10. Sudden Cardiac Arrest in Women with Migraine — 82
    *Poonam Malhotra*

## Section 2: Endocrinology
### Gagan Priya

1. Diabetes, Women, and Pregnancy — 89
   *Belinda George, Ankia Coetzee*

2. **Thyroid Dysfunction in Women** — 100
   Vaishali Deshmukh, Dina Shreshtha

3. **Polycystic Ovary Syndrome: A Multifaceted Endocrinopathy** — 114
   Savita Jain, Sarah Nadeem, Gagan Priya

4. **Contraception and Women's Health** — 126
   Arundhati Dasgupta, Faria Afsana

5. **Health Issues during Menopausal Transition** — 135
   Tejal Lathia, Than Than Aye

## Section 3: Rheumatology
*Mohanjeet Kaur, Vikas Gupta*

1. **Pertinent Rheumatological Issues in Women** — 147
   Benzeeta Pinto, Ramya Janardana

2. **Risk of Cardiovascular Events in the Presence of Autoimmune Diseases** — 155
   Nupoor Acharya, Debasish Mishra

## Section 4: Neurology
*Monika Singla, Aastha Takkar Kapila*

1. **Epilepsy in Women** — 163
   Anuja Patil, Sita Jayalakshmi

2. **Specific Issues of Stroke in Women** — 173
   Sucharita Ray, MV Padma Srivastava

3. **Movement Disorders: Gender Issues and Management Strategies** — 180
   Roopa Rajan, Asha Kishore

4. **Headache Disorders: Are They Different in Women?** — 187
   Monika Singla, Sulena, Aastha Takkar Kapila

5. **Neuroimmunology: Special Considerations in Women** — 195
   Aastha Takkar Kapila, Anu Gupta, Julie Sachdeva, Monika Singla

## Section 5: Gastroenterology
*Vandana Midha*

1. **Gender Divide: Common Gastrointestinal Disorders in Women** — 213
   Shobna Bhatia, Sridhar Sundaram

2. **Gut Microbiome and Obesity: Ladies Corner** — 220
   Usha Dutta, Shubra Mishra

3. **Gastrointestinal and Liver Disorders in Pregnancy** — 230
   Vandana Midha, Harmeet Kaur

4. Hepatobiliary Disorders in Females ............................................................................. 238
   *Shivani Mehta, Neha Berry, Praneet Wander*

5. Does Gender Matter in Liver Transplantation? ............................................................ 244
   *Mayank Jain, Chandan Kumar Kedarisetty, Tamarai Selvan,*
   *Senthil Kumar, Jayanthi Venkataraman*

## Section 6: Oncology
### Shibba Takkar Chhabra, Mohanjeet Kaur

1. Breast and Gynecological Cancers: An Overview ......................................................... 253
   *Jaya Gosh, Davinder Paul*

2. Pertinent Hemato-oncological Issues in Women .......................................................... 264
   *Shruti Kakkar*

## Section 7: Nephrology
### Simran Kaur, Suman Sethi

1. Hypertensive Disorders in Pregnancy ........................................................................... 273
   *Suman Sethi, Nitin Sethi*

2. Lupus Nephritis: What's New? ........................................................................................ 282
   *Simran Kaur, Vikas Makkar*

3. Acute Kidney Injury in Pregnancy .................................................................................. 291
   *Jasmine Das*

4. Challenges of Urinary Tract Infections in Females ....................................................... 298
   *Harmeet Riyait*

5. Challenges of Renal Transplant in Females .................................................................. 306
   *Suceena Alexander, Elenjickal Elias John, Santosh Varughese*

## Section 8: Pulmonology
### Shibba Takkar Chhabra, Akashdeep Singh

1. Pulmonology: Salient Issues in Women ........................................................................ 313
   *Battu Chaithanya, Jayasri Helen Gali*

## Section 9: Infectious Diseases
### Mohanjeet Kaur

1. HIV in Women ................................................................................................................... 327
   *Harbir Kaur Rao, Rajinder Singh Gupta, Rahul Purbey*

2. Approach to Fever in a Pregnant Women .................................................................... 334
   *Savita Kapila, Ena Sharma, Jeji Pukhraj*

3. Vaccination in Adolescent Girls and Women — 343
*Mary John*

4. Tuberculosis in Women: Unaddressed Issues — 350
*Mohanjeet Kaur, Rupinder Kaur, Jyoti Jindal*

## Section 10: Miscellaneous
*Anubha Rathi*

1. Women and Eye Health — 357
*Anubha Rathi, Madhushmita Mahapatra, Supriya Sharma, Namrata Sharma*

2. Dry Eye in Women — 366
*Manpreet Kaur, Swapna Shanbhag, Anubha Rathi, Namrata Sharma*

3. Uveitis in Women — 373
*Supriya Arora, Anubha Rathi, Somashiela Murthy*

4. Otolaryngorhinology in Women — 379
*Bhumika Sharma, Neha Chauhan*

5. Ear, Nose, and Throat Disorders in Pregnancy — 383
*Neha Chauhan, Bhumika Sharma*

6. Women and Mental Health — 387
*Navkiran Mahajan*

7. Women and Skin Ailments — 394
*Aditi Jha, Parul Verma, Divya Seshadri*

8. Medical Ailments in Adolescent Girls — 402
*Puneet A Pooni, Sujata Bhatti*

9. Sex Education of Adolescent Girls — 407
*Ruchita Shah, Sana Yumnam Devi*

10. Medical Problems in Women Undergoing Infertility Treatment — 414
*Suman Puri, Rupinder Kaur*

11. Dental Health in Women — 423
*Ena Sharma, Amit Lakhani, Savita Kapila, Divya Arora*

12. Women and Transfusion Medicine — 426
*Kusum Thakur*

13. Challenges for Lady Physicians in India — 431
*Roopali Khanna, Vinita Mani Daniel*

*Index* — 435

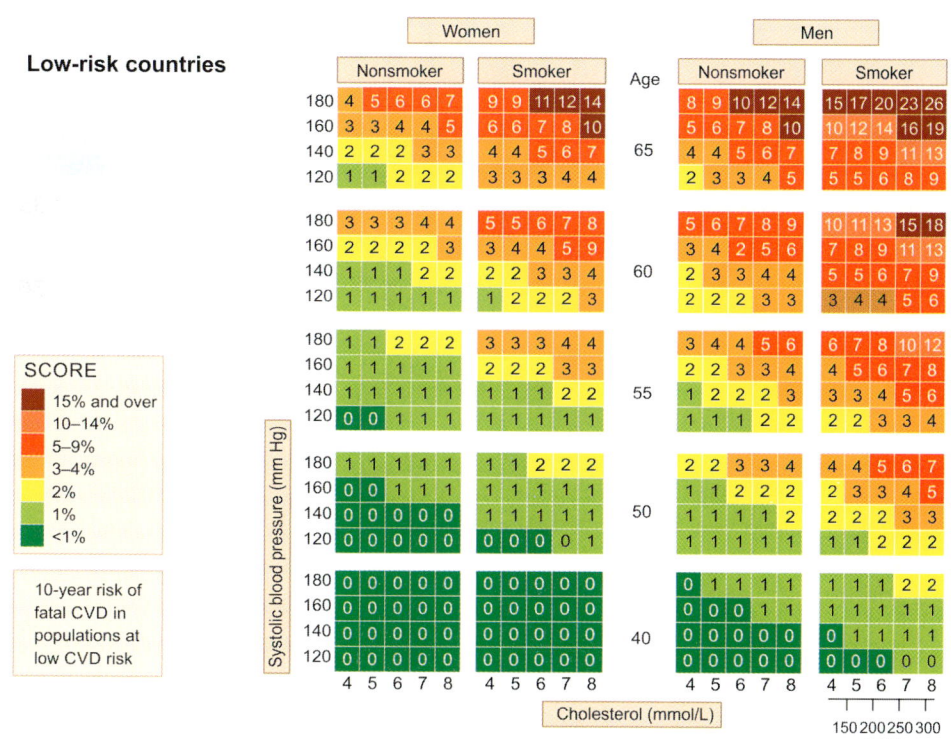

(CVD: cardiovascular disease; SCORE: Systematic Coronary Risk Evaluation)

**FIG. 1:** SCORE calculation in low-risk countries. *(Section 1, Chapter 2)*
(*Source:* Tomasik T et al.)

# PLATE 2

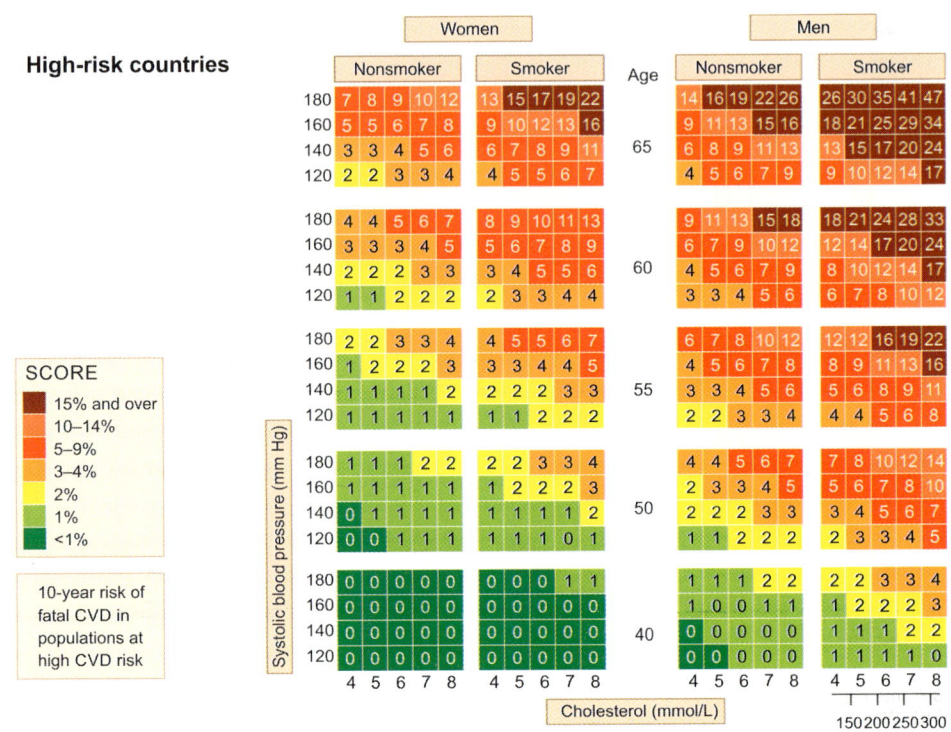

(SCORE: Systematic Coronary Risk Evaluation)

**FIG. 2:** SCORE calculation in high-risk countries. *(Section 1, Chapter 2)*
(*Source:* Tomasik T et al.)

# PLATE 3

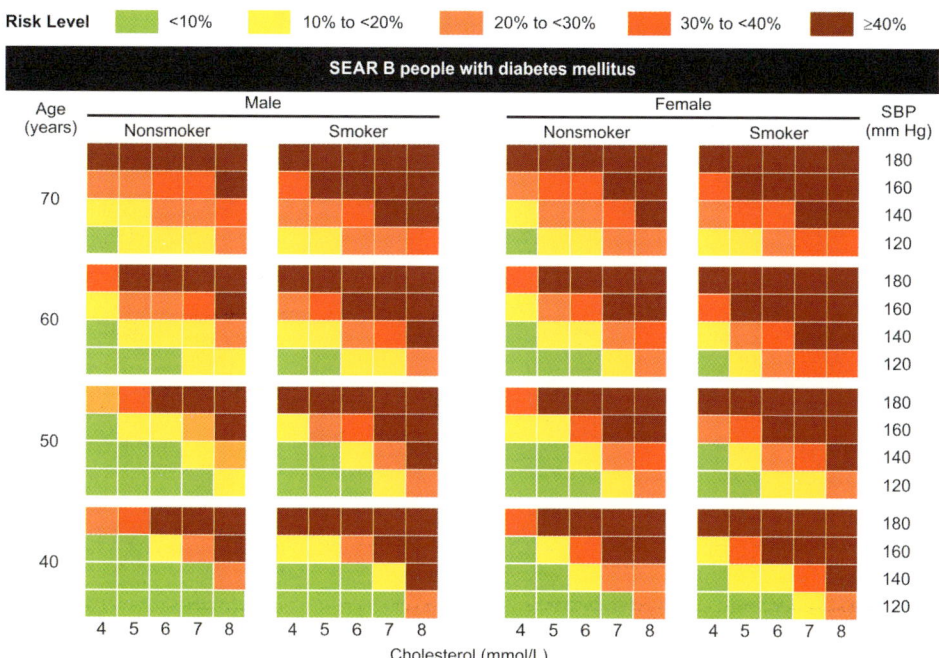

(ISH: International Society of Hypertension; SEAR: Southeast Asia subregions; SBP: systolic blood pressure; WHO: World Health Organization)

**FIG. 3:** WHO/ISH risk prediction chart SEAR B with Diabetes. *(Section 1, Chapter 2)*

# PLATE 4

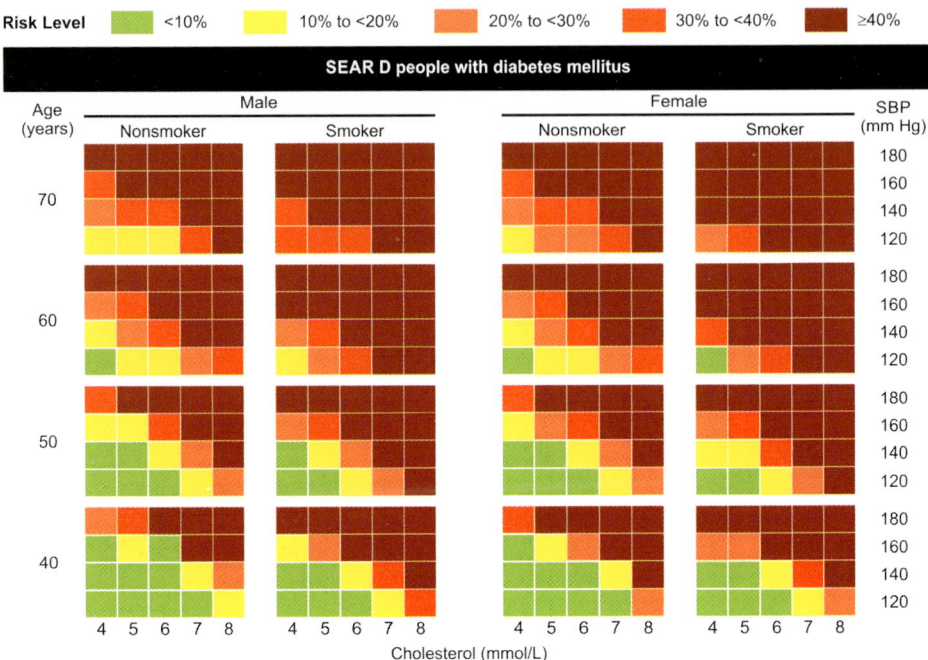

(ISH: International Society of Hypertension; SEAR: Southeast Asia subregions; SBP: systolic blood pressure; WHO: World Health Organization)

**FIG. 4:** WHO/ISH risk prediction chart SEAR D with Diabetes. *(Section 1, Chapter 2)*

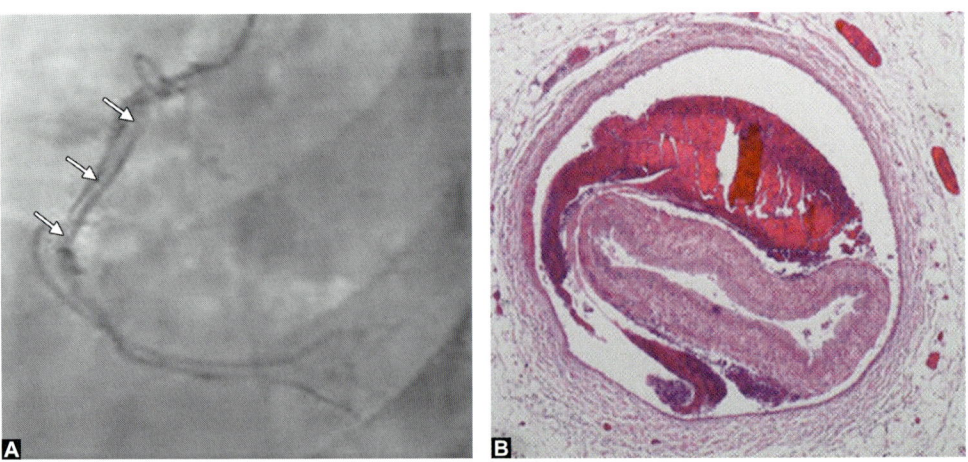

**FIGS. 1A AND B:** (A) Coronary angiogram and (B) microscopic appearance of spontaneous coronary artery dissection (SCAD). *(Section 1, Chapter 5)*

*Source*: Hussaini A, Adlam D. Spontaneous coronary artery dissection. Heart. 2017;103:1043-51.

# PLATE 5

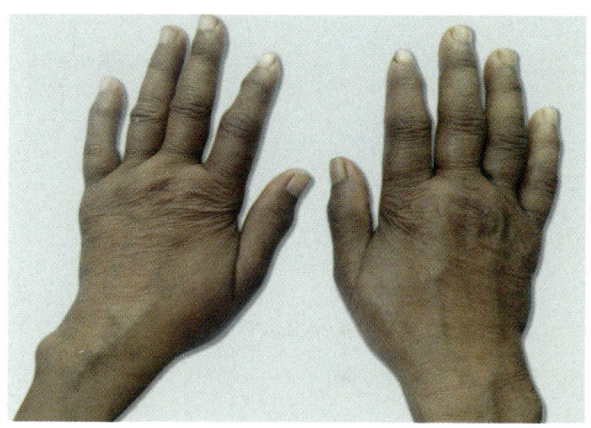

**FIG. 1:** Both hands showing swelling of proximal interphalangeal joints and wrists without deformities. *(Section 3, Chapter 1)*

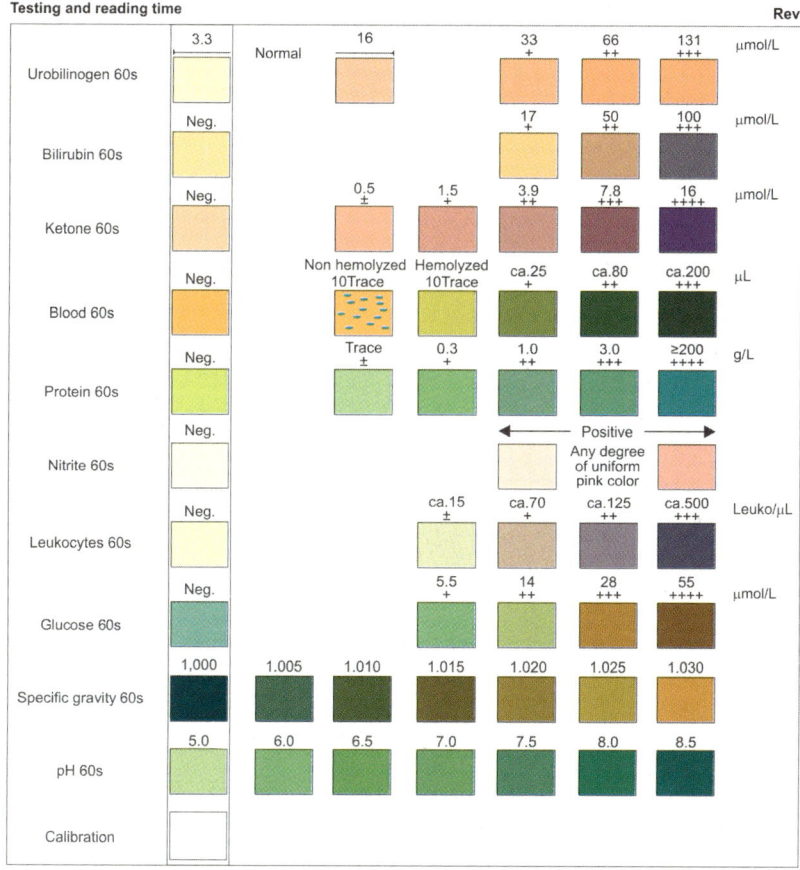

**FIG. 3:** Total 10 parameter urine dipstick. *(Section 7, Chapter 4)*

# PLATE 6

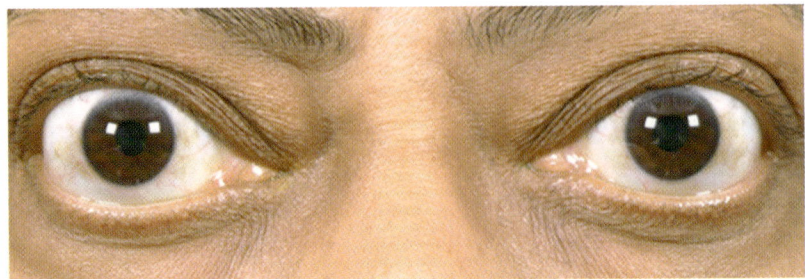

**FIG. 1:** Clinical photograph of bilateral axial proptosis in a woman with thyroid eye disease (TED). *(Section 10, Chapter 1)*

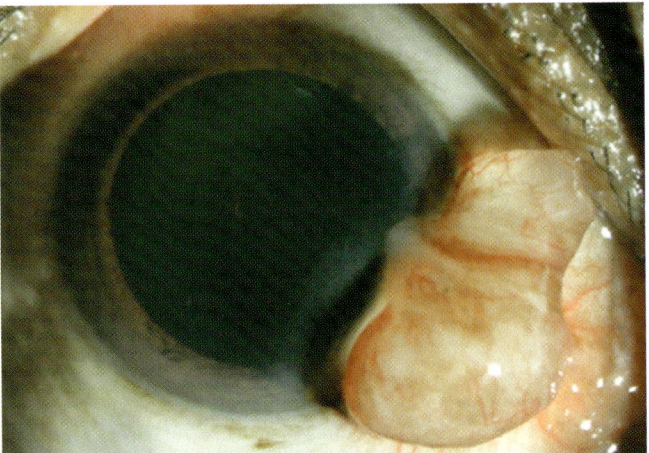

**FIG. 2:** Clinical photograph of pterygium with cystic degeneration. *(Section 10, Chapter 1)*

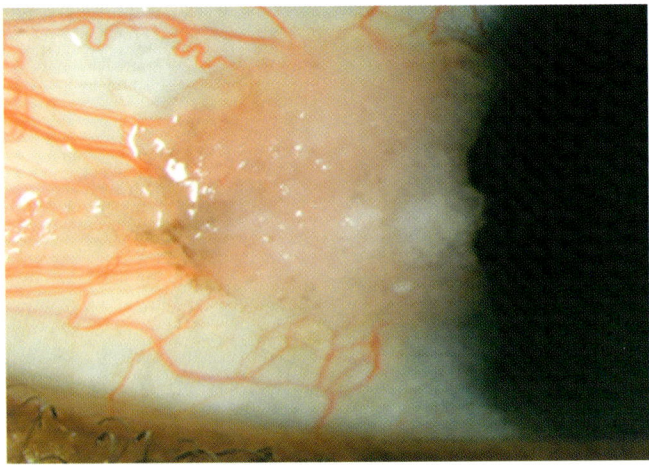

**FIG. 3:** Clinical photograph of an eye with ocular surface squamous neoplasia (OSSN). *(Section 10, Chapter 1)*

# PLATE 7

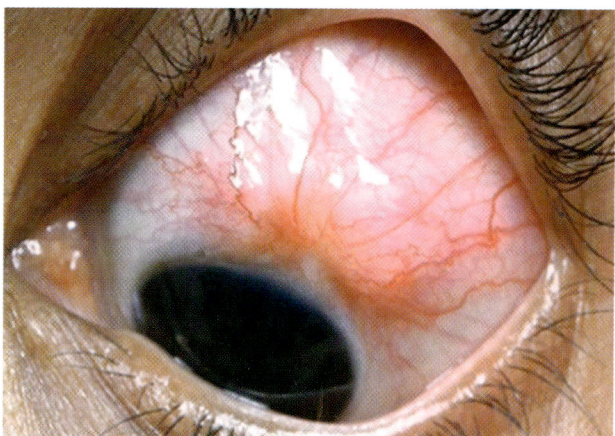

**FIG. 4:** Clinical photograph of an eye with nodular scleritis. *(Section 10, Chapter 1)*

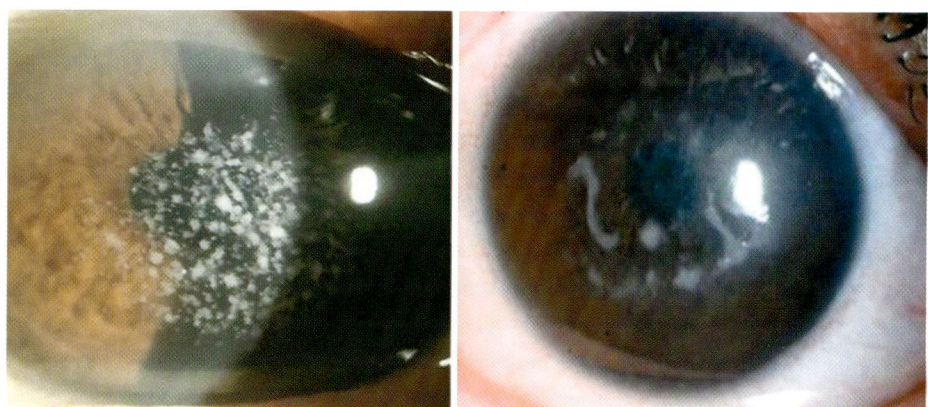

**FIG. 5:** Clinical photograph of eyes with corneal dystrophies. *(Section 10, Chapter 1)*

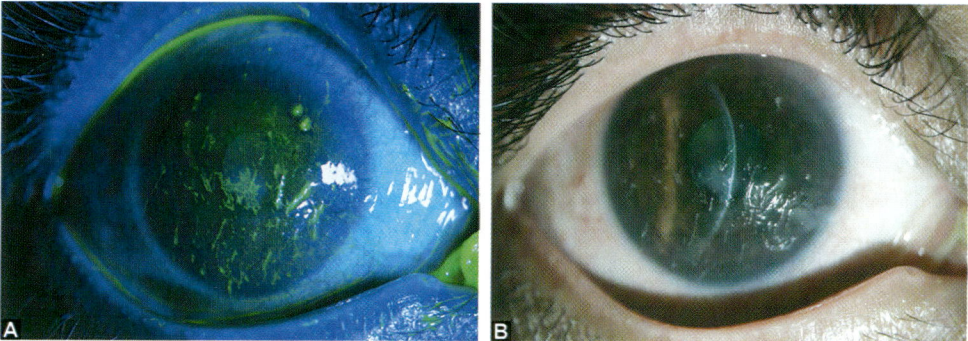

**FIG. 2:** (A) Clinical photograph of an eye with severe dryness after fluorescein staining under cobalt blue filter; (B) Clinical photograph of an eye with severe dryness showing a lustreless cornea. *(Section 10, Chapter 2)*

## PLATE 8

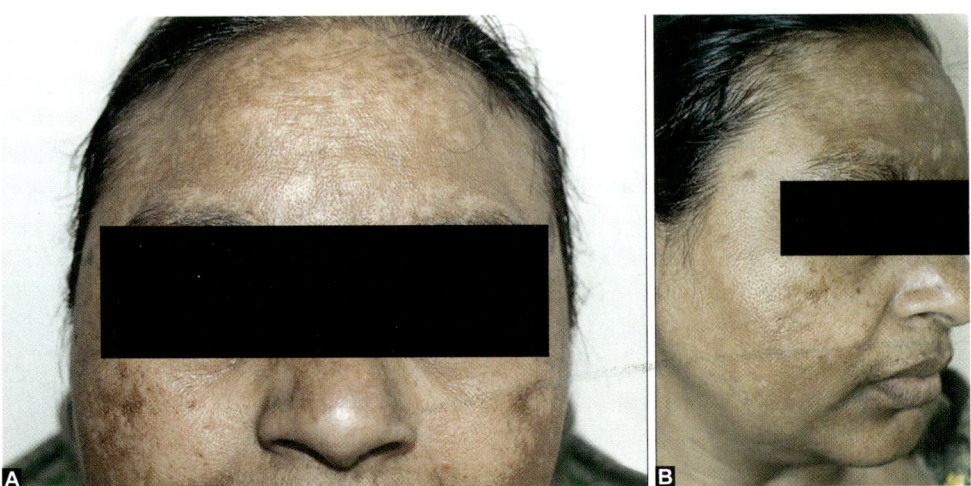

**FIGS. 1A AND B:** Well-demarcated brownish macules present over the forehead and malar areas of a middle age female with melasma. *(Section 10, Chapter 7)*

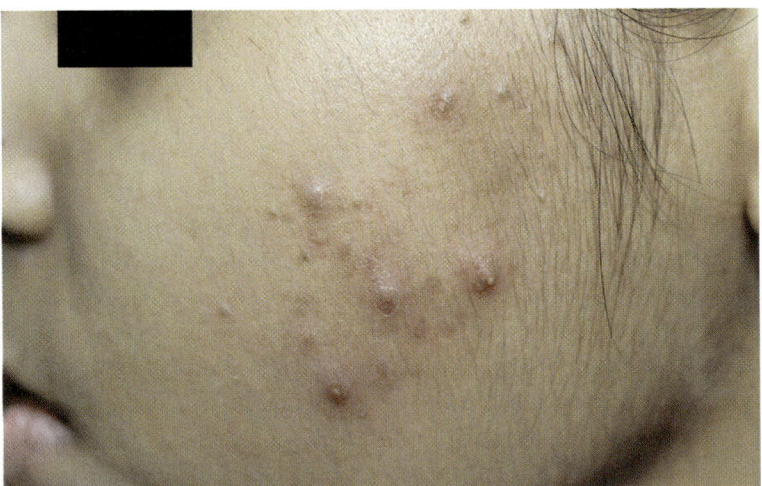

**FIG. 2:** Comedones, erythematous papules, and pustules on the cheeks of an adolescent female with acne vulgaris. *(Section 10, Chapter 7)*

# SECTION 1

# Cardiology

**SECTION EDITORS**
Shibba Takkar Chhabra, Gurbhej Singh

# CHAPTER 1

# Role of Women in Development of Cardiology in India

*IB Vijayalakshmi*

## ABSTRACT

Women in cardiology have been outnumbered by their male colleagues not only in India but all over the universe. The present review highlights the role of pertinent women who have been instrumental in development of cardiology in India. Their struggle has paved way for several young lady cardiologists who now tread the path with confidence and zeal.

## INTRODUCTION

Dr Helen Brooke Taussig, a pediatrician at Johns Hopkins, was the codeveloper of first successful "Blue Baby" operation at Johns Hopkins Hospital. The two great Indian pioneers of pediatric cardiology in India, Dr Kamala I Vytilingam and Dr S Padmavati both were trained in Johns Hopkins hospital, under Dr Helen Brooke Taussig, "Mother of pediatric cardiology." The journey of cardiology in India started with toddlers steps of pediatric cardiology by women! Thus, it has been truly fascinating and full of challenges, determination, and dedication by many illustrious women. So much so that once great cardiac anatomist and a world authority, Bob Anderson once exclaimed during world congress of pediatric cardiology to Dr IB Vijayalakshmi- "Oh Vijay I thought you were a man!!. We have laid the solid foundation for structural heart diseases, now it is to the young Indian pediatric cardiologist to build it further." The remarkable journey of cardiology in India has many women luminaries who have brightened the path of future cardiologists.

## HISTORY OF BEGINNING OF CARDIOLOGY IN INDIA

The first formal department of cardiology in India was started in Christian Medical College (CMC) Hospital, Vellore in 1957 by Dr Kamala I Vytilingam, after training at Johns Hopkins Hospital, Baltimore. The DM cardiology training course was initiated in CMC in 1965. The birth of the specialty of pediatric cardiology in India took place at Vellore under Dr Reeve Betz who started the first cardiothoracic surgery department at Vellore in 1949. Dr T Thomas and Dr Gopinath joined Dr Betz subsequently and initiated the first open heart surgery program in 1960. Late Dr Vytilingam established one of the

**SECTION 1:** Cardiology

earliest cardiac catheterization laboratories in India. Butreal interventional cardiology started only in 1985.

## PIONEERS IN CARDIOLOGY

### Dr S Padmavati

Dr Sivaramakrishna Iyer Padmavati, widely regarded as the doyenne of cardiology in India. She is India's first woman cardiologist and woman of many firsts! The first Indian doctor who completed training in pediatric cardiology is Dr S Padmavati who studied CHD as a fellow with Dr Helen Taussig from 1948 to 1951 and subsequently in pediatric cardiology department in Boston at the Massachusetts general hospital. She had rare privilege of publishing a paper "Results of Operation for Pulmonary Stenosis and Atresia Transactions" with Dr Helen Taussig in Association of American Physicians in 1951. On her return to India, she was amazed to find the wards full of young women and children with acute rheumatic fever (ARF) and rheumatic heart disease (RHD). As she did not have access to surgical management of pediatric cardiac patients, she had to predominantly look after adults. She opened a cardiac clinic in Lady Hardinge hospital where there were a lot of children with CHD. In 1980, she published her paper "Congenital Heart Disease in Delhi School Children."

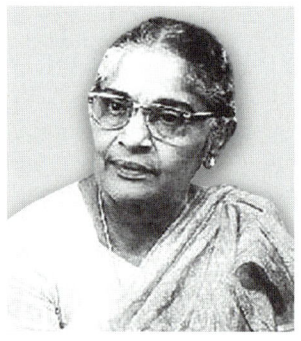

Dr Kamala I Vytilingam

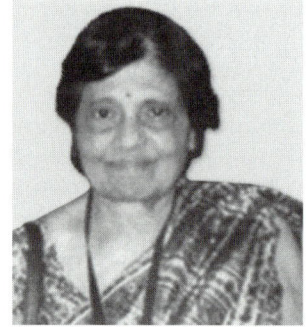

Dr S Padmavati

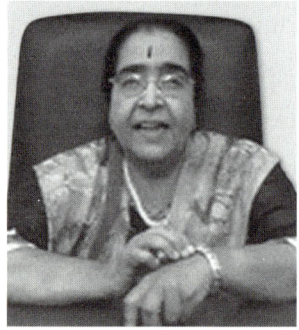

Dr P S Sreemathi

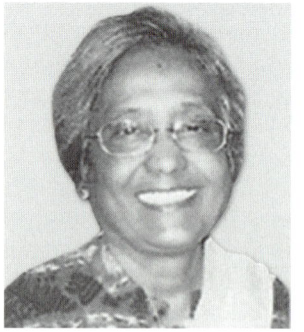

Dr Savitri Shrivastava

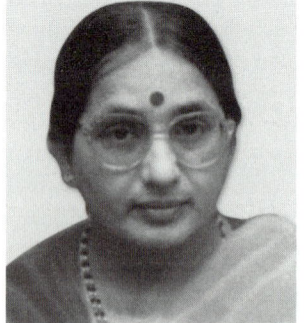

Dr (Mrs) Ramesh Arora

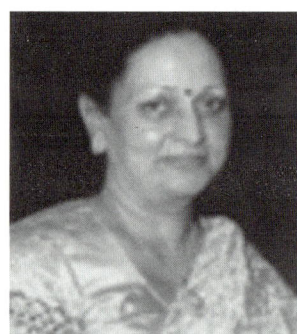

Dr Lekha Pathak

## Dr Kamala I Vytilingam

The first formal Department of Cardiology in India, was started in Christian Medical College (CMC) Hospital, Vellore in 1957, by Dr Kamala I Vytilingam, who brought modern cardiology to India after a period of training at Johns Hopkins Hospital, Baltimore in the early 1950s. She did a year's training with Dr Helen Taussig in 1961. The availability of surgical help allowed her to look after both adult as well as pediatric patients. She established one of the earliest cardiac catheterization laboratories in India.

## Dr Savitri Shrivastava

Professor Savitri Shrivastava did her MBBS from GRM College, Gwalior, Agra University in 1957 and MD (Medicine) at GRM College, Vikram University in 1961. She did her DM (Cardiology) at All India Institute of Medical Sciences, Delhi, India in 1971. Subsequently between 1975 and 1976, she did her fellowship in pediatric cardiology at University of Minnesota, Minneapolis, USA. She came back to AIIMS. Her special achievement in field of interventional cardiology described for the first time in the world was an original technique of balloon dilatation of the atrial septum (static balloon) in transposition of great vessels. This was published in Indian Heart Journal in 1988. She also reported for the first time in the world "Percutaneous catheter commissurotomy in rheumatic mitral stenosis" in the New England Journal of Medicine in 1985. She was also instrumental in doing a lot of procedures for the first time in India at AIIMS. The procedures were balloon valvuloplasty for pulmonary valve, aortic valve, balloon dilation of aortic coarctation, aortoarteritis, peripheral pulmonary arteries, coil occlusions of BT Shunt, coronary AV fistula, and aortopulmonary collaterals. She was awarded "PICS Achievement Award" at the Annual PICS (Pediatric Interventional Cardiology Symposiums) meeting held in Miami, Florida on January 21, 2013. This is a great honor for an Indian. After her retirement from AIIMS, the good work is being continued at present by Dr Anitha Saxena who did school surveys for RHD disease with mobile echo machine and Dr Shyam Kothari who has worked on pulmonary hypertension.

## Dr (Mrs) Ramesh Arora (Fig. 1)

She established a registry of transcatheter noncoronary interventional procedures in the country and was awarded with national interventional council of CSI award for development of noncoronary interventional cardiology in India (1999). She started nonsurgical (device) closure of patent ductus arteriosus (PDA) in 1987 by using Rashkind umbrella device for the first time in the country.

For valvular lesions specially percutaneous transvenous mitral commissurotomy (PTMC) in children was done in 1987 by her using double Mansfield balloon technique and in 1990 with Inoue balloon. Nonsurgical closure of atrial septal defect (ASD) was first time attempted in the country by using various sizes of Sideris devices (1993), followed by Starflex, Cardioseal, and Amplatzer devices (1998). She started devices closure of ventricular septal defect (VSD), both perimembranous and muscular by using Rashkind umbrella device in 1995 and this was replaced by muscular Amplatzer VSD device in 1999. First human use of specially designed perimembranous VSD device was done in

December 2000 by Dr Ramesh Arora. Various other rare cardiac lesions were attempted like coronary arteriovenous (AV) fistula, ruptured sinus of valsalva pulmonary AV fistula, PA to LA fistula, etc. She made all Indians proud by having done the highest number of PTMC and perimembranous VSD closure by device in the world, at a particular time! She is a bundle of energy and enthusiasm for innovations. So much so when Dr IB Vijayalakshmi showed her the booklet with the diagram of Amplatzer device drawn by Kurt himself she had jumped with joy!

## Dr Lekha Pathak

Dr Lekha Pathak is the Director and Head of the Cardiology Department at Nanavati Super Speciality Hospital, Mumbai, India. She completed MBBS from Netaji Subhash Chandra Bose Medical College, Jabalpur in 1965, and MD-General Medicine from Netaji Subhash Chandra Bose Medical College, Jabalpur in 1968, DM-Cardiology from King Edward Memorial Hospital and Seth Gordhandas Sunderdas Medical College in 1971. She has done over 10,000 interventional procedures for past 10 years. Dr Lekha Pathak has been awarded with Lifetime Achievement Award by Ex-President APJ Abdul Kalam for outstanding contribution in the field of cardiology 2008, Priyadarshini award in 2008, Doctor of Science (DSc) by University of Loyola, Chicago, USA in 2012 and many more. She is a member of Maharashtra University of Health Sciences, Padmashree Dr D Y Patil University-Member Management Council, Association of Physicians of India (API) and Indian College of Physician. Some of the services provided by the doctor are carotid angioplasty and stenting, coronary and noncoronary interventions, angioplasty and stenting, interventional procedures and minimally invasive cardiac surgery. She is the second woman to be president of CSI after Dr Padmavathi. She is a cardiologist in Vile Parle West, Mumbai and has an experience of 47 years in this field.

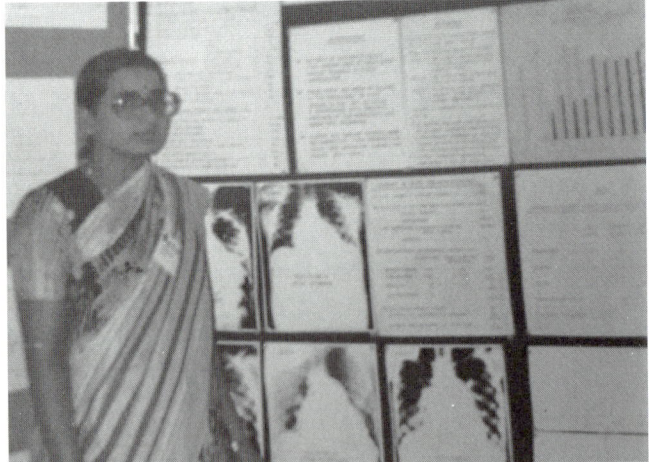

**FIG. 1:** Dr Ramesh Arora is seen presenting on rheumatic fever and rheumatic heart disease (RHD) in June 1980 in London in the first world congress of pediatric cardiology.

## Dr Anitha Saxena

She was born in November 1956, presently serving as full professor of cardiology since 1998, at the All India Institute of Medical Sciences, New Delhi, a very high volume tertiary care public hospital catering primarily to northern, central, and eastern parts of India. Her responsibilities include teaching, research, and patient-related clinical work. She is regularly teaching postgraduate fellows and residents who are undergoing 3 years structured training programs in cardiology and has served as guide/co-guide for thesis for over 50 postdoctoral students.

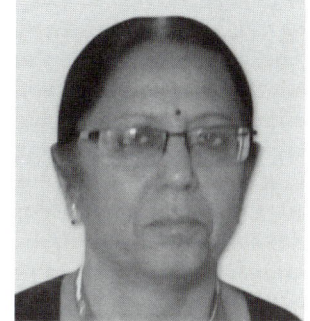

She completed her education with MBBS, MD, and DM degrees, all from University of Delhi, and has been a gold medalist throughout the academic carrier. She has over 33 years of experience in the subspecialty of pediatric cardiology and adults with CHD. She has many publications with over 312 research articles in reputed national and international journals. Some of the landmark articles are frequently cited in literature and textbooks. She has been the principle investigator for a number of community-related research projects on public health issues related to cardiology. Some of her publications on community research, related primarily to rheumatic and CHD, have been widely cited.

She is actively engaged in the formulation of national guidelines for the management of CHD and RHD and has published extensively on status and management of CHD in India. She is also a member of several international groups dealing with global burden of RHD and the co-chair of the Working Group of Task Force on Rheumatic Heart Disease, set up by the World Heart Federation, Geneva. She is frequently invited as an expert group member by the Ministry of Health and Family Welfare, Government of India, for formulation of policies and guidelines related to the specialty of cardiology. The Indian Council of Medical Research has also been regularly inviting her as one of the experts for evaluation of research projects and for policymaking decisions, related to the specialty of cardiology.

She has held important positions in several national and international academic organizations including President of Asia Pacific Pediatric Cardiac Society, Pediatric Cardiac Society of India, and National Rheumatic Heart Consortium. She has been awarded Fellow of American College of Cardiology.

## Dr IB Vijayalakshmi (Figs. 2 and 3)

On November 14, 1998 for the first time in South India government set up pediatric cardiology department was started in Sri Jayadeva Institute of Cardiology. Dr IB Vijayalakshmi, first lady cardiologist of Karnataka, who headed the department, was the first one to use Amplatzer septal occluder and Amplatzer duct occluder (ADO) on January 27, 1999 in South India. Thanks to Children's Heart link, Minnesota, she was trained in four best centers in USA: (1) Fairview University Children's Hospital (Minneapolis), (2) St. Mary's Hospital (Rochester), teaching hospital of Mayo Clinic Medical School, (3) Children's Hospital Medical Centre (Boston, Massachusetts), teaching hospital of Harvard University in 1998, and later was (4) trained at Children's Hospital at Chicago University in 2002 under Dr Ziyad Hijazi.

Thanks to the excellent training that she received, she went on to do several interventions for the first time in the world. One such case was a 4-year-old child with non-compaction of left ventricle with the aorto-left ventricular tunnel (ALVT) closed with Amplatzer device in 2001. When the first ALVT was closed surgically by Evalon plug from aortic end by Dr Lillehei Minnesota, Dr Kurt Amplatz was part of that great team! So Kurt was excited about the ALVT being closed by his device. He donated three devices to be tried for this case and wrote "Nobody can advise you, as no one has any experience, use your clinical acumen and all the best." True to his words, the two sizes of VSDs were too big and compressing on the aortic valve, the third, 16 × 14 largest ADO was a bit small to block the aneurysmally dilated extra cardiac portion of the tunnel, leading to hemolysis for 5 days. This case was presented at 37th Annual Scientific meeting and AGA Medical 4th International Symposium at Porto, Portugal, on 15 May, 2002 and published in pediatric cardiology journal. And also in the same meeting, the first case of isolated dextrocardia with mid-muscular VSD closed through the jugular approach with 16 mm Amplatzer device was presented by her.

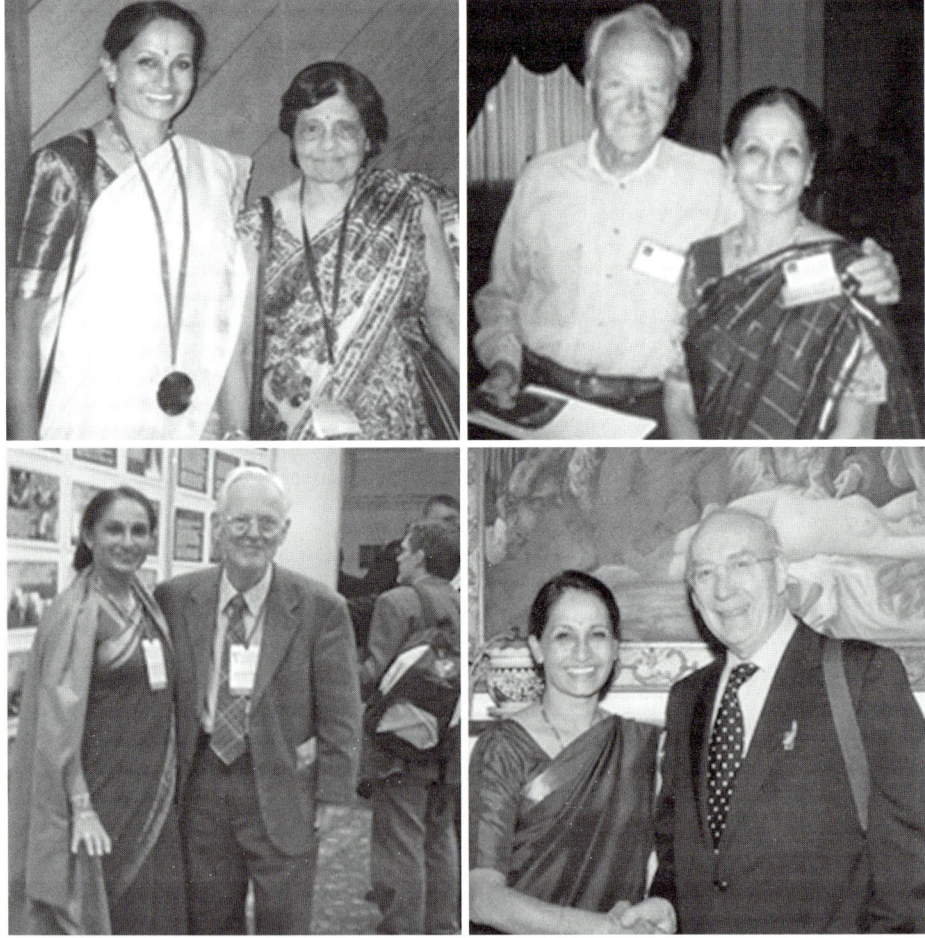

**FIG. 2:** From left to right Dr IB Vijayalakshmi with her source of inspiration Dr S Padmavati, Dr Kurt Amplatz, Dr Richard Van Praagh, and Dr Fontan.

# CHAPTER 1: Role of Women in Development of Cardiology in India

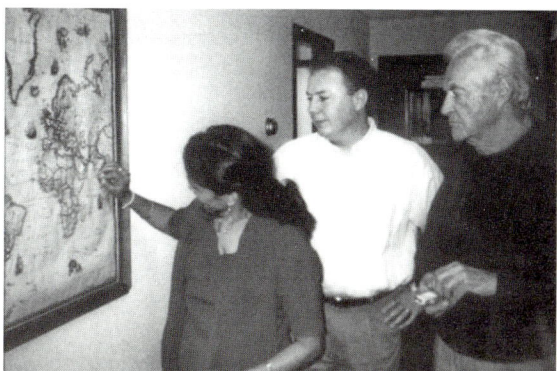

**FIG. 3:** Dr IB Vijayalakshmi is seen putting the red pin on Bengaluru to mark the centers using Amplatzer device. Dr Kurt Amplatz and his son-in-law watching the global map in the head office of AGA in 1998.

When it was explained to Dr Kurt, that the available Amplatzer devices require larger French sheaths to introduce and hence it was difficult to do the device closure in emaciated low-weight Indian children, he came out with innovative "modified Amplatzer device" in which only one layer of polyester material was stitched, instead of three layers! Thanks to this alteration, a large PDA in a 3.9 kg infant was closed with 10 × 8 ADO in 2002 and was presented in PICS-VI at Chicago, USA in September, 2002 and initial experience in 10 infants was published in 2006. This was done when nobody was doing device closure in children weighing <6 kg. When the angiogram of a PDA larger than aorta in a 4.5 kg infant was mailed to Dr Kurt, he came out with the custom made angled PDA device which had no polyester material at all in it! These custom made angled devices became the prototype for ADO II additional size (ADO II AS) which were used in infants and newborns later! For the first time in the world, a case of sickle cell anemia with ASD was closed with device closure in 2005. This was presented in World Congress in Buenos Aires, Argentina. Thanks to the low profile and easy trackability of ADO II, first time in the world a case of left coronary cameral fistula to RV was closed with ADO II in 2011, which topped the top 20 publications in noncoronary section in 2013. For the first time in the world, a case of aorto-right ventricular tunnel (ARVT) (only the 17th case) was closed with ADO II in 2013. For the first time in India, the workshop of PDA closure with Nit Occlud was done in 2002 with Dr Lee. For the first time, ADO II was used to close Gerbode defects with no complete heart block.

Dr IB Vijayalakshmi has written four textbooks for the cardiologists, (1) A monogram on "Acute Rheumatic fever and Rheumatic heart Disease," (2) "Step by Step to Echo in Congenital Heart Disease," (3) Chief editor of a textbook "A Comprehensive Approach to Congenital Heart Disease" for which the book review has been written by Dr Crystal R Bonnichsen of Mayo clinic and published in European Heart Journal. Dr Crystal writes "As stated in the epilogue, the editors used the approach of "A Lifelong Journey" to describe the management of congenital heart disease through the various stages, often called the "womb to tomb" approach. The editors undertook a formidable challenge by covering all aspects of congenital heart disease at all stages of life". For the first time in the world, she has proposed and published "*Vijaya's Echo criteria*" for diagnosis of carditis in ARF. In the recently revised Jones criteria, her two studies are cited and echo features are incorporated. Her study has been quoted in latest editions of standard pediatric cardiology textbooks like Heart Diseases in Infants and Children by Moss and Adams' and Park's Pediatric Cardiology for Practitioners.

**SECTION 1:** Cardiology

## Dr Suman Rao

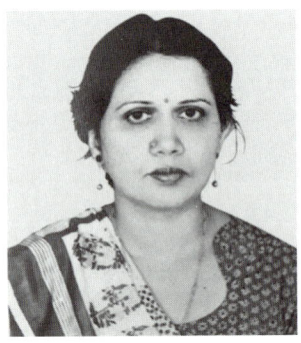

Dr Suman Rao, the first cardiologist of Himachal Pradesh, born on May 3, 1946, did her MD (medicine) as well as DM in cardiology from PGIMER, Chandigarh. She is a WHO fellow from cardiovascular institute, Mount Sinai, New York, USA. She worked as professor and head of the department of cardiology at IGMC Shimla for 12 years. She held post of director of medical education in the state of Himachal Pradesh and has been advisor to the state government. She is principal of Tanda Medical College. She has number of publications in national journals on cardiac status at high altitudes. In addition, she has a number of publications in national and international journals of cardiology. She is the recipient of DP Basu Complimentary Award at CSI Conference and has taken active part in national and international conferences of cardiology.

## JOURNEY OF CATHETER-BASED INTERVENTIONS BY WOMEN

The various pediatric cardiac catheter interventions initiated in India are:
- Rashkind balloon septostomy in d-TGA in early 1970s—CMCH, Vellore.
- Balloon pulmonary valvotomy in 1985 by Dr M Khalilullah and Dr Ramesh Arora at GB Pant Hospital, New Delhi.
- Balloon aortoplasty of coarctation of the aorta (CoAo) 1985 by Dr M Khalilullah and Dr Ramesh Arora, New Delhi.
- The first PTMC in rheumatic mitral stenosis was done in 1985 by legendary Dr Savitri Shrivastava.
- Balloon aortic valvuloplasty in 1986 by Dr M Khalilullah and Dr Ramesh Arora, New Delhi.
- Procedure of balloon dilatation of the atrial septum in transposition of great vessels by static balloon was introduced in 1988 by Dr Savitri Shrivastava and followed by Dr Ramesh Arora.
- Dr Ramesh Arora started nonsurgical (device) closure of PDA in 1988 by using Rashkind umbrella device for the first time in the country.
- Device closure of PDA in 1988 by Dr Ramesh Arora at GB Pant Hospital, New Delhi and subsequently by using Amplatzer devices (1998).
- Nonsurgical transcatheter closure of ASD was first time attempted in the country by using various sizes of Sideris devices (1993), followed by Starflex, Cardioseal by Dr Ramesh Arora.
- Dr Ramesh Arora also did the first device closure of VSD, both perimembranous and muscular by using Rashkind umbrella device in 1995 and this was replaced by muscular Amplatzer VSD device in 1999.
- Later for the first time in India, various Amplatzer devices were used to close ASD and PDA by Dr Ramesh Arora in North India and Dr IB Vijayalakshmi in South India in January 1999.
- The valvular lesions, especially PTMC in children, was done in 1987 by using double Mansfield balloon technique and in 1990 with Inoue Balloon by Dr Savitri Shrivastava, Dr Satyvan Sharma, and Dr Ramesh Arora.
- For the first time, transcatheter noncoronary interventional procedures council was established in 1999 in the country and Dr Ramesh Arora was awarded the national

interventional council of CSI award for development of noncoronary interventional cardiology in India.
- First human use of specially designed perimembranous VSD device was done in December 2000 by Dr Ramesh Arora.
- Along with Dr Ramesh Arora, Dr IB Vijayalakshmi did the first PDA closure with specially designed angled device in neonates (2003). Incidentally, this was the first case in the world in whom 8.6 mm PDA larger than aorta (8.2 mm) was closed in 4.5 kg infant.

Various other rare cardiac lesions were attempted like coronary AV fistula, ruptured sinus of valsalva pulmonary AV fistula, PA to LA fistula, etc., by Dr Ramesh Arora and Dr IB Vijayalakshmi.

For the first time in the country, a national policy for CHD was proposed by Dr IB Vijayalakshmi in 2004. Since then many centers started coaching fellows in pediatric cardiology. Now, DNB itself has identified 11 centers training 22 fellows in pediatric cardiology and two centers in India offering DM in pediatric cardiology.

## CONCLUSION

The situation is not very different in India from west where 20% of cardiologists are women, though there is no compiled data available. More women are now heart specialists in India. The journey of cardiology started virtually with only three centers having just M-mode echocardiograms in India. But the cardiac catheterization laboratory has clearly transformed from a diagnostic facility to a place for providing definitive treatment to nearly 65% of simple CHDs without scar on the chest. So fascinating is the history of interventional cardiology. Many surprises are bound to come as gifted minds toil night and day to make this world a better place with less suffering. Thanks to medical tourism, today India is the destination for interventions in cardiology and women are contributing a great deal in taking care of hearts of ailing patients.

*"One hundred years from now, it will not matter what kind of car I drove, what kind of house I lived in, how much was my bank account, nor what my clothes looked like. BUT the world may be a little better because I was important in the life of a child"*— Anonymous

## SUGGESTED READING

1. Tandon R. Development of Pediatric Cardiology in India.
2. Taussig HB, King JT, Bauersfeld R, Padvamati-Iyer S. Results of operation for pulmonary stenosis and atresia; (report of 1000 cases). Trans Assoc Am Physicians. 1951;64:67-73.
3. Shrestha NK, Padmavati S. Congenital heart disease in Delhi school children. Indian J Med Res. 1980;72:403-7.
4. Shrivastava S, Radhakrishnan S, Dev V, Singh LS, Rajani M. Balloon dilatation of atrial septum in complete transposition of great artery--a new technique. Indian Heart J. 1987;39(4):298-300.
5. Lock JE, Khalilullah M, Shrivastava S, Bahl V, Keane JF. Percutaneous catheter commissurotomy in rheumatic mitral stenosis. N Engl J Med. 1985;313:1515-8.
6. Arora R, Jain P, Rajagopal S, Nair M, Keane JK, Khalilullah M. Transcatheter closure of patent ductus arteriosus: preliminary experience with five patients. Indian Heart J. 1988;40(4):253-7.
7. Arora R, Nair M, Rajagopal S, Sethi KK, Mohan JC, Nigam M, et al. Percutaneous balloon mitral valvuloplasty in children and young adults with rheumatic mitral stenosis. Am Heart J. 1989;118 (5 Pt 1):883-7.
8. Arora R, Nair M, Kalra GS, Sethi KK, Mohan JC, Nigam M, et al. Non-surgical mitral valvuloplasty for rheumatic mitral stenosis. Indian Heart J. 1990;42:329-34.

## SECTION 1: Cardiology

9. Arora R, Trehan VK, Kalra GS, Chawla R, Jhamb U, Nigam M, et al. Transcatheter closure of atrial septal defect using buttoned device--Indian experience. Indian Heart J. 1996;48(2):145-9.
10. Kalra GS, Verma PK, Dhall A, Singh S, Bhardwaj S, Arora R. Transcatheter closure of secundum atrial septal defect with atrial septal defect occlusion system (ASDOS): initial experience and short-term follow-up. Indian Heart J. 1998;50(4):409-13.
11. Kalra GS, Verma PK, Dhall A, Singh S, Arora R. Transcatheter device closure of ventricular septal defects: immediate results and intermediate-term follow-up. Am Heart J. 1999;138(2 Pt 1):339-44.
12. Bass JL, Kalra GS, Arora R, Masura J, Gavora P, Thanopoulos BD, et al. Initial human experience with the Amplatzer perimembranous ventricular septal occluder device. Catheter Cardiovasc Interv. 2003;58(2):238-45.
13. Vijayalakshmi IB, Chitra N, Prabhu Deva AN. Use of an Amplatzer duct occluder for closing an aortico-left ventricular tunnel in a case of noncompaction of the left ventricle. Pediatr Cardiol. 2004;25:77-9.
14. Vijayalakshmi IB, Chitra N, Rajasri R, Vasudevan K. Initial clinical experience in transcatheter closure of large patent arterial ducts in infants using the modified and angled Amplatzler duct occluder. Cardiol Young. 2006;16(4):378-84.
15. Vijayalakshmi IB, Chitra N, Praveen J, Prasanna SR. Challenges in device closure of a large patent ductus arteriosus in infants weighing less than 6 kg. J Interv Cardiol. 2013;26:69-76.
16. Vijayalakshmi IB, Narasimhan C, Agarwal A. Transcatheter closure of left coronary cameral fistula With Amplatzer Duct Occluder II. J Invasive Cardiol. 2013;25:265-7.
17. Vijayalakshmi IB, Narasimhan C, Agarwal A. Closure of aorto-right ventricular tunnel with Amplatzer Duct Occluder II. J Invasive Cardiol. 2013;25(4):E75-7.
18. Vijayalakshmi IB, Natraj Setty HS, Chitra N, Manjunath CN. Amplatzer duct occluder II for closure of congenital Gerbode defects. Catheter Cardiovasc Interv. 2015;86(6):1057-62.
19. Vijayalakshmi IB, Narasimhan C, Singh B, Manjunath CN. Treatment of congenital non-ductal shunt lesions with the Amplatzer duct occluder II. Catheter Cardiovasc Interv. 2017;89(6):85-E193.
20. Gewitz MH, Baltimore RS, Tani LY, Sable CA, Shulman ST, Carapetis J, et al. Revision of the Jones Criteria for the diagnosis of acute rheumatic fever in the era of Doppler echocardiography: a scientific statement from the American Heart Association. Circulation. 2015;131(20):1806-18.
21. Vijayalakshmi IB, Chitra N, Rajasri R, Prabhudeva AN. Amplatzer angled duct occluder for closure of patent ductus arteriosus larger than the aorta in an infant. Pediatr Cardiol. 2005;26:480-3.
22. Vijayalakshmi S, Prabhudev N. Coronary heart disease in Indian women—change the gender bias. In: Rao GH, Kakkar VV (Eds). Coronary artery disease in South Asians. New Delhi: Jaypee Brothers Medical Publishers Pvt Ltd; 2001. p. 92.

# CHAPTER 2

# Cardiovascular Risk Assessment and Primary Prevention Strategies in Women

*Jyotsana, Naveen Kumar, Lalitha Nimani*

## ABSTRACT

Several risk assessment models have been developed for the estimation of cardiovascular disease (CVD) risk. Despite the vast knowledge of understanding of the pathophysiology of coronary heart disease (CHD), an ideal risk assessment tool is still nonexistent. Moreover, females owing to their phenotypic and genotypic variations to men need a special risk assessment model. The present chapter highlights the available tools for CVD risk assessment along with their advantages and limitations. Also, a new risk model for women with special emphasis on female-specific risk factors has been proposed.

## INTRODUCTION

Women are a different subset than men as regards their cardiovascular disease (CVD) risk. The present chapter discusses the available and suggested risk scores for CVD risk assessment. It also highlights the components of primary and secondary prevention strategies in females.

## FRAMINGHAM RISK SCORE

Among the many studies that contributed to the understanding of cardiovascular (CV) risk factors, the FHS (Framingham Heart Study) was a landmark achievement. The FHS gave a simple coronary disease prediction algorithm, FRS (Framingham Risk Score), using categorical variables, which allows physicians to predict multivariate coronary heart disease (CHD) risk in patients without overt CHD and provides a 10-year estimate of CVD risk.

### Factors Included

Several risk factors were identified as strong independent predictors of CHD in the FHS. These include age, sex, total cholesterol, high-density lipoprotein cholesterol (HDL-C) level, blood pressure (BP), cigarette smoking, and diabetes.

The importance of the FRS is underscored by its inclusion in guidelines as the NCEP ATP III (National Cholesterol Education Program Adult Treatment Panel III) in 2001. Those individuals with two or more above-mentioned risk factors were recommended to get their FRS calculated. FRS of >20% was considered to be at risk of developing CHD.

## Interpretation of the Framingham Risk Score

**Table 1** represents the correlation of FRS to heart disease risk percentage.

## Limitations of Framingham Risk Score

Though a rich source of information regarding risk assessment, FRS is not without limitations. It can only predict the development of CHD and not other vascular diseases. Young patients were underrepresented in the cohort of FHS, and the young patients in the study had few events, thereby making FRS an unreliable tool in young patients. While it was found to be a useful risk assessment tool in white males and females, it failed to do so in the subsequent studies in Japanese American men and women, Hispanics, and Native American men and women and north and south European populations, where it overestimated the prevalence of CHD. Diabetes considered as a coronary disease equivalent, is not given the importance it deserves in FHS as it is not devised for the diabetic population. Another potential limitation is that FHS did not take a family history of coronary artery disease (CAD) into account as a risk factor.

> Even though short-term cardiovascular risk is less in women, lifetime cardiovascular risk is high.

**TABLE 1:** Interpretation of Framingham Risk Score (FRS) for coronary heart disease (CHD) risk assessment.

| FRS points | Heart diseases risk percentage over 10 years |
|---|---|
| <0 | 0% |
| 0–8 | <1% |
| 9–12 | 1% |
| 13–14 | 2% |
| 15 | 3% |
| 16 | 4% |
| 17 | 5% |
| 18 | 6% |
| 19 | 8% |
| 20 | 11% |
| 21 | 14% |
| 22 | 17% |
| 23 | 22% |
| 24 | 27% |
| ≥25 | >30% |

In an attempt to improve the accuracy of FHS, high-sensitivity C-reactive protein (hs-CRP) was incorporated into the FRS by Wilson and associates, who found that it did not add further prognostic information. While it is challenging to improve predictive accuracy substantially, new models that include family history and coronary artery calcium assessment are forthcoming. Even though short-term CV risk is less in women, lifetime CV risk is high. Many important female-specific factors such as pregnancy-related risk or family history or subclinical CVD were not included in CV risk estimation.

## SCORE RISK CHARTS

By using FRS, CAD risk was overestimated in Danish and German people, and then the European Society of Cardiology (ESC) did a project based on a large pool of representative European data sets. This led to the establishment of the SCORE (Systematic COronary Risk Evaluation) project.

The SCORE project in liaison with the Third Joint Taskforce developed a system of risk estimation for clinical use in Europe. It pooled a dataset of cohort studies from 12 European countries. Thus being derived from a heterogeneous population, it could accommodate more parameters and widened its range of application to different populations.

### Advantages of SCORE over FRS

It gave the 10-year risk of fatal CVD events for 400 combinations for the high-risk and low-risk populations in the form of charts for both males and females. This has the main advantage of calculating the total CV risk apart from the CHD risk, the major setback of FRS. Unlike FRS, where only low-density lipoprotein cholesterol (LDL-C) is given primary importance, low HDL-C was given equal importance in these charts. Hence, the risk estimation is given with the help of two charts in relation to cholesterol and cholesterol/HDL ratio.

### Assessment of Risk by SCORE

These risk assessment scores as there are designed for detection high- or intermediate- or low-risk category from the general population and not applicable to already known as high-risk categories, such as known CVD or CHD, and type 2 diabetes mellitus (T2DM) or type 1 diabetes mellitus (T1DM) with target organ damage.

The important thing about this score is that these charts show (**Figs. 1** and **2**) the relative risk but not the absolute risk in the form of percentages. For example, a young woman with low total CV risk may not have a low relative risk. This can be known only when relative charts are applied. As the age of the women increases, then this high relative risk will translate into a high total risk. So, this particular woman requires intense lifestyle advice from the first time testing (at a younger age), not after the increase in the total CV risk in the advanced age.

The second approach to detect the risk in younger women is by determining the CV risk age. For example, a 50-year female, hypertensive with severe dyslipidemia and smoker, has 2% 10-year risk of CAD, which is the same as a 65-year female without any risk factors, so her risk age is 65. This risk can be modified by controlling the BP and lipid abnormality along with the cessation of smoking.

# SECTION 1: Cardiology

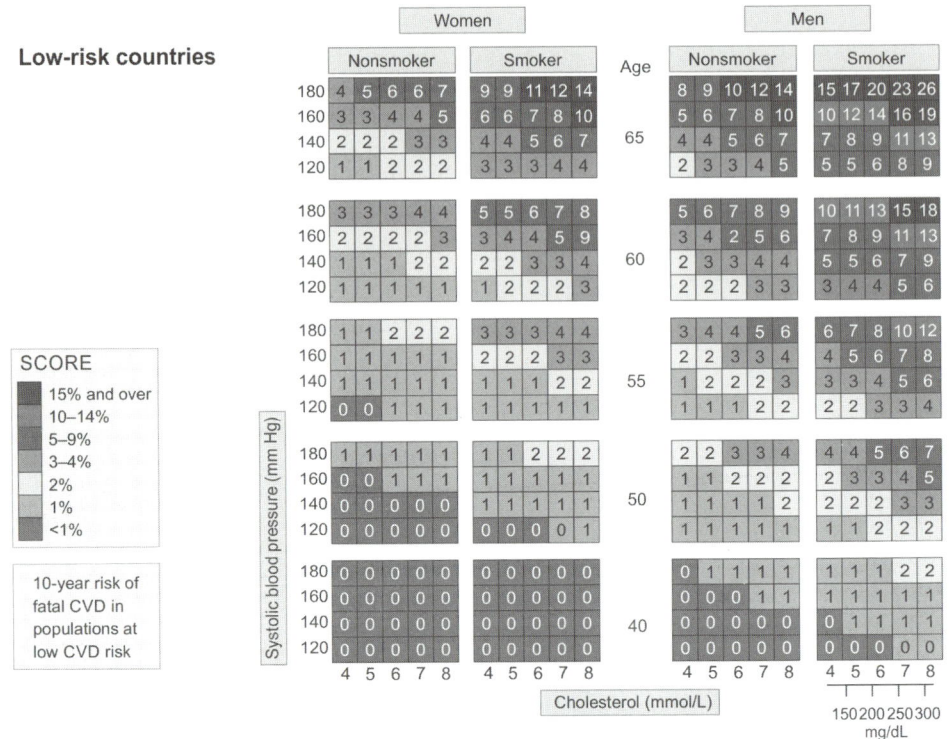

(CVD: cardiovascular disease; SCORE: Systematic Coronary Risk Evaluation)

**FIG. 1:** SCORE calculation in low-risk countries. *(For color version, see Plate 1)*
(*Source:* Tomasik T et al.)

## RISK ESTIMATION USING SCORE

This SCORE should be applied with caution by physicians and have to give be important to the local conditions. In CAD-declining countries, this score may overestimate the risk, whereas, in CAD-epidemic countries, this underestimates the risk. The risk in females is about 10 years older than males. At any given age, the risk appears lower for women than men.

This SCORE may be higher in sedentary or obese persons or persons with a strong family history of premature atherosclerosis or in ethnic minorities. This SCORE should use only in people with diabetes without end-organ damage.

## Limitations of SCORE

Despite making up for a few drawbacks of FRS, SCORE charts are not without limitations. Some of them such as, diabetes is not included in the risk function. It takes into account only fatal events; nonfatal events were not endpoints while creating the risk charts. Factors, with uncertain accuracies such as a strong family history of early-onset CVD, milder degrees of impaired glucose regulation, triglycerides, and fibrinogen, were not given the status of risk factors.

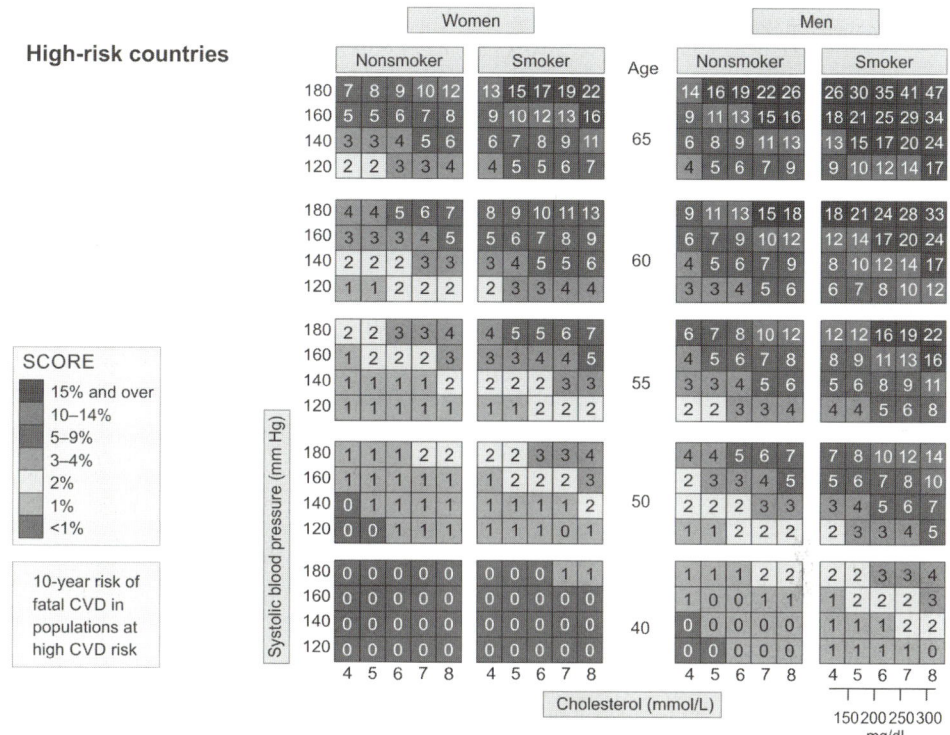

(CVD: cardiovascular disease; SCORE: Systematic Coronary Risk Evaluation)

**FIG. 2:** SCORE calculation in high-risk countries. *(For color version, see Plate 2)*
(*Source:* Tomasik T et al.)

# WORLD HEALTH ORGANIZATION/INTERNATIONAL SOCIETY OF HYPERTENSION RISK CHARTS

Instead of other guidelines, which focused on single risk factors, the World Health Organization (WHO) and International Society of Hypertension (ISH), gave an integrated and cost-effective approach for managing risk factors in the guidelines published in 2007. They addressed both coronary and noncoronary vascular events. These guidelines took into consideration some important facts—that multiple risk factors are responsible for cardiovascular events that these risk factors and determinants of coronary and noncoronary events were very similar, and therefore prevention approaches are similar.

The WHO/ISH risk prediction charts indicate a 10-year total CV risk for fatal and nonfatal events. These are two sets of charts from 14 epidemiological subregions that are meant to be used in low-income and middle-income countries, where predefined charts do not exist.

These charts classify an individual at high risk (maroon and red), medium risk (orange and yellow), or low risk (green) risk for coronary heart disease, stroke, or other atherosclerotic diseases. Not only does this predict a CV risk, but these guidelines also suggested prevention strategies. Though applied and studied in various populations and individual levels, the application of these charts in women, in particular, is not validated extensively.

The revision of these charts with extension to 21 global regions has been validated recently and is now available for use. Its application in women can be an advance toward CVD risk assessment in women. For example, here we are mentioning the charts for Southeast Asia subregions (SEAR). The WHO subregions SEAR B and SEAR D charts in color for use in settings where total blood cholesterol can be measured (**Figs. 3** and **4**).

## COMPARISON OF FRS, SCORE, AND WHO/ISH MODELS

Four CV risk prediction models were assessed in an Asian population. The WHO/ISH model performed poorly for CV risk stratification. The Framingham and SCORE models could stratify risk in Asian men and women. The SCORE-high model accurately predicted risk for men, but not women. The Framingham model stratified risk better than the SCORE models in women.

## REYNOLDS RISK SCORE

The Reynolds Risk Score was calculated from nearly 25,000 Americans. With a better understanding of underlying biological processes, more and more novel inflammatory markers were incorporated into the prediction algorithms; the better validated was of Reynolds Risk Score. Probably the only risk assessment score, which was studied in two separate cohorts of men and women. It included hs-CRP and family history but excluded diabetes as it considers diabetes in itself as a high risk for prediction of CVD.

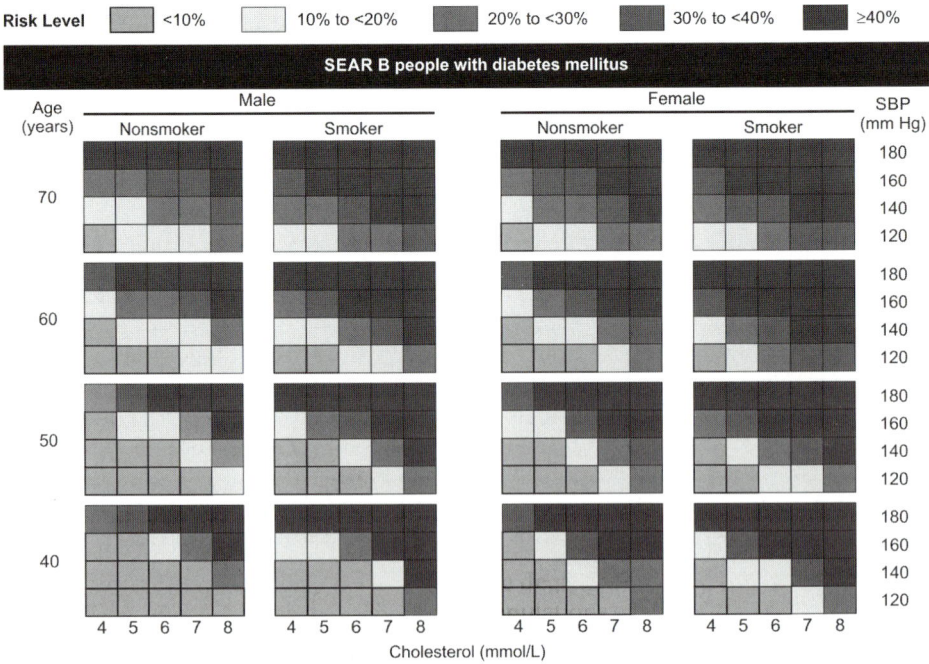

(ISH: International Society of Hypertension; SEAR: Southeast Asia subregions; SBP: systolic blood pressure; WHO: World Health Organization)

**FIG. 3:** The WHO/ISH risk prediction chart SEAR B with Diabetes. *(For color version, see Plate 3)*

CHAPTER 2: Cardiovascular Risk Assessment and Primary Prevention Strategies in Women

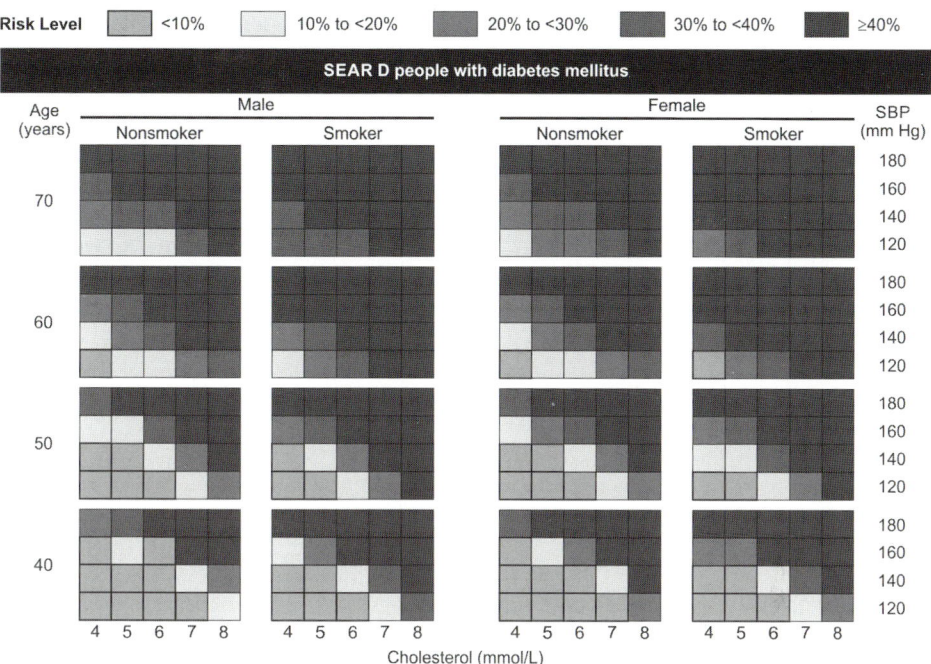

(ISH: International Society of Hypertension; SEAR: Southeast Asia subregions; SBP: systolic blood pressure; WHO: World Health Organization)

**FIG. 4:** The WHO/ISH risk prediction chart SEAR D with Diabetes. *(For color version, see Plate 4)*

High-sensitivity C-reactive protein, by its role as an acute phase reactant, can be elevated in trivial conditions making it a less reliable marker in low- and middle-income countries with a high incidence of subclinical infections. Nevertheless, Reynolds Score can be a handy tool in women, especially with chronic inflammation (atherosclerosis).

## 2011 EFFECTIVENESS-BASED GUIDELINES FOR THE PREVENTION OF CAD IN WOMEN

The American Heart Association (AHA) published its women-specific clinical recommendations for the prevention of CVD in 1999. The update in 2004 classified women into high risk, intermediate risk, lower risk, and optimal risk—this is completely based on clinical criteria and FRS. The latter update in 2007 classified women into high risk, at-risk, or at optimal risk. These guidelines questioned the conventional thinking that women should be treated the same as men, quoting the lack of adequate representation of women in clinical trials.

The 2011 guidelines are a significant evolution in comparison to earlier updates in that substantial role was given to the effectiveness of preventive therapies, thereby transforming it to "effective-based" guidelines for the prevention of CVD in women.

This identifies women's ideal cardiovascular health, at-risk, or high-risk for CVD so that those appropriate preventive strategies can be planned.

## 2013 ATHEROSCLEROTIC CARDIOVASCULAR DISEASE POOLED COHORT RISK EQUATIONS

The Working group ACC (American College of Cardiology)/AHA guidelines of 2013 made a dramatic turnover in the risk prediction by giving gender-specific pooled cohort equations for establishing the 10-year risk for the development of the first atherosclerotic CVD (ASCVD) event. They included the data from different ethnic groups, from geographically different populations and study patients of Atherosclerosis Risk in Communities (ARIC) and the Coronary Artery Risk Development in Young Adults (CARDIA). However, this data did not include the Indians and Hispanic whites.

## UNITED KINGDOM PROSPECTIVE DIABETES STUDY CARDIAC RISK SCORE

This scoring system was mainly derived from the UK population (UK Prospective Diabetes Study). This includes the gender, age, duration of diabetes, smoking status, HbA1c, systolic BP, total cholesterol/HDL, and urinary microalbumin levels.

## OTHER RISK ASSESSMENT SCORES

Apart from the risk scores mentioned earlier, The PROCAM (Prospective Cardiovascular Münster) study is based on a sample of industrial employees; it may be considered somewhat underpowered for risk estimation for women. The QRISK, QRISK2 and QRISK3 systems are different because they are based on databases of general practice attendees and are, therefore, not random representative samples of the population. However, the advantage of using these data is substantially larger numbers that can be included. QRISK3 (the most recent version of QRISK) is a prediction algorithm for (CVD) that uses traditional risk factors together with body mass index (BMI), ethnicity, measures of deprivation, family history, chronic kidney disease (CKD), rheumatoid arthritis, atrial fibrillation (AF), diabetes mellitus, and antihypertensive treatment.

## EMERGING RISK FACTORS: IMPLICATION FOR RISK ASSESSMENT IMAGING-BASED RISK SCORES

### Coronary Artery Calcification

Many studies {US MESA (Multi-Ethnic Study of Atherosclerosis), German HNR, [Heinz-Nixdorf Recall (Risk Factors, Evaluation of Coronary Calcium, Lifestyle)], Rotterdam study group, CARDIA studies} proved that coronary artery calcium (CAC) by CT scan without contrast was well correlated with the presence (extent of atherosclerotic plaque burden) of CAD by angiogram, but not with the degree of luminal narrowing. This effect was shown in a wide variety of asymptomatic populations of all ages, people with diabetes, and smokers. A study concentrating only on postmenopausal women was done under the Women's Health Initiative. Even though recent trails created the controversies of the effectiveness of calcium score as a predictor of CAD risk, depending on the MESA study, calcium score was incorporated in the CAD risk model for the prediction of CAD risk at 10 years. However, this risk score does not consider the stroke and all forms of ASCVD.

The degree of progression, CAC = 0 to >0 less in females, but the rate and degree of the progression are not important risk factors for the CAD risk calculation.

Proposed guideline using 10-year ASCVD risk estimate plus CAC scoring (CACS) to guide statin therapy:
- *ASCVD risk <5%:* Statin is not recommended regardless of CACS.
- *ASCVD risk 5–7.5% + CACS = 0:* Statin not recommended or CACS >1 consider statin.
- *ASCVD risk >7.5–20% + CACS = 0:* Statin not recommended or CACS >0 recommend statin.
- *ASCVD risk >20%:* Recommend statin regardless of CACS.
- *Less than 5% and >20%:* CACS not effective for this population.

## Breast Calcification with Coronary Calcium Score

Breast arterial calcification (BAC) with CAC on CT scan are proposed as a sex-specific tool to predict CAD risk in asymptomatic women.

## Mitral Annular Calcification

Mitral annular calcification (MAC), along with metabolic syndrome, was associated with an increase in CAD.

## Carotid Artery Imaging

Intima medial thickness assessment is associated with CVD risk.

## Coronary Artery Wall Thickness

Magnetic resonance imaging (MRI)-derived coronary artery wall thickness in women was proved to be a marker for CAD.

## Biomarkers

### lncRNA ANRIL

The expression of the long non-coding RNA (lncRNA) antisense non-coding RNA in the INK4 locus (ANRIL) represented good diagnostic value for CAD, and its high expression was associated with increased stenosis degree, raised inflammation, and poor outcomes in CAD patients.

## UNFOCUSED RISK FACTORS: IMPLEMENTATION IN RISK ASSESSMENT

Even though anemia or level of hemoglobin was included in the risk assessment for women, it may be important to incorporate this factor also, as precipitation of coronary events occurs by anemia.

Similarly, pregnancy-related complications, oral contraceptive ingestion, surgical intervention for obesity, MAC are also important in the generation of CAD, so important for risk assessment.

As there are advantages and disadvantages of each of these risk scores, conclusively, we cannot say that a single risk score is an ideal one for all. Present risk score modification requires the inclusion of a few more clinical and laboratory parameters.

## PROPOSED NEW RISK MODELS FOR WOMEN

Gender-specific risk factors for women are pregnancy-related problems (preterm delivery, hypertensive disorders of pregnancy, gestational diabetes, abruptio placenta, spontaneous coronary artery dissection, mother with low birth weight baby, and peripartum cardiomyopathy), breast cancer-related treatment, polycystic ovary diseases, menstrual irregularities including functional hypothalamic amenorrhea, and usage of oral contraceptive are associated with subsequent development of CAD latter in the life. Furthermore, some of the risk factors more frequent in females such as depression and stress, autoimmune diseases, physical inactivity, and metabolic syndromes are also associated with CVD risk. According to Lalita et al. (unpublished, personal communication), additional risk factors for later development of CAD are early menarche (<12 years) and early menopause (≤45 years), history of pregnancy complication and loss of pregnancy. Early age at first pregnancy (≤18 years) and multiparity (≥3) also contribute to the risk of later CVD.

So, there is a need for a new scoring system, including the gender-specific and frequent risk factors for females. We are proposing a new model for the risk assessment in women. At present, we are able to say that below suggested risk factors be included in the new model, but we require specific projects give the exact scoring.

### Primary Prevention of Cardiovascular Diseases

Cardiovascular disease, which includes CHD, stroke, and peripheral artery disease, remains the leading cause of death in men and women. CVD is becoming the leading cause of death worldwide.

*Rationale for primary prevention of CVD:*
The following have been identified as major risk factors for CVD, are modifiable, and should be considered for intervention in all adults:
- Smoking
- Overweight and obesity
- Unhealthy diet
- Physical inactivity
- Dyslipidemia
- Hypertension
- Diabetes mellitus (considered in some guidelines as CHD risk equivalent).

Globally, up to 90% of the stroke burden may be attributable to modifiable risk factors, and up to 75% of this burden may be reduced by specifically addressing lifestyle and metabolic risk factors. Additionally, in the descriptive INTERHEART study of patients from 52 countries, nine potentially modifiable factors accounted for over 90% of the population-attributable risk of a first myocardial infarction (MI). These included cigarette smoking, dyslipidemia, hypertension, diabetes, abdominal obesity, and psychosocial factors. In addition, factors that were associated with lowered risks included regular physical activity, daily consumption of fruits and vegetables, and daily consumption of small amounts of alcohol.

In descriptive data from a nationally representative survey, five modifiable risk factors for CVD (elevated cholesterol, diabetes, hypertension, obesity, and smoking) accounted for one half of CVD deaths in United States adults aged 45–79 years from 2009 to 2010. The preventable fraction of CVD mortality associated with these risk factors was 54% for men and 50% for women.

The deleterious consequences of multiple risk factors are, at least, additive. In the FHS of over 5,000 men and women, those with five risk factors had a 10-year risk of a first CHD event of 25–30%, which is comparable to the absolute risk of a recurrent event for many patients who have survived a prior MI or occlusive stroke.

The majority of the risk factors for CVD and stroke are modifiable by preventive measures, including both therapeutic lifestyle changes (TLCs) and adjunctive drug therapies of proven benefit. In the United States, since 1975, CVD mortality has declined overall, although men and black people continue to experience higher absolute mortality rates at earlier ages than their female and white counterparts. However, since 2011, the rates of decline have slowed and are no longer evident. It has been estimated that nearly half of the decline is due to earlier diagnosis and more aggressive treatment of modifiable risk factors, especially of lipids and BP with adjunctive drug therapies, including statins, aspirin, angiotensin-converting enzyme (ACE) inhibitors, and beta-blockers. The remaining half of the decline in CVD mortality is attributable to favorable TLCs, such as avoidance and cessation of cigarette smoking.

Further supporting the benefits of the primary prevention of CVD by maintaining a healthy lifestyle was the Nurse's Health Study, a large prospective cohort study of over 120,000 female nurses followed for over 20 years. Women who maintained desirable body weight ate a healthy diet, exercised regularly, and did not smoke cigarettes experienced and 84% reduction in risk of clinical CVD events. Additionally, in the Women's Health Study of almost 40,000 female health professionals, practicing healthy lifestyle behaviors was associated with a 55% lower risk of stroke.

## Major Components of Primary Prevention of Cardiovascular Disease
### *Healthy Diet*
Individuals who self-select for a healthy diet have significantly lower risks CVD, including both CHD and stroke. Components of a healthy diet include intakes of:
- Fruits and vegetables
- Fiber, including cereals
- Foods with a low glycemic index and low glycemic load.
- Monounsaturated fat rather than trans-fatty acids or saturated fats.
- Omega-3 fatty acids (from fish, plant sources, or supplements).

Observational studies have consistently shown that individuals consuming diets high in vegetables and fruits, such as the Mediterranean diet, have a reduced risk of CVD. It is possible that the apparent benefit may be due to specific compounds in vegetables and fruits. It is also likely that people who eat more vegetables and fruits tend to eat less meat and saturated fat.

Basic research has suggested mechanisms of benefit, and observational studies have shown that individuals who self-select diets high in antioxidant vitamins or supplements have lower risks. Nonetheless, the most reliable data from large-scale randomized trials have not shown significant benefits of antioxidant vitamin supplementation in the primary prevention of CVD.

### *Smoking Avoidance and Cessation*
Cigarette smoking remains the leading avoidable cause of premature death and a major avoidable cause of premature disability. The totality of evidence indicates that the amount of cigarettes currently smoked increases morbidity and mortality from CVD, and benefits of cessation begin to appear after only a few months and reach that of the nonsmoker in several years, even among older adults. Thus, for CVD, it is never too late to quit, whereas,

for cancer, it is never too early, as the risks relate largely to duration rather than the amount currently smoked.

All smokers should be counseled to quit on a regular basis. A number of approaches, including behavioral therapy, nicotine replacement therapy, and other pharmacologic therapies, are available.

## *Hypertension Control*

Hypertension is a well-established risk factor for CVD, including morbidity and mortality from stroke, CHD, heart failure (HF), and sudden death.
- *Definition*: Hypertension is defined in the 2017 AHA/ACC guidelines as systolic pressure ≥130 mm Hg or a diastolic pressure ≥80 mm Hg.
- *Goal BP*: Goal BP may depend in part upon comorbidities (e.g., diabetes, and chronic kidney disease) and estimated CV risk.
- *Nonpharmacologic measures*: All patients with hypertension or elevated BP should practice nonpharmacologic TLCs, which include weight reduction if overweight or obese, salt restriction, and avoidance of excess alcohol intake.
- *Pharmacologic therapy*: Antihypertensive drugs are necessary for patients with persistent hypertension, despite TLCs. Most patients will require multiple antihypertensive drug therapies to achieve their BP goals.

## *Dyslipidemia*

Several large-scale randomized trials and their meta-analyses of statins in high-, moderate-, and low-risk primary prevention subjects without clinical evidence of CHD have demonstrated clinical benefits on CVD, including MI, stroke, and CVD death as well as total mortality.

All primary prevention subjects, especially those with dyslipidemia, should be counseled to achieve and maintain desirable body weight, engage in regular physical activity, and eat a prudent diet.

## *Physical Activity*

A number of observational studies have shown that individuals who self-select for increased physical activity have lower morbidity and mortality from CHD.

Regular physical activity is recommended in the early school years and throughout life. Common recommendations include moderate-intensity exercise for 150 minutes a week, vigorous-intensity exercise for 75 minutes a week, or an equivalent combination of these activities. Adults with limited exercise capacity due to comorbidities should stay as physically active as their condition allows. Even the modest amounts of regular physical activity, such as brisk walking for 20 minutes daily, are associated with significant benefits on the risk of CHD.

## *Weight Loss*

Overweight and obesity increase risk for several major risk factors for CVD, including hypertension, dyslipidemia, and insulin resistance, while weight loss has been shown to improve these parameters. Data from large prospective cohort studies have consistently shown that individuals with higher body weights have a linear increase in morbidity and mortality from CHD, after appropriate adjustment for smoking and other confounders.

The selection of treatment for overweight subjects is based upon an initial risk assessment. All should be evaluated for their willingness and ability to adapt therapeutic lifestyle changes as well as other interventions of proven benefit. All individuals who are willing, ready, and able to lose weight should receive information about behavior modification, diet, and increased physical activity.

## *Management of Type 2 Diabetes Mellitus*

There is a pandemic of T2DM, which is strongly associated with overweight and obesity. Morbidity and mortality from diabetes include both macrovascular (CHD, stroke, and peripheral artery disease) as well as microvascular complications (retinopathy, nephropathy, and neuropathy).

To reduce macrovascular complications, multifactorial interventions are crucial, especially weight reduction, increased physical activity, and control of BP, lipids, and glucose.

For microvascular complications, tight glycemic control reduces microvascular complications in both T1DM and T2DM. Tight glycemic control may also reduce risks of macrovascular complications in patients with T1DM and T2DM. The target A1c levels in patients with diabetes should be tailored to the individual by weighing the benefits on morbidity and mortality against the risk of hypoglycemia.

## *Aspirin*

In primary prevention trials of individuals at the low absolute risk of a first CHD event, aspirin confers a statistically significant and clinically important reduction in risk of nonfatal MI but no benefit on all-cause mortality and nonfatal stroke. The decision to recommend aspirin should be based upon an individual clinical judgment that includes an assessment of the magnitude of both the absolute CVD risk reduction and the absolute increase in major bleeding.

## *Fish Oil*

Fish oil supplementation may provide benefit in primary CVD prevention, although data from randomized trials are limited. In a randomized trial of 25,871 men and women without known CVD (VITAL trial), after a median of 5.3 years, low-dose n-3 polyunsaturated fatty acid (PUFA; 1 g/day) did not reduce the primary endpoint of major cardiovascular events, which included both heart disease and stroke [hazard ratio (HR) 0.92, 95% CI 0.80–1.06]. Among secondary outcomes, there was a reduction in total MI (HR 0.72, 95% CI 0.59–0.90), percutaneous intervention (HR 0.78, 95% CI 0.63–0.95), total CHD (HR 0.83, 95% CI 0.71–0.97), and death from MI (HR 0.50, 95% CI 0.26–0.97). The results of these secondary outcomes and subgroup analyses are compatible with the hypothesis that low-dose n-3 PUFA supplements may benefit CHD but not stroke, in primary prevention. However, further primary prevention trials with CHD or MI as a primary endpoint are needed as there is inadequate evidence to recommend the use of fish oil in primary CVD prevention.

*Benefits and risks of small amounts of daily alcohol*: In numerous case-control and prospective cohort studies, individuals who consume small amounts of alcohol have lower risks of morbidity and mortality from CHD than nondrinkers. The benefit seems related to the small amount of alcohol consumed rather than the type of alcoholic beverage. In some, but not the majority of analytic studies, individuals who consume red wine tend to have lower risks than those who consume other types of alcohol. This inconsistent finding may be due to other components in red wine or confounding by social class. A meta-analysis of nearly 600,000 individuals in 83 prospective studies who consumed alcohol found the lowest risk of all-cause mortality occurred at alcohol intake of about 100 g/week (approximately six drinks/week). In this analysis, small amounts of daily alcohol intake were associated with a decreased risk of mortality from MI but not from other causes. Thus, any benefit of daily alcohol intake for CAD must be weighed against the risks, which include hypertension, cerebral hemorrhage, and breast cancer.

## Lifestyle Changes

In primary prevention, modification of multiple major risk factors will produce additive reductions in risk of CHD and stroke.

A European prospective cohort study of 2,339, including 1,507 men and 832 women aged 70–90 years without CVD or cancer at baseline, assessed whether self-selection for a Mediterranean diet, being physically active, having small to moderate alcohol intake daily, and/or not smoking reduced all-cause and cause-specific mortality. After a mean follow-up of 10 years, compared with those who adopted zero or one lifestyle change, those who self-selected for all four therapeutic lifestyle changes had a 67% lower risk of CVD mortality and a 65% lower risk of total mortality.

A prospective cohort study of over 20,000 Swedish men aged 45–79 years without cancer, CVD, or CVD risk factors assessed whether individuals who self-selected for all of the five low-risk factors (healthy diet, moderate alcohol consumption, not smoking, being physically active, and having no abdominal adiposity) had lower risks of MI. During the 11-year follow-up, these men who practiced a healthy lifestyle had an 86% lower risk for MI (95% CI 0.04–0.43).

Similar results for primary prevention of stroke were seen in combined data from two large prospective cohorts, the Health Professionals Follow-up Study (43,685 men) and Nurses' Health Study (71,243 women), in which a low-risk lifestyle was defined as not smoking, BMI <25 kg/m$^2$, ≥30 min/day of moderate activity, modest alcohol consumption, and scoring in the top 40% on a healthy diet score. Compared with participants having none, men and women with all five low-risk factors had significantly lower risks of stroke (relative risks 0.31 in men and 0.21 in women).

## Polypill

Polypills to reduce CVD contains various combinations of statins, antihypertensive medications, and aspirin. Potential advantages of polypills include increased compliance and decreased costs. As such, they may be useful as a population-based strategy in resource-limited settings. Potential disadvantages include increased adverse effects, individual patient variability concerning the optimal combination of medications, and difficulty in titration.

A 2017 systematic review of 13 randomized trials concluded that the effects of polypills on mortality or CVD events are inconclusive. However, most of the included trials evaluated changes in risk factors rather than CVD events. In some but not all individual randomized trials, polypills increased adherence and decreased BP and cholesterol but increased adverse events.

In a subsequent cluster-randomized trial of a daily polypill conducted among 6,818 persons older than age 50 years in Iran, 11% of whom had CVD, compared with the educational intervention group, those assigned to the polypill group had fewer major CVD events (defined as hospitalization for acute coronary syndrome, fatal MI, sudden death, HF, coronary artery revascularization, and nonfatal and fatal stroke) at 5 years (5.9 vs. 8.8%; adjusted HR 0.66, 95% CI 0.55–0.80), without an increase in adverse events. The polypill contained hydrochlorothiazide 12.5 mg, aspirin 81 mg atorvastatin 20 mg and enalapril 5 mg; participants who developed a cough were switched to a polypill containing valsartan 40 mg instead of enalapril. The polypill demonstrated efficacy in both primary and secondary prevention. The intervention produced a 1.5 mm Hg reduction in systolic and diastolic BP and a 20 mg/dL reduction in LDL-C.

The use of polypills has been proposed as a strategy to decrease CVD in underserved communities. In an open-label trial among 303 low-income adults in Alabama without CVD, 96% of whom were black, those randomized to receive a polypill containing atorvastatin (10 mg), amlodipine (2.5 mg), losartan (25 mg), and, hydrochlorothiazide (12.5 mg) had a greater decrease in mean BP (9 vs. 2 mm Hg, 7 mm Hg difference, 95% CI −12 to −2), and LDL-C levels (15 vs. 4 mg/dL, 11 mg/dL difference, 95% CI −18 to −5) at 1 year compared with those in the usual care group. Adherence at 1 year was 86%.

## CONCLUSION

Women are a different subset than men as regards their CVD risk. Risk assessment in females should include their different anatomical and physiological variations. Primary and secondary prevention of CAD in women should be based on gender-specific risk factors. The role of biomarkers and newer imaging modalities should be considered for risk analysis.

## SUGGESTED READING

1. Wilson P, D'Agostino R, Levy D, Belanger AM, Silbershatz H, Kannel WB. Prediction of coronary heart disease using risk factor categories. Circulation. 1997;97(18):1837-47.
2. Expert Panel on Detection, Evaluation, and Treatment of High Blood Cholesterol in Adults. Executive Summary of The Third Report of The National Cholesterol Education Program (NCEP) Expert Panel on Detection, Evaluation, and Treatment of High Blood Cholesterol In Adults (Adult Treatment Panel III). JAMA. 2001;285(19):2486-97.
3. D'Agostino RB Sr, Grundy S, Sullivan LM, Wilson P. Validation of the Framingham coronary heart disease prediction scores: results of a multiple ethnic groups investigation. JAMA. 2001; 286(2):180-7.
4. Empana JP, Ducimetiere P, Arveiler D, Ferrières J, Evans A, Ruidavets JB, et al. Are the Framingham and PROCAM coronary heart disease risk functions applicable to different European populations? The PRIME Study. Eur Heart J. 2003;24(21):1903-11.
5. Wilson PW, Nam BH, Pencina M, D'Agostino RB Sr, Benjamin EJ, O'Donnell CJ. C-reactive protein and risk of cardiovascular disease in men and women from the Framingham Heart Study. Arch Intern Med. 2005;165(21):2473-8.
6. World Health Organization. (2007). Prevention of cardiovascular disease: Guidelines for assessment of cardiovascular risk. [online] Available from https://apps.who.int/iris/handle/10665/43685. [Last accessed February, 2020].
7. WHO CVD Risk Chart Working Group. World Health Organization cardiovascular disease risk charts: revised models to estimate risk in 21 global regions. Lancet Glob Health. 2019;7(10):e1332-45.
8. Selvarajah S, Kaur G, Haniff J, Cheong KC, Hiong TG, van der Graaf Y, et al. Comparison of the Framingham Risk Score, SCORE and WHO/ISH cardiovascular risk prediction models in an Asian population. Int J Cardiol. 2014;176(1):211-8.
9. Ridker P, Buring JE, Rifai N, Cook NR. Development and validation of improved algorithms for the assessment of global cardiovascular risk in women: The Reynolds Risk Score. JAMA. 2007;297(6):611-9.
10. Mosca L, Grundy SM, Judelson D, King K, Limacher M, Oparil S, et al. Guide to preventive cardiology for women: AHA/ACC Scientific Statement Consensus panel statement. Circulation. 1999;99(18):2480-4.
11. Mosca L, Appel LJ, Benjamin EJ, Berra K, Chandra-Strobos N, Fabunmi RP, et al. Evidence-based guidelines for cardiovascular disease prevention in women. Circulation. 2004;109(5):672-93.
12. Kavaric N, Klisic A, Ninic A. Cardiovascular Risk Estimated by UKPDS Risk Engine Algorithm in Diabetes. Open Med. 2018;13:610-7.
13. Assmann G, Cullen P, Schulte H. Simple scoring scheme for calculating the risk of acute coronary events based on the 10-year follow-up of the Prospective Cardiovascular Munster (PROCAM) study. Circulation. 2002;105(3):310-5.
14. Hippisley-Cox J, Coupland C, Vinogradova Y, Robson J, May M, Brindle P. Derivation and validation of QRISK, a new cardiovascular disease risk score for the United Kingdom: prospective open cohort study. BMJ. 2007;335:136.

## SECTION 1: Cardiology

15. Hippisley-Cox J, Coupland C, Vinogradova Y, Robson J, Minhas R, Sheikh A, et al. Predicting cardiovascular risk in England and Wales: prospective derivation and validation of QRISK2. BMJ 2008;336(7659):1475-82.
16. Goff DC, Lloyd-Jones DM, Bennett G, Coady S, D'Agostino RB, Gibbons R, et al. 2013 ACC/AHA guideline on the assessment of cardiovascular risk: a report of the American College of Cardiology/American Heart Association Task Force on Practice Guidelines. Circulation. 2014;129(25 Suppl 2):S49-73.
17. Gill EA, Blaha MJ, Guyton JR. JCL roundtable: Coronary artery calcium scoring and other vascular imaging for risk assessment. J Clin Lipidol. 2019;13(1):4-14.
18. Ryan AJ, Choi AD, Choi BG, Lewis JF. Breast arterial calcification association with coronary artery calcium scoring and implications for cardiovascular risk assessment in women. Clin Cardiol. 2017;40(9):648-53.
19. Gorantla P, Kapoor A, Maddury J. Mammographically detected Breast Arterial Calcification—A Marker of Coronary Artery Disease in Women. Ind J Car Dis Wom. 2017;02(04):082-5.
20. Aksoy F, Guler S, Kahraman F, Kuyumcu MS, Bagcı A, Bas HA, et al. The relationship between mitral annular calcification, metabolic syndrome and thromboembolic risk. Braz J Cardiovasc Surg. 2019;34(5):535-41.
21. Li Y, Zhu G, Ding V, Jiang B, Boothroyd D, Rodriguez F, et al. Carotid artery imaging is more strongly associated with the 10-year atherosclerotic cardiovascular disease score than coronary artery imaging. J Comput Assist Tomogr. 2019;43(5):679-85.
22. Ghanem AM, Matta JR, Elgarf R, Hamimi A, Muniyappa R, Ishaq H, et al. Sexual dimorphism of coronary artery disease in a low- and intermediate-risk asymptomatic population: association with coronary vessel wall thickness at mri in women. Radiology: Cardiothoracic Imaging. 2019;1(1).
23. Hu Y, Hu J. Diagnostic value of circulating lncRNA ANRIL and its correlation with coronary artery disease parameters. Braz J Med Biol Res. 2019;52(8):e8309.
24. Araujo LF, Soeiro ADM, Fernandes JL, Pesaro AE, Serrano Jr CV. Coronary artery disease in women: a review on prevention, pathophysiology, diagnosis, and treatment. Vasc Health Risk Manag. 2006;2(4):465-75.
25. Maddury J, Achukatla K. Long-term cardiovascular effects of pregnancy-related disorders. Ind J Car Dis Wom. 2018;03(02/03):167-83.
26. Romundstad PR, Magnussen EB, Smith GD, Vatten LJ. Hypertension in pregnancy and later cardiovascular risk: common antecedents? Circulation. 2010;122(6):579-84.
27. Nemani L. Hypertensive Disorders in Pregnancy. Ind J Car Dis Wom. 2018;03(02/03):068-78.
28. Goueslard K, Cottenet J, Mariet AS, Giroud M, Cottin Y, Petit JM, et al. Early cardiovascular events in women with a history of gestational diabetes mellitus. Cardiovasc Diabetol. 2016;15:15.
29. Bradshaw PT, Stevens J, Khankari N, Teitelbaum SL, Neugut AI, Gammon MD. Cardiovascular disease mortality among breast cancer survivors. Epidemiology. 2016;27(1):6-13.
30. Coviello AD, Sam S, Legro RS, Dunaif A. High prevalence of metabolic syndrome in first-degree male relatives of women with polycystic ovary syndrome is related to high rates of obesity. J Clin Endocrinol Metab. 2009;94(11):4361-6.
31. Shaw LJ, Bairey Merz CN, Azziz R, Stanczyk FZ, Sopko G, Braunstein GD, et al. Postmenopausal women with a history of irregular menses and elevated androgen measurements at high risk for worsening cardiovascular event-free survival: results from the National Institutes of Health–National Heart, Lung, and Blood Institute sponsored Women's Ischemia Syndrome Evaluation. J Clin Endocrinol Metab. 2008;93(4):1276-84.
32. Merz CN, Johnson BD, Berga S, Braunstein G, Reis SE, Bittner V, et al. Past oral contraceptive use and angiographic coronary artery disease in postmenopausal women: data from the National Heart, Lung, and Blood Institute-sponsored Women's Ischemia Syndrome Evaluation. Fertil Steril. 2006;85(5):1425-31.
33. Prasad M, Hermann J, Gabriel SE, Weyand CM, Mulvagh S, Mankad R, et al. Cardiorheumatology: Cardiac involvement in systemic rheumatic disease. Nat Rev Cardiol. 2015;12(3):168-76.
34. Sinicato NA, da Silva Cardoso PA, Appenzeller S. Risk factors in cardiovascular disease in systemic lupus erythematosus. Curr Cardiol Rev. 2013;9(1):15-19.
35. Prabhakaran D, Chaturvedi V, Shah P, Manhapra A, Jeemon P, Shah B, et al. Differences in the prevalence of metabolic syndrome in urban and rural India: a problem of urbanization. Chronic Illn. 2007;3(1):8-19.

36. Feigin VL, Krishnamurthi RV, Parmar P, Norrving B, Mensah GA, Bennett DA, et al. Update on the Global Burden of Ischemic and Hemorrhagic Stroke in 1990-2013: The GBD 2013 Study. Neuroepidemiology. 2015;45(3):161-6.
37. Yusuf S, Hawken S, Ounpuu S, Dans T, Avezum A, Lanas F, et al. Effect of potentially modifiable risk factors associated with myocardial infarction in 52 countries (the INTERHEART study): case-control study. Lancet. 2004;364(9438):937-52.
38. Anderson KM, Odell PM, Wilson PW, Kannel WB. Cardiovascular disease risk profiles. Am Heart J. 1991;121(1 Pt 2):293-8.
39. Capewell S, Beaglehole R, Seddon M, McMurray J. Explanation for the decline in coronary heart disease mortality rates in Auckland, New Zealand, between 1982 and 1993. Circulation. 2000;102(13):1511-6.
40. Stampfer MJ, Hu FB, Manson JE, Rimm EB, Willett WC. Primary prevention of coronary heart disease in women through diet and lifestyle. N Engl J Med. 2000;343(1):16-22.
41. Kurth T, Moore SC, Gaziano JM, Kase CS, Stampfer MJ, Berger K, et al. Healthy lifestyle and the risk of stroke in women. Arch Intern Med. 2006;166(13):1403-9.
42. Sotos-Prieto M, Bhupathiraju SN, Mattei J, Fung TT, Li Y, Pan A, et al. Changes in Diet quality scores and risk of cardiovascular disease among us men and women. Circulation. 2015;132(23):2212-19.
43. Guirguis-Blake JM, Evans CV, Senger CA, O'Connor EA, Whitlock EP. Aspirin for the Primary Prevention of Cardiovascular Events: A Systematic Evidence Review for the U.S. Preventive Services Task Force. Ann Intern Med. 2016;164(12):804-13.
44. Manson JE, Cook NR, Lee IM, Christen W, Bassuk SS, Mora S, et al. Marine n-3 fatty acids and prevention of cardiovascular disease and cancer. N Engl J Med. 2019;380(1):23-32.
45. Leening MJ, Berry JD, Allen NB. Lifetime Perspectives on Primary Prevention of Atherosclerotic Cardiovascular Disease. JAMA. 2016;315(14):1449-50.
46. Knoops KT, de Groot LC, Kromhout D, Perrin AE, Moreiras-Varela O, Menotti A, et al. Mediterranean diet, lifestyle factors, and 10-year mortality in elderly European men and women: the HALE project. JAMA. 2004;292(12):1433-9.
47. Akesson A, Larsson SC, Discacciati A, Wolk A. Low-risk diet and lifestyle habits in the primary prevention of myocardial infarction in men: a population-based prospective cohort study. J Am Coll Cardiol. 2014;64(13):1299-306.
48. Chiuve SE, Rexrode KM, Spiegelman D, Logroscino G, Manson JE, Rimm EB. Primary prevention of stroke by healthy lifestyle. Circulation. 2008;118(9):947-54.
49. Bahiru E, de Cates AN, Farr MR, Jarvis MC, Palla M, Rees K, et al. Fixed-dose combination therapy for the prevention of atherosclerotic cardiovascular diseases. Cochrane Database Syst Rev. 2017;3:CD009868.
50. Selak V, Elley CR, Bullen C, Crengle S, Wadham A, Rafter N, et al. Effect of fixed dose combination treatment on adherence and risk factor control among patients at high risk of cardiovascular disease: randomised controlled trial in primary care. BMJ. 2014;348:g3318.
51. Castellano JM, Sanz G, Peñalvo JL, Bansilal S, Fernández-Ortiz A, Alvarez L, et al. A polypill strategy to improve adherence: results from the FOCUS project. J Am Coll Cardiol. 2014;64(20):2071-82.
52. Yusuf S, Pais P, Afzal R, Xavier D, Teo K, Eikelboom J, et al. Effects of a polypill (Polycap) on risk factors in middle-aged individuals without cardiovascular disease (TIPS): a phase II, double-blind, randomised trial. Lancet. 2009;373(9672):1341-51.
53. Muñoz D, Uzoije P, Reynolds C, Miller R, Walkley D, Pappalardo S, et al. Polypill for cardiovascular disease prevention in an underserved population. N Engl J Med. 2019;381:1114-23.
54. Roshandel G, Khoshnia M, Poustchi H, Hemming K, Kamangar F, Gharavi A. Effectiveness of polypill for primary and secondary prevention of cardiovascular diseases (PolyIran): a pragmatic, cluster-randomised trial. Lancet. 2019; 394(10199):672-83.
55. Gutierrez J, Ramirez G, Rundek T, Sacco RL. Statin therapy in the prevention of recurrent cardio-vascular events: A sex-based meta-analysis. Arch Intern Med. 2012;172(12):909-19.
56. Truong QA, Murphy SA, McCabe CH, Armani A, Cannon CP. Benefit of intensive statin therapy in women: Results from PROVE IT-TIMI 22. Circ Cardiovasc Qual Outcomes. 2011;4(3):328-36.
57. Kostis WJ, Cheng JQ, Dobrzynski JM, Cabrera J, Kostis JB. Meta-analysis of statin effects in women versus men. J Am Coll Cardiol. 2012;59(6):572-82.
58. Zhang H, Plutzky J, Skentzos S, Morrison F, Mar P, Shubina M, et al. Discontinuation of statins in routine care settings. Ann Intern Med. 2013;158(7):526-34.

59. Preiss D, Seshasai SR, Welsh P, Murphy SA, Ho JE, Waters DD, et al. Risk of incident diabetes with intensive-dose compared with moderate-dose statin therapy: A meta-analysis. JAMA. 2011;305(24):2556-64.
60. Mosca L, Benjamin EJ, Berra K, Bezanson JL, Dolor RJ, Lloyd-Jones DM, et al. Effectiveness-based guidelines for the prevention of cardiovascular disease in women—2011 update: A guideline from the American Heart Association. Circulation. 2011;123(11):1243-62.
61. Randomised trial of intravenous streptokinase, oral aspirin, both, or neither among 17,187 cases of suspected acute myocardial infarction: ISIS-2. ISIS-2 (Second International Study of Infarct Survival) Collaborative Group. Lancet. 1988;2(8607):349-60.
62. Graham I, Atar D, Borch-Johnson K, Boysen G, Burell G, Cifkova R, et al. European guidelines on cardiovascular disease prevention in clinical practice: executive summary. Atherosclerosis. 2007;194(1):1-45.
63. Zinman B, Wanner C, Lachin JM, Fitchett D, Bluhmki E, Hantel S, et al. Empagliflozin, cardiovascular outcomes, and mortality in type 2 diabetes. N Engl J Med. 2015;373(22):2117-28.
64. Fitchett D, Zinman B, Wanner C, Lachin JM, Hantel S, Salsali A, et al. Heart failure outcomes with empagliflozin in patients with type 2 diabetes at high cardiovascular risk: results of the EMPA-REG OUTCOME trial. Eur Heart J. 2016;37(19):1526-34.
65. Marso SP, Daniels GH, Brown-Frandsen K, Kristensen P, Mann JF, Nauck MA, et al. Liraglutide and cardiovascular outcomes in type 2 diabetes. N Engl J Med. 2016;375(4):311-22.
66. Neal B, Perkovic V, Mahaffey KW, de Zeeuw D, Fulcher G, Erondu N, et al. Canagliflozin and cardiovascular and renal events in type 2 diabetes. N Engl J Med. 2017;377:644-57.
67. American Heart Association. Aspirin and Heart Disease. [online] Available from https://www.heart.org/en/health-topics/heart-attack/treatment-of-a-heart-attack/aspirin-and-heart-disease. [Last accessed February, 2020].
68. US Preventive Services Task Force. Aspirin for the prevention of cardiovascular disease: U.S. Preventive Services Task Force recommendation statement. Ann Intern Med. 2009;150(6):396-404.
69. Vandvik PO, Lincoff AM, Core JM, Gutterman DD, Sonnenberg FA, Alonso-Coello P, et al. Primary and secondary prevention of cardiovascular disease: Antithrombotic Therapy and Prevention of Thrombosis, 9th ed: American College of Chest Physicians Evidence-Based Clinical Practice Guidelines. Chest. 2012;141(2 Suppl):e637S-68S.
70. Bell AD, Roussin A, Cartier R, Chan WS, Douketis JD, Gupta A, et al. The use of antiplatelet therapy in the outpatient setting: Canadian Cardiovascular Society Guidelines Executive Summary. Can J Cardiol. 2011;27(2):208-21.

# CHAPTER 3

# IHD in Women: Epidemiology, Presentation, Diagnosis and Management Strategies

*Shibba Takkar Chhabra, Jyoti Jindal, Pooja Tandon*

## ABSTRACT

Ischemic heart disease is the number one killer in women. Women have varied atypical presentations, diagnostic dilemmas, and distinct responses to therapeutic interventions. Women in age group 40–70 more often have nonobstructive coronary artery disease (NOCAD) and coronary vasomotor disorders compared with traditional obstructive CAD seen in men. In addition to traditional risk factors, women-specific risk factors are gestational diabetes, insulin resistance/polycystic ovarian disease, pregnancy-induced hypertension, preeclampsia, eclampsia, menopause, mental stress, autoimmune diseases, etc. Differences in underlying pathophysiology lead to varied presentation of angina symptoms necessitating a more gender sensitive diagnostic and therapeutic approach.

## INTRODUCTION

Cardiovascular disease (CVD) is the number one killer of women. Women as well as their treating physicians continue to undermine the significance of CVD as the leading cause of mortality and morbidity. CVD mortality in women is more than mortality by all the cancers (endometrial, breast, ovarian) combined together. Women have varied atypical presentations, diagnostic dilemmas, and distinct responses to therapeutic interventions. The present review attempts to identify the varied clinical presentations and management strategies in this gender.

## EPIDEMIOLOGY

Although there has been a reduction in the death rate from CVD since 1980, it accounted for 22% of all-cause mortality in women in 2013. Between the ages of 45 and 64, one in nine women develops symptoms of some form of CVD. After age 65, the ratio increases to one in three women. One in five women dies from heart disease versus one in 30 with breast cancer. Also, 1-year mortality post myocardial infarction (MI) is 42% in women versus 24% in men. There is 8-fold higher CAD mortality in Asian Indian women (30–39 years) than Chinese and white women. In a Canadian angiographic study, Asian Indian women were twice as likely to have left main or three vessels CAD compared to white women.

The WISE (Women's Ischemia Syndrome Evaluation) study, analyzing the ischemic symptoms of women affirmed more atypical symptoms, usually at rest and stress related. Also, 60% of women had nonobstructive coronary artery disease (NOCAD). Shaw et al. identified coronary microvascular and endothelial dysfunctions in women with ischemic heart disease (IHD). Hormonal alterations coupled with pro-atherogenic risk factors result in higher prevalence of coronary microvascular dysfunction in women and were responsible for the observed ischemia paradox; despite having higher prevalence of angina, they tend to have lower prevalence of obstructive CAD and worse prognosis when compared with men.

## CLINICAL PRESENTATION

Clinical presentation in women is varied and often nonspecific or atypical. The symptom spectrum might be less severe and inclusive of shortness of breath, arm, shoulder, back, jaw or epigastric pain, palpitations, indigestion, profuse sweating, giddiness, fatigue, presyncope or syncope. In a meta-analysis of 69 studies, more women with acute coronary syndrome (ACS) presented without chest pain or chest discomfort as compared with men (37 vs. 27%). About 42% of MI in women versus 31% in men present without any chest pain. Hospital mortality differences and absence of chest pain tend to decline with rising age.

In the VIRGO (Variation in Recovery: Role of Gender on Outcomes) study, women presented with more symptoms, waited more than a week to seek healthcare than men and were more likely to not think that their symptoms were heart related. Because of these features, it was hypothesized that women who present to the emergency department with new-onset angina undergo less rigorous evaluation than men. Varied presentation in women instigated the VIRGO classification in MI patients (**Table 1**) with a new taxonomy for patients with MI. One in eight women (n = 54) presenting with acute MI (<55 years) fell in unclassified group by the 3rd universal definition for MI (**Flowchart 1**).

*The Ischemia with NOCAD (INOCA)*: Women with INOCA represent a very different group, regarding the extent of atherosclerosis, the presence of risk factors, symptoms, and functional impairment. Women with symptoms of angina have twice as often ischemia with NOCAD (INOCA) compared with men. The combination of INOCA with vasomotor disorders frequently occurs in young and middle-aged women. Unawareness and gender differences lead to delaying in recognition of angina in women. Despite having a higher

**TABLE 1:** The VIRGO classification system in myocardial infarction (MI) patients.

| Class I | Plaque-mediated culprit lesion |
|---|---|
| Class IIa | Obstructive CAD with evidence for supply demand mismatch |
| Class IIb | Obstructive CAD without evidence for supply demand mismatch |
| Class IIIa | Nonobstructive CAD with evidence for supply demand mismatch |
| Class IIIb | Nonobstructive CAD without evidence for supply demand mismatch |
| Class IV | Other, nonatherosclerotic pathophysiologic mechanism |
| Class V | Indeterminate |

(CAD: coronary artery disease; VIRGO: Variation in Recovery: Role of Gender on Outcomes)

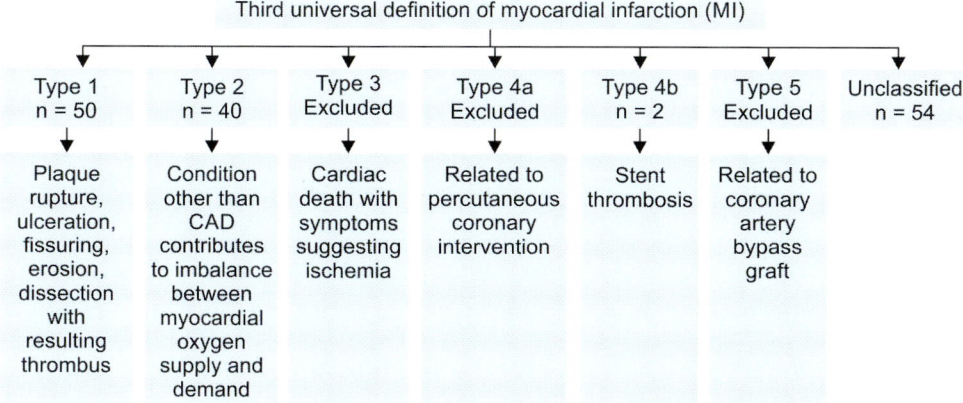

(CAD: coronary artery disease; VIRGO: Variation in Recovery: Role of Gender on Outcomes)

**FLOWCHART 1:** Number of VIRGO female patients classified by the 3rd universal definition for MI. n = number of VIRGO female patients classified by the 3rd universal definition of myocardial infarction. About 54 patients remained unclassified leading to new VIRGO classification system in MI patients.

prevalence of NOCAD, women even in the absence of critical lesions not only continue to have symptoms while on anti-ischemic therapy but also have 2.5% yearly risk of major adverse cardiac events (MACEs).

*Microvascular angina (Former Syndrome X)*: Women with chest pain and no evidence of atherosclerotic coronary artery disease on coronary angiography may have cardiac syndrome X or more rarely takotsubo cardiomyopathy or coronary dissection.

*The MI in nonobstructive coronary artery (MINOCA)*: MINOCA is common in women especially the younger women. Women with MINOCA usually have underlying traditional risk factors though dyslipidemia is not as frequent. Though low all-cause mortality in MINOCA is significant in comparison to obstructive CAD (in-hospital mortality rate 1.1 vs. 3.2%, $p = 0.001$; 1-year mortality rate 6.7 vs. 3.5%, $p = 0.03$). The proposed etiological factors of MINOCA include subendocardial ischemia, spontaneous coronary artery dissection, coronary vasospasm myocarditis, and takotsubo or hypertrophic cardiomyopathy.

With microvascular angina and functional disorder of coronary (micro) circulation predominating in women, clinically relevant sex differences in plaque morphology need to be identified in women. Fewer calcifications, less focal obstruction, more diffuse pattern of atherosclerosis, and outward remodeling with soft plaques are usually seen in women.

For evaluation of NOCAD, it is needed to develop better tools for assessment of functional CAD in coronary microvasculature (IVUS/FFR/IFR, etc.). Hence, it is needed to divert from traditional stenotic thought process and visualize female pattern of IHD. Also, important is to identify the relationship between the microvascular dysfunction and epicardial atherosclerosis as a single process where the response to endothelial injury varies in relation to the gender-directed vascular remodeling and reactivity.

*Yentl syndrome*: Female pattern IHD characterized by relatively low obstructive CAD burden and preserved left ventricular ejection fraction (LVEF) represent a Yentl syndrome whereby women's CAD is under diagnosed and under treated. Coined in 2001 by Bernadine Healy, this calls attention to paradox of adverse outcomes.

## SECTION 1: Cardiology

## DIAGNOSIS

Female patients often have atypical presentation and this makes it difficult to diagnose IHD in female patients. Women with suspected CAD, that means who present with chest discomfort or ischemic equivalents have been classified to low, low intermediate, intermediate high, and high-risk IHD (**Flowchart 2**).

Broadly, all symptomatic premenopausal women are considered as low risk and such patients routinely do not require any test exceptionally in some cases electrocardiography (ECG) is required.

- *Low to intermediate risk:* Symptomatic female in fifth decade performing activities of daily living (ADL'S).
- *Intermediate risk:* Symptomatic females in fifth decade and not performing ADL'S. All those 60 years or more than considered as intermediate risk.
- *High-risk:* Age 70 years or older considered as high-risk.

For symptomatic patients at intermediate risk with normal baseline ECG, an exercise ECG stress test should be initial diagnostic test if functional capacity is >5 metabolic equivalents (METs).

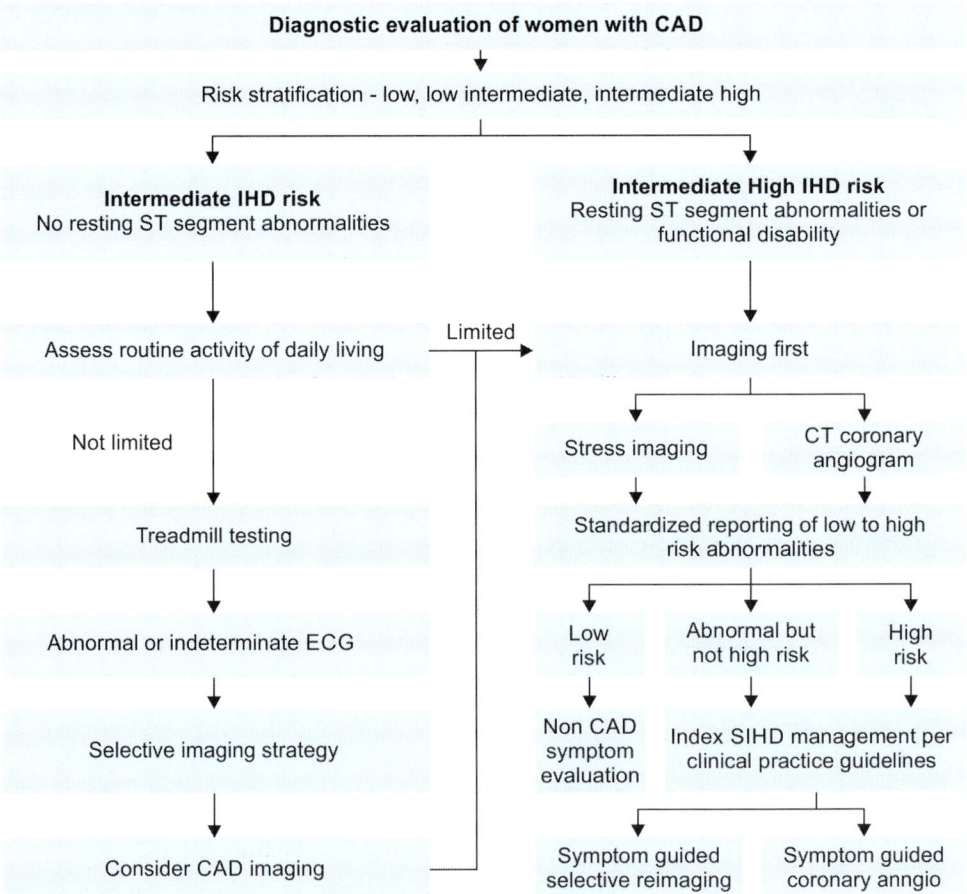

(IHD: ischemic heart disease; SIHD: stable ischemic heart disease)

**FLOWCHART 2:** Diagnostic evaluation of women with coronary artery disease (CAD).

**TABLE 2:** The predictive value of noninvasive testing in women with coronary artery disease (CAD). Stress tests have high likelihood of false positive reports and have a high negative predictive value.

| Type of study | Sensitivity | Specificity | Likelihood ratio for positive test | Likelihood ratio for negative test |
|---|---|---|---|---|
| Myocardial perfusion imaging | 0.77<br>0.69–0.81 | 0.71<br>0.69–0.78 | 2.54<br>1.95–3.32 | 0.36<br>0.28–0.46 |
| Exercise echo | 0.82<br>0.73–0.89 | 0.60<br>0.48–0.71 | 2.06<br>1.53–2.77 | 0.29<br>0.18–0.47 |
| Type of study | Sensitivity | Specificity | Positive predictive value | Negative predictive value |
| Treadmill testing | 031–0.71 | 0.66–0.86 | ~0.47 | 0.78 |

Those at intermediate high risk with abnormal resting ECG, next step is noninvasive imaging.

Higher false positive rate and diminished accuracy of exercise ECG in women can be due to resting ST-T wave changes, lower ECG voltage, and hormonal functions (indigenous estrogen in premenopausal and hormonal replacement therapy in postmenopausal women).

WOMEN (What is Optimal Method for Ischemia Evaluation in Women?) trial on 824 symptomatic women revealed similar outcomes in functionally capable women whether randomized to exercise ECG or myocardial perfusion imaging (MPI) (p = 0.59).

The predictive value of noninvasive testing in women with CAD is depicted in **Table 2**.

Amount of radiation exposure warrants special attention while treating women. The risk benefit ratio needs to be considered and individualization as regards risk stratification is of utmost importance. While low-risk premenopausal women may be subjected to tests without radiation exposure (e.g., treadmill testing) or no testing strategy in intermediate or high-risk women where diagnosing IHD is of paramount significance, diagnostic procedure exposing women to ionizing radiation (stress MPI, CT coronary angiogram, CAG) may be warranted. The guidelines justifying the use and dose reduction optimization should be adhered to limit radiation exposure and cancer risk in women.

Stress echocardiography can be used as a diagnostic and prognostic tool in patients with either abnormal ECG at baseline or those who cannot exercise. Stress MPI, PET has better image quality and increased diagnostic accuracy for detection of obstructive CAD in obese women. Coronary computed tomography angiography (CCTA) diagnostic accuracy is similar among men and women.

## TREATMENT OF ISCHEMIC HEART DISEASE

The medical management guidelines for IHD remains the same for both sexes across the spectrum of ST-segment elevation myocardial infarction (STEMI)/non-ST segment elevation myocardial infarction (NSTEMI) and chronic stable angina. However, women not only receive less intensive pharmacological regimen but also delayed and less aggressive cardiac intervention culminating into poor outcomes. Bangalore et al. in their data of 31,555 STEMI patients found increased mortality rates and duration of hospitalization in all women. Women above 45 years of age were less likely to receive ACE inhibitors, β-blockers, and clopidogrel + aspirin at discharge; had lesser LDL levels checked and received less β-blockers in first 24 hours of hospitalization. The door to thrombolytic time <30 minutes was achieved less in women especially in the younger group (<45 years) who also had higher in hospital deaths.

Lesser women receive stents than men with ACS and lesser women achieve the door to balloon time of 90 minutes. The benefit of cardiac intervention was more in women with positive biomarkers versus men which had no such difference. Also, higher mortality post percutaneous coronary intervention (PCI) was seen in the females. Post fibrinolysis, however, women demonstrated lower 30 day mortality. The bleeding risk was also higher in women receiving GPIIb/IIIa inhibitors during PCI which was attributed to body surface area and renal functions.

Significant gender disparities were also recognized in a meta-analysis of 731,213 patients with consistent excessive mortality in women by Hyon Jae Lee, Sameer Mehta et al. Post coronary artery bypass graft surgery (CABG) women also have higher morbidity and mortality. Post CABG women also suffer higher depression rates and poor quality of life. Off-pump CABG was associated with lower mortality rates in women.

## CONCLUSION

Cardiovascular disease is the leading cause of death in women. Women have varied atypical presentations, diagnostic dilemmas, and distinct responses to therapeutic interventions. NOCAD, MINOCA, YENTL syndrome, etc., are seen in women highlighting the fact of nonobstructive but prognostically worse microvascular coronary artery disease. Gender bias is also prevalent in duration of presentation, physician referral, and management strategies of women. Moreover, pregnancy and pregnancy-related events mimic a stress test and are harbinger of future CVD in women. Future studies should be focused on further elucidation of the link between pregnancy related events and CVD. Guidelines-directed medical therapy should be used effectively for symptom and ischemia management. Enrollment of women in large cardiovascular prevention and intervention trials is needed to gain greater understanding.

## SUGGESTED READING

1. Mosca L, Hammond G, Mochari-Greenberger H, Towfighi A, Albert M. American Heart Association Cardiovascular Disease and Stroke in Women and Special Populations Committee of the Council on Clinical Cardiology, Council on Epidemiology and Prevention, Council on Cardiovascular Nursing, Council on High Bloo. Fifteen-year trends in awareness of heart disease in women: results of a 2012 American Heart Association National Survey. Circulation. 2013;127(11):1254-63.
2. Roger VL, Go AS, Lloyd-Jones DM, Adams RJ, Berry JD, Brown TM, et al. Heart disease and stroke statistics—2011 update: a report from the American Heart Association. Circulation. 2011;123(4):e18–209.
3. Leading Causes of Death in Females, 2013 United States. Centers for Disease Control and Prevention, 2013. https://www.cdc.gov/women/lcod/2013/index.htm (Accessed on June 14, 2017).
4. Merz CNB, Kelsey SF, Pepine CJ, Reichek N, Reis SE, Rogers WJ, et al. The Women's Ischemia Syndrome Evaluation (WISE) study: protocol design, methodology and feasibility report. J Am Coll Cardiol. 1999;33(6):1453-61.
5. Shaw LJ, Bugiardini R, Merz CNB. Women and ischemic heart disease: evolving knowledge. J Am Coll Cardiol. 2009;54(17):1561-75.
6. Merz CNB. Women and ischemic heart disease. JACC Cardiovasc Imaging. 2011;4(1).
7. Kennedy JW, Killip T, Fisher LD, Alderman EL, Gillespie MJ, Mock MB. The clinical spectrum of coronary artery disease and its surgical and medical management, 1974–1979. The Coronary Artery Surgery study. Circulation. 1982;66(5 pt 2):III16-23.

8. Diamond GA, Staniloff HM, Forrester JS, Pollock BH, Swan H. Computer-assisted diagnosis in the noninvasive evaluation of patients with suspected coronary artery disease. J Am Coll Cardiol. 1983;1(2):444-55.
9. Douglas PS, Hoffmann U, Patel MR, Mark DB, Al-Khalidi HR, Cavanaugh B, et al. Outcomes of anatomical versus functional testing for coronary artery disease. N Engl J Med. 2015;372(14):1291-1300.
10. Hemal K, Pagidipati NJ, Coles A, Dolor RJ, Mark DB, Pellikka PA, et al. Sex differences in demographics, risk factors, presentation, and noninvasive testing in stable outpatients with suspected coronary artery disease: insights from the PROMISE Trial. JACC Cardiovasc Imaging. 2016;9(4):337-46.
11. Bucholz EM, Strait KM, Dreyer RP, Lindau ST, Onofrio GD', Geda M, et al. Sex differences in young patients with acute myocardial infarction: a VIRGO study analysis. Eur Heart J Acute Cardiovasc Care. Epub 2016 Aug 2.
12. Spatz ES, Curry LA, Masoudi FA, Zhou S, Strait KM, Gross CP, et al. The Variation in Recovery: Role of Gender on Outcomes of Young AMI Patients (VIRGO) Classification System: A Taxonomy for Young Women With Acute Myocardial Infarction. Circulation. 2015;132(18):1710-8.
13. Bellasi A, Raggi P, Merz CB, Shaw LJ. New insights into ischemic heart disease in women. Cleve Clin J Med. 2007;74(8):585.
14. Pepine CJ, Anderson RD, Sharaf BL, Reis SE, Smith KM, Handberg EM, et al. Coronary microvascular reactivity to adenosine predicts adverse outcome in women evaluated for suspected ischemia results from the National Heart, Lung and Blood Institute WISE (Women's Ischemia Syndrome Evaluation) study. J Am Coll Cardiol. 2010;55(25):2825-32.
15. Ghadri JR, Sarcon A, Diekmann J, Bataiosu DR, Cammann VL, Jurisic S, et al. Happy heart syndrome: role of positive emotional stress in takotsubo syndrome. Eur Heart J. 2016;37(37):2823-29.
16. Gulati M, Cooper-DeHoff RM, McClure C, Johnson BD, Shaw LJ, Handberg EM, et al. Adverse cardiovascular outcomes in women with NOCAD: a report from the Women's Ischemia Syndrome Evaluation Study and the St James Women Take Heart Project. Arch Intern Med. 2009;169(9):843-50.
17. Pasupathy S, Air T, Dreyer RP, Tavella R, Beltrame JF. Systematic review of patients presenting with suspected myocardial infarction and nonobstructive coronary arteries. Circulation. 2015;131(10):861-70.
18. Merz CNB. The Yentl syndrome is alive and well. Eur Heart J. 2011;32:1313-5.
19. Mieres JH, Gulati M, Bairey Merz N, Berman DS, Gerber TC, Hayes SN, et al. Role of Noninvasive Testing in the Clinical Evaluation of Women With Suspected Ischemic Heart Disease: A Consensus Statement From the American Heart Association. Circulation 2014;130:350-79.
20. Fazel R, Dilsizian V, Einstein AJ, Ficaro EP, Henzlova M, Shaw LJ. Strategies for defining an optimal risk-benefit ratio for stress myocardial perfusion SPECT. J Nucl Cardiol. 2011;18(3):385-92.
21. Blomkalns AL, Chen AY, Hochman JS, Peterson ED, Trynosky K, Diercks DB, et al. Gender disparities in the diagnosis and treatment of non–ST-segment elevation acute coronary syndromes: Large-scale observations from the CRUSADE (Can Rapid Risk Stratification of Unstable Angina Patients Suppress Adverse Outcomes with Early Implementation of the American College of Cardiology/American Heart Association Guidelines) National Quality Improvement Initiative. J Am Coll Cardiol. 2005;45:832-37.
22. Boersma E, Harrington RA, Moliterno DJ, White H, Théroux P, Van de Werf F, et al. Platelet glycoprotein IIb/IIIa inhibitors in acute coronary syndromes: a meta-analysis of all major randomised clinical trials. Lancet. 2002;359(9302):189-98.
23. Cho L, Topol EJ, Balog C, Foody JM, Booth JE, Cabot C, et al. Clinical benefit of glycoprotein IIb/IIIa blockade with Abciximab is independent of gender: pooled analysis from EPIC, EPILOG and EPISTENT trials. Evaluation of 7E3 for the Prevention of Ischemic Complications. Evaluation in Percutaneous Transluminal Coronary Angioplasty to Improve Long-Term Outcome with Abciximab GP IIb/IIIa blockade. Evaluation of Platelet IIb/IIIa Inhibitor for Stent. J Am Coll Cardiol. 2000;36(2):381-6.
24. Hemingway H, McCallum A, Shipley M, Manderbacka K, Martikainen P, Keskimäki I. Incidence and prognostic implications of stable angina pectoris among women and men. JAMA. 2006;295(12):1404-11.
25. Vaccarino V, Lin ZQ, Kasl SV, Mattera JA, Roumanis SA, Abramson JL, et al. Sex differences in health status after coronary artery bypass surgery. Circulation. 2003;108(21):2642-7.
26. Vaccarino V, Abramson JL, Veledar E, Weintraub WS. Sex differences in hospital mortality after coronary artery bypass surgery: evidence for a higher mortality in younger women. Circulation. 2002;105(10):1176-81.

# CHAPTER 4

# Women with Heart Failure: Etiopathogenesis, Clinical Presentation, Diagnostic, and Management Strategies

*Neelam Dahiya, Krishna Prasad, Basant*

## ABSTRACT

Heart failure (HF) is a clinical syndrome in which there are characteristic signs and symptoms, such as edema, breathlessness and fatigue, due to an underlying abnormality of cardiac function. HF is significant cause of morbidity in women, and about 50% of women have HF with preserved ejection fraction (HFpEF). Peripartum cardiomyopathy (PPCM) is rare cause of HF in young females. Women have different responses to HF in terms of gene expression. Women often present with atypical symptoms of HF as they have multiple comorbidities. Women are represented less in various HF trial. Though trials have shown women have equal benefits with HF medications, they are less likely to get guidelines-directed medications. Even though device therapy for HF have shown equal benefits in men and women, women gets fewer devices. Fewer women have received cardiac transplant. Hence, there is need for more women specific HF trials to cater specific needs of women.

## INTRODUCTION

Heart failure (HF) is a clinical syndrome characterized by typical symptoms (e.g., breathlessness, fatigue, and ankle swelling) that may be accompanied by signs (e.g., pulmonary crackles, elevated jugular venous pressure, and peripheral edema) caused by a structural and/or functional cardiac abnormality, resulting in a reduced cardiac output and/or elevated intracardiac pressures at rest or during stress.

## TYPES OF HEART FAILURE (TABLE 1)

On the basis of ejection fraction (EF), HF can be divided into:
- HF with preserved ejection fraction (HFpEF)
- HF with mid-range ejection fraction (HFmrEF)
- HF with reduced ejection fraction (HFrEF)

**TABLE 1:** Types of heart failure with their signs and symptoms.

| HFpEF | HFmrEF | HFrEF |
|---|---|---|
| Sign and symptoms | Sign and symptoms | Sign and symptoms |
| LVEF >50% | LVEF 40–49% | LVEF <40% |
| • Elevated levels of natriuretic peptides<br>• At least one additional criteria<br>• Relevant structural heart disease<br>• Diastolic dysfunction | • Elevated levels of natriuretic peptides<br>• At least one additional criteria<br>• Relevant structural heart disease<br>• Diastolic dysfunction | |

(HFpEF: heart failure with preserved ejection fraction; HFmrEF: heart failure with mid-range ejection fraction; HFrEF: heart failure with reduced ejection fraction; LVEF: left ventricular ejection fraction)

## EPIDEMIOLOGY

### Global

Women-specific global prevalence of HF is difficult to estimate, as there are no specific registries related to women especially in developing countries. According to the 2019 American Heart Association (AHA) Heart Disease and Stroke Statistics Update, 3.2 million adult females have HF. There were 505,000 adult females with HF in 2014, and 42,932 females died of HF in 2016.

The lifetime risk of developing HF is 1 in 5 after 40 years of age in both men and women, however, women at an older age are at greater risk than men. Incidence rates of HF in men approximately doubles with each 10-year increase in age from 65 to 85 years; however, the HF incidence rate triples for women between ages 65 to 74 and 75 to 84 years. The incidence of HF is lowest in white women and highest in black females.

### India

It is difficult to estimate the true prevalence of HF in women in India as we are lacking proper HF registries. According to INDUS (INDia Ukieri Study), the prevalence of HF at age <30 years, 30–50 years, and >50 years was 22.53%, 24.29%, and 14.91% respectively. The mean age of presentation was 39 ± 16 years. The most common reason for HF was rheumatic heart disease in this study which explains the higher prevalence of HF in young. In the Trivandrum HF registry, the most common etiology was coronary artery disease. Women present late in life with HF and have more comorbidities.

Rheumatic heart disease and dilated cardiomyopathy are the main causes of HF in women. More women have HFpEF than men. India has the highest reported mortality up to 30% in HF patients. In most Indian studies, representation of women has been very low. Three-fourths of cardiovascular clinical trials in India do not report sex-specific results making implementation of these trial results to women difficult than men. **Table 2** shows some HF studies in India and the representation of men and women.

## STAGES OF HEART FAILURE

The ACC/AHA guideline has proposed four stages of HF:
*Stage A*: Patients are with risk factors of HF but without structural heart disease.
*Stage B*: Patients have structural heart disease but without signs or symptoms of HF.

**TABLE 2:** Representation of women in different heart failure studies.

| Study | Men% | Women% |
| --- | --- | --- |
| INDUS | 57 | 43 |
| Asian HF | 75.5 | 24.5 |
| PIQIP | 77 | 23 |
| THFR | 69 | 31 |
| Inter-CHF | 62 | 38 |
| Medanta registry | 83 | 17 |

(CHF: congestive heart failure; HF: heart failure; INDUS: INDia Ukieri Study; PIQIP: PINNACLE India Quality Improvement Program; THFR: Trivandrum Heart Failure Registry)

*Stage C*: Patients have structural heart disease with prior or current symptoms of HF.
*Stage D*: Patients have refractory HF requiring specialized intervention.

## ETIOLOGY OF HEART FAILURE

Among myriad causes of HF, most common causes of HF are coronary artery disease, hypertension, idiopathic cardiomyopathy, and valvular heart disease. Less common causes are arrhythmia, collagen vascular disease, endocrine/metabolic disorders (e.g., thyroid disease, diabetes mellitus,), hypertrophic cardiomyopathy, myocarditis, pericarditis, postpartum cardiomyopathy, restrictive cardiomyopathies, and toxic cardiomyopathy (e.g., alcohol, cocaine, radiation chemotherapeutic agents). Various precipitating factors that can decompensate stable HF are anemia, atrial fibrillation, volume overload, infections, and poor drug compliance.

Hypertension, valvular heart disease, diabetes, and coronary artery disease are common causes of HF in women. Hypertension, diabetes, and obesity are the most common causes of HFpEF in women.

Peripartum cardiomyopathy (PPCM) occurs more commonly in premenopausal women and is rare. Stress-induced cardiomyopathy or takotsubo cardiomyopathy occurs more commonly in postmenopausal women. HF due to autoimmune disorders and collagen vascular diseases are more common in females.

According to HERS, atrial fibrillation, history of myocardial infarction, creatinine clearance <40 mL/minute, systolic blood pressure >120 mm Hg, active smoking, BMI >35 kg/m$^2$, left bundle branch block, left ventricular hypertrophy, and diabetes were most common factors associated with the development of HF in women.

## PATHOGENESIS

Any structural or functional insult to the heart leads to the initiation of an adaptive mechanism that maintains heart function for the short-term (compensatory phase). However, if stress to heart prevails for long, this adaptive mechanism becomes mal-adaptive, leading to cardiac remodeling. Persistent wall stress leads to cardiac myocyte hypertrophy, apoptosis, and myocyte regeneration. This process of cardiac remodeling can be eccentric or concentric depending on the type of stress or cause of HF. Eventually, this leads to decreased cardiac contractile function and reduced cardiac output initiating a cascade of neurohormonal and vascular responses.

Decreased renal perfusion activates the renin–angiotensin–aldosterone system (RAAS) and sympathetic nervous system (SNS). RAAS activation leads to vasoconstriction, the increased workload to cardiac muscles. SNS activation causes increased heart rate and enhanced cardiac contractility. All of these mechanisms will further cause negative remodeling and worsen the left ventricular function, causing symptoms of HF.

The pathogenesis of HFpEF includes increased cardiac wall thickness and mass, concentric left ventricular hypertrophy, leading to increased myocardial stiffness, reduced compliance, abnormal filling pressures, and diastolic dysfunction.

## THE DIFFERENCE IN PATHOPHYSIOLOGY OF HEART FAILURE IN MEN AND WOMEN

As compared to men, women have lower left ventricular mass, greater contractility, lower rate of apoptosis, higher heart rate, and lower blood pressure. Women are less responsive to catecholamines. Differential gene expression has been proposed at the new onset of HF by Heidecker and colleague. GATAD1, SLC2A12, and PDE6B are prevalent in females in new-onset HF, while men express more KCNK1, CD24, and PLEKHA8.

## SIGNS AND SYMPTOMS

Typical symptoms of HF are breathlessness, edema, orthopnea, paroxysmal nocturnal dyspnea, and fatigue. Other symptoms are less typical and include nocturnal cough, wheezing, dizziness, palpitation, and syncope. Elderly people present with atypical symptoms such as confusion and depression. Specific signs include third heart sound, elevated jugular venous pressure, hepatojugular reflex, while weight gain, murmur, lung crepitations, tachycardia, irregular pulse, hepatomegaly, tachypnea are less specific signs for HF.

Although symptoms are similar in both males and females but women complain more of edema, more functional limitations, and more dyspnea with similar left ventricular function. Women have worse quality of life and are more depressed then men.

### Diagnostic Workup

Diagnosis of HF can be difficult in women in view of different symptomatology and the presence of obesity in females. Hence, diagnostic workup includes a careful detailed history and necessary investigations. Natriuretic peptides (NPs) levels are more in women and peak VO2 during cardiopulmonary exercise is less in women.

## INVESTIGATION

- *Blood test*:
    - Complete blood count
    - Serum electrolytes
    - Renal and liver function test
    - Blood glucose
    - Thyroid function test
    - Serum iron profile

- *Electrocardiography (ECG)*: It should be done in all patients. Common findings include sinus tachycardia, bundle branch blocks, atrial fibrillation, and repolarization abnormalities.
- *Chest X-Ray*: A chest X-ray is of limited use in the diagnostic work-up of patients with suspected HF, probably most useful in identifying an alternative explanation for a patient's symptoms and signs, i.e., pulmonary malignancy and interstitial pulmonary disease. In acute HF, chest X-ray will show signs of pulmonary venous congestion in the form of Batwing appearance. In chronic HF cardiomegaly and
- *Echocardiography*: A thorough and comprehensive echocardiogram is the most important investigation in HF. In women, LV size, mass, and volume should be indexed to body surface area.

## Biomarkers

Measurement of brain natriuretic peptide (BNP) or N-terminal pro-brain natriuretic peptide (NT proBNP) for diagnosis and prognosis has been recommended in various guidelines. These biomarkers have high negative predictive value and the positive predictive value is low. BNP levels >35 pg/mL and NT proBNP >125 pg/mL is suggestive of HF in chronic HF, in the acute setting, higher values should be used (BNP 100 pg/mL, NT-proBNP 300 pg/mL). High levels of NP despite HF are seen in increasing age, acute coronary syndrome, renal insufficiency, right ventricular dysfunction, atrial fibrillation, pulmonary hypertension, pulmonary embolism, pneumonia, anemia, and sepsis. Lower levels than expected can be seen in flash pulmonary edema, pericarditis, cardiac tamponade, genetic polymorphism, end-stage cardiomyopathy, and obesity. Other biomarkers of potential use in HF are high-sensitivity troponins, sST2, procalcitonin, galectin-3, cystatin C, and neutrophil gelatinase-associated lipocalin (NGAL).

## Other Diagnostic Tests

- Exercise electrocardiogram (treadmill test)
- Single-photon emission computed tomography (SPECT)
- Cardiac magnetic resonance (CMR)
- Cardiac computed tomography
- Positron emission tomography (PET)
- Coronary angiography
- Endomyocardial biopsy (EMB)

*Management includes:*
- Patient education and counseling
- Nonpharmacological therapy
- Pharmacological therapy
- Advance therapy such as device implantation namely cardiac resynchronization therapy (CRT) and implantable cardioverter defibrillator (ICD), revascularization, mechanical circulatory support, and cardiac transplantation.

*Pharmacological management:*
The drugs that have been shown to have mortality reduction in HFrEF are angiotensin-converting enzyme (ACE) inhibitor, angiotensin receptor blockers (ARBs) (class effect), Mineralocorticoid receptor antagonist (MRA) (eplerenone and spironolactone), angiotensin receptor neprilysin inhibitor (ARNI) (sacubitril-Valsartan), and beta-blockers

(sustained release metoprolol, carvedilol, bisoprolol). All the trials have showed similar benefits in males and females with guideline-directed medical therapy (GDMT) still women are under prescribed. Women treated by a male physician are least likely to get full dosage while the female physician is more likely to prescribe the full target dose in women. ACE inhibitors improve survival, decrease hospitalization in women as in men, however, women are undertreated with ACE inhibitors. ACE inhibitors are contraindicated in pregnancy. Beta-blockers have a similar benefit in women as in men, as is with MRA. However, women have shown increased mortality with digoxin, because of the smaller body surface area and increased mean serum concentration. Women are prescribed less of anticoagulant despite similar benefit as in men.

## Device Therapy

The CRT and ICD have shown equal benefit in women. Women show a better response to CRT, still among eligible women only 27% of them received CRT, and only 20–30% underwent ICD implantation. In the INTERMACS registry, 401 women received left ventricular assist device (LVAD), and there were 1,535 men receiving LVAD. In India, about 70 patients underwent LVAD implantation, among them about half were Indian patients and only three women from India received LVAD. Complications and outcomes were similar in both. Women have smaller body frames and these devices have specific requirements for implantation, so lesser eligible women are receiving these devices.

According to the International Society for Heart and Lung Transplantation, only about 23% of heart transplant recipients were women and had lesser 1 year survival rates. In AIIMS, less than one-third of cardiac transplant recipients were women. A recent meta-analysis showed that men were a three times more likely to be enrolled in cardiac rehabilitation (CR) compared with women.

## MANAGEMENT OF ACUTE HEART FAILURE

- *Identification of precipitating factors*: Acute coronary syndrome, arrhythmias, infection, and poor drug compliance are the main causes of decompensation in stable HF. These should be recognized and managed accordingly.
- *Oxygen and ventilatory support*: Patients should be assessed for the need for supplemental oxygen. According to clinical status, oxygen can be given via mask, noninvasive ventilation or in severe cases invasive ventilation by endotracheal intubation can be given.
- *Drugs*: Diuretics relieve congestion and provide symptomatic relief, and are an essential part of therapy. If the patient has the blood pressures are >100 mm Hg then vasodilators are recommended, if blood pressures are <90 mm Hg then inotropic support is required. ACE inhibitors should be started if blood pressure allows, beta-blockers are not recommended in acute conditions and should be started once the patient is stable. Other drugs that can be useful sometimes are vasopressors, digoxin, and amiodarone.
- *Mechanical circulatory support*: In severe cases refractory to medical management or in cardiogenic shock mechanical circulatory support devices such as intra-aortic balloon pump, ventricular assist devices are helpful.

*Heart failure with preserved ejection fraction*: Diagnosis of HFpEF can be challenging in view of normal LV size and EF and the presence of multiple comorbidities. According to ESC guidelines, following criteria should be fulfilled for diagnosis:

- Signs and symptoms of HF.
- Elevated natriuretic peptide levels (BNP ≥35 pg/mL or NT-proBNP level ≥125 pg/mL).
- A preserved EF [left ventricular ejection fraction (LVEF ≥50%)].
- Additional alteration to cardiac structure and/or function:
  - Left atrial volume index >34 mL/m$^2$
  - Left ventricular mass index ≥115 g/m$^2$ for males and ≥95 g/m$^2$ for females.
  - E to E' ratio ≥13
  - Mean E' septal and lateral wall <9 cm/s.

## MANAGEMENT OF HEART FAILURE WITH PRESERVED EJECTION FRACTION

Most pharmacological and many of nonpharmacological therapies have been studied and proved beneficial in HFrEF. However, in HFpEF management is difficult as none has proven to show reduced mortality. Patients with HFpEF should be managed as follows:
- Risk factor management such as adequate control of hypertension, diabetes, and arrhythmias. SPRINT did show a 37% reduction in HF with intense blood pressure control.
- Lifestyle modification such as exercise and calorie restriction has shown improvement in symptoms of HF.
- ACE inhibitors except for candesartan, beta-blocker, and statins have not shown any promising results in HFpEF. Spironolactone has shown a reduction in HF hospitalization in selective population. Diuretics provide symptomatic relief.
- Device-based therapies are also being tested in HFpEF including interatrial shunt devices and minimally invasive pericardial modification.
- Drugs that target cardiometabolic functional abnormalities are currently under investigation for the treatment of HFpEF such as:
  - *Partial adenosine A1-agonists*: Capadenoson and neladenoson,
  - *Carnitine palmitoyltransferase-1 inhibitors*: Etomoxir and perhexiline,
  - *Fatty acid oxidation inhibitor*: Trimetazidine,
  - *Mitochondrial enhancer*: Elamipretide

## PREGNANCY AND HEART FAILURE

Heart failure in pregnancy can be because of PPCM or de novo because of other etiologies. PPCM is defined as HF that develops in the last month of gestation or up to 5 months postpartum period with LVEF <45% or fractional shortening <30%, or both. Risk factors for PPCM include women <30 years of age, multiple gestations, primigravida, preeclampsia, eclampsia, presence of other cardiovascular risk factors, and use of tocolytics. PPCM has a genetic predisposition, also the role of prolactin, placental angiogenic factor, and autoimmunity has been described as etiology. Recent studies report improvement in left ventricular function in 50–80% of women in the first 6 months after diagnosing PPCM. Women with known HF should have preconceptional counseling. Pregnancy should be supervised by the multidisciplinary team as hemodynamic changes can worsen symptoms of HF. Patients should be managed as per guidelines, but ACE inhibitors, ARBs, and mineralocorticoids antagonist should be avoided in pregnancy. ARNIs should not be used, beta 1 selective blocker such as metoprolol should be used. Diuretics can be used if congestive symptoms are present. Other drugs that can be used are digoxin, hydralazine, and nitrates. Role of prolactin inhibitors, antisense therapy against microRNA-146a,

VEGF agonism and removal of anti-angiogenic proteins, serelaxin, perhexiline, and pentoxifylline are being explored as emerging therapy in PPCM.

## PROGNOSIS

According to recent study, global survival in HF patients at 1, 5, 10, 15 years were 75.5%, 45.4%, 24.5%, and 12.7% respectively. Women had worse short- and long-term outcomes than men with 1 and 15-year survival in women versus men were 74.5% versus 77.2% and 11.0% versus 14.1% respectively. Overall 1-year survival has improved by 6.6% from 2000 to 2016 and 5-year survival has improved by 7.2%. Women with diabetes and HF have a worse prognosis than without diabetes. Trivandrum Heart Failure Registry from India has shown the worse outcomes. The in-hospital mortality rate was 9.7% in HFrEF and 4.8% in HFpEF. After 3 years, 44.8% study population died. Such high mortality can be explained by more ischemic causes of HF. The INTER-CHF study has reported the highest 1-year mortality in India and Africa.

## CONCLUSION

Heart failure is an important cause of morbidity and mortality in women. Women show considerable differences in the etiopathogenesis, progression, and outcome of HF. HFpEF is more common in women. Current guidelines do not endorse sex-specific recommendations. Even then, women receive suboptimal therapy as compared to men. Also, women are represented less in clinical trials and further gender specific studies are needed to evaluate and improve outcomes of HF in the fair sex.

## SUGGESTED READING

1. Ponikowski P, Voors AA, Anker SD, Bueno H, Cleland JGF, Coats AJS et al. 2016 ESC Guidelines for the diagnosis and treatment of acute and chronic heart failure: The Task Force for the diagnosis and treatment of acute and chronic heart failure of the European Society of Cardiology (ESC) developed with the special contribution of the Heart Failure Association (HFA) of the ESC. Eur Heart J. 2016;37(27):2129-200.
2. Benjamin EJ, Blaha MJ, Chiuve SE, Cushman M, Das SR, Deo R, et al. Heart disease and stroke statistics-2017 update: A Report From the American Heart Association. Circulation. 2017;135(10):e146-603.
3. Mozaffarian D, Benjamin EJ, Go AS, Arnett DK, Blaha MJ, Cushman M, et al. Heart Disease and Stroke Statistics-2016 Update: A Report From the American Heart Association. Circulation. 2016;133(4):e38-360.
4. Lloyd-Jones DM, Larson MG, Leip EP, Beiser A, D'Agostino RB, Kannel WB, et al. Lifetime risk for developing congestive heart failure: the Framingham Heart Study. Circulation. 2002;106(24):3068-72.
5. Chaturvedi V, Parakh N, Seth S, Bhargava B, Ramakrishnan S, Roy A, et al. Heart failure in India: The Indus (India Ukieri Study) study. J Pract Cardiovasc Sci. 2016;2(1):28-35.
6. Masoudi FA, Havranek EP, Smith G, Fish RH, Steiner JF, Ordin DL, et al. Gender, age, and heart failure with preserved left ventricular systolic function. J Am Coll Cardiol. 2003;41(2):217-23.
7. Huffman MD, Prabhakaran D. Heart failure: Epidemiology and prevention in India. Natl Med J India. 2010;23(5):283-8.
8. Lam CS, Anand I, Zhang S, Shimizu W, Narasimhan C, Park SW, et al. Asian Sudden Cardiac Death in Heart Failure (ASIAN-HF) registry. Eur J Heart Fail. 2013;15(8):928-36.
9. Kalra A, Glusenkamp N, Anderson K, Kalra RN, Kerkar PG, Kumar G, et al. American College of Cardiology (ACC)'s PINNACLE India Quality Improvement Program (PIQIP)-Inception, progress and future direction: A report from the PIQIP Investigators. Indian Heart J. 2016;68(Suppl 3):S1-4.

10. Sanjay G, Jeemon P, Agarwal A, Viswanathan S, Sreedharan M, Vijayaraghavan G, et al. In-Hospital and Three-Year Outcomes of Heart Failure Patients in South India: The Trivandrum Heart Failure Registry. J Card Fail. 2018;24(12):842-8.
11. Dokainish H, Teo K, Zhu J, Roy A, AlHabib KF, ElSayed A, et al. Global mortality variations in patients with heart failure: results from the International Congestive Heart Failure (INTER-CHF) prospective cohort study. Lancet Glob Health. 2017;5:6650-72.
12. Chopra VK, Mittal S, Bansal M, Singh B, Trehan N. Clinical profile and one-year survival of patients with heart failure with reduced ejection fraction: The largest report from India. Indian Heart J. 2019;71(3):242-8.
13. Hunt SA, Abraham WT, Chin MH, Feldman AM, Francis GS, Ganiats TG, et al. 2009 focused update incorporated into the ACC/AHA 2005 guidelines for the diagnosis and management of heart failure in adults: a report of the American College of Cardiology Foundation/American Heart Association Task Force on Practice Guidelines. J Am Coll Cardiol. 2009;53:e1-90.
14. Bibbins-Domingo K, Lin F, Vittinghoff E, Barrett-Connor E, Hulley SB, Grady D, et al. Predictors of heart failure among women with coronary disease. Circulation. 2004;110(11):1424-30.
15. Lee CS, Tkacs NC. Current concepts of neurohormonal activation in heart failure: mediators and mechanisms. AACN Adv Crit Care. 2008;19:364-85.
16. Paulus WJ, Tschöpe C. A novel paradigm for heart failure with preserved ejection fraction: comorbidities drive myocardial dysfunction and remodeling through coronary microvascular endothelial inflammation. J Am Coll Cardiol. 2013;62(4):263-71.
17. Carroll JD, Carroll EP, Feldman T, Ward DM, Lang RM, McGaughey D, et al. Sex- associated differences in left ventricular function in aortic stenosis of the elderly. Circulation. 1992;86(4):1099-107.
18. Heidecker B, Lamirault G, Kasper EK, Wittstein IS, Champion HC, Breton E, et al. The gene expression profile of patients with new-onset heart failure reveals important gender-specific differences. Eur Heart J. 2010;31(10):1188-96.
19. Riedinger MS, Dracup KA, Brecht ML, Padilla G, Sarna L, Ganz PA. Quality of life in patients with heart failure: do gender differences exist? Heart Lung. 2001;30(2):105-16.
20. Gottlieb SS, Khatta M, Friedmann E, Einbinder L, Katzen S, Baker B, et al. The influence of age, gender, and race on the prevalence of depression in heart failure patients. J Am Coll Cardiol. 2004;43(9):1542-9.
21. McKee PA, Castelli WP, McNamara PM, Kannel WB. The natural history of congestive heart failure: the Framingham study. N Engl J Med. 1971;285(26):1441-6.
22. Wang TJ, Larson MG, Levy D, Leip EP, Benjamin EJ, Wilson PW, et al. Impact of age and sex on plasma natriuretic peptide levels in healthy adults. Am J Cardiol. 2002;90(3):254-8.
23. Daida H, Allison TG, Johnson BD, Squires RW, Gau GT. Comparison of peak exercise oxygen uptake in men versus women in chronic heart failure secondary to ischemic or idiopathic dilated cardiomyopathy. Am J Cardiol. 1997;80(1):85-8.
24. Lang RM, Badano LP, Mor-Avi V, Afilalo J, Armstrong A, Ernande L, et al. Recommendations for cardiac chamber quantification by echocardiography in adults: an update from the American Society of Echocardiography and the European Association of Cardiovascular Imaging. J Am Soc Echocardiogr. 2015;28(1):1-39.
25. Baumhäkel M, Müller U, Böhm M. Influence of gender of physicians and patients on guideline-recommended treatment of chronic heart failure in a cross-sectional study. Eur J Heart Fail. 2009;11:299-303.
26. Ghali JK, Pina IL, Gottlieb SS, Deedwania PC, Wikstrand JC. Metoprolol CR/XL in female patients with heart failure: analysis of the experience in Metoprolol Extended-Release Randomized Intervention Trial in Heart Failure (MERIT-HF). Circulation. 2002;105(13):1585-91.
27. Pitt B, Zannad F, Remme WJ, Cody R, Castaigne A, Perez A, et al. The effect of spironolactone on morbidity and mortality in patients with severe heart failure. Randomized Aldactone Evaluation Study Investigators. N Engl J Med. 1999;341(10):709-17.
28. The Digitalis Investigation Group. The effect of digoxin on mortality and morbidity in patients with heart failure. N Engl J Med. 1997;336(8):525-33.
29. Chatterjee NA, Borgquist R, Chang Y, Lewey J, Jackson VA, Singh JP, et al. Increasing sex differences in the use of cardiac resynchronization therapy with or without implantable cardioverter-defibrillator. Eur Heart J. 2017;38(19):1485-94.

30. Stevenson LW, Pagani FD, Young JB, Jessup M, Miller L, Kormos RL, et al. INTERMACS profiles of advanced heart failure: the current picture. J Heart Lung Transplant. 2009;28:535-41.
31. Taylor DO, Stehlik J, Edwards LB, Aurora P, Christie JD, Dobbels F, et al. Registry of the International Society for Heart and Lung Transplantation: Twenty-sixth Official Adult Heart Transplant Report-2009. J Heart Lung Transplant. 2009;28(10):1007-22.
32. Airan B, Singh SP, Seth S, Hote MP, Sahu MK, Rajashekar P, et al. Heart transplant in India: Lessons learned. J Pract Cardiovasc Sci. 2017;3:94-9.
33. Samayoa L, Grace SL, Gravely S, Scott LB, Marzolini S, Colella TJ. Sex differences in cardiac rehabilitation enrollment: a meta-analysis. Can J Cardiol. 2014;30:793-800.
34. Wright JT Jr, Williamson JD, Whelton PK, Snyder JK, Sink KM, Rocco MV, et al. A randomized trial of intensive versus standard blood-pressure control. N Engl J Med. 2015;373:2103-16.
35. Kitzman DW, Brubaker P, Morgan T, Haykowsky M, Hundley G, Kraus WE, et al. Effect of caloric restriction or aerobic exercise training on peak oxygen consumption and quality of life in obese older patients with heart failure with preserved ejection fraction: a randomized clinical trial. JAMA. 2016;315:36-46.
36. Pfeffer MA, Swedberg K, Granger CB, Held P, McMurray JJ, Michelson EL, et al. Effects of candesartan on mortality and morbidity in patients with chronic heart failure: the CHARM-Overall programme. Lancet. 2003;362(9386):759-66.
37. Pfeffer MA, Claggett B, Assmann SF, Boineau R, Anand IS, Clausell N, et al. Regional variation in patients and outcomes in the treatment of preserved cardiac function heart failure with an aldosterone antagonist (TOPCAT) Trial. Circulation. 2015;131:23-42.
38. Hasenfuss G, Hayward C, Burkhoff D, Silvestry FE, McKenzie S, Gustafsson F, et al. A transcatheter intracardiac shunt device for heart failure with preserved ejection fraction (REDUCE LAP-HF): a multicentre, open-label, single-arm, phase 1 trial. Lancet. 2016;387:1298-304.
39. Borlaug BA, Carter RE, Melenovsky V, DeSimone CV, Gaba P, Killu A, et al. Percutaneous pericardial resection: A novel potential treatment for heart failure with preserved ejection fraction. Circ Heart Fail. 2017;10(4):e003612.
40. Greene SJ, Sabbah HN, Butler J, Voors AA, Albrecht-Kupper BE, Dungen HD, et al. Partial adenosine A1 receptor agonism: a potential new therapeutic strategy for heart failure. Heart Fail Rev. 2016;21(1):95-102.
41. Elkayam U. Clinical characteristics of peripartum cardiomyopathy in the United States: diagnosis, prognosis, and management. J Am Coll Cardiol. 2011;58:659-70.
42. Daubert MA, Yow E, Dunn G, Marchev S, Barnhart H, Douglas PS, et al. Novel mitochondria-targeting peptide in heart failure treatment: a randomized, placebo-controlled trial of elamipretide. Circ Heart Fail. 2017;10(12):e004389.
43. Pearson GD, Veille JC, Rahimtoola S, Hsia J, Oakley CM, Hosenpud JD, et al. Peripartum cardiomyopathy: National Heart, Lung, and Blood Institute and Office of Rare Diseases (National Institutes of Health) workshop recommendations and review. JAMA. 2000;283:1183-8.
44. Kao DP, Hsich E, Lindenfeld J. Characteristics, adverse events, and racial differences among delivering mothers with peripartum cardiomyopathy. JACC Heart Fail. 2013;1:409-16.
45. Fett JD, Sundstrom BJ, Etta King M, Ansari AA. Mother-daughter peripartum cardiomyopathy. Int J Cardiol. 2002;86:331-2.
46. Hilfiker-Kleiner D, Kaminski K, Podewski E, Bonda T, Schaefer A, Sliwa K, et al. A cathepsin D-cleaved 16 kDa form of prolactin mediates postpartum cardiomyopathy. Cell. 2007;128:589-600.
47. Liu J, Wang Y, Chen M, Zhao W, Wang X, Wang H, et al. The correlation between peripartum cardiomyopathy and autoantibodies against cardiovascular receptors. PLoS One. 2014;9:e86770.
48. Haghikia A, Kaya Z, Schwab J, Westenfeld R, Ehlermann P, Bachelier K, et al. Evidence of autoantibodies against cardiac troponin I and sarcomeric myosin in peripartum cardiomyopathy. Basic Res Cardiol. 2015;110:60.
49. Elkayam U, Akhter MW, Singh H, Khan S, Bitar F, Hameed A, et al. Pregnancy-associated cardiomyopathy: clinical characteristics and a comparison between early and late presentation. Circulation. 2005;111:2050-5.
50. Regitz-Zagrosek V, Roos-Hesselink JW, Bauersachs J, Blomström-Lundqvist C, Cífková R, De Bonis M, et al. 2018 ESC Guidelines for the management of cardiovascular diseases during pregnancy. Eur Heart J. 2018;39:3165-241.

51. Halkein J, Tabruyn SP, Ricke-Hoch M, Haghikia A, Nguyen NQ, Scherr M, et al. MicroRNA-146a is a therapeutic target and biomarker for peripartum cardiomyopathy. J Clin Invest. 2013;123:2143-54.
52. Patten IS, Rana S, Shahul S, Rowe GC, Jang C, Liu L, et al. Cardiac angiogenic imbalance leads to peripartum cardiomyopathy. Nature. 2012;485:333-8.
53. Teerlink JR, Cotter G, Davison BA, Felker GM, Filippatos G, Greenberg BH, et al. Serelaxin, recombinant human relaxin-2, for treatment of acute heart failure (RELAX-AHF): a randomised, placebo-controlled trial. Lancet. 2013;381(9860):29-39.
54. Cappola TP. Perhexiline: lessons for heart failure therapeutics. JACC Heart Fail. 2015;3:212-3.
55. Sliwa K, Skudicky D, Candy G, Bergemann A, Hopley M, Sareli P. The addition of pentoxifylline to conventional therapy improves outcome in patients with peripartum cardiomyopathy. Eur J Heart Fail. 2002;4:305-9.
56. Taylor CJ, Ordóñez-Mena JM, Roalfe AK, Lay-Flurrie S, Jones NR, Marshall T, et al. Trends in survival after a diagnosis of heart failure in the United Kingdom 2000-2017: population-based cohort study. BMJ. 2019;364:l223.

# CHAPTER 5

# Coronary Intervention in Women: How is it Different?

Hetan C Shah, Rajesh Matta

## ABSTRACT

Cardiovascular disease (CVD) is a leading cause of mortality and morbidity in both men and women globally. However, women are underdiagnosed, undertreated, and the scope of the problem is underestimated. Only 20% turn up for evaluation and treatment. Biologic differences between sexes account for the variation in the natural history and management of coronary artery disease (CAD). Management of CAD during pregnancy involves special challenges for interventional cardiologists.

Here, we explore the special considerations that need to be taken into account when managing CAD in women. Gender differences exist with respect to clinical presentation, comorbid conditions, access for percutaneous coronary intervention (PCI), coronary anatomy and pathology, hardware required for the procedure, and medical management.

## INTRODUCTION

The risk of death from heart disease in women is eight times higher than dying from breast cancer. A recent study in Kerala (Krishnan MN et al.) showed that the prevalence of coronary artery disease (CAD) in women was 14.3% compared to 9.8% in men.

Despite the evidence of advances in the management of CAD, there seems to be a discrepancy in the outcomes for women compared to men. According to recent systematic review and meta-analysis, mortality was significantly lower in male patients at all follow-up time points—immediate and long-term mortality. This indicates that this issue remains relevant to contemporary practice for the interventional cardiologist.

## CLINICAL AND DEMOGRAPHIC PROFILE OF FEMALES WITH CAD

Clinical presentation of CAD is atypical in women which leads to its underdiagnosis. Moreover, they tend to have a high prevalence of hypertension, diabetes, and other comorbidities. The earlier statistics showed that the presentation of CAD in women is generally 10 years later compared to men, however, the current modern lifestyle, the presentation is at a relatively younger age. They are more likely to present with unstable angina and heart failure due to delayed presentation and comorbidities and especially have poor outcomes with coexisting diabetes mellitus (DM).

Oral contraceptive pills (OCPs) use as a risk factor for developing acute coronary syndrome (ACS) requires a special mention. Various studies have confirmed the association between 2nd generation OCP and increased risk of ACS among young women even without concomitant existence of prothrombotic mutations. However, this risk is still unclarified with the use of 3rd generation OCP.

## MANAGEMENT OF CAD IN WOMEN

### Acute Coronary Syndrome in Women

Atypical chest pain and more associated symptoms are common presentations in a woman with ACS. In Woman the reason for chest pain is not only obstructive epicardial CAD but it can also be caused by printzmetal angina, syndrome X, and mitral valve prolapse and a significant percentage is attributed to spontaneous coronary artery dissection (SCAD). The presentation is usually Non-ST segment elevation of acute coronary syndrome (NTSE-ACS) rather than ST-elevation myocardial infarction (STEMI). Women usually receive suboptimal medical management and do not receive guideline-based therapy.

#### Intervention in NSTE-ACS

Non-ST-segment elevation of acute coronary syndrome in women receives less invasive treatment compared to man, due to late presentation (atypical symptoms), patient preference, and less reference for invasive treatment by physician. It has poor outcomes compared to men mostly due to delayed presentation, less body mass index (BMI), and associated comorbidities.

Meta-analysis of eight ACS trials, has shown that an early invasive strategy was safe and effective in reducing major adverse cardiac events (MACEs) for women with raised biomarkers. However, in women with negative biomarkers, such invasive strategy did not reduce MACE and showed higher rates for death or myocardial infarction (MI).

#### Intervention in STEMI

Primary percutaneous coronary intervention (PCI) for STEMI as per guidelines is the modality of treatment. Women are less likely to receive early invasive therapy in STEMI. Studies have shown that women have higher mortality due to older age and high-risk profile. Prolonged ischemic times (associated with longer symptom to balloon and door to balloon time) and higher PCI failure rates in women are partly responsible for such adverse outcomes.

#### Intervention in Stable Angina

In women with stable angina, the current recommendations include a combination therapeutic approach with antiplatelets, nitrates, beta-blockers, statins, angiotensin-converting enzyme (ACE) inhibitors/angiotensin receptor blockers (ARBs), and/or calcium channel blockers (CCBs) for long-term symptom control and cardiovascular risk reduction. In stable angina according to EURO Heart Survey, women are likely to receive suboptimal medical therapy (Aspirin: 73% vs. 81%; Statin: 45% vs. 51%). Invasive therapy leads to higher mortality (49% vs. 31%).

## Challenges During Intervention

### Vascular Access

Women have 1.5–4 times higher risk of vascular complications. Although femoral access usually has higher risk, radial artery size in females is smaller and is more prone to develop spasm.

In the SAFE-PCI (Study of Access Site for Enhancement of PCI for Women) trial, it was seen that the radial artery access was not seen to reduce bleeding or vascular complications in women undergoing PCI. It was noted that access site crossover occurred more frequently in women assigned to radial access. The use of lower sheath sizes and hydrophilic coating improves the procedural outcome with minimal complication and crossover. However, there have been no gender-specific data on arterial vascular puncture closure devices.

## Anticoagulation During PCI

Women are at higher risk of bleeding during PCI, hence weight-based dosing of anticoagulants is particularly essential. In the SYNERGY (Superior Yield of the New Strategy of Enoxaparin, Revascularization and Glycoprotein IIb/IIIa Inhibitors) trial, no statistically significant difference in MACE was found in women treated with enoxaparin versus unfractionated heparin (UFH). Bivalirudin as an alternative antithrombotic therapy during PCI lowers the bleeding events compared with heparin and a glycoprotein (GP) IIb/IIIa inhibitors. The CRUSADE registry showed excess bleeding for women treated with a GP IIb/IIIa inhibitor. It identified women as a vulnerable group, susceptible to excess dosing. So, caution should be used when administering these agents to female patients during or immediately after PCI. It is preferable to postpone elective PCI in women with active heavy menstrual bleeding.

## CORONARY ARTERY ANATOMY AND CAD PATTERN IN WOMEN

The coronary caliber is relatively small with a more diffuse pattern of CAD, ostial involvement being more common. The paradox of ischemic heart disease in women though women have higher rates of myocardial ischemia and mortality, they have less obstructive CAD. Thus, the "Female-pattern" IHD implies a relatively lower obstructive CAD burden and preserved left ventricular function. A study done among Indian women undergoing coronary angiography showed a greater proportion of women having triple vessel disease (TVD) (39.6%). Women with double vessel disease (DVD) (12.9%) or single-vessel disease (SVD) (15.8%) were lesser as compared to TVD. Another study done estimated that involvement of left anterior descending artery (LAD) 35.2% women, left circumflex artery (LCX) in 25.6% women, right coronary artery (RCA) in 26% women, and left main coronary artery (LMCA) in 3.4% women.

In addition, women with ACS are more likely to have normal angiograms or demonstrate no obstructive CAD. Infact, a registry showed that the odds of obstructive CAD are 50% lower for women undergoing coronary angiography. Other ACS registries have demonstrated more frequent nonobstructive CAD in women (10–25% of women vs. 6–10% of men) although this does not carry a benign prognosis.

*The myocardial infarction with nonobstructive coronary arteries (MINOCA):* The increasing recognition of MINOCA occurs more frequently in women, particularly younger women. There are multiple causes for MINOCA including subendocardial ischemia (coronary

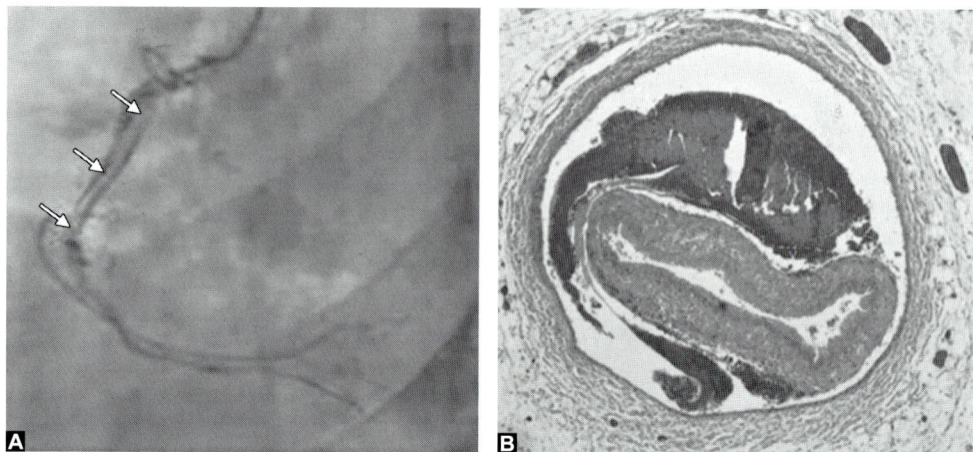

**FIGS. 1A AND B:** (A) Coronary angiogram and (B) microscopic appearance of spontaneous coronary artery dissection (SCAD). *(For color version, see Plate 4)*
*Source*: Hussaini A, Adlam D. Spontaneous coronary artery dissection. Heart. 2017;103:1043-51.

microvascular disease), myocarditis, coronary vasospasm, Takotsubo cardiomyopathy, hypertrophic cardiomyopathy, and SCAD.

*Spontaneous coronary artery dissection* (**Figs. 1A and B**): Recent data indicate that SCAD is responsible for 22–31% of ACS in women under the age of 60, and up to 43% of pregnancy-related ACS. Intracoronary imaging modalities including optical coherence tomography (OCT) and intravascular ultrasound (IVUS) should be considered to confirm diagnosis. Dissection of the coronary intimal or medial layer or rupture of the vasa vasorum can lead to intramural hematoma formation, which can ultimately result in various degrees of coronary occlusion. At-risk patients are generally young females in their peripartum state with recent intensive emotional stress or those with connective tissue disorder. Management is predominantly conservative with standard ACS therapy, although revascularization might be considered in persistently symptomatic patients despite optimized medical management.

## PCI-RELATED COMPLICATIONS IN WOMEN

Vascular complications include subcutaneous hematoma formation, pseudoaneurysm, retroperitoneal bleeding have a higher incidence in women.

Bleeding increases morbidity and mortality among patients undergoing PCI. This can be attributed to shock in acute settings. In the long run, it might lead to anemia and hence increase morbidity in patients. The occurrence of a bleeding event may result in cessation of dual antiplatelet therapy (DAPT), which increases the risk of stent thrombosis and MI. The high bleeding rates in women can be attributed to modifiable and nonmodifiable sex-associated risk factors. The excess risk of complications may be secondary to nonmodifiable sex-associated factors, such as the presence of a lower BMI and lower creatinine clearance, and anatomic differences, such as smaller vessel size. With the growing number of premenopausal females suffering an ACS and subsequent PCI, concerns about heavy menstrual bleeding following PCI require special mention. This warrant detailed and thorough evaluation to rule out local uterine pathology as well as reconsideration of antiplatelet therapy. To minimize the risk of bleeding events, drug dosing should be based on renal function and the use of anticoagulant strategies may be individualized according to the above-mentioned factors.

It is to be mentioned here that there does not exist a convincing evidence to suggest that women are at risk of developing other complications during PCI such as a significant increase in postprocedural stroke in a single study (OR 3.2, 95% CI 1.4–7.4, p <0.01). Some studies found that complications such as coronary perforation and tamponade were more common in women. However, in a large review of grade III coronary perforations, female gender was not found to be a significant predictor, however, predictors in PCI were rotablation, complex lesions, and IVUS-guided procedures.

## ANTIPLATELET THERAPY IN WOMEN AFTER PCI

Aspirin has been the mainstay of antiplatelet therapy in patients with CAD as well as in patients following PCI. Women have been seen to have greater aspirin resistance than in men. HOPE (Heart Outcome Prevention Evaluation) trial evaluated the relationship between aspirin resistance and the risk of the adverse cardiovascular outcomes, indicated that women may be more aspirin resistant (p = 0.0004). However, aspirin for secondary prevention in women has been well established. Still, aspirin continues to be underutilized in women.

The P2Y12 inhibitors, when given in addition to aspirin, these agents reduce the rates of subacute stent thrombosis after stent implantation. The PCI-CURE (Clopidogrel in Unstable Angina to Prevent Recurrent Events) study enrolled ACS patients treated with PCI, of whom 30.2% were women and found that clopidogrel for up to 12 months was superior to aspirin alone. A trend toward benefit was seen in women (RR 0.77, 95% CI 0.52–1.15) compared with the statistically significant benefit seen in men (RR 0.65, 95% CI 0.48–0.87). In the CREDO (Clopidogrel for Reduction of Events During Observation) trial, 29% were women, benefits of clopidogrel for up to 12 months after elective PCI in women did not reach statistical significance.

Nonetheless, DAPT with aspirin and P2Y12 inhibitor is recommended following PCI for a finite duration even in women.

## PREGNANCY AND CORONARY INTERVENTION

During pregnancy an ACS is rare and estimated at 3–6/100,000 deliveries. Maternal mortality after ACS is estimated at 5–10% and is highest during the peripartum period. A study found that in pregnant women with ACS, 38% occurred in the antepartum, 21% occurred in the intrapartum, and 41% occurred in the 6-week postpartum period.

The risk factors for acute myocardial infarction (AMI) such as DM, smoking, advanced maternal age, dyslipidemia, significant family history, and hypertension are also commonly seen in pregnancy. Additionally, risk factors such as black race, eclampsia, preeclampsia, anemia, migraine headaches, and thrombophilia have been identified during pregnancy. Historically, SCAD was often regarded as a disease of pregnancy that carried a high risk of fatal MI. Repeated pregnancies and the use of hormonal therapies such as selective estrogen receptor modulators or hormone replacement therapy are believed to increase the risk of SCAD in women.

In the management of atherothrombotic ACS, early coronary revascularization and reperfusion of ischemic myocardium through PCI has improved short-term outcomes, and long-term prognosis to a significant extent. Early invasive approach is preferred in high-risk ACSs as it identifies the culprit lesion and a decision for management may be made immediately. Studies have shown limited technical success in patients with SCAD.

Most of the current data for PCI during pregnancy is available for bare metal stents. ACE inhibitors, ARBs, and renin inhibitors are contraindicated during pregnancy. Beta-blockers and low dose acetylsalicylic acid have been considered to be relatively safe, while this is unknown for thienopyridines. Clopidogrel should, therefore, only be used during pregnancy when strictly needed. A multidisciplinary approach including obstetrician and cardiologist must be a norm while managing such patients.

*Radiation hazards*: There is a gap in the literature regarding estimated fetal radiation exposure during a cardiac intervention. However, carefully performed cardiac interventions can reduce the radiation exposure to less than a CT. Besides, other preventive measures such as the use of lower frame rates, beam collimator, and use of wedge filters must be adopted. The use of external shielding of abdomen and pelvis is a common practice however, of a limited significance. This is because the fetal exposure from fluoroscopy is more from a scatter from thoracic tissues, rather than direct fetal irradiation from the primary X-ray beam.

## CONCLUSION

Women differ compared to men in a significant manner with respect to CAD risk factors. Clinical presentation includes the timing of initial presentation to medical personnel, to a choice of invasive versus conservative management as well as to CAD distribution and pattern. Certain specific entities such as SCAD are almost certainly more commonly seen in women which might warrant further investigation. The timing of coronary intervention differs significantly in women, so does the access site and its associated issues, the hardware used for the procedure, the intraprocedural medications, procedural success, and its complications. Bleeding and vascular site complications warrant a special mention in this respect. The postprocedural DAPT and its underprescription are important impediments to the long-term success of PCI in all patients, especially women. The outcomes of PCI are significantly affected by all the aforementioned factors. An interventionist is expected to be aware of all these possible loopholes in the management of women undergoing PCI and make necessary effort in the direction to minimize adverse outcomes in women, which comprise at least half of the patients referred for PCI.

## SUGGESTED READING

1. The top 10 causes of death. https://www.who.int/. [online] Available from https://www.who.int/news-room/fact-sheets/detail/the-top-10-causes-of-death. (Last accessed January, 2020).
2. Krishnan MN, Zachariah G, Venugopal K, Mohanan PP, Harikrishnan S, Sanjay G, et al. Prevalence of coronary artery disease and its risk factors in Kerala, South India: a community-based cross-sectional study. BMC Cardiovasc Disord. 2016;16:12.
3. Jacobs AK. Coronary revascularization in women in 2003: Sex revisited. Circulation. 2003;107(3):375-7.
4. O'Donoghue M, Boden WE, Braunwald E, Cannon CP, Clayton TC, de Winter RJ, et al. Early invasive vs conservative treatment strategies in women and men with unstable angina and non-ST-segment elevation myocardial infarction: A meta-analysis. JAMA. 2008;300(1):71-80.
5. Shaw LJ, Shaw RE, Merz CN, Brindis RG, Klein LW, Nallamothu B, et al. Impact of ethnicity and gender differences on angiographic coronary artery disease prevalence and in-hospital mortality in the American College of Cardiology-National Cardiovascular Data Registry. Circulation. 2008;117(14):1787-801.
6. Ezhumalai B, Jayaraman B. Angiographic prevalence and pattern of coronary artery disease in women. Indian Heart J. 2014; 66:422-4.

7. Hochman JS, Tamis JE, Thompson TD, Weaver WD, White HD, Van de Werf F, et al. Sex, clinical presentation, and outcome in patients with acute coronary syndromes. Global Use of Strategies to Open Occluded Coronary Arteries in Acute Coronary Syndromes IIb Investigators. N Engl J Med. 1999;341:226-32.
8. Elkayam U, Jalnapurkar S, Barakkat MN, Khatri N, Kealey AJ, Mehra A, et al. Pregnancy-associated acute myocardial infarction: a review of contemporary experience in 150 cases between 2006 and 2011. Circulation. 2014;129(16):1695-702.
9. Chan MY, Sun JL, Wang TY, Lopes RD, Jolicoeur ME, Pieper KS, et al. Patterns of discharge antiplatelet therapy and late outcomes among 8,582 patients with bleeding during acute coronary syndrome: a pooled analysis from PURSUIT, PARAGON-A, PARAGON-B, and SYNERGY. Am Heart J. 2010;160:1056-64, 1064.e2.
10. Lazar JM, Uretsky BF, Denys BG, Reddy PS, Counihan PJ, Ragosta M. Predisposing risk factors and natural history of acute neurologic complications of left-sided cardiac catheterization. Am J Cardiol. 1995;75(15):1056-60.
11. Fasseas P, Orford JL, Panetta CJ, Bell MR, Denktas AE, Lennon RJ, et al. Incidence, correlates, management, and clinical outcome of coronary perforation: analysis of 16,298 procedures. Am. Heart J. 2004;147(1):140-5.
12. Al-Lamee R, Ielasi A, Latib A, Godino C, Ferraro M, Mussardo M, et al. Incidence, predictors, management, immediate and long-term outcomes following grade III coronary perforation. JACC Cardiovasc. Interv. 2011;4(1):87-95.
13. Ladner HE, Danielsen B, Gilbert WM. Acute myocardial infarction in pregnancy and the puerperium: a population-based study. Obstet Gynecol. 2005;105(3):480-4.
14. James AH, Jamison MG, Biswas MS, Brancazio LR, Swamy GK, Myers ER. Acute myocardial infarction in pregnancy: a United States population-based study. Circulation. 2006;113(12):1564-71.

# CHAPTER 6

# Structural Heart Disease in Women: Age-based Presentation, Medical, and Interventional Strategies

*Tripti Deb, Shashank S Telang, Sandeep Kaur, Rajiv Gupta*

## ABSTRACT

Last two decades have seen emerging therapy for management of structural heart diseases. Most of the development in this field has occurred in the form of newer devices and evolution of deployment techniques. Structural heart disease in women needs discussion in view of gender based differences in physiology and haemodynamics. In addition, pregnancy affects body hemodynamics thus altering pathophysiology of structural heart diseases. Therefore, these need to be discussed before a definite management plan is formulated in females with structural heart diseases.

## INTRODUCTION

In 1999, Martin Leon primarily developed and announced the term "Structural heart disease" at the Transcatheter Cardiovascular Therapeutics meeting so as to cover noncoronary cardiac diseases and developing interventional strategies. In fact, the preliminary study in 1952 by Rubio-Alvarez and Limon regarding critical pulmonic valve stenosis led to the triggering of breakthrough in procedure and technology. This progress paved way for treatment and cure of structural heart disease.

There is a strong belief that cardiovascular disease (CVD) chiefly affects men. Hence, the women affected with CVD are mostly under-diagnosed and not managed correctly. Multiple susceptibility parameters regarding gender-based risk have surfaced; however, dearth in clinical application causes misdiagnosis and improper treatment of women affected by CVD. For this reason, it becomes essential to tackle symptoms particular to the gender combined with risk factors so as to develop the required strategy of therapy apart from affecting the morbidity and mortality in this set of patients positively.

## SPECTRUM OF STRUCTURAL HEART DISEASE

### Atrial Septal Defect

Atrial septal defect (ASD), a prevalent congenital heart defect, can affect patients at any age. Secundum ASDs affect primarily women with a percentage of 65–75%. On the other hand, sinus venosus and ostium primum ASDs show equal occurrence among both sexes. Many patients are asymptomatic and diagnosed on routine examination; however, symptomatic patients present with palpitations, fatigue, atrial fibrillation, shortness of breath, right-sided heart failure or recurrent respiratory infection.

Atrial septal defect is most common adult congenital lesion to be treated with percutaneous technique . The type of the defect based on its anatomy decides the mode of treatment of ASDs. While surgery is the choice of therapy for septum primum or sinus venosus, percutaneous closure is the recommended mode of therapy for managing septum secundum defects. Amplatzer device is frequently used in percutaneous closure. Closure of ASD is recommended in the following cases:
- Symptomatic patient
- Large size of the defect resulting in considerable left-to-right shunt.
- Qp (= pulmonary blood flow) to Qs (= systemic blood flow) ratio of >1.5.
- Considerable enlargement of right atrium and ventricles.

## Patent Foramen Ovale

Foramen ovale is an integral part of normal fetal circulation as it provides a link between the two atria. Normally, closure of the septae happens soon after birth and in most of them, they merge by 2 years. Nevertheless, a minute persisting defect called as patent foramen ovale (PFO) is present in above 35% of children, and in adult, the occurrence of PFO has been reported to be >27% as per autopsy studies.

Many studies have reported on the safety and efficacy of percutaneous PFO closure since the first report by Bridges et al. in 1992, and various equipment to manage PFO are still under different levels of making and commercialization. With either medical or surgical therapy, annual risk of recurrent cryptogenic stroke decreases to 2–4% and complete elimination of recurrence is not seen with either approach. Few small-scale researches have shown beneficial outcomes with PFO closure when compared to treatment with drugs in limiting recurrent events in cryptogenic stroke cases. Extensive endorsement of regular PFO closure is yet to take place.

## Ventricular Septal Defect

Ventricular septal defect (VSD) is an interventricular septal defect. Most of the VSDs are perimembranous. VSD's occur equally in both males and females. It is common in pediatric age group. Symptoms include infective endocarditis, recurrent respiratory infection, arrhythmias, pulmonary hypertension, aortic regurgitation, failure to thrive, and congestive heart failure (CHF).
Closure of VSD is done in symptomatic patients and (Qp:Qs >1.5).

For treatment, percutaneous closure is more challenging but has lower morbidity compared to surgical closure. Amplatzer occluders [membranous, muscular, and muscular postmyocardial infarction (MI)] are available for VSD closure.

In a potential research comprising 83 procedures in 75 different muscular VSD cases, the device could be positioned in about 86.7%. Mainly 10.7% (8/75) of the subjects reportedly encountered considerable complication related to device or procedure. The follow-up after 1 year presented a closure rate of almost 93%.

An additional nonrandomized potential research conducted on 100 subjects with the mean age of 9 years showed an outcome that VSD closure is a safe and effective management procedure in contrast to surgery.

## Patent Ductus Arteriosus

Ductus arteriosus is a vessel leading from bifurcation of pulmonary artery to aorta, just distal and opposite the origin of left subclavian artery. The ductus permits oxygenated blood to travel from the pulmonary artery into the aorta avoiding the lungs, which are not fully developed. Spontaneous closure of the ductus occurs in most children soon after birth; nonetheless, it continues to be evident in about 1 out of 2,000 births. Maternal rubella in first trimester predisposes to persistent ductus arteriosus. PDA is seen more commonly in females with ration of 2 to 3:1. In older patients it is even more frequently diagnosed in females.

Closure of patent ductus arteriosus (PDA) is done in symptomatic patients with left-to-right shunt.

Method of closure is transcatheter technique, in which an occlude is placed from either the pulmonary artery or the aorta. The Amplatzer Ductal Occluder is mostly used in closure in adult patients now-a-days.

## Left Atrial Appendage

Left atrial thrombi are associated with embolic stroke in patients with nonvalvular atrial fibrillation. In 90% of cases, the left atrial appendage (LAA) is the site of formation of thrombus and the source of embolism as per autopsy studies and echocardiography.

Watchman and the Amplatzer ACP devices are LAA occluder devices. A randomized trial was done in which the Watchman device versus anticoagulation were compared in 707 patients. The efficacy of percutaneous closure of the LAA with this device was equal to that of anticoagulation therapy.

## Left Ventricular Aneurysm

Left ventricular (LV) aneurysm is a critical condition that can form after a transmural MI. The consequence could be (CHF), thrombus formation, and ventricular arrhythmias or may prove fatal also. In left ventricular aneurysm, intervention aims at enhanced systolic function by rectifying the left ventricular structure so as to decrease tension on its walls and paradoxical movement.

Surgical therapy is the main choice of management to achieve left ventricular reduction/restoration. Percutaneous implantation of devices can also be performed; however, hardly few cases claim favorable percutaneous implantation of a device till now. A novel device (Parachute, Cardiokinetix), which is currently under study, has been especially developed for LV aneurysm.

## Valvular Heart Disease

### Mitral Stenosis

Inoue et al. in 1984, first described clinical application of percutaneous mitral balloon valvuloplasty (PTMV) in mitral stenosis (MS) which has become the treatment of choice. In contrast to rheumatic mitral stenosis, where there is a female predilection, congenital mitral stenosis is more common in males. Indications of PTMV are symptomatic patients (NYHA II-IV), isolated moderate to severe MS, mild MS with pulmonary hypertension. When performed on appropriately selected patients with favorable anatomy, acute and long-term results of PTMV are excellent.

## Mitral Regurgitation

Mitral regurgitation (MR) results from disease or abnormality of any one or more than five functional components of complex mitral valve apparatus, which include the mitral valve leaflets, annulus, chordae, papillary muscles, and ventricle. All the guidelines proposed by ACC/AHA aid the practitioner to improve the timing of surgery in acute MR patients. There is increased mortality in cases with severe MR regardless of symptoms.

Multiple devices are being innovated to manage MR; these are presently in various levels of progress for percutaneous treatment.

The edge-to-edge repair method (Alfieri stitch) is similar to a surgical technique. A Mitra-Clip is embedded through the trans-septal approach to approximate the anterior and posterior leaflets of the mitral valve, decrease the back flow opening, and reduce the acuteness of MR.

## Aortic Stenosis

For severe aortic stenosis, surgical treatment is gold standard, but patients who are high risk for surgery, less invasive measures, i.e., percutaneous aortic valve implantation is an effective alternative.

Alain Cribier initially did the valve implantation in 2002. Many important advances aim at simplifying the technique and decreasing the morbidity and mortality related to the procedure.

# HYPERTROPHIC OBSTRUCTIVE CARDIOMYOPATHY

Hypertrophic obstructive cardiomyopathy (HOCM) is a primary disorder marked by left ventricle hypertrophy. It is mostly familial or genetically determined condition that occurs in absence of causative hemodynamic factor such as hypertension, aortic valve disease or systemic infiltrative or storage disease. Incidence of HOCM is about 1 for 500 cases. About 25% of these cases report different levels of dynamic blockage of left ventricular outflow tract.

Less invasive treatments have been tried for HOCM which include prescribing drugs such as beta-blockers, verapamil or disopyramide and use of dual chamber pacemakers.

In patients with severe medically refractive symptoms surgical myectomy or alcohol septal ablation may be effective. It seems that both the choices of management offer similar hemodynamic and clinical outcomes; nevertheless, there is absence of random research that differentiates percutaneous and surgical septal ablation.

# OTHER STRUCTURAL HEART INTERVENTIONS

The percutaneous methods are increasingly being used in adult patients for the following:
- Pulmonary valve implantation
- Closure of sinus of Valsalva aneurysm rupture
- Treatment of vascular fistulae

# CHALLENGES

There are three basic challenges in the treatment of structural heart disease:
1. The function of imaging and preprocedural evaluation in the management of percutaneous technique in these diseases depends primarily on hemodynamic and fluoroscopic evaluation.

2. Patient and procedural volume. Many institutes may not do structural heart interventions, while few do for only one or some forms of structural heart disease.
3. Wide spectrum of variability in each structural heart disease.

## FUTURE DIRECTIONS

Structural heart diseases are frequently being treated by catheter-based techniques for almost a decade. However, it must be known that the occurrence of most structural heart diseases is usually quite less.

Potential patients who require structural heart interventions cannot be compared to those needing percutaneous therapy for coronary heart disease.

An optimization has to exist between the prospective advancements like catheterization and the cost-effectiveness of the treatment. In high surgical risk patients, less invasive alternatives are desired.

Due to the above-mentioned issues, it is clear that percutaneous therapy is evolving and will persistently amend the approach toward structural heart disease.

A combination of different new devices/methods, ideas, and skills of therapeutic strategies is essential in order to get the best results through a percutaneous approach.

## CONCLUSION

Last decade has witnessed increase in the number of structural cardiac interventions. As we evolve technically, there is a simultaneous evolution in imaging and device deployment techniques. Understanding the anatomical details of structural heart diseases is vital for success of interventions.

## SUGGESTED READING

1. Rubio-Alvarez V, Limon R, Soni J. Intracardiac valvulotomy by means of a catheter. Arch Inst Cardiol Mex. 1953;23:183-92.
2. Webb G, Gatzoulis MA. Atrial septal defects in the adult: recent progress and overview. Circulation. 2006;114(15):1645-53.
3. Mas JL, Zuber M. Recurrent cerebrovascular events in patients with patent foramen ovale, atrial septal aneurysm, or both and cryptogenic stroke or transient ischemic attack. French Study Group on Patent Foramen Ovale and Atrial Septal Aneurysm. Am Heart J. 1995;130: 1083-8.
4. Bridges ND, Hellenbrand W, Latson L, Filiano J, Newburger JW, Lock JE. Transcatheter closure of patent foramen ovale after presumed paradoxical embolism. Circulation. 1992;86:1902-8.
5. Windecker S, Wahl A, Nedeltchev K, Arnold M, Schwerzmann M, Seiler C, et al. Comparison of medical treatment with percutaneous closure of patent foramen ovale in patients with cryptogenic stroke. J Am Coll Cardiol. 2004;44:750-8.
6. Thanopoulos BV, Dardas PD, Karanasios E, Mezilis N. Transcatheter closure versus medical therapy of patent foramen ovale and cryptogenic stroke. Catheter Cardiovasc Interv. 2006;68:741-6.
7. Wechsler LR. PFO and stroke: What are the data? Cardiol Rev. 2008;16:53-7.
8. Steinberg DH, Pichard AD, Satler LF, Slack MC, Wunderlich N, Majunke N, et al. Patent foramen ovale closure: past, present and future. Expert Rev Cardiovasc Ther 2007;5:881–91.
9. Neumayer U, Stone S, Somerville J. Small ventricular septal defects in adults. Eur Heart J. 1998;19:1573-82.
10. Gabriel HM, Heger M, Innerhofer P, Zehetgruber M, Mundigler G, Wimmer M, et al. Long-term outcome of patients with ventricular septal defect considered not to require surgical closure during childhood. J Am Coll Cardiol. 2002;39:1066-71.

11. Hijazi ZM, Hakim F, Haweleh AA, Madani A, Tarawna W, Hiari A, et al. Catheter closure of perimembranous ventricular septal defects using the new Amplatzer membranous VSD occluder: initial clinical experience. Catheter Cardiovasc Interv. 2002;56(4):508-15.
12. Holzer R, Balzer D, Cao QL, Lock K, Hijazi ZM. Device closure of muscular ventricular septal defects using the Amplatzer muscular ventricular septal defect occluder: immediate and mid-term results of a U.S. registry. J Am Coll Cardiol. 2004;43(7):1257-63.
13. Holzer R, de Giovanni J, Walsh KP, Tometzki A, Goh T, Hakim F, et al. Transcatheter closure of perimembranous ventricular septal defects using the amplatzer membranous VSD occluder: immediate and midterm results of an international registry. Catheter Cardiovasc Interv. 2006;68:620-8.
14. Carlgren LE. The incidence of congenital heart disease in children born in Gothenburg 1941–1950. Br Heart J. 1959;21:40-50.
15. Mitchell SC, Korones SB, Berendes HW. Congenital heart disease in 56,109 births. Incidence and natural history. Circulation. 1971;43:323-32.
16. Pas D, Missault L, Hollanders G, Suys B, De Wolf D. Persistent ductus arteriosus in the adult: clinical features and experience with percutaneous closure. Acta Cardiol. 2002;57:275-8.
17. Portsmann W, Wierny L, Warnke H. Closure of persistent ductus arteriosus without thoracotomy. Ger Med Mon. 1967;12:259-61.
18. Masura J, Walsh KP, Thanopoulous B, Chan C, Bass J, Goussous Y, et al. Catheter closure of moderate-to large-sized patent ductus arteriosus using the new Amplatzer duct occluder: immediate and short-term results. J Am Coll Cardiol. 1998;31:878-82.
19. Bilkis AA, Alwi M, Hasri S, Haifa AL, Geetha K, Rehman MA, et al. The Amplatzer duct occluder: experience in 209 patients. J Am Coll Cardiol. 2001;37:258-61.
20. Pass RH, Hijazi Z, Hsu DT, Lewis V, Hellenbrand WE. Multicenter USA Amplatzer patent ductus arteriosus occlusion device trial: initial and one-year results. J Am Coll Cardiol 2004;44:513-9.
21. Blackshear JL, Odell JA. Appendage obliteration to reduce stroke in cardiac surgical patients with atrial fibrillation. Ann Thorac Surg. 1996;61:755-9.
22. Holmes DR, Reddy VY, Turi ZG, Doshi SK, Sievert H, Buchbinder M, et al. Percutaneous closure of the left atrial appendage versus warfarin therapy for prevention of stroke in patients with atrial fibrillation: a randomised non-inferiority trial. Lancet. 2009;374(9689):534-42.
23. Block PC, Burstein S, Casale PN, Kramer PH, Teirstein P, Williams DO, et al. Percutaneous left atrial appendage occlusion for patients in atrial fibrillation suboptimal for warfarin therapy: 5-year results of the PLAATO (Percutaneous Left Atrial Appendage Transcatheter Occlusion) Study. JACC Cardiovasc Interv. 2009;2:594-600.
24. Clift P, Thorne S, de Giovanni J. Percutaneous device closure of a pseudoaneurysm of the left ventricular wall. Heart. 2004;90:e62.
25. Harrison W, Ruygrok PN, Greaves S, Wijesinghe N, Charleson H, Wade C, et al. Percutaneous closure of left ventricular free wall rupture with associated false aneurysm to prevent cardioembolic stroke. Heart Lung Circ. 2008;17:250-3.
26. Chen YT, Kan MN, Chen JS, Lin WW, Chang MK, Hu WS, et al. Detection of prosthetic mitral valve leak: a comparative study using transesophageal echocardiography, transthoracic echocardiography, and auscultation. J Clin Ultrasound. 1990;18(7):557-61.
27. Linden BC, Schumacher CW, MacIver RH, Mrachek JP, Bianco RW. Paravalvular leaks around prosthetic valves implanted in the mitral position: technical refinements of the ovine model. J Heart Valve Dis. 2003;12(3):400-5.
28. Safi AM, Kwan T, Afflu E, Al Kamme A, Salciccioli L. Paravalvular regurgitation: a rare complication following valve replacement surgery. Angiology. 2000;51(6):479-87.
29. Shapira Y, Hirsch R, Kornowski R, Hasdai D, Assali A, Vaturi M, et al. Percutaneous closure of perivalvular leaks with Amplatzer occluders: feasibility, safety, and short-term results. J Heart Valve Dis. 2007;16(3):305-13.
30. Pate GE, Al Zubaidi A, Chandavimol M, Thompson CR, Munt BI, Webb JG. Percutaneous closure of prosthetic paravalvular leaks: case series and review. Catheter Cardiovasc Interv. 2006;68(4):528-33.
31. Crenshaw BS, Granger CB, Birnbaum Y, Pieper KS, Morris DC, Kleiman NS, et al. Risk factors, angiographic patterns, and outcomes in patients with ventricular septal defect complicating acute myocardial infarction. GUSTO-I (Global Utilization of Streptokinase and TPA for Occluded Coronary Arteries) Trial Investigators. Circulation. 2000;101:27-32.

## SECTION 1: Cardiology

32. Birnbaum Y, Fishbein MC, Blanche C, Siegel RJ. Ventricular septal rupture after acute myocardial infarction. N Engl J Med. 2002;347:1426-32.
33. Radford MJ, Johnson RA, Daggett WM Jr, Fallon JT, Buckley MJ, Gold HK, et al. Ventricular septal rupture: a review of clinical and physiologic features and an analysis of survival. Circulation. 1981;64:545-53.
34. Holzer R, Balzer D, Amin Z, Ruiz CE, Feinstein J, Bass J, et al. Transcatheter closure of postinfarction ventricular septal defects using the new Amplatzer muscular VSD occluder: results of a U.S. Registry. Catheter Cardiovasc Interv. 2004;61:196-201.
35. Thiele H, Kaulfersch C, Daehnert I, Schoenauer M, Eitel I, Borger M, et al. Immediate primary transcatheter closure of postinfarction ventricular septal defects. Eur Heart J. 2009;30:81-8.
36. Martinez MW, Mookadam F, Sun Y, Hagler DJ. Transcatheter closure of ischemic and post-traumatic ventricular septal ruptures. Catheter Cardiovasc Interv. 2007;69:403-7.
37. Inoue K, Owaki T, Nakamura T, Kitamura F, Miyamoto N. Clinical application of transvenous mitral commissurotomy by a new balloon catheter. J Thorac Cardiovasc Surg. 1984;87:394-402.
38. Ben Farhat M, Ayari M, Maatouk F, Betbout F, Gamra H, Jarra M, et al. Percutaneous balloon versus surgical closed and open mitral commissurotomy: seven-year follow-up results of a randomized trial. Circulation. 1998;97(3):245-50.
39. Palacios IF, Sanchez PL, Harrell LC, Weyman AE, Block PC. Which patients benefit from percutaneous mitral balloon valvuloplasty? Prevalvuloplasty and postvalvuloplasty variables that predict long-term outcome. Circulation. 2002;105:1465-71.
40. Bonow RO, Carabello BA, Kanu C, de Leon AC Jr, Faxon DP, Freed MD, et al. ACC/AHA 2006 guidelines for the management of patients with valvular heart disease: a report of the American College of Cardiology/American Heart Association Task Force on Practice Guidelines (writing committee to revise the 1998 Guidelines for the Management of Patients With Valvular Heart Disease): developed in collaboration with the Society of Cardiovascular Anesthesiologists: endorsed by the Society for Cardiovascular Angiography and Interventions and the Society of Thoracic Surgeons. Circulation. 2006;114:e84-231
41. Enriquez-Sarano M, Avierinos JF, Messika-Zeitoun D, Detaint D, Capps M, Nkomo V, et al. Quantitative determinants of the outcome of asymptomatic mitral regurgitation. N Engl J Med. 2005;352(9):875-83.
42. Masson JB, Webb JG. Percutaneous mitral annuloplasty. Coron Artery Dis. 2009;20(3):183-8.
43. Cribier A, Eltchaninoff H, Bash A, Borenstein N, Tron C, Bauer F, et al. Percutaneous transcatheter implantation of an asortic valve prosthesis for calcific aortic stenosis: first human case description. Circulation. 2002;106:3006-8.
44. Wigle ED, Rakowski H, Kimball BP, Williams WG. Hypertrophic cardiomyopathy. Clinical spectrum and treatment. Circulation. 1995;92(7):1680-92.
45. Maron BJ, McKenna WJ, Danielson GK, Kappenberger LJ, Kuhn HJ, Seidman CE, et al. American College of Cardiology/European Society of Cardiology clinical expert consensus document on hypertrophic cardiomyopathy. A report of the American College of Cardiology Foundation Task Force on Clinical Expert Consensus Documents and the European Society of Cardiology Committee for Practice Guidelines. J Am Coll Cardiol. 2003;42(9):1687-713.
46. Maron BJ, Maron MS, Wigle ED, Braunwald E. The 50-year history, controversy, and clinical implications of left ventricular outflow tract obstruction in hypertrophic cardiomyopathy from idiopathic hypertrophic subaortic stenosis to hypertrophic cardiomyopathy: from idiopathic hypertrophic subaortic stenosis to hypertrophic cardiomyopathy. J Am Coll Cardiol. 2009;54:191-200.
47. Qin JX, Shiota T, Lever HM, Kapadia SR, Sitges M, Rubin DN, et al. Outcome of patients with hypertrophic obstructive cardiomyopathy after percutaneous transluminal septal myocardial ablation and septal myectomy surgery. J Am Coll Cardiol. 2001;38:1994-2000.
48. Firoozi S, Elliott PM, Sharma S, Murday A, Brecker SJ, Hamid MS, et al. Septal myotomy-myectomy and transcoronary septal alcohol ablation in hypertrophic obstructive cardiomyopathy. A comparison of clinical, haemodynamic and exercise outcomes. Eur Heart J. 2002;23(20):1617-24.
49. Oosterhof T, Hazekamp MG, Mulder BJ. Opportunities in pulmonary valve replacement. Expert Rev Cardiovasc Ther. 2009;7:1117-22.
50. Zhao SH, Yan CW, Zhu XY, Li JJ, Xu NX, Jiang SL, et al. Transcatheter occlusion of the ruptured sinus of Valsalva aneurysm with an Amplatzer duct occluder. Int J Cardiol. 2008;129:81-5.
51. Girona J, Marti G, Betrian P, Gran F, Casaldaliga J. Percutaneous embolization of vascular fistulas using coils or Amplatzer vascular plugs. Rev Esp Cardiol. 2009;62:765-73.

# CHAPTER 7

# A to Z of Rheumatic Heart Disease in Women

*Arati Dave Lalchandani*

## ABSTRACT

Rheumatic heart disease (RHD) is caused by Group A Beta-hemolytic Streptococcal infection which initially causes acute rheumatic fever (RF) leading to chronic valvular heart disease known as RHD. Pregnancy and the peripartum period are accompanied by significant cardiocirculatory alterations which are responsible for pronounced clinical worsening in the women suffering from heart disease. The prevalent valvular abnormal condition that can affect pregnant women is rheumatic mitral stenosis (MS); the condition can probably be accompanied by other symptoms including pulmonary congestion, edema, and atrial arrhythmias during pregnancy period or immediately following delivery. The higher volume load and higher cardiac output during the pregnancy period result in elevated left atrial volume and pressure, increased pulmonary venous filling pressure dyspnea, and lower exercise tolerance. The elevation in the maternal heart rate causes lowering of the diastolic filling period thereby leading to enhanced left atrial pressure. Mortality may possibly occur in pregnant women who show very few symptoms, but the rate of occurrence is not even 1%. Women affected by RF and RHD, particularly the poorer community and those living in completely unhygienic situations, experience a greatly decreased life span and acutely morbid complications because of valvular heart disease and heart failure. Nevertheless, there are preventive measure easily available very soon and at a lower cost.

## INTRODUCTION

Rheumatic heart disease (RHD) is caused by Group A Beta-hemolytic Streptococcal infection which initially causes acute rheumatic fever (RF) leading to a chronic valvular heart disease known as RHD. It is the most commonly acquired heart disease in young people usually beginning in childhood as a streptococcal sore throat with migratory arthritis of typically knee and ankle joints which show complete recovery within a few days. However, sooner than later the heart gets involved as a pancarditis.

There is pericarditis which recovers without much effusion.

There is myocarditis which can result in heart failure.

There is endocarditis—valvulitis which may result in regurgitant valve lesions typically aortic and mitral regurgitation (MR) which may recover or progress to organic heart valve destruction leading to mitral stenosis (MS), MR, aortic stenosis, aortic regurgitation, rarely tricuspid stenosis, and tricuspid regurgitation. Other clinical features of acute RF are chorea, subcutaneous nodules, and erythema marginatum.

The epidemiology of RF and RHD shows a sharp contrast between the developed and the developing countries. In the developing countries, the prevalence of RHD may still be 0.1–4.58/1,000 (Lalchandani A et al. 2004) whereas, in developed countries it is <5/100,000 school children and even eradicated in most developed countries (Nova PK 1994).

## RHEUMATIC HEART DISEASE IN FEMALES

Aly A Hasav et al. (1997) in their study at Omany reported a prevalence rate of RHD of 8/10,000 with no significant difference between the sexes 9.07/1,000 for males and 7.28/1,000 for females. Ravisha MS et al. (2003) in their study of RF and RHD at Mumbai found a ratio of 1.15 to 1 male versus female.

## RHEUMATIC HEART DISEASE IN PREGNANCY

In a study (Mane SV, Gharpure VP, Merchant RH 1993) on pregnant cardiac patients at Bombay, 82.3% of patients were having a cardiac disease of rheumatic origin, while in 17.7% cases it was of nonrheumatic in origin. About 25.7% of cases of the rheumatic disease were graded as Class III or IV as per NYHA classification. Thilen U and Olssan SB in 1997 did a review of pregnancy with heart disease and found that about 1% of the happening pregnancies are associated with maternal heart disease thus causing significant effect on the maternal and fetal health. The 2002 research on RHD in pregnant women conducted by Lim ST presented acute RF and rheumatic valvular disease as one among the prevalent etiologies of heart diseases during pregnancy; MS being the most commonly affecting rheumatic valvular lesion. In case of the disease being mildly severe, it is recommended that the lesions be corrected and the patient stabilized before conception.

Naidu DP et al. in 2002 performed a study over maternal deaths due to pre-existing cardiac disease and found RHD in pregnancy is an uncommon problem in the developed world but reaches a significant prevalence in poor countries. RHD is cause of mortality in a significant proportion of patients due to heart disease with MS encountered frequently. Several preventable factors that precipitated decompensation were identified which might have contributed to the high mortality rates.

Bhatla N et al. in 2003 while evaluating the maternal and fetal outcomes of pregnancies complicated by cardiac disease in developing countries found that RHD in 88% with isolated MS was the predominant cardiac problem seen.

Asghar F et al. carried out a study in 2005 on a pregnant patients with heart disease and found that RHD (66%) with MS was predominant lesion.

Abdel Hady ES, El Shamy M et al. (2005) in their study found that RHD was predominant cardiac disease accounting for 89.5% in pregnant patients.

## CARDIOVASCULAR PHYSIOLOGY DURING PREGNANCY AND PUERPERIUM

Important changes in cardiac and circulatory system occur during pregnancy the hemodynamics of pre-existing cardiac pathology. These are discussed below:

*Blood volume:* Blood volume is considerably very high in pregnancy, beginning from the initiation as early as from the 6th week and increasing steeply till the mid-pregnancy period after which the increase happens gradually, at a controlled pace (Elkayam U et al. 1998) and averages 50%. This higher blood volume corresponds to placental mass, the weight of the products of conception, and maternal and neonatal weight.

*Cardiac output, stroke volume, and heart rate:* Cardiac output begins rising in pregnancy and is expected to become higher by about 50%. The increase happens by about the 5th week and the rise is steep till the 24th week after which it sustains and settles or increases mildly. Caval compression by the gravid uterus while in the third trimester reduces the venous return to the heart thereby the body position largely affecting the cardiac output. It is seen to increase in the lateral position and declines in the supine position. The increase in cardiac output seen during early pregnancy is contributed by an increase in the stroke volume, whereas, in the third trimester it is largely due to an accelerated heart rate. Heart rate peaks during the third trimester with an average increase of 10–20 beats per minute (Clapp JF III et al. 1997).

*Blood pressure and systemic vascular resistance*: Systemic arterial pressure begins to fall during the first trimester. This decline in systemic vascular resistance is related to reduced vascular tone, probably mediated by: (1) Increased levels of circulating prostaglandin and atrial natriuretic peptides as well as endothelial nitric oxide, (2) Increased heat production by the developing fetus, and (3) The creation of a low resistance circulation in the pregnant uterus. This fall in systemic arterial pressure reaches a nadir during mid-pregnancy and returns toward pregestational levels before term. There is widening of pulse pressure as the diastolic blood pressure decreases substantially more than systolic pressure.

*Hemodynamic changes during labor and delivery:* With the onset of labor the cardiac output rises substantially secondary to pain, uterine contractions, and anxiety. The oxygen consumption increased 3-fold. The cardiac output is gradually escalating while labor due to the elevation of stroke volume and heart rate. Contractions during labor cause a noticeable rise in systolic and diastolic blood pressure, which is significantly enhanced as the second stage sets in.

*Hemodynamic effects of cesarean section:* It is very common to perform a cesarean section instead of a normal vaginal delivery in those women suffering from cardiac disease so as to avert unforeseen hemodynamic changes. But, there are chances of significant hemodynamic alterations to occur in cesarean type of delivery as well, substantially associated with anesthesia and drugs. Additional factors including considerable blood loss, the relief of caval compression, extubation, and postoperative awakening probably enhance the hemodynamic alterations.

*Hemodynamic changes in postpartum*: Postpartum includes movement of uterine blood volume into circulation and relieving the caval compression. This sudden spurt in the total blood volume happens though there is blood loss while delivering. The rise in blood volume leads to large increase in ventricular filling pressure, stroke volume, and cardiac output thereby causing clinical deterioration (Hameed AP et al. 2001).

However, heart rate and cardiac output are back to normal or prelabor values within 1 hour postdelivery while it takes 24 hours for mean blood pressure and stroke volume values to return to normalcy following delivery. Hemodynamic alterations that happened during pregnancy period continue after delivery and slowly come back to prepregnancy values in about 12–24 weeks following delivery.

## SPECIFIC VALVULAR LESIONS DURING PREGNANCY

### Mitral Stenosis

Rheumatic MS can be regarded as the prevalent clinically notable valvular disorder in pregnant women. The hemodynamic changes during pregnancy include an elevated stroke volume and heart rate; these parameters probably cause reduced diastolic filling period, also enhancing left atrial pressure and increase in pulmonary capillary wedge pressures resulting in clinical deterioration. However, pregnant women with very limited symptoms present mortality rate of not even 1% (Clark S 1991). If the pregnant woman with MS present multiple symptoms, then the effects are acute. Indicators of severe maternal complications comprise a decreased mitral valve area (<1.5 cm$^2$) and an disorderly functional class before pregnancy (Barbosa PJ et al. 2000). Fetal mortality is more when the maternal functional capacity is declining; almost 30% fetal mortality is reported associated with NYHA Class IV disease in the mother.

Pregnant women with a history of surgical management with balloon mitral valvuloplasty (BMV) or valve surgery before conception manage pregnancy with limited consequences though they encountered acute symptoms (NYHA Class III or IV) or severe MS (a valve area of <1.0 cm$^2$) when compared to those women who received medical management. Pregnant women encountering acute symptoms have been reported to deliver normally with very good fetal results if successful percutaneous BMV was done during their second trimester.

Balloon mitral valvuloplasty is recommendedly done under transesophageal echocardiographic guidance, so as to avoid the susceptibility of the fetus to radiation exposure. Cardiac surgery in women experiencing severe MS reports identical consequences in both pregnant and nonpregnant women; however, about 10-30% pregnant women report fetal loss.

### Mitral Regurgitation

Mitral regurgitation causes decrease in systemic vascular resistance; this is the cause for the condition to be routinely well tolerated during pregnancy. Women who present with symptoms of MR are advised favorably for mitral valve surgery, especially repair, before planning a conception. The consequence of pregnancy can be associated significantly or can be predicted with left ventricular function. Left ventricular dysfunction combined with MR corresponds to enhanced susceptibility in pregnant women.

The occurrence of RHD is almost the same in both sexes; yet it is common for women to postpone help, seek delayed medical assistance and they have lesser approach to medical care, additional burden for women including pregnancy worsen their outcomes and form the cause of increased morbidity and mortality in them.

Global maternal mortality ratio has declined by 45% from 1990; however, in few areas as in South Africa, the maternal mortality has been increasing from since 2000. The history of previous cardiac disease is the key factor that is instrumental in maternal mortality especially in underdeveloped countries; RHD reportedly being the most prevalent reasons. A systematic review performed in South Africa documented that rheumatic MS, MR, and previous surgical mitral valve repair contributed to 71-84% of antenatal heart disease.

Rheumatic heart disease and pregnancy outcomes-the reports Registry Of Pregnancy And Cardiac Disease (ROPAC) estimated the massive prospective cohort of pregnant women n = 390 with RHD till today. It reiterates that women who encountered mild mitral valve disease with limited symptoms generally tolerated pregnancy in a better way. MS is not as tolerated as MR and is accompanied with enhanced chances of heart failure and the requirement for hospitalization. The probability of heart failure was 49.1% and 31.8% in severe and moderate MS, respectively. Reports suggest that women having mixed valve disease show acute adverse consequences similar to those suffering from moderate-to-severe regurgitation and stenosis and severe MS. Severe MS is an independent susceptibility factor resulting in for adverse fetal consequences like premature delivery and low birth weight. The global REMEDY study global RHD registry documented about 25% of adult women with RHD showed limited left ventricular function and 20% experienced antenatal heart failure. In a total of 56 patients who had mixed moderate-to-severe regurgitation and stenosis, about 9% showed antenatal atrial fibrillation, 48% of them reported increased pulmonary artery systolic pressure, 28% encountered heart failure while another 10%, of them had peripartum atrial fibrillation. Repair of rheumatic MR is the best option otherwise the choice between mechanical and bioprosthetic valve is difficult to make in young women of childbearing age. With mechanical valve replacement data from REMEDY registry showed increased maternal morbidity and mortality especially in lower-income countries due to difficulty in anticoagulation and monitoring of PT INR. Complications related to anticoagulation result in increased maternal and fetal mortality even beyond 1 week postpartum.

## CONCLUSION

Rheumatic fever and RHD in females especially those who are poor and live in deplorable hygienic conditions results in a very shortened life span and great morbidity due to valvular heart disease and heart failure. However, prevention is cheap readily available and cost-effective.

## SUGGESTED READING

1. Noah PK. Trends in acute rheumatic fever. The Barbados experience. J Trop Pediatr. 1994,40(2):94-6.
2. Hasab AA, Jaffar A, Riyani AM. RHD among Omani School Children. East Mediterr Health J. 1999;3(1):17-23.
3. Ravisha MS, Tullu MS, Kamat JR. Rheumatic fever and rheumatic heart disease: Clinical Profile of 550 cases in India. Arch Med Res. 2003;34(5):382-7.
4. Mane SV, Gharpure VP, Merchant RM. Maternal heart disease and perinatal outcome. Indian Pediatr. 1993;30(12):1407-11.
5. Thilen U, Olsson SB. Pregnancy and heart disease: a review. Eur J Obstet Gynecol Reprod Biol. 1997;75(1):43-50.
6. Lim ST. Rheumatic heart disease in pregnancy. Ann Acad Med Singapore. 2002;31:340-8.
7. Naidu DP, Desai DK, Moodley J. Maternal deaths due pre-existing cardiac disease. Cardiovas J S Afr. 2002;13(1):1326-31.
8. Bhatla N, Lal S, Bahera G, Kriplani A, Mittal S. Agarwal N, et al. Cardiac disease in pregnancy. Int J Gynaecol Obstet. 2003;82(2):153-9.
9. Asghar F, Kokab H. Evaluation of outcome of pregnancy complicated by heart disease. J Pak Med Assoc. 2005;55(10):416-9.
10. Abdel Hady ES, EL-Shamy M, El-Rifai AA, Goda H, Abdel-Samad A, Moussa S. Maternal and perinatal outcome of pregnancies complicating cardiac diseases. Int J Gynaecol Obstet. 2005;90(1):21-5.
11. Elkayam U, Gleicher N. Hemodynamic and cardiac function during normal pregnancy and puerperium. In: Elkayam U, Gleicher N (Eds.). Cardiac Problems in Pregnancy, 3rd edition. New York: Wiley–Liss;1998. pp. 3-20.
12. Clapp JF III, Capeless E. Cardiovascular function before, during and after the 1st and subsequent pregnancy. Am J Cardiol. 1997;80:1469-73.

13. Hameed AP, Karaalp IS, Tummala PP, Wani OR, Canetti M, Akhter MW, et al. The effect of valvular heart disease on maternal and fetal outcome in pregnancy. J Am Coll Cardiol. 2001;37:893.
14. Clark SL. Cardiac disease in pregnancy. Crit Care Clin. 1991;7:777-97.
15. Barbosa PJ, Lopes AA, Feitosa GS, Almeida RV, Silva RM, Brito JC, et al. Prognostic factors of rheumatic mitral stenosis during pregnancy and puerperium. Arq Bras Cardiol. 2000:75(3):215-24.
16. French CA, Poppas A. Rheumatic heart disease in pregnancy. Circulation. 2018;137:817-9.
17. Lalchandani AD. Azithromycin (ARMOR) must replace benzathine penicillin for treatment and prophylaxis of rheumatic fever. J Clin Exp Cardiolog.
18. Lalchandani AD. ARMOR Regime for management of rheumatic fever and rheumatic heart disease easy and painless. Journal of Internal Medicine of India. 2018;12(1).

# CHAPTER 8

# Congenital Heart Disease: Pertinent Issues in the Fair Sex

*Anita Saxena, Nidhi Bhim Sain*

## ABSTRACT

Unlike coronary artery disease, there are few studies reporting gender differences for congenital heart disease (CHD) in terms of outcomes. The influence of specific environmental factors, hormones, pregnancy, etc., is likely to further contribute toward sex differences in the prevalence, symptomatology, and prognosis of CHD. The fair sex has much higher risk of pulmonary hypertension (PH), idiopathic, or that associated with large left to right cardiac shunts. Also, the maternal mortality for pregnant females with PH is prohibitively high. Pregnancy is not advisable in women with other serious cardiac ailments such as severe symptomatic aortic stenosis, severe coarctation of aorta, etc. Moreover, underutilization of healthcare for girls as compared to boys has been reported in several studies requiring urgent corrective measures.

## INTRODUCTION

Congenital heart disease (CHD) is the most frequently occurring congenital disorder, responsible for 28% of all congenital birth defects. The birth prevalence of CHD is reported to be 8–12/1,000 live births. Considering a rate of 9/1,000, about 1.35 million babies are born with CHD each year globally. Gender differences are well described for most cardiovascular diseases, including coronary artery disease; the data for CHD is sparse and ill defined. It is believed that the total number of deaths due to cardiovascular disease is higher for women than for men. Sudden cardiac death due to myocardial infarction is also higher in females, perhaps due to nonspecific symptoms and the general belief that coronary artery disease is more common in men. While chest pain is more prominent in men, women can often have shortness of breath, weakness, fatigue, and bloating as prominent symptoms of coronary artery disease. This can lead to challenges in diagnosis. Women tend to have higher heart rates and longer QT intervals compared with men. Association of arrhythmias with menstrual cycles has been recognized in some studies.

Despite similar overall prevalence rate of CHD in males and females, certain CHDs are more common in females as compared to males. The outcomes and complications of CHD are also reported to be different between the two genders. For example, females develop pulmonary hypertension (PH) more frequently than males. These differences could be partly related to basic biological differences between females and males. Pregnancy, labor, and contraception are other factors influencing the clinical picture and outcomes in women with CHD. Some of the CHDs are associated with higher risk for the pregnant mothers. In this article, the important issues related to female patients with CHD are described in detail.

## BIOLOGICAL DIFFERENCES BETWEEN MEN AND WOMEN

Important sex-specific differences in the normal anatomy and physiology of the myocardium exist. It is essential to consider these differences in assessing the meaning of cardiac symptoms in men and women and in constructing strategies for the prevention and treatment of cardiovascular illnesses.

Some of these differences are due to real biological differences resulting from difference in gene expression from sex chromosome, and are called sex differences. Sex differences are frequently reproducible in animal models. On the other hand, differences arising out of sociocultural processes such as different behaviors of women and men; exposure to specific influences of the environment; different forms of nutrition, lifestyle, or stress; or attitudes toward treatments and prevention are called gender differences and are unique to humans. Both of these are very important in influencing human development.

A woman's heart is generally smaller than a man's heart. This is perhaps related to the smaller body surface area. Women have also been reported to have smaller coronary arteries. This may be responsible for higher complication rates following percutaneous revascularization for coronary artery disease. It is not clear, whether inflammatory mediated autoimmune factors play an important part in the pathogenesis of atherosclerosis in women, akin to its role in diseases such as systemic lupus erythematosus and thyroiditis.

The response of the myocardium to increased work (e.g., due to aortic stenosis) varies between males and females. Both increase myocardial muscle mass, but women respond by developing concentric hypertrophy of the left ventricle and men increase muscle mass more by left ventricular dilatation.

Women have a faster resting heart rate than men; this is not due to differences in autonomic tone but to a difference in exercise capacity between the sexes. Hormonal influences are also not likely to be responsible as faster heart rate is apparent in female children as young as 5 years of age.

The QTc interval is same in boys and girls till puberty, but is longer for postpubertal females. This difference again disappears by about 50 years of age. Longer QTc in females may be responsible for much higher incidence of Torsades de pointes type of arrhythmia in response to antiarrhythmic drugs.

## GENDER DIFFERENCES IN BIRTH PREVALENCE OF CONGENITAL HEART DISEASE

Most congenital cardiac lesions are equally distributed between males and females. However, slight female preponderance is seen in patients with atrial septal defect, patent ductus arteriosus (when not associated with congenital Rubella syndrome), and mitral valve prolapse. Left ventricular outflow tract obstructions have clear predilection for males (**Table 1**). Transposition of great arteries and double outlet left ventricle are also less common in females when compared with men. Other studies have shown male

**TABLE 1:** Prevalence of common congenital heart diseases in males and females.

| Congenital heart disease | Male to female ratio |
|---|---|
| Patent ductus arteriosus | 1/1.7 |
| Atrial septal defect | 1/1.5 |
| Ebstein anomaly | 1/1.6 |
| Pulmonary stenosis/atresia | 1/1.6 |
| Hypoplastic left heart syndrome | 2.6/1 |
| Aortic stenosis | 1.95/1 |
| Coarctation of aorta | 1.3/1 |
| Transposition of great arteries | 2.2/1 |
| Double outlet right ventricle | 2.7/1 |

dominance in univentricular hearts, Fallot's tetralogy, and total anomalous pulmonary venous drainage. In adulthood, CHD may be more common in men overall, due to the high prevalence of male-dominated aortic stenosis in this age group.

# GENDER DIFFERENCES IN OUTCOMES OF CONGENITAL HEART DISEASE

Evidence for gender differences in outcomes is scanty. Response to various drugs used in management of CHD is different in females. This may be due to lower body weight, higher proportion of body fat, lower glomerular filtration rate, and endogenous hormone levels in the postpubertal age group. In general, women's heart is more sensitive to drug side effects. Physician's perception of lower risk of heart disease in females leads to reduced attention to signs and symptoms in females. The females may be therefore treated suboptimally; this gender bias is labeled as "Yentl syndrome".

The mortality and outcomes of various CHD differ in women when compared with those in men. Factors affecting CHD outcomes related to gender are poorly understood. Some of these may be primarily related to biological differences and the type of CHD seen in women. However, a number of social factors including healthcare behavior and utilization of health facilities may be important determinants of gender-related outcomes of CHD. Pregnancy and contraception also influence outcomes, especially for significant CHDs, which are unrepaired. Most of the gender differences in relation to CHD have been reported in adults and from high-income countries. These may not be strictly applicable to low- and middle-income countries, where a large proportion of adults with CHD are unrepaired or unoperated and have native heart defect.

## Pulmonary Hypertension

The association of PH with female gender is well described and is difficult to explain. Idiopathic PH is much more common in females (2.5:1). A number of genetic mutations and polymorphisms have been found to be associated with idiopathic PH, none appear to be sex-linked. Female patients with CHD, associated with large left to right shunts, develop earlier and more aggressive pulmonary vascular obstructive disease (PVOD) secondary to PH. In the Dutch nationwide CONCOR national registry for adults with CHD, women were 33% more likely to present with PH.

Eisenmenger syndrome (reversal of shunt due to advanced PVOD), which is established for unknown reasons in childhood and puberty, may be equally common in males and females. However, a significant number of females with Eisenmenger syndrome die during pregnancy and labor as the maternal mortality is as high as 30–50%. In one study from Mayo Clinic, conducted on 4,000 adult patients with CHD presenting to clinic, isolated secundum atrial septal defect with Eisenmenger syndrome in women exceeds that in men by 28:1.

Without doubt, being female carries special risks when there is serious pulmonary vascular disease in comparison to males with comparable disease and defects. The female tendency to develop pulmonary vascular injury may relate to hormonal factors, but remains unproven. Pregnancy further precipitates pulmonary vascular disease, especially in women previously exposed to higher pulmonary artery pressures.

## Aortic Stenosis and Coarctation of Aorta

Aortic lesions are more common in males as compared to females. Women are better for the same degree of disease, even during pregnancy. Women with aortic aneurysm have a 33% lower risk of adverse outcomes (odds ratio 0.67), mainly due to smaller aorta in females and, therefore, lower rates of surgery. Fatal aortic rupture rate, though rare, is more common in females with a worse surgical outcome and higher mortality. This may be related to delayed surgery for females, as the same cut off values of aortic dimensions are used for females as for males when referring for surgery.

## Tetralogy of Fallot

This is the most common cyanotic CHD with a slight preponderance in males. No gender difference has been reported for surgical morbidity or mortality. However, sudden unexpected death following repair of tetralogy of Fallot was more common in males as compared to females. On the other hand, females with repaired Fallot had a higher incidence of death related to pulmonary vascular disease after palliative shunts. This was not encountered in males.

## Univentricular Hearts

Overall risk of major cardiovascular complications, including mortality, is higher in males as compared to females receiving a Fontan type of surgery. Male patients with Fontan type surgery are at an increased risk of progressive aortic dilatation and aortic regurgitation.

## Other Outcomes

Studies have shown lower risk of infective endocarditis in women. In a study of adults with CHD, 71% of patients with infective endocarditis were males. Better dental hygiene and lower rates of smoking and intravenous drug abuse may be responsible for lower rates of infective endocarditis in women.

The CONCOR registry showed that men were more likely to receive implantable cardioverter defibrillators (ICDs) even though the frequency of ventricular arrhythmia was similar in men and women. Women are more likely to refuse ICD implants than men. Also, more women are considered ineligible for these implants.

The longevity of homografts has been shown to be longer in women. Smoking and higher body mass index in males seem to be the risk factor for accelerated conduit degeneration. On the other hand, female gender is associated with more likelihood of conduit regurgitation of right ventricular to pulmonary artery conduit in those undergoing Ross operation.

## Mortality

Centers for Disease Control and Prevention demonstrated lower mortality rates in female children and adults with CHD when compared with male patients. This could result from difference in sex distribution of CHD at birth, milder lesions in female subjects born with CHD, or differences in mortality related to CHD surgical or medical outcomes. In another study from USA on sex differences in mortality in children undergoing CHD surgery, 54.7% of 33,848 hospitalizations for CHD surgery were males. Males were more likely to have CHD surgery in infancy, high-risk CHD surgery, and multiple CHD procedures than females. Females had more major noncardiac structural anomalies and more low-risk procedures. However, the adjusted risk of in-hospital death was higher in females (odds ratio 1.21, 95% confidence interval 1.08–1.36) on account of the subgroup with high-risk surgeries who were <1 year of age. Data for CHD in adults (18–45 years) also showed lower 30-day in-hospital mortality for nonpregnant females.

## PREGNANCY AND CONGENITAL HEART DISEASE: AN IMPORTANT ISSUE IN WOMEN

The influence of pregnancy on CHD cannot be undermined. Since CHD further adds to the hemodynamic burden of normal pregnancy, many women with CHD become symptomatic for the first time during pregnancy. In general, the risk and complications of pregnancy in a mother with CHD are directly proportional to the severity of underlying CHD and the symptom status of the patient. In a study from United Kingdom, 20% of cardiac deaths during pregnancy between the year 2000 and 2002 were secondary to CHD. In a retrospective study of 100 pregnancies with heart disease reported from India, maternal CHD was present in 36%. Cardiac complications were seen in 32% of 100 women, especially in those who were in functional New York Heart Association (NYHA) class III or IV at presentation.

A number of hemodynamic changes occur during pregnancy. These changes start in early first trimester and gradually increase to plateau at around 28 weeks of gestation. Further changes occur at the time of labor. Pregnancy can also result in formation of ascending aortic aneurysms or even dissection of aorta in predisposed women, e.g., women with Marfan syndrome, bicuspid aortic valve, or coarctation of aorta. Presence of cyanosis and PH in mother poses risk not only to mother but also to fetus.

Pregnancy is contraindicated in patients with severe PH. If PH is detected while pregnant, termination of pregnancy should be offered to these women. Conditions such as severe symptomatic aortic stenosis, Marfan syndrome with aortic dilatation of >45 mm, bicuspid aortic valve with aortic dilatation of >50 mm, and native severe coarctation of aorta are other conditions where pregnancy is associated with very high-risk to mother. Cyanotic CHD with maternal saturation of <85% is associated with higher complications and significant fetal wastage. Pregnancy should be discouraged in such patients, but if already pregnant, they should be advised to restrict physical activity and use compression stockings to prevent venous stasis (to avoid paradoxical embolism). Thromboprophylaxis with low-molecular weight heparin should be considered, if there are no contraindications.

Those with ideal Fontan circuit may tolerate pregnancy with slightly increased risk of atrial arrhythmias and worsening of functional class. Patients with presence of ventricular dysfunction and atrioventricular valve regurgitation are particularly vulnerable to complications.

Congenital heart diseases such as atrial septal defect, small-to-moderate ventricular septal defect or patent ductus arteriosus, mild or moderate pulmonary or aortic stenosis, mild or moderate degree of atrioventricular valve regurgitation are usually well tolerated during pregnancy and are not a contraindication to pregnancy.

Offspring complications, including mortality (4%), are more frequent in women with CHD than in the general population. Maternal and neonatal events are highly correlated. The risk of miscarriage is also increased in women with CHD. The risk of prematurity, low birth weight is related to severity of maternal heart disease. Fetal outcome is generally dependent on uteroplacental blood flow, which may be compromised in women with CHD. Neonatal survival rates are 87–89% in mothers with severe PH, a condition that has a very high-risk for the mother. Cyanosis poses a significant risk to the fetus, a live birth is unlikely, if arterial oxygen saturation is <85%. The fetal loss is <10%, if maternal arterial saturation is >90%. In mothers with a Fontan circulation, the offspring risk includes premature birth, small for gestational age, and fetal death in up to 50% of cases. Risk of neonatal events is increased in mothers with left heart obstruction, mechanical heart valve prosthesis, use of oral anticoagulants, and, most importantly, high maternal NYHA class.

*Recurrent risk of CHD in offspring*: On an average, the recurrent risk is about 3–5%. The risk is higher in mothers having left ventricular outflow tract obstruction. Similarly, CHDs associated with syndromes such as Noonan, 22q11 microdeletion, and Holt–Oram have almost 50% recurrence risk. Fetal risk is 50% in mothers with Marfan syndrome (**Table 2**).

Prepregnancy assessment should also include careful review of medications. Spironolactone and angiotensin-converting enzyme inhibitors such as enalapril, ramipril, and angiotensin receptor blockers (ARBs) are contraindicated during pregnancy. One may have to advise to stop these medicines, if considered safe for the mother, before conception.

**TABLE 2:** Risk of congenital heart disease (CHD) recurrence in the fetus.

| Type of CHD in mother | Risk of recurrence |
| --- | --- |
| Tetralogy of Fallot | 2.0–4.5 |
| Patent ductus arteriosus | 4.1 |
| Coarctation of aorta | 4.1–6.3 |
| Atrial septal defect | 4.6–11 |
| Pulmonary stenosis | 5.3–6.5 |
| Ventricular septal defect | 6.0–15.6 |
| Atrioventricular septal defect | 7.9–13.9 |
| Aortic stenosis | 8.0–13.9 |
| Marfan syndrome | 50 |
| 22q11 deletion syndrome | 50 |

Vaginal delivery, often with epidural analgesia is the preferred mode of delivery in majority of women with CHD. Assistance during second stage of labor can decrease the hemodynamic load of labor.

Patient with CHD should receive good care in peripartum period, as fatal events are known to occur during this period as in Eisenmenger syndrome. Cardiac rhythm and saturation should be monitored in high-risk patients. Good hydration must be maintained especially in patients with cyanotic CHD and for this, intravenous fluid administration may be necessary. Symptoms and signs of apparently minor problems must be taken seriously and managed promptly. Ergometrine is best avoided in third stage of labor. Patients should be monitored for at least 72 hours to 1 week postpartum. In low-risk cases, lactation may be encouraged.

## GENDER DIFFERENCES IN UTILIZATION OF HEALTHCARE

Gender disparity in access to healthcare is widely prevalent across the world. Girls and women from developing countries appear to be underinvestigated, underdiagnosed, and undertreated. Women are less likely to receive thrombolysis and angiography as compared to men for coronary artery disease even in developed world. However, gender inequality in utilization of healthcare systems for children has been evaluated only in a small number of studies. In a retrospective study from Hong Kong, significant gender disparity was found but was suggested to be due to male vulnerability to diseases. There was no gender disparity in acyanotic CHD-related admissions. Very few studies have reported gender disparity in utilization of healthcare for children with CHD.

Parental preference for male children exists in many sections of Indian society where girls with CHD are not provided with the same treatment opportunities as boys. Gender bias can be seen across a number of domains, including nutrition, immunization, school attendance, treatment facility utilization, and child mortality. In all these parameters, girls finish a poor second.

Given the almost equal overall prevalence of CHD in males and females, it is alarming that not only are relatively fewer girls brought to the tertiary centers for CHD but fewer still are having corrective procedures. In a large study of 15,066 children undergoing cardiac interventions in Narayana Hrudayalaya, Bangalore, boys predominated with a ratio of 1.4:1. Another study from a public hospital tertiary care center in North India provides even greater cause for concern by revealing that of the 405 consecutive pediatric referrals aged under 12 years, only 134 were girls. One year later, 70% of the boys but only 44% of the girls had undergone surgery. In the subgroup of girls, socioeconomic status was an important determinant of surgery status (p <0.002). The percentage of patients undergoing surgery progressively declined from the "upper" class (90%) to the "upper-lower" class (21.3%). Lower educational level of the head of the household was also associated with poorer compliance with surgery (p = 0.001). In a developing country such as India, the healthcare sources are limited and the vulnerable sections of the society are marginalized. Not only was the acceptance of surgical pediatric cardiac care lower among girls, but the access to such care was also lower. In a similar study published in 2015, where of 519 children with CHD or rheumatic heart disease who underwent an intervention, only 37.6% were girls (male to female ratio of 1.66:1). No difference was found between urban and rural populations in terms of gender disparity.

An analysis of the Indian national sample survey published in 2004 suggested that households facing financial constraints are more likely to spend their meagre resources on hospitalization of boys than girls. The results of a small study among parents of newborn infants also suggested that the perception of illness and spending on health were lower for newborn girls than boys. These socioeconomic factors are primarily responsible for underutilization of healthcare facilities by girl child and may be operative in some other countries also.

## CONCLUSION

It has long been recognized that total deaths from cardiovascular disease are higher in females as compared to males. However, most of such data is for coronary artery disease. Very few studies have reported on gender differences for CHDs in terms of outcomes. Women differ from men in normal anatomy and physiology of heart. In addition, the influence of specific environmental factors, hormones, pregnancy, etc., is likely to further contribute toward sex differences in the prevalence, symptomatology, and prognosis of CHD. In general, females have much higher risk of PH, idiopathic, or that associated with large left to right cardiac shunts. The prevalence of aortic diseases is lower in females. The maternal mortality for pregnant females with PH is prohibitively high. Women with other serious heart diseases such as severe symptomatic aortic stenosis and severe coarctation of aorta are also advised against getting pregnant. The recurrent risk in fetus is 3–5 times in women with CHD. A number of studies from India have shown inferior utilization of healthcare for girls as compared to boys. The reasons are both economic and social and require urgent corrective measures.

## SUGGESTED READING

1. Saxena A. Congenital heart disease in India: A status report. Indian Pediatr. 2018;55(12):1075-82.
2. Hoffman JIE. The global burden of congenital heart disease. Cardiovascular J Africa. 2013;24(4):141-45.
3. Hoffman JIE. Incidence of congenital heart disease: I. Postnatal incidence. Pediatr Cardiol. 1995;16(3):103-13.
4. Peterson ED, Lansky AJ, Kramer J, Anstrom K, Lanzilotta MJ. Effect of gender on the outcomes of contemporary percutaneous coronary intervention. Am J Cardiol. 2001;88(4):359-64.
5. Yarnoz MJ, Curtis AB. More reasons why men and women are not the same (gender differences in electrophysiology and arrhythmias). Am J Cardiol. 2008;101(9):1291-6.
6. Mercuroa G, Bassareoa PB, Mariuccib E, Deiddaa M, Zeddaa AM, Bonvicinib M. Sex differences in congenital heart defects and genetically induced arrhythmias. J Cardiovasc Med. 2014;15(12):855-63.
7. Warnes CA. Sex Differences in Congenital Heart Disease Should a Woman Be More Like a Man? Circulation. 2008;118:3-5.
8. Verheugt CL, Uiterwaal CSPM, van der Velde ET, Meijboom FJ, Pieper PG, Vliegen HW, et al. Gender and Outcome in Adult Congenital Heart Disease. Circulation. 2008;118(1):26-32.
9. Nollert GD, Däbritz SH, Schmoeckel M, Vicol C, Reichart B. Risk factors for sudden death after repair of tetralogy of Fallot. Ann Thorac Surg. 2003;76(6):1901-5.
10. Schilling C, Dalziel K, Nunn R, Du Plessis K, Shi WY, Celemajer D, et al. The epidemic population projections from the Australia and New Zealand Fontan Registry. Int J Cardiol. 2016;219:14-9.
11. Tutarel O, Alonso-Gonzalez R, Montanaro C, Schiff R, Uribarri A, Kempny A, et al. Infective endocarditis in adults with congenital heart disease remains a lethal disease. Heart. 2018;104(2):161-5.
12. D'Alto M, Budts W, Diller GP, Mulder B, Egidy Assenza G, Oreto L, et al. Does gender affect the prognosis and risk of complications in patients with congenital heart disease in the modern era? Int J Cardiol. 2019;290:156-61.
13. Gilboa SM, Salemi JL, Nembhard WN, Fixler DE, Correa A. Mortality resulting from congenital heart disease among children and adults in the United States, 1999 to 2006. Circulation. 2010;122(22):2254-63.
14. Marelli A, Gauvreau K, Landzberg M, Jenkins K. Sex differences in mortality in children undergoing congenital heart disease surgery: a United States population-based study. Circulation. 2010;122(11 Suppl):S234-40.

15. Lewis G, Drife JO. Why mothers die 2000-2002: The sixth report of confidential enquiries into maternal deaths in the United Kingdom. London: RCOG Press; 2004.
16. Subbaiah M, Sharma V, Kumar S, Rajeshwari S, Kothari SS, Roy KK, et al. Heart disease in pregnancy: cardiac and obstetric outcomes. Arch Gynecol Obstet. 2013;288(1):23-7.
17. Bedard E, Dimopoulos K, Gatzoulis MA. Has there been any progress made on pregnancy outcomes among women with pulmonary arterial hypertension? Eur Heart J. 2009;30(3):256-65.
18. Hon KL, Nelson EA. Gender disparity in paediatric hospital admissions. Ann Acad Med Singapore. 2006;35(12):882-8.
19. Kiran VS, Nath PP, Maheshwari S. Spectrum of paediatric cardiac diseases: a study of 15,066 children undergoing cardiac intervention at a tertiary care centre in India with special emphasis on gender. Cardiol Young. 2011;21(1):19-25.
20. Ramakrishnan S, Khera R, Jain S, Saxena A, Kailash S, Karthikeyan G, et al. Gender differences in the utilization of surgery for congenital heart disease in India. Heart. 2011;97(23):1920-5.
21. Chhabra ST, Masson S, Kaur T, Gupta R, Sharma S, Goyal A, et al. Gender bias in cardiovascular healthcare of a tertiary care centre of North India. Heart Asia. 2016;8(1):42-5.
22. Asfaw A, Lamanna F, Klasen S. Gender gap in parents' financing strategy for hospitalization of their children: evidence from India. Health Econ. 2010;19(3):265-79.
23. Willis JR, Kumar V, Mohanty S, Singh P, Singh V, Baqui AH, et al. Gender difference in perception and care seeking for illness of newborns in rural Uttar Pradesh, India. J Health Popul Nutr. 2009;27(1):62-71.

# CHAPTER 9

# Pregnancy and The Heart

*Asha Moorthy, Jain T Kallarakkal*

## ABSTRACT

A thorough knowledge of the underlying defect and hemodynamic changes during pregnancy is mandatory. Besides rheumatic heart disease, other ailments of major concern are congenital heart diseases and acquired diseases inclusive of myocardial infarction, aortic dissection, and various cardiomyopathies. Moreover, pregnancy is like a stress test for women. Pregnancy-induced hypertension, preeclampsia, eclampsia, gestational diabetes, maternoplacental syndrome, etc., can be harbinger of future cardiovascular events.

## INTRODUCTION

Pregnancy related complications, especially hypertensive disorders of pregnancy and pregnancy related diabetes mellitus are identified as risk factors for cardiovascular disease. These pregnancy related complications help in identifying women at risk for developing cardiovascular disease early. Women with pre-existing cardiovascular disease need proper care and prepregnancy evaluation.

## HEMODYNAMIC CHANGES

Rise in plasma volume begins in 6th week and approaches above 50% of baseline in second trimester. During this period, rise in red cell mass is slightly lesser leading to relative anemia. Baseline heart rate increases by 20% during this period. Uterine blood flow gradually increases, peripheral resistance slightly reduces and hence blood pressure decreases. Increase in venous pressure leads to pedal edema. Cardiac output reaches 30–50% by the end of second trimester. Mothers with pre-existing cardiac illness should be monitored closely during this period.

In labor, up to 500 mL of blood is released into the circulation with each contraction. Cardiac output may increase above 50% of baseline during the second stage and hence it should be reduced in patients with heart disease. Hemodynamic burden to the parturient is high with cesarean section as the blood loss approaches 800 mL. After delivery venous return abruptly increases, leading to pulmonary edema in a diseased heart. In most cases, a vaginal delivery is preferable. However, cesarean section is indicated in anticoagulated patients, patients with dilated unstable aorta, severe pulmonary hypertension, and severe aortic stenosis. Antibiotic prophylaxis should be considered in patients with cyanotic heart disease and prosthetic valves.

## EVALUATION OF THE PATIENT

Heart rate increases and usually pulse is bounding. Because of volume overload and reduced peripheral resistance, jugular pressure is elevated with brisk descents. Pedal edema may be present. Auscultation may reveal loud first sound, accentuation of second heart sound, presence of a third heart sound, and an ejection systolic murmur.

Chest X-ray is usually not recommended due to the radiation exposure to the fetus. Transthoracic echocardiogram is the investigation of choice. As the velocities increase across cardiac valves, careful assessment is required to differentiate it from organic disease. Transesophageal echo is not routinely performed, but may be carried out safely in suspected endocarditis. CT is not recommended and limited data is available on magnetic resonance imaging is probably safe but gadolinium should be avoided.

B type natriuretic peptide (BNP) is usually normal. Its elevation suggests an underlying cardiac disease. A normal BNP levels has a good negative predictive value for adverse cardiac events.

## HIGH-RISK PREGNANCIES

Patients with severe pulmonary hypertension, dilated cardiomyopathy with severe left ventricular systolic dysfunction, symptomatic obstructive lesions, cyanotic congenital heart diseases, Marfan's syndrome with aortic root dilatation >40 mm, and those with mechanic prosthetic valves are at high risk from pregnancy and if occurs may need to consider termination of pregnancy. Cardiac surgery should be avoided, as there is a high risk for fetal malformation or loss.

## ACYANOTIC CONGENITAL HEART DISEASE

Ostium secundum atrial septal defect is usually well tolerated unless complicated by pulmonary hypertension or atrial fibrillation. Special attention should be given to look for deep vein thrombosis as it can precipitate paradoxical embolism.

Patients with small ventricular septal defect (VSD) usually tolerate pregnancy well, large VSD with pulmonary hypertension is a high-risk pregnancy.

*Patent ductus arteriosus (PDA)*: Small PDA with normal pressures withstands pregnancy well. But a large ductus may precipitate LV failure and patients with pulmonary hypertension are at high risk.

*Congenital aortic stenosis*: Mild-to-moderate aortic stenosis is well tolerated. Patients with severe aortic stenosis should be counseled not to have pregnancy. They may require beta-blockers and an early delivery. Aorta should be looked into for dilatation. Patients with a root dilatation >40 mm and aortic dilatation >50 mm are at high-risk. Percutaneous aortic balloon valvuloplasty is considered safe for those with suitable valves.

*Coarctation of aorta*: Anti hypertension management, small-for-dates babies, and fetal loss are the major issues to be taken care. Percutaneous stenting of coarctation and surgical options may be considered for appropriate patients.

*Pulmonary stenosis*: Usually well tolerated in patients with sinus rhythm and those with right ventricular pressures <70% of systemic pressures. Patients with severe stenosis may be considered for balloon valvotomy.

## CYANOTIC HEART DISEASE

*Ebstein's anomaly*: Outcome depends on right ventricle size, its function, degree of tricuspid regurgitation, atrial communication, and presence of atrial arrhythmias.

*Congenitally corrected transposition*: These patients usually have a successful pregnancy if they have a normal LV systolic function. However, outcome may be compromised in presence of VSD, pulmonary stenosis, and complete heart block.

## VALVULAR HEART DISEASE

Stenotic lesions are less well tolerated than regurgitant lesions. Most commonly encountered lesions include bicuspid aortic valve and mitral stenosis which worsen during pregnancy due to increased cardiac output and heart rate. Beta-blockade and judicious use of diuretics are the cornerstones of therapy. Balloon valvotomy are reserved for patients who are refractory to medical therapy with favorable valve anatomy. Surgical intervention is reserved for patients who are not suitable for balloon valvotomy. Mild-to-moderate regurgitant lesions are fairly well tolerated during pregnancy.

## CARDIOMYOPATHIES

Peripartum cardiomyopathy is a form of idiopathic dilated cardiomyopathy diagnosed by otherwise unexplained left ventricular systolic dysfunction, confirmed echo-cardiographically, presenting during the last antepartum month or in the first five postpartum months. It usually manifests as heart failure, although arrhythmias and embolic events also occur. Many affected women will show improvement in functional status and ventricular function postpartum, but others may have persistent or progressive dysfunction.

## ARRHYTHMIAS

Arrhythmias in the form of premature atrial or ventricular beats are common in normal pregnancy, although sustained tachyarrhythmias have also been reported. In those with pre-existing arrhythmias, pregnancy may exacerbate their frequency or hemodynamic severity. Pharmacological treatment is usually reserved for patients with severe symptoms or when sustained episodes are poorly tolerated in the presence of ventricular hypertrophy, ventricular dysfunction or valvar obstruction. Sustained tachyarrhythmias such as atrial flutter or atrial fibrillation should be treated promptly, avoiding teratogenic antiarrhythmic drugs. Digoxin and blockers are antiarrhythmic drugs of choice in view of their known safety profiles.

## CORONARY ARTERY DISEASE

Coronary artery disease is not common in pregnancy, but may occur in the setting of diabetes mellitus and smoking. In acute coronary syndromes, coronary angiography followed by percutaneous coronary intervention may be considered. Thrombolysis is also preferred because of possibilities of coronary dissection.

## HYPERTENSION

Hypertensive pregnancy disorders cover a spectrum of conditions, including preeclampsia/eclampsia, gestational hypertension, chronic hypertension, and preeclampsia superimposed on chronic hypertension. Hypertensive pregnancy disorders represent the most significant complications of pregnancy and contribute significantly to maternal and perinatal morbidity and mortality. Most of the current recommendations for the treatment of these disorders are based on expert opinion and observational studies, with a lack of evidence from randomized controlled trials. The overall strategy in the treatment of hypertension in pregnancy is to prevent maternal cerebrovascular and cardiac complications, while preserving the uteroplacental and fetal circulation and limiting medication toxicity to the fetus.

## CONCLUSION

Pregnancy encompasses several hemodynamic changes which have a bearing in physiological as well as pathological state. The ailments of major concern are rheumatic heart disease (stenotic lesions especially worsening during pregnancy), congenital heart diseases and women may present with myocardial infarction (spontaneous coronary artery dissection), aortic dissection, and peripartum cardiomyopathy. Pregnancy, a stress test for women, can be harbinger of future cardiovascular events. Hence, women suffering from pregnancy-induced hypertension, preeclampsia, eclampsia, gestational diabetes, maternoplacental syndrome, etc., need close follow-up and monitoring.

## SUGGESTED READING

1. Siu SC, Sermer M, Harrison DA, Grigoriadis E, Liu G, Sorensen S, et al. Risk and predictors for pregnancy-related complications in women with heart disease. Circulation. 1997;96:2789-94.
2. Rossiter J, Repke J, Morales A, Murphy EA, Pyeritz RE. A prospective longitudinal evaluation of pregnancy in the Marfan syndrome. Am J Obstet Gynecol. 1995;173:1599-606.
3. Bonow RO, Carabello B, de Leon AC Jr, Edmunds LH Jr, Fedderly BJ, Freed MD, et al. Guidelines for the management of patients with valvular heart disease: executive summary. A report of the American College of Cardiology/American Heart Association task force on practice guidelines (committee on management of patients with valvular heart disease). Circulation. 1998;98:1949-84.
4. Presbitero P, Somerville J, Stone S, Aruta E, Spiegelhalter D, Rabajoli F. Pregnancy in cyanotic congenital heart disease. Outcome of mother and fetus. Circulation. 1994;89:2673-6.
5. Weiss BM, von Segesser LK, Alon E, Seifert B, Turina MI. Outcome of cardiovascular surgery and pregnancy: a systematic review of the period 1984-1996. Am J Obstet Gynecol. 1998;179:1643-53.

# CHAPTER 10

# Sudden Cardiac Arrest in Women with Migraine

*Poonam Malhotra*

## ABSTRACT

Migraine predisposes to the risk of ischemic heart disease, shock, and sudden cardiac death in women during third and fourth decades of life. Conditions with increased risk of platelet aggregation and atherosclerosis such as hypertension, hyperlipidemia, and preeclampsia are colinked to migraine. It is also seen that arrhythmias and patent foramen ovale are much more prevalent in patients with chronic migraine. We discuss the migraine in women and association to cardiovascular manifestations.

## INTRODUCTION

The pathophysiology of migration is linked to vascular system and the potential mechanisms involved are endovascular dysfunction, enhanced clotting tendency, increased incidence of vascular complications, genetic markers, depolarization from the brain, and inflammation. Most of the above mechanisms are also involved as risk factors in cardiac disease events, migraine can thus be considered as a prognostic marker for any cardiovascular disease (CVD). Few studies have shown increased risk of ischemic heart disease in young patients with migraine. This is important because if a link does exist between migraine and cardiac death, it will have great public health importance, especially in younger patients.

Migraine is a chronic and highly debilitating condition with symptoms such as weakness, numbness, visual changes, vertigo, and difficulty in speaking. Of its various subtypes, migraine with aura is the most common type. Migraine affects women three times more than men (**Fig. 1**).

## POTENTIAL BIOLOGICAL MECHANISMS INVOLVED IN MIGRAINE

There are several mechanisms that are said to be involved in migraine and are also implicated in increased risk of CVD, such as increased thrombogenic susceptibility, shared genetic markers, and inflammation processes. In women with migraine, hypertension, higher body mass index, and hypercholesterolemia are common. Migraine can also be considered as a systemic disorder affecting the endovascular system.

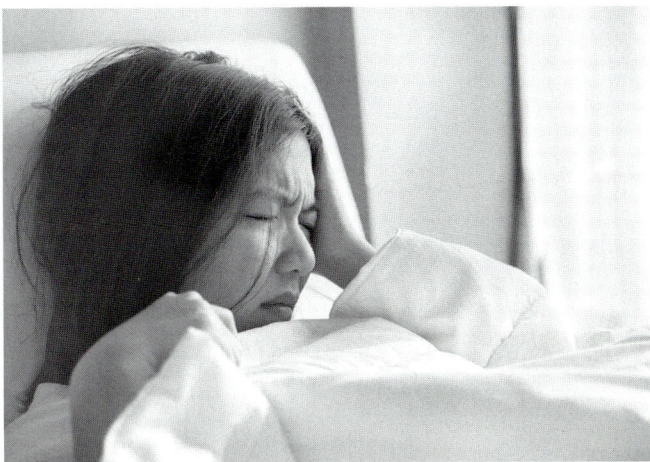

**FIG 1:** A migraine attack leaves us lonely and unable to join work.

## RISK FACTORS FOR MIGRAINE ARE MULTIFACTORIAL

In young men and women with sudden cardiac death, cardiac arrhythmias have been implicated during a migraine attack. It is seen that there is coronary artery bridging which leads to ischemia and infarction, ventricular tachycardia, and then sudden cardiac death. Brainstem area is seen with migraine, which gives rise to stroke and sudden cardiac death, may be even in sleep. High incidence of hypertension, hyperlipidemia, endothelial dysfunction, and increased platelet aggregation is also seen in preeclampsia pregnant patients, who also have migraine as a common symptom during pregnancy (**Fig. 2**).

In patients who suffer from migraine with aura, the underlying pathophysiological mechanism for the aura is thought to be related to cortical spreading depression, which is a slowly propagating wave of depolarization, resulting in the suppression of brain activity. Spreading depression is also the major mechanism for neuronal damage in the context of large vessel cerebrovascular occlusion (e.g., middle cerebral artery). A wave of depolarization markedly increases interstitial glutamate and paves the way for excitotoxic neuronal death. If brain perfusion is normal, astrocytes are able to take up glutamate rapid enough to prevent neuronal injury (**Fig. 2**).

Multiple meta-analyses have also confirmed these associations. In three meta-analyses that focused on ischemic stroke, the consistent finding was that migraine was associated with 2-fold increase in the adjusted risk of ischemic stroke (**Table 1**). This association was observed only in women but not in men.

## IMPLICATIONS OF FINDINGS FROM LITERATURE SO FAR

The mechanism behind association of migraine and increased risk of CVD and mortality has not been clearly identified. There is also a lack of enough data to prove that prevention and management of migraine can reduce this risk. The National Health and Nutrition Examination Survey and a randomized clinical trial observed that a statin and vitamin D, when used together, can reduce the burden of migraine. This is attributed to their anti-inflammatory action.

# SECTION 1: Cardiology

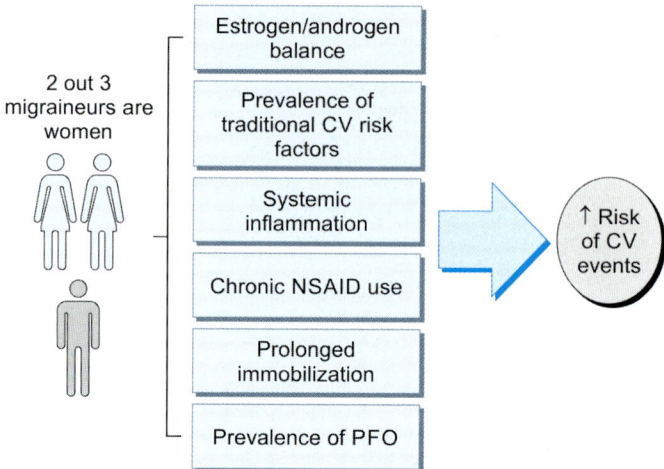

(CV: cardiovascular; NSAID: nonsteroidal anti-inflammatory drug; PFO: patent foramen ovale)

**FIG. 2:** Summary for the pathophysiological mechanisms involved in migraine.

**TABLE 1:** Cohort studies reporting the cardiovascular events for the subgroup of migraine with aura among women.

| Studies | Outcomes of migraine attacks | Adjusted hazard ratio [95% confidence interval (CI)] |
| --- | --- | --- |
| Kurth et al. | • Ischemic stroke<br>• Myocardial infarction<br>• Cardiac mortality | • 1.91 (1.17–3.10)<br>• 2.08 (1.30–3.31)<br>• 2.33 (1.21–4.51) |
| Peng et al. | • Ischemic stroke | • 1.60 (1.08–2.38) |
| Gudmundsson et al. | • All-cause mortality<br>• Cardiac mortality | • 1.21 (1.09–1.33)<br>• 1.18 (1.00–1.40) |

More research is needed to have a clear understanding of the mechanisms involved and hence developing management strategies.

**Is calcitonin gene-related peptide the "targeted therapy" in migraine treatment?**
Calcitonin gene-related peptide (CGRP) is a molecule that is synthesized in neurons (nerve cells in the brain and spinal cord). It acts as vasodilator and is involved in different pain pathways including that of migraine. Preventing it from getting activated at the initiation of the migraine, it can be used as an abortive treatment plan. Antagonists to CGRP can lead to reduction in migraine pain as shown in some studies, but their use has been associated with adverse effects like hepatotoxicity.

## MONOCLONAL ANTIBODIES: CUTTING-EDGE TRANSLATIONAL SCIENCE FOR MIGRAINE PROPHYLAXIS

They are easy to administer and have less frequent dosing (usually monthly). Moreover, trials have shown statistically significant decrease in number of days of migraine. These new molecules are being developed by four drug companies. Two versions are already in process of approval from the Food and Drug Administration (FDA).

## FUTURE OF MIGRAINE PROPHYLAXIS

The suitable candidates for migraine prophylaxis are those who do not respond to the standard treatment or have intolerable adverse effects such as hypotension and cognitive dysfunction. For them, CGRP monoclonal antibodies are safe and well tolerated.

The association of migraine frequency with risk of CVD is still unclear. Studies have shown that the risk of ischemic stroke increases with increase in migraine frequency among women with migraine with aura. However, there is paucity of data regarding association of migraine frequency with major ischemic vascular events, including myocardial infarction (MI).

Case reports have suggested a link between anticoagulant warfarin use and improvement in the symptoms of migraine headache, there could be a platelet-induced vasoconstrictor effect leading to migraine as well according to Nilsson B et al. The sue of lasmiditan is seen to improve acute symptoms of the migraine headache, but are all under trial phase.

## CONCLUSION

As observed in literature, migraine is a common, upcoming medical condition particularly in women. Venous thromboembolisms due to enhance immobilization are associated with migraine. All these cardiovascular events may lead to sudden death. A paradoxical emboli as an etiology could be coincidental or pathophysiological in patients with cryptogenic stroke. Estrogen rise could be a contributing factor as well, but no known treatment exists to lower cardiovascular risk in women with migraine. CGRP antagonists did show good results in aborting a migraine, but due to serious side effects like liver toxicity, its use was limited. A detailed cardiovascular history is essential to finalize treatment in migraine patients.

## SUGGESTED READING

1. Sacco S, Ornello R, Ripa P, Pistoia F, Carolei A. Migraine and hemorrhagic stroke: a meta-analysis. Stroke. 2013;44:3032-8.
2. Scher AI, Terwindt GM, Picavet HSJ, Verschuren WM, Ferrari MD, Launer LJ. Cardiovascular risk factors and migraine: the GEM population-based study. Neurology. 2005;64:614-20.
3. Wang YC, Lin CW, Ho YT, Huang YP, Pan SL. Increased risk of ischemic heart disease in young patients with migraine: a population-based, propensity score-matched, longitudinal follow-up study. Int J Cardiol. 2014;172:213-6.
4. Schürks M, Rist PM, Bigal ME, Buring JE, Lipton RB, Kurth T. Migraine and cardiovascular disease: systematic review and meta-analysis. BMJ. 2009;339:b3914.
5. Gudmundsson LS, Scher AI, Aspelund T, Eliasson JH, Johannsson M, Thorgeirsson G, et al. Migraine with aura and risk of cardiovascular and all-cause mortality in men and women: prospective cohort study. BMJ. 2010;341:c3966.
6. Monroe DJ. Sudden cardiac death in a young man with migraine associated arrhythmia. 2015;60:1633-6.
7. Lee ST, Chu K, Jung KH, Kim DH, Kim EH, Choe VN, et al. Decreased number and function of endothelial progenitor cells in patients with migraine. Neurology. 2008;70:1510-7.
8. Mawet J, Kurth T, Ayata C. Migraine and stroke: in search of shared mechanisms. Cephalalgia. 2015;35:165-81.

9. Kurth T, Schürks M, Logroscino G, Gaziano JM, Buring JE. Migraine, vascular risk, and cardiovascular events in women: prospective cohort study. BMJ. 2008;337:a636.
10. Liman TG, Bachelier-Walenta K, Neeb L, Rosinski J, Reuter U, Böhm M, et al. Circulating endothelial microparticles in female migraineurs with aura. Cephalalgia. 2015;35:88-94.
11. Mahmoud AN, Mentias A, Elgendy AY, Qazi A, Barakat AF, Saad M, et al. Migraine and the risk of cardiovascular and cerebrovascular events: a meta-analysis of 16 cohort studies including 1,152,407 subjects. BMJ Open. 2018;8:e020498.
12. Dreier JP, Reiffurth C. The stroke-migraine depolarization continuum. Neuron. 2015;86:902-22.
13. Peng KP, Chen YT, Fuh JL, Tang CH, Wang SJ. Migraine and incidence of ischemic stroke: A nationwide population-based study. Cephalalgia. 2017;37(4):327-35.
14. Spector JT, Kahn SR, Jones MR, Jayakumar M, Dalal D, Nazarian S. Migraine headache and ischemic stroke risk: an updated meta-analysis. Am J Med. 2010;123:612-24.
15. Burch RC, Loder S, Loder E, Smitherman TA. The prevalence and burden of migraine and severe headache in the United States: updated statistics from government health surveillance studies. Headache. 2015;55:21-34.
16. Longoni M, Ferrarese C. Inflammation and excitotoxicity: role in migraine pathogenesis. Neurol Sci. 2006;27:S107-10.
17. Bigal ME, Kurth T, Santanello N, Buse D, Golden W, Robbins M, et al. Migraine and cardiovascular disease: a population-based study. Neurology. 2010;74:628-35.
18. Buettner C, Burstein R. Association of statin use and risk for severe headache or migraine by serum vitamin D status: a cross-sectional population-based study. Cephalalgia. 2015;35:757-66.
19. Tietjen GE, Al-Qasmi MM, Athanas K, Utley C, Herial NA. Altered hemostasis in migraineurs studied with a dynamic flow system. Thromb Res. 2007;119:217-22.
20. Malik R, Freilinger T, Winsvold BS, Anttila V, Heiden JV, Traylor M, et al. Shared genetic basis for migraine and ischemic stroke: A genome-wide analysis of common variants. Neurology. 2015;84:2132-45.
21. Longoni M, Ferrarese C. Inflammation and excitotoxicity: role in migraine pathogenesis. Neurol Sci. 2006;27:S107-10.
22. Nilsson B, Back V, Wei R, Plane F, Jurasz P, Bungard TJ. Potential Antimigraine Effects of Warfarin: An Exploration of Biological Mechanism with Survey of Patients. TH Open. 2019;3:e180-9.
23. Shapiro RE, Hochstetler HM, Dennehy EB, Khanna R, Doty EG, Berg PH, et al. Lasmiditan for acute treatment of migraine in patients with cardiovascular risk factors: post-hoc analysis of pooled results from 2 randomized, double-blind, placebo controlled, phase 3 trials. J Headache Pain. 2019;20:90.
24. Elgendy IY, Nadeau SE, Merz CNB, Pepine CJ, American College of Cardiology Cardiovascular Disease in Women Committee. Migraine Headache: An Under-Appreciated Risk Factor for Cardiovascular Disease in Women. J Am Heart Assoc. 2019;8:e014546.

# SECTION 2

# Endocrinology

**SECTION EDITOR**
Gagan Priya

# CHAPTER 1

# Diabetes, Women, and Pregnancy

*Belinda George, Ankia Coetzee*

## ABSTRACT

As we witness an alarming rise of obesity and type 2 diabetes mellitus (T2DM) in the younger generation, the incidence of pregnant women with diabetes is rapidly increasing over time. It is imperative that those patients with pre-existing diabetes be identified early, screened for complications, managed with appropriate drugs, and we ensure that glycemic control is excellent prior to conception. It is equally important to identify patients who develop diabetes during the course of pregnancy. A combination of lifestyle measures along with insulin and close glucose monitoring is the most preferred strategy for optimal glycemic management. Care for such women should extend from the beginning of reproductive age group to preconception care, management during pregnancy, and continued care in the postpartum period and thereafter.

## INTRODUCTION

The alarming rate at which diabetes and obesity is affecting our young population will translate into higher number of pregnant women presenting with pre-existing diabetes mellitus (DM) as well as gestational diabetes mellitus (GDM). The estimates provided by the International Diabetes Federation (IDF) suggest that diabetes affects around 415 million people across the world and this number is projected to further increase to 642 million people by the year 2040. The estimates also suggest an equally high burden of pre-diabetes, affecting approximately 318 million people; and is likely to increase to around 481 million people by the year 2040.

In any given population, the prevalence of hyperglycemia in pregnancy (HIP) parallels the occurrence of overweight, obesity, pre-diabetes, and type 2 diabetes mellitus (T2DM) in that population. Data collected by the World Health Organization (WHO) in 2014 revealed that more than half of the world's population is either obese (13%) or overweight (39%), and this estimate included 42 million pregnant women.

Data obtained from several countries across the world including the USA, UK, Scotland, and Sweden demonstrate a clear increase in the percentage of cases with DM complicating pregnancy over the past two decades, largely driven by increasing prevalence of both GDM and T2DM in the younger age group. A study by Sheshaiah et al. from South India reported a prevalence of 18.9% for HIP (16.3% were GDM and 2.6% were pre-existing or newly diagnosed overt diabetes in pregnancy), with increasing age and body mass index (BMI) emerging as independent risk factors.

Globally, the estimates by IDF suggest that 1 in 6 live births (16.8%) occur in women with some form of HIP, 2.5% driven by overt diabetes, and the remaining 14.3% (1 in 7 pregnancies) by GDM. Bearing in mind that the exposure to hyperglycemia in utero plays a central role in the self-perpetuating nature of diabetes by metabolic imprinting, the detection of any degree of HIP offers an opportunity to stop the "diabesity" cycle.

## CLASSIFICATION OF HYPERGLYCEMIA IN PREGNANCY

The definition and diagnostic criteria for pregnancy with diabetes have been revised over the decades and significant heterogeneity exists among various guidelines. The International Association of Diabetes and Pregnancy Study Groups (IADPSG) evaluated the available evidence and put forth new criteria based on the level of maternal glucose associated with adverse pregnancy outcomes. The 2013 WHO guidelines on pregnancy has clearly defined various categories of dysglycemia that may be encountered during pregnancy, as depicted in **Flowchart 1**. Hyperglycemia in pregnancy can be divided as diabetes predating the current pregnancy (type 1, type 2 or other forms of DM) and hyperglycemia first detected in pregnancy (HFDP). Hyperglycemia first detected in pregnancy is further classified as diabetes in pregnancy (DIP) or GDM, based on the degree of hyperglycemia at diagnosis, as outlined in **Table 1**. GDM is diagnosed using the IADPSG criteria using any one of three cut off values: Fasting plasma glucose (FPG) ≥92 mg/dL (5.1 mmol/L); 1-hour value post 75 g glucose ≥180 mg/dL (10.5 mmol/L) and 2-hour value post 75 g glucose ≥153 mg/dL (8.5 mmol/L). If the plasma glucose values exceed the threshold for the diagnosis of diabetes that is used outside of pregnancy; i.e.,

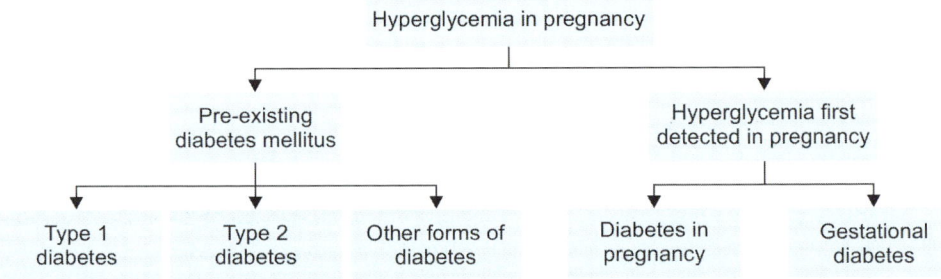

**FLOWCHART 1:** Classification of hyperglycemia in pregnancy.

**TABLE 1:** Diagnostic criteria for gestational diabetes mellitus and diabetes in pregnancy.

|  | Overt diabetes mellitus | Gestational diabetes mellitus |
| --- | --- | --- |
| Fasting plasma glucose (mg/dL) | ≥126 | ≥92 |
| 1-h post 75 g glucose plasma glucose (mg/dL) |  | ≥180 |
| 2-h post 75 g glucose plasma glucose (mg/dL) | ≥200 | ≥153 |
| Random plasma glucose (mg/dL) | ≥200 with symptoms |  |
| HbA1c (%) | ≥6.5 |  |

(HbA1c: glycosylated hemoglobin)

FPG ≥126 mg/dL (7 mmol/L), 2-hour post-glucose value ≥200 mg/dL (11.1 mmol/L), random plasma glucose ≥200 mg/dL with symptoms or glycosylated hemoglobin (HbA1c) ≥6.5%, a diagnosis of overt diabetes or DIP is made.

Depending on their clinical phenotype, women with overt DM or DIP may be classified as probable type 1 diabetes mellitus (T1DM) (presence of ketoacidosis or other features), T2DM (features of insulin resistance) or rarely, maturity onset diabetes of the young (MODY). MODY is a subgroup of diabetes caused by single gene defects and accounts for <5% of all cases of diabetes. It is often misdiagnosed due to lack of awareness and low index of suspicion; also, the clinical phenotype may share considerable similarities with T1DM or T2DM. One study from India reported that 18% of women with HIP tested positive for MODY on selective genetic screening of women with dominant family history of diabetes.

In resource-limited environment, optimal screening and management of non-communicable diseases such as T2DM rarely occurs in the general population. In these settings, universal screening for GDM is ideal and should be implemented at all antenatal clinics. Thus, hyperglycemia is often first detected in pregnancy and glucose abnormalities first detected in pregnancy, thus include a wide spectrum ranging from mild to overt hyperglycemia.

## PATHOPHYSIOLOGY OF HYPERGLYCEMIA IN PREGNANCY

Many profound physiological changes occur in pregnancy in all organ systems in order to best accommodate and ensure sustainability of the fetoplacental unit. The metabolism of a pregnant mother is modified to ensure optimal and continued nutrient delivery to the growing fetus.

### Early Pregnancy

Early pregnancy is characterized by an anabolic phase, wherein the mother accumulates and stores energy as adipose tissue. This phase is facilitated by an increase in appetite and nutrient intake, increased triglyceride synthesis and lipogenesis. This phase is mediated by an increase in both insulin secretion and insulin sensitivity early in pregnancy, followed by progressive increase in insulin resistance in later half. The factors regulating increased insulin secretion and beta cell hyperplasia are not well known. It is postulated that one of the mediators may be the growth factor, human placental lactogen (HPL). Insulin levels are higher both in the fasting and postprandial states in normal pregnancy and FPG concentrations are lower as a result. This lower physiological blood glucose is due to increased storage of glucose as glycogen, increased tissue utilization of glucose, and decreased gluconeogenesis in early pregnancy.

### Late Pregnancy

The latter half of pregnancy is often described as a catabolic phase, during which there occurs increased hepatic gluconeogenesis, adipose tissue lipolysis, and ketogenesis. These metabolic adaptations ensure an uninterrupted supply of nutrients, primarily glucose, to the growing fetus. One of the key factors mediating these changes in the mother is a physiological rise in insulin resistance. Maternal insulin resistance is a normal phenomenon that begins in the second trimester and peaks in the third. It results from increased secretion of placental growth hormone, corticotropin-releasing hormone (CRH) which drives the release of cortisol, human chorionic somatotropin (HCS), and

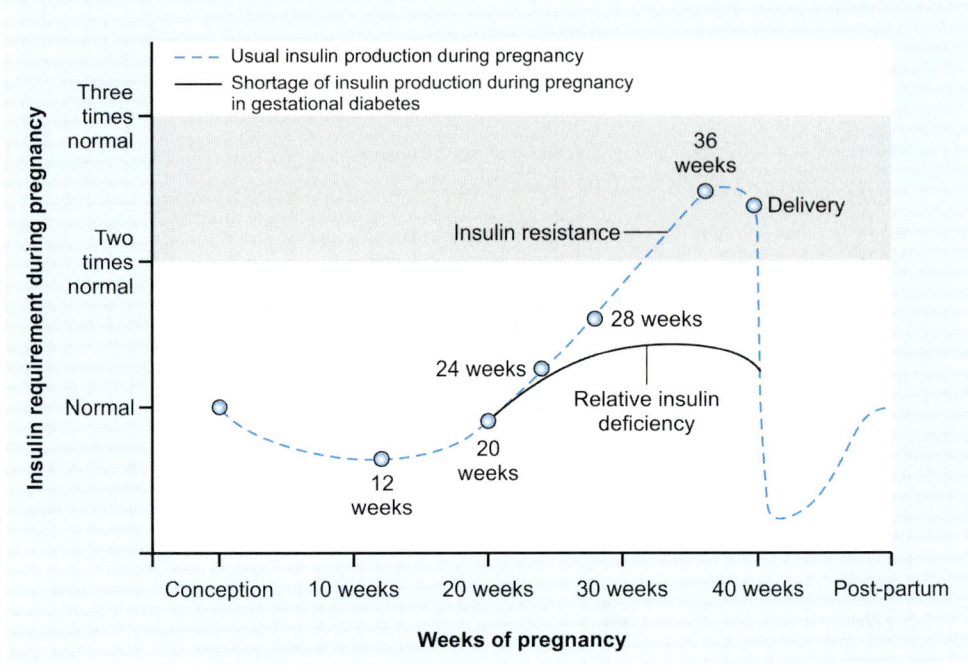

**FIG. 1:** Pathogenesis of gestational diabetes mellitus.

progesterone from the placenta. Maternal insulin resistance aims to reserve and direct glucose transplacentally toward the growing fetus. The fasted state is one of accelerated starvation in which alternative fuels such as lipids are made available to the mother, while glucose is reserved for the fetus. Due to these reasons, maternal glucose homeostasis shows important differences from the nonpregnant state. This gives rise to transient maternal hyperglycemia after meals due to insulin resistance and transient hypoglycemia in the fasting state due to the continuous fetal shunting of glucose. The mother's β-cells, when normal, are able to compensate for the insulin resistant state and GDM occurs only when a woman's pancreatic function is not sufficient to overcome or to compensate for the insulin resistance, as depicted in **Figure 1**.

## After Delivery

The pregnancy-associated insulin resistance rapidly decreases during labor, since the production of HCS, which has a short half-life, is terminated with the delivery of the placenta. It is therefore implied that in GDM, by removing the factors that create the insulin resistant state in the mother, she should return to a normoglycemic state shortly after delivery pregnancy if it is, in fact, true GDM. Early postpartum screening can, therefore, be indicative of prediabetes or overt diabetes which manifests in pregnancy due to the demand on the β-cells brought about by the increase in insulin resistance. Early postpartum screening may therefore identify women with a particularly high-risk of persistent DM.

In patients with DM, especially type 1, this adaptation of carbohydrate and lipid metabolism is abnormal due to deficiency of insulin, which can lead to uncontrolled glycemia, ketoacidosis, and death. The increase in insulin dose necessary in pregnant women with T1DM required to match the needs of increased caloric intake, increasing adiposity, decreasing physical activity, and increasing levels of counter-regulatory hormones can be as high as 3-fold toward the third trimester.

## ADVERSE OUTCOMES ASSOCIATED WITH DIABETES IN PREGNANCY

Overt diabetes in pregnancy is associated with adverse outcomes for both the mother and the fetus, and may impact future pregnancies as well. It is strongly associated with an increased risk of congenital anomalies as early development occurs in an unfavorable environment for embryonic and fetoplacental growth. Fetal structural defects due to maternal pregestational diabetes, enlisted in **Table 2**, are three to four times higher as compared to nondiabetic pregnancies. These include congenital heart defects (atrial or ventricular septal defect, patent ductus arteriosus, truncus arteriosus, etc.), central nervous system (anencephaly, encephalocele, spina bifida, cleft lip/palate, etc.), musculoskeletal (caudal regression syndrome), and genitourinary defects (omphalocele, bilateral renal agenesis, etc.,) among others. The risk of birth defects is proportional to the severity of maternal hyperglycemia. This calls for a need for strict glycemic control in the periconceptional period.

Maternal hyperglycemia at any time during the gestational period increases the risk of adverse fetal and maternal outcomes, as summarized in **Table 3**. Glucose is transported freely across the placenta by facilitated diffusion; in the presence of maternal hyperglycemia

**TABLE 2:** Structural birth defects caused by uncontrolled maternal hyperglycemia in early pregnancy in women with pregestational diabetes.

| Organ system | Birth anomaly |
|---|---|
| Cardiovascular | • Transposition of great vessels |
| | • Patent ductus arteriosus |
| | • Atrial or ventricular septal defects |
| | • Coarctation of aorta |
| | • Dextrocardia |
| | • Single ventricle/hypoplastic right heart |
| | • Pulmonary hypoplasia |
| Central nervous system | • Neural tube defects such as anencephaly, meningomyelocele |
| | • Hydranencephaly |
| | • Holoprosencephaly |
| | • Midline facial defects (cleft lip/palate) |
| | • Microtia/anotia |
| Musculoskeletal system | • Caudal regression syndrome |
| | • Sacral agenesis with hypoplastic pelvis |
| | • Femoral hypoplasia |
| | • Clubfoot |
| Genitourinary system | • Renal agenesis |
| | • Hydronephrosis |
| | • Ureteral duplication |
| Gastrointestinal system | • Omphalocele |
| | • Duodenal atresia |
| | • Anorectal atresia |

**TABLE 3:** Adverse maternal and fetal outcomes associated with hyperglycemia in pregnancy.

| Maternal complications | Fetal and neonatal complications |
|---|---|
| • Polyhydramnios | • Congenital birth defects |
| • Preterm labor | • Macrosomia/large-for-gestational age |
| • Pregnancy-induced hypertension/ preeclampsia | • Birth injury |
| • HELLP syndrome | • Neonatal hypoglycemia |
| • Cesarean section | • Neonatal hyperbilirubinemia |
| • Perineal injuries | • Polycythemia |
| • Hypoglycemia | • Hypocalcemia |
| • Increased insulin requirements | • Respiratory distress |
| • Infections: Urinary tract infection | • Intrauterine growth restriction |
| • Diabetic ketoacidosis | • Preterm delivery |
| • Worsening of diabetic nephropathy or retinopathy | • Long-term risk of obesity and cardiometabolic disease |
| • Long-term risk of overt diabetes and cardiovascular disease | |

(HELLP: hemolysis, elevated liver enzymes, and low platelet count)

large amounts of glucose reach the fetus which leads to fetal hyperinsulinemia that causes fetal overgrowth and/or macrosomia, stillbirth, and preterm delivery. Macrosomia occurring in children of mothers with diabetes is classically dysmorphic with a greater growth of shoulders and abdomen in relation to head which increases the risk of several obstetric complications, such as cesarean section, shoulder dystocia, perineal lacerations, and postpartum hemorrhage. Hypoglycemia is the most common neonatal complication that occurs in diabetic pregnancies. It can be asymptomatic or be accompanied by lethargy, agitation, and even convulsions.

Mothers with pregestational or unknown overt diabetes first diagnosed in pregnancy are at risk of progression of microvascular complications during pregnancy. Therefore, they should be screened for possible diabetes-related complications such as retinopathy and nephropathy in the index pregnancy. If present, it has major implications for the pregnancy and needs to be addressed promptly and appropriately. Other maternal complications during pregnancy include gestational hypertension, pregnancy-induced hypertension, hemolysis, elevated liver enzymes and low platelets (HELLP) syndrome, and worsening of any degree of a pre-existing renal insufficiency and retinopathy. To improve the outcome of the pregnancy, overt diabetes in pregnancy should be detected as early as possible in order to provide an adequate opportunity to implement intervention strategies.

The adverse perinatal outcomes associated with diabetes in pregnancy shows a linear and continuous relationship with plasma glucose values as demonstrated in the HAPO (Hyperglycemia and Adverse Pregnancy Outcome) study. Importantly, the risk for adverse outcome was without a clear inflection point. The degree of hyperglycemia, the duration of exposure to elevated plasma glucose values, and the onset of exposure in the course of pregnancy all play significant role in contributing to these adverse outcomes.

Early exposure overlapping with placentation and organogenesis is associated with more severe and long-lasting effects that extend into the adult life of the offspring. Undiagnosed pre-existing diabetes at the time of conception transmits the worst prognosis with high rates of miscarriages and congenital malformations. Similarly, outcomes associated with pre-existing diabetes are slightly worse in comparison with gestational-onset diabetes due to the duration of exposure. Pre-existing diabetes may cause either macrosomia or intrauterine growth retardation (IUGR). Exposure to elevated plasma glucose early on in the pregnancy may prime the fetal β-cells and lead to increased β-cell mass that can contribute to persistent fetal hyperinsulinemia even if the glycemic control is appropriate later in pregnancy. On the contrary, pre-existing diabetes can lead to IUGR through its effect on placental development. Hence, diabetes may be associated with both small for gestational age (SGA) or large for gestational age (LGA) babies in approximately 20% and 30% of pregnancies, respectively.

## PREPREGNANCY PLANNING

Compared with women who do not have DM, pregnant women with pre-existing diabetes have worse outcomes and a higher risk of pregnancy complications. The recognition of increased incidence of congenital malformations in infants born to diabetic mothers was first documented more than four decades ago. Most congenital defects occur during early gestational period during embryonic development before the seventh week of gestation. There is enough evidence to prove that good peri-conceptional control of glycemia is associated with better outcomes with regards to congenital malformation and perinatal mortality.

There are two distinct components to prepregnancy planning in patients with pre-existing diabetes—preconception counseling and prepregnancy care. Preconception counseling consists of educating every woman in the reproductive age regarding pregnancy, contraception, and importance of glycemic control before conceiving. It should ideally be done at regular intervals during her reproductive years and should include the following—target HbA1c before conception, adverse outcomes of hyperglycemia in pregnancy, how these effects can be mitigated by good glycemic control, use of folic acid supplements before and during pregnancy, and avoidance of drugs such as statins and angiotensin converting enzyme inhibitors/angiotensin receptor blockers during early pregnancy.

Prepregnancy care includes additional interventions necessary to prepare a woman with diabetes for pregnancy. It starts from ensuring appropriate contraception until optimal HbA1c is achieved, to ensuring all drugs taken during the periconception period are known to be safe and screening for co-morbid diseases. The risk benefit ratios of antidiabetes medication and commonly used antihypertensives should be carefully scrutinized and if warranted, the drug withdrawn in this period. Patients with increased BMI could also be guided toward appropriate lifestyle modification to facilitate weight loss. Due to the strong association between glycemic status and congenital malformations, it is imperative that patient is counseled to defer pregnancy till target HbA1c is achieved. As per ADA guidelines, HbA1c in women with pre-existing diabetes should be preferably <6.5% at the time of conception, as this level is associated with the lowest risk for congenital malformations. Achieving this target may not be possible, especially in patients with T1DM where hypoglycemia is often the limiting factor. However, the aim of getting the HbA1c as close to normal range without increasing the risk of hypoglycemia should always be deliberated.

## MANAGEMENT OF HYPERGLYCEMIA IN PREGNANCY

The management of women with either pregestational diabetes, overt diabetes or GDM involves a multimodality approach with close liaison between the patient and her family, diabetes care specialist, obstetrician, and nutritionist. While lifestyle modification remains the cornerstone of GDM management in most women, women with overt diabetes and quite often those with GDM require pharmacological treatment.

## Restricting Weight Gain

As per recommendations of the Institute of Medicine (IOM), the gestational weight gain should be adjusted according to the prepregnancy BMI in order to promote appropriate fetal growth. The recommended numbers are: About 12.5–18 kg for underweight women; 11.5–16 kg for normal weight women; 7–11.5 kg for overweight women; and 5–9 kg for obese women. In women with HIP, the lower end of this recommendation would be more appropriate, i.e., 7 kg weight gain for a woman that is overweight and 5 kg for women who is obese. The weekly increment in weight is higher after 20 weeks of gestation and women with HIP who have gained excessive weight throughout pregnancy usually exhibit higher weekly weight gain even before 20 weeks. Consequently, it is important to address the issue of weight gain early in the course of pregnancy, monitor it closely, and take corrective measures promptly.

## Dietary Changes

In pregnancy, dietary changes are necessary to match the increased energy requirements of the growing fetus and the physiological adaptive responses like accelerated starvation. Small frequent meals with monitored carbohydrate intake is the ideal approach to ensure optimal gestational weight achievement. The IOM recommends additional intake of 35 g of carbohydrate per day during pregnancy. In women with HIP, the recommended minimum total daily carbohydrate intake is 175 g, which includes 150 g from main carbohydrate sources (rice, roti, bread, whole grain, dairy products, fruits, potatoes, pasta, etc.), and 25 g from other sources (vegetables). Consumption of refined carbohydrates including sweets should be avoided or minimized. The carbohydrate content may be distributed as 20 g, 40 g, and 40 g consumed at breakfast, lunch, and dinner; and 10–20 g as snacks taken 2–4 times a day. Importantly, the recommended upper limit of carbohydrate content should be evenly distributed and should not exceed the allowed amount at each time point. Preference for carbohydrates with low glycemic index will limit postprandial glycemic excursions.

All women with HIP should be referred to a qualified dietitian who individualizes a nutritional plan that is feasible early in the course of pregnancy. This holds true for women with or at risk of pre-existing diabetes, and as soon as identified for those with GDM. Though carbohydrate counting is not a practical option in India, several smartphone applications are available which may be utilized for the same. In the Western Cape Province of South Africa, a non-block food recommendation list assists woman who remain hungry between meals with food suggestions that do not contribute to carbohydrate load. This list includes foods readily available at low cost such as unsalted nuts, avocado, pear etc.

## Physical Activity

Women should be encouraged to engage in moderate intensity physical activity until the latter stages of pregnancy. Most pregnant women can safely engage in moderate aerobic activity such as brisk walking, jogging, running, dancing or regular sports. Exercises that increase the risk of falling or abdominal trauma should be avoided.

## Therapeutic Targets

Women should be advised regarding regular self-monitoring of blood glucose (SMBG) with testing of fasting, preprandial, and postprandial glucose values. Recommended targets for fasting, 1 hour postprandial and 2-hour postprandial glucose values are ≤95 mg/dL,

≤140 mg/dL, and ≤120 mg/dL, respectively. HbA1c is a retrospective target and should not be a substitute for SMBG that can be used as a prompt guide to make therapeutic decisions.

## Insulin Therapy

Pharmacological therapy should be promptly initiated in women with significant hyperglycemia, those who do not attain glycemic targets within 1–2 weeks of initiation of lifestyle modification, and in those who demonstrate features of macrosomia on fetal ultrasound (estimated fetal weight or abdominal circumference >70th percentile). The most preferred and approved pharmacological agent for use in HIP is insulin.

The most favored insulin regimen during pregnancy is multiple subcutaneous insulin injections (MSII) with basal and bolus components titrated accordingly to SMBG profile. For basal insulin, the intermediate-acting Neutral Protamine Hagedorn (NPH) or insulin detemir are preferred. The long-acting insulin analog detemir acts for 24 hours with a peakless profile and has significantly lesser risk of hypoglycemia than NPH. However, insulin glargine can also be used, especially in individuals who were on glargine prior to pregnancy. The choice of prandial insulin includes regular human insulin and the rapid-acting insulin analogs, lispro and aspart, which are approved for use during pregnancy. Rapid acting analogs score over conventional insulin regular as they have faster onset, shorter duration of action, and a lower risk of hypoglycemia.

The ideal regimen would include rapid-acting analogs for prandial doses and long-acting insulin analog for basal coverage given as multiple daily injections in women with T2DM and GDM. Many women with GDM may require only prandial doses for management of mealtime glucose excursions or require relatively smaller doses of basal insulin. The dose plan should be guided by SMBG. Insulin pump therapy is an alternative option, especially in women with T1DM.

In resource-limited settings, very similar results can be achieved using conventional insulin regularly used as prandial doses and NPH insulin given for basal requirement with slightly increased risk of hypoglycemia necessitating close glucose monitoring.

## Oral Hypoglycemic Agents

According to most guidelines, insulin is the preferred drug for management of hyperglycemia in pregnancy. Treatment with oral hypoglycemic agents, including sulfonylureas, metformin, and other agents are best avoided as these drugs may cross the placenta and exert direct effects on the growing fetus. Ideally, women with pre-existing diabetes treated with these agents should be switched to insulin while planning conception, or at least immediately after conceiving. Though offspring safety data is available for metformin use in pregnancy, currently, the Indian Health ministry guidelines advise limiting the use of metformin in pregnancy to after 20 weeks of gestation. Glyburide is the other oral drug that has been used in pregnancy; but has been associated with higher incidence of neonatal hypoglycemia and increased birth weight when compared to women treated with insulin.

## Additional Strategies

Continuous glucose monitoring systems have seen tremendous improvement with technological advancements and the new flash glucose monitoring without repeated needle pricks is likely to change the way we track glycemic changes, especially during pregnancy. The most popular method being used now is the repeated timed self-monitoring of blood glucose with glucometers.

It is also important to screen the woman for hypertension, progression of kidney disease, and retinal changes during pregnancy. Appropriate pharmacological management of hypertension is an essential component of diabetes care during pregnancy. Routine supplementation with folic acid is recommended and should begin in the preconceptional period. Low-dose aspirin prophylaxis is considered in women at high-risk of preeclampsia, to be started before 16 weeks of gestation and continued until delivery.

## POSTPARTUM CARE

There occurs a sharp decline in insulin resistance soon after delivery, and most women with GDM do not require continued pharmacological treatment. In the patient with pregestational DM, hyperglycemia is unlikely to subside after delivery and evaluation and treatment of diabetes after pregnancy should be established early postpartum. Insulin dose requirements fall substantially in the postpartum period as insulin sensitivity is further improved with lactation and insulin should be titrated accordingly. Oral hypoglycemic agents are not recommended as routine in lactating women.

Gestational diabetes mellitus strongly predisposes to T2DM after pregnancy and shares many of the same risk factors. Postpartum risk stratification and detection of impaired fasting glucose (IFG) and/or impaired glucose tolerance (IGT) also provides an opportunity for timeous intervention to delay the onset of diabetes through diet, physical activity, weight management, and/or pharmacological intervention. Therefore, routine postpartum evaluation of pregnant women with GDM is advocated by all the major guidelines. It includes early (4–12 weeks) screening with an oral glucose tolerance test and ongoing (1 yearly followed by 3 yearly) screening.

Type 2 diabetes mellitus has a unique collection of undesirable complications and needs to be prevented or delayed as far and as long as possible. The hypothesis that T2DM is preventable by lifestyle intervention in patients at high-risk for T2DM is supported by large observational studies and clinical trials. The incidence of T2DM in patients with prediabetes was reduced by 58% with only lifestyle change versus 31% reduction with the antidiabetic agent metformin. When the persistence of these effects was investigated 10 years thereafter, the risk for developing T2DM was reduced by 34% in the lifestyle group and 18% in the metformin group compared with placebo in nonpregnant patients. Women with prior GDM had a larger reduction in the development of T2DM (55%) with lifestyle only. Metformin was also more effective in the GDM cohort, with a 50% risk reduction, compared with 14% in the non-GDM matched group.

Thus, the identification and intervention strategies in patients with prior GDM constitute a unique window of opportunity for early detection, intervention, and reduction of the future burden of T2DM, over and above detecting women erroneously classified as GDM with T2DM.

## CONCLUSION

As we witness an alarming rise of obesity and T2DM in the younger generation, the incidence of HIP including GDM is only going to increase with time. It is imperative that those patients with pre-existing diabetes be identified early, managed with appropriate drugs and ensure that glycemic control is excellent prior to conception. It is equally important to identify patients who develop diabetes during the course of pregnancy. A combination of lifestyle measures along with insulin and close glucose monitoring is the most preferred strategy in the management. It is also important to identify other comorbidities and act appropriately.

## SUGGESTED READING

1. Lawrence JM, Contreras R, Chen W, Sacks DA. Trends in the prevalence of pre-existing diabetes and gestational diabetes mellitus among a racially/ethnically diverse population of pregnant women, 1999–2005. Diabetes Care. 2008;31(5):899-904.
2. Wilmot EG, Mansell P. Diabetes and pregnancy. Clin Med. 2014:14(6):677-80.
3. Sacks DA, Hadden DR, Maresh M, Deerochanawong C, Dyer AR, Metzger BE, et al. For the HAPO Study Cooperative Research Group frequency of gestational diabetes mellitus at collaborating centers based on IADPSG Consensus Panel–Recommended Criteria The Hyperglycemia and Adverse Pregnancy Outcome (HAPO) Study. Diabetes Care. 2012;35(3):526-8.
4. Omori Y, Jovanovic L. Proposal for the reconsideration of the definition of gestational diabetes. Diabetes Care. 2005;28:2592-3.
5. Coustan DR, Lowe LP, Metzger BE, Dyer AR. The HAPO Study: Paving the way for new diagnostic criteria for GDM. Am J Obstet Gynecol. 2010;202(6):654.e1-654.e6.
6. Maegawa Y, Sugiyama T, Kusaka H, Mitao M, Toyoda N. Screening tests for gestational diabetes in Japan in the 1st and 2nd trimester of pregnancy. Diabetes Res Clin Pract. 2003;62(1):47-53.
7. Butte NF. Carbohydrate and lipid metabolism in pregnancy: normal compared with gestational diabetes mellitus. Am J Clin Nutr. 2000;71(5 Suppl):1256S-61S.
8. Homko CJ, Sivan E, Albert Reece E, Boden G. Fuel metabolism during pregnancy. Semin Reprod Med. 1999;17(2):119-25.
9. Handwerger S, Freemark M. The roles of placental growth hormone and placental lactogen in the regulation of human fetal growth and development. J Pediatr Endocrinol Metab. 2000;13(4):343-56.
10. Yamashita H, Shao J, Friedman JE. Physiologic and molecular alterations in carbohydrate metabolism during pregnancy and gestational diabetes mellitus. Clin Obstet Gynecol. 2000;43(1):87-98.
11. Schaefer UM, Songster G, Xiang A, Berkowitz K, Buchanan TA, Kjos SL. Congenital malformations in offspring of women with hyperglycemia first detected during pregnancy. Am J Obstet Gynecol. 1997;177:1165-71.
12. Gabbay-Benziv R, Reece EA, Wang F, Yang P. Birth defects in pregestational diabetes: defect range, glycemic threshold and pathogenesis. World J Diabetes. 2015;6(3):481-8.
13. Vambergue A, Fajardy I. Consequences of gestational and pregestational diabetes on placental function and birth weight. World J Diabetes. 2011;2(11):196-203.
14. Negrato CA, Mattar R, Gomes MB. Adverse pregnancy outcomes in women with diabetes. Diabetol Metab Syndr. 2012;4:41.
15. Priya G, Kalra B, Grewal E, et al. Premarriage counseling in type 1 diabetes. Indian J Endocrinol Metab. 2018;22(1):126-31.
16. NICE Guidelines. Diabetes in pregnancy: management from preconception to the postnatal period. [online] Available from nice.org.uk/guidance/ng3. [Last accessed January, 2020].
17. Metzger BE, Buchanan TA, Coustan DR, de Leiva A, Dunger DB, Hadden DR, et al. Summary and recommendations of the Fifth International Workshop-Conference on Gestational Diabetes Mellitus. Diabetes Care. 2007;30 (Suppl 2):S251-60.
18. Priya G, Kalra S. Metformin in the management of diabetes during pregnancy and lactation. Drugs Context. 2018;7:212523.
19. Kitzmiller JL, Dang-Kilduff L, Taslimi MM. Gestational diabetes after delivery: short-term management and long-term risks. Diabetes Care. 2007 Jul;30(Suppl 2):S225-35.
20. O'Reilly SL. Prevention of diabetes after gestational diabetes: better translation of nutrition and lifestyle messages needed. Healthcare (Basel). 2014:2:468-91.
21. Ferrara A, Peng T, Kim C. Trends in postpartum diabetes screening and subsequent diabetes and impaired fasting glucose among women with histories of gestational diabetes mellitus: a report from the Translating Research Into Action for Diabetes (TRIAD) Study. Diabetes Care. 2009 02;32(2):269-74.
22. Curtis L, Burgess C, McCord N, Masding MG. Early postpartum glycemic assessment in patients with gestational diabetes. Pract Diab. 2017,34:89-91.

# CHAPTER 2

# Thyroid Dysfunction in Women

*Vaishali Deshmukh, Dina Shreshtha*

## ABSTRACT

Thyroid disorders are one of the most common endocrinopathies that affect women in the reproductive age group. The prevalence of hypothyroidism across all ages in women remains higher than men and it has a significant impact on their reproductive health and fertility as well as maternal and fetal outcomes during pregnancy. This calls for a need for greater vigilance for thyroid dysfunction in women than men with case-specific screening and prompt initiation of appropriate therapy, especially in women of reproductive age. The need for thyroxine replacement in overt hypothyroidism is well-established; quite often, subclinical hypothyroidism in women also requires treatment. There is a need to further evaluate the role of thyroxine in women who have high titers of antithyroid autoantibodies but are otherwise euthyroid. The management of hyperthyroidism in women also requires greater vigilance and poses unique challenges, specifically relating to the woman's desire for pregnancy. Hyperthyroidism per se, thyroid-stimulating hormone (TSH) receptor antibodies, and antithyroidal drugs can all impact fetal outcomes. Therefore, there is a need for patient-centered approach keeping in mind the desire for pregnancy, size of the goiter, severity of hyperthyroidism, and the titers of TSH-receptor stimulating antibodies. Management of Graves' disease during pregnancy offers unique challenges and should be carefully supervised to minimize risk to both the mother and the fetus.

## INTRODUCTION

Thyroid disease is the most common endocrine condition affecting women of reproductive age. Thyroid hormones play a crucial role in metabolism and their secretion is intricately regulated by the hypothalamic-pituitary-thyroid (HPT) axis as depicted in **Figure 1**. The thyroid gland controls the rate of metabolic processes and also affects growth and development via the production of two hormones, triiodothyronine (T3) and thyroxine (T4). Changes in thyroid function can impact multiple organ systems including reproductive function before, during, and after conception.

# CHAPTER 2: Thyroid Dysfunction in Women

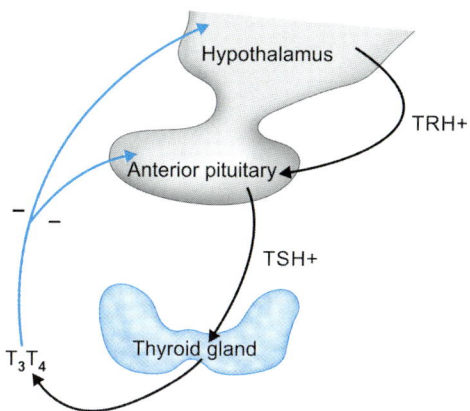

**FIG. 1:** Regulation of thyroid hormone release. The hypothalamus secretes thyrotropin-releasing hormone (TRH) that stimulates the secretion of thyroid-stimulating hormone (TSH) from the anterior pituitary. In turn, TSH acts via TSH receptors on the thyroid gland to stimulate the synthesis and secretion of triiodothyronine (T3) and thyroxine (T4). Thyroid hormones exert a negative feedback on the secretion of TRH and TSH through thyroid hormone receptors situated in the hypothalamus and anterior pituitary. A decrease in thyroid hormone secretion leads to an increase in the secretion of TSH while an excess of thyroid hormones suppresses TSH secretion.

Over the last few decades, there has been an increase in the prevalence of thyroid disorders. There is a distinct female preponderance, with female-to-male ratio of 4–6:1 for autoimmune thyroid disorders (AITD) and about 3–4:1 for thyroid nodules. For papillary thyroid carcinoma (PTC), the female-to-male ratio is greatest during reproductive age and drops from >5 in patients aged 20–24 years to one in patients over 80 years age. Hypothyroidism is the most common AITD and is caused by autoimmune thyroiditis (Hashimoto's thyroiditis), iodine deficiency or following surgery or radioiodine therapy. Thyrotoxicosis has a prevalence of 2% in women and 0.2% in men. Graves' disease predominates in younger women, while thyroid autonomy with nodules is more common in elderly women.

The effects of female gonadal hormones (estrogen and prolactin) and X chromosome inactivation on thyroid gland and immune system greatly contribute to the female predilection of AITD. Estrogen regulates the functions of nearly all immunocyte subsets through direct action and therefore, may contribute to the development of AITD. In addition, local expression of estrogen receptor (ER) subtypes may lead to goiter, thyroid nodule formation, and cancer in women.

In this chapter, we discuss unique issues in relation to thyroid dysfunction in women and also discuss pregnancy-specific management of thyroid disorders.

## HOW DOES THYROID FUNCTION AFFECT FEMALE LIFECYCLE?

### Puberty and Menstruation

Thyroid disorders can cause either early or delayed puberty. Historically, Kendle reported precocious puberty in a young girl with severe hypothyroidism in 1905.

Thyroid dysfunction can also cause light or heavy menstrual bleeding, irregular cycles, or even amenorrhea.

## Reproduction

Thyroid dysfunction may affect ovulation, leading to subfertility/infertility or bad obstetric outcomes. Hypothyroidism may be associated with increased risk for ovarian cyst development, hyperprolactinemia, and galactorrhea.

## Pregnancy and Postpartum

Thyroid disorders during pregnancy may be associated with adverse fetal and maternal outcomes and risk of postpartum thyroiditis. The impact of hypothyroidism and thyrotoxicosis on pregnancy is discussed in later section of this chapter.

## Menopause

Thyroid disorders may cause premature or early menopause. Thyrotoxicosis symptoms may mimic symptoms often attributed to menopause such as absent or irregular menstruation, hot flashes, mood swings, and sleep disturbances. Therefore, a high index of suspicion should be maintained. Treatment of hyperthyroidism may help alleviate vasomotor symptoms associated with menopause and may also prevent early cessation of menstrual cycles. Hypothyroidism may occur in perimenopausal women; one in five postmenopausal women tends to have thyroid dysfunction.

# FUNCTIONAL THYROID DISORDERS IN WOMEN

Abnormal thyroid function, including both hypothyroidism and hyperthyroidism, can result from a wide variety of causes as enlisted in **Table 1**. The interpretation of thyroid functions and evaluation of abnormal thyroid function tests are summarized in **Table 2**. A subset of women may have high titers of antithyroid autoantibodies, but are biochemically euthyroid.

## Hypothyroidism in Women

Hypothyroidism is common, with overt hypothyroidism affecting 0.5% of women and subclinical hypothyroidism 2–4% of women in reproductive age. Symptoms of hypothyroidism in adults can be vague, including weight gain, fatigue, dry skin, constipation, or memory loss, but many patients may be asymptomatic. Women may present with irregular or missed cycles, altered bleeding patterns, galactorrhea, or bad obstetric history such as subfertility or miscarriages. Neonates and children may present with prolonged neonatal jaundice, delayed milestones, growth delay or short stature, obesity, mental retardation, pubertal or menstrual disorders.

While routine universal screening of all women for thyroid dysfunction is not recommended, evaluation for thyroid dysfunction should be considered in women with suspicious or concerning features and in those with risk factors for thyroid disease, as enlisted in **Box 1**.

Hypothyroidism can affect the pulsatile secretion of gonadotropin-releasing hormone (GnRH) that maintains the cyclical secretion of anterior pituitary hormones, follicle-stimulating hormone (FSH) and luteinizing hormone (LH). Therefore, it can result

**TABLE 1:** Causes of thyroid dysfunction in women.

| Hypothyroidism | Thyrotoxicosis |
|---|---|
| Primary hypothyroidism<br>• Autoimmune disease:<br>  ○ Atrophic thyroiditis<br>  ○ Hashimoto's thyroiditis<br>• Iatrogenic:<br>  ○ Radioiodine therapy<br>  ○ Thyroidectomy<br>  ○ External irradiation<br>  ○ Antithyroid drugs<br>• Transient:<br>  ○ Subacute (de Quervain's) thyroiditis<br>  ○ Postpartum thyroiditis<br>• Iodine deficiency | Hyperthyroidism with increased radioiodine uptake<br>• Autoimmune:<br>  ○ Grave's disease<br>• Toxic nodular Goiter<br>• Toxic adenoma<br>• Drugs—iodine, amiodarone, chemotherapy |
| Secondary hypothyroidism<br>• Hypopituitarism<br>• Pituitary tumor<br>• Sheehan's syndrome<br>Tertiary hypothyroidism<br>• Hypothalamic failure | Thyrotoxicosis with absent radioiodine uptake<br>• Subacute thyroiditis<br>• Painless thyroiditis<br>• Postpartum thyroiditis<br>• Iodine therapy<br>• Drugs—amiodarone, lithium, interferons |

**TABLE 2:** Interpretation of thyroid function tests.

| TSH | T4 | T3 | Diagnosis | What next? |
|---|---|---|---|---|
| Decreased<br><0.4 IU/mL | ↑<br>N<br>↓ | ↑<br>N<br>↓ | Thyrotoxicosis<br>Subclinical thyrotoxicosis<br>Central hypothyroidism | Thyroid Scan<br>Anti TPO antibodies<br>Pituitary imaging |
| Increased<br>>4.5 IU/mL | ↓<br>N<br>↑ | ↓<br>N<br>↑ | Primary hypothyroidism<br>Subclinical hypothyroidism<br>Central hyperthyroidism | Anti TPO antibodies<br>Treat<br>Pituitary imaging |

(T3: triiodothyronine; T4: thyroxine; TPO: thyroid peroxidase; TSH: thyroid-stimulating hormone)

in ovulatory dysfunction. When hypothyroidism develops in young or adolescent girls, there may occur a delay in growth and puberty with delay in sexual maturation. Rapid thyroxine replacement in such girls can lead to accelerated puberty. In adult women, hypothyroidism often presents with menstrual abnormalities such as oligo/amenorrhea or menorrhagia.

Treatment of hypothyroidism in women requires special considerations. Higher serum thyroid-stimulating hormone (TSH) levels have been observed in women with menstrual disturbances, anovulatory cycles, and subfertility. Elevated TSH is often associated with subfertility and suboptimal response to assisted reproductive technology. In fact, pregnancy rates have been reported to be reduced even at serum TSH levels above 2.5 mU/L. Levothyroxine replacement in such women resulted in better rates of implantation, pregnancy, and live births. This has not only been demonstrated

## SECTION 2: Endocrinology

> **BOX 1**    **Risk factors for thyroid dysfunction.**
> - History of thyroid dysfunction/thyroid surgery
> - Family history of thyroid disease
> - Clinical symptoms/signs of hypothyroidism or thyrotoxicosis
> - Goiter
> - Positive thyroid autoantibodies
> - Type 1 diabetes mellitus
> - Other autoimmune disorders
> - History of miscarriage/preterm delivery
> - History of subfertility
> - History of therapeutic head or neck irradiation
> - Age ≥30 years
> - Morbid obesity
> - Previous treatment with amiodarone
> - Previous treatment with lithium
> - Recent exposure to iodinated radiological contrast agents

in women who have overt hypothyroidism but also subclinical hypothyroidism. However, egg number and fertilization rates and the rates of successful implantation, confirmed pregnancy, and live births remains lower than euthyroid controls.

The replacement dose of thyroxine is based on body weight and usual dose in adults is 1.6 µg/kg/day. However, it is the fat-free mass that is particularly important. Therefore, doses are slightly higher in men than women. Care should also be taken not to overtreat women who are more prone to bone loss and fracture risk, especially as they reach menopause.

## Thyroid Autoantibodies

Thyroid autoimmunity is thought to be present in up to 25% of the general population and has been implicated in subfertility and reproductive concerns. Presence of thyroid autoantibodies may be associated with increased risk of other autoimmune disorders such as antiphospholipid antibody (APLA) syndrome, diabetes mellitus, and systemic lupus erythematosus.

The most common cause of hypothyroidism in women is autoimmune thyroid disease (AITD) or Hashimoto's disease. Almost all women with Hashimoto's thyroiditis have elevated titers of antithyroid autoantibodies, most commonly antithyroid peroxidase antibodies (TPOAb). Almost two-thirds of women with postpartum thyroid dysfunction and a significant number of women with Graves' disease also have antithyroid antibodies. Almost 5–10% of euthyroid women may also have elevated antithyroid autoantibodies, especially women with subfertility, polycystic ovary syndrome, endometriosis, and poor obstetric outcomes.

Presence of antithyroid autoantibodies has been presumed to be an early marker of lymphocytic infiltration of the thyroid gland and may predict the onset of thyroid disease even when serum TSH is normal. Several mechanisms have been postulated to explain subfertility in such women including T-cell infiltration of endometrium, cross-reaction of polyclonal B-cells with trophoblastic tissue, hyperactivity of natural killer cells, cross-reactivity of thyroid antibodies with placental and zona pellucida antigens, presence of vitamin D deficiency or other concurrent autoimmune diseases.

## Hyperthyroidism in Women

Hyperthyroidism, both clinical and subclinical, has been reported in 1.5% of women. Presentation may be with history of weight loss, fatigue, heat intolerance, restlessness or agitation, excess sweating, palpitations, tremors, or frequent stools. On physical examination, there may be tachycardia, systolic hypertension, tremors, hyperpyrexia with vasodilatation (flushing), goiter, thyroid bruit, exophthalmos or other features of Graves' ophthalmopathy. In severe cases, there may be features of congestive heart failure, atrial fibrillation, altered sensorium, delirium or coma.

Women with hyperthyroidism may complain of hypomenorrhea or polymenorrhea. While the mechanism leading to menstrual disturbances in hyperthyroidism is not so well understood, it could result from increased sensitivity to GnRH with increased secretion of LH. A rise in the levels of sex hormone-binding globulin (SHBG) further contributes to a hyperestrogenic state. However, most hyperthyroid women continue to have ovulatory cycles.

Diagnosis involves the biochemical documentation of thyrotoxicosis and evaluation for specific etiology. While in many cases, the differentiation between thyrotoxicosis due to destructive thyroiditis and Graves' disease or autonomous nodules can be made on clinical grounds, many patients will require further evaluation with radioiodine or technetium scintigraphy and estimation of TSH receptor antibodies (TRAb).

While most patients with hyperthyroidism are initially treated with antithyroid drugs, the choice of therapy should take into account the desire to attain pregnancy in the near future. A trial of antithyroid drugs can be continued for 12–18 months, but definitive therapy is advisable in those who have large goiter, very high titers of TRAb or require high doses of antithyroid drugs. Methimazole or carbimazole are preferred over propylthiouracil as the latter is associated with increased risk of serious hepatoxicity.

## ANATOMICAL THYROID DISORDERS IN WOMEN

### Thyroid Nodules

Thyroid nodules are commonly seen in adult women and may affect up to 50% of women, but only 5–15% of those are malignant. Nodules may be:
- *Benign nodules*: These include colloid nodule, follicular adenoma, thyroid cysts, inflammatory nodules or thyroiditis.
- *Autonomously functioning nodules*: These are usually benign and cause hyperthyroidism.
- Thyroid cancer

Many nodules do not cause symptoms until they are large enough to affect the surrounding tissues and organs or to be visible on the neck. Symptoms may include visible and/or palpable swelling of the neck, pain, difficulty in swallowing, hoarseness of voice, features of thyrotoxicosis or hypothyroidism or facial congestion. Diagnosis requires careful local and systemic physical examination, especially documenting the characteristics of the nodules, presence of other nodules, and lymph nodes.

The primary concern when evaluating nodules is to differentiate benign nodules from malignant ones. Ultrasound evaluation of thyroid nodules can provide important information. Suspicious ultrasound findings should be followed up with fine-needle aspiration (FNA) evaluation of the nodule. Other investigations that may assist in diagnosis include thyroid function testing, computed tomography, and radionuclide scans.

Treatment depends on the type and cause of the nodule. Surgery is required if the nodules are malignant or suspicious. In others, watchful observation and regular follow-up is all that is needed.

## Thyroid Cancer

Thyroid malignancies constitute the third most common cancer in women. Most common thyroid cancers include differentiated nonaggressive tumors that are highly treatable, even when there is metastatic spread to lymph nodes with a 98–99% survival rate at 20 years. Total thyroidectomy with removal of any suspicious lymph node is the preferred treatment. Postoperative radioactive iodine ablation to destroy cancer cells and supplementation with thyroxine in suppressive doses is able to achieve high cure rates even in those with residual disease in most cases.

# THYROID DISORDERS DURING PREGNANCY

Pregnancy has a profound effect on thyroid gland function as summarized in **Table 3**. During pregnancy, the thyroid gland increases in size by 10–20% and the demand of thyroid hormones increases to about 30–50%. In a way, pregnancy can be considered as a stress test for the thyroid gland. Therefore, pregnant women are more susceptible to a derangement in thyroid function especially if they have underlying overt or subclinical thyroid dysfunction.

## Changes in Thyroid Physiology during Pregnancy

Serum levels of βhCG increase sharply in early pregnancy. Since this is structurally closely related to TSH, high levels of βhCG can cross-react with TSH receptor and stimulate the secretion of thyroid hormones. A rise in the secretion of thyroid hormones is associated with a parallel decrease in TSH levels in the first trimester. As pregnancy progresses, serum βhCG levels begin to decline and TSH levels return back to baseline. Another important physiological change in thyroid physiology in a pregnant woman involves the progressive rise in the secretion of thyroid-binding globulin (TBG) in response to estrogen. The clearance of TBG is also reduced. This is accompanied by a progressive rise in the levels of total T3 and total T4, beginning from 8 weeks, and these plateau in later half of gestation. Pregnancy is also associated with increased renal plasma flow and increased renal clearance of iodine as well as free thyroid hormones. The net result is an increased demand for thyroid hormone synthesis.

An understanding of these physiological alterations in thyroid physiology during pregnancy is important from many aspects. Maternal iodine requirements are estimated to be 250 µg/day during pregnancy and lactation. Maternal iodine deficiency may be associated with maternal as well as fetal goiter, low birth weight, fetal loss, congenital hypothyroidism, and impaired neurological development. On average, mothers should be supplemented with 100–150 µg/day of iodine.

Fetal thyroid gland develops after 12th week of gestation whereas thyroid hormones are vital to fetal brain development in early first trimester. Regular fetal T4 secretion does not occur until 18–20 weeks of gestation. Therefore, fetus relies exclusively on maternal thyroid hormone supply in early pregnancy.

## CHAPTER 2: Thyroid Dysfunction in Women

**TABLE 3:** Changes in thyroid physiology during pregnancy.

| | Physiological changes in the mother | Changes in maternal thyroid function |
|---|---|---|
| Thyrotropic effect of placental hCG | Placental hCG increases with a peak at the end of the first trimester and then declines to plateau in second and third trimesters. This results in a transient increase in thyroid hormone production in first trimester | • TSH is lower in the first trimester. It reaches a trough around 11–14 weeks and slightly rises later<br>• There is a simultaneous rise in free T4 toward the end of first trimester, which then decreases during latter half of pregnancy<br>• Total T3 and total T4 increase from 6–8 weeks due to increased TBG levels, starting from early pregnancy to approximately 1.5 times at 16th week of gestation and then plateau<br>• Free T4 assays may be unreliable due to high TBG levels. Significant reduction in free T4 in third trimester may be seen in automated immunoassays. More accurate methods such as equilibrium dialysis or ultrafiltration are more expensive |
| Increased TBG levels | TBG increases, beginning at 6–8 weeks with 2–3 fold rise by 20th week of gestation. This results from increased production due to effect of estradiol and decreased renal clearance of more sialylated forms | |
| Increased iodine demand | Increased renal filtration of iodine, transplacental transfer of iodine to developing fetus and increased demand for thyroid hormone production | |
| Transplacental transfer of thyroid hormones | Approximately 50% increase in thyroid hormone demand and transfer to fetus for skeletal growth and neurological development | |
| Placental deiodinases | Increased intraplacental breakdown of T4 and T3 by placental deiodinases (D3) | |
| Immune modulation | Period of immunosuppression during pregnancy and rebound increase in immunity after delivery. May affect the course of autoimmune Graves' disease with relative quiescence during pregnancy and increased risk of relapse postpartum | |

(T3: triiodothyronine; T4: thyroxine; hCG: human chorionic gonadotropin; TBG: thyroid-binding globulin; TSH: thyroid-stimulating hormone)

When thyroid gland is functioning normally, it is able to compensate for the increased pregnancy demands with an appropriate increase in thyroid hormone production. However, any underlying abnormality can get unmasked during pregnancy and lead to thyroid dysfunction. Any abnormality in thyroid function, whether it is hypothyroidism or hyperthyroidism, can adversely affect reproductive health of women, and result in lower rates of conception, increased rates of miscarriages, and adverse maternal and fetal outcomes during pregnancy.

## Interpretation of Thyroid Functions during Pregnancy

The interpretation of thyroid functions is obviously different during pregnancy than in nonpregnant individuals. Due to sequential changes in serum TSH, total T3 and total T4 and free T4 levels during pregnancy, it is important to use assay-specific, trimester-specific, and population-specific reference ranges for these hormones. These levels are determined using data from healthy pregnant women who do not have thyroid dysfunction, goiter or risk factors, are negative for thyroid autoantibodies, have sufficient iodine intake, are not taking medications that may affect thyroid function, and have singleton pregnancies. If such reference range is not available, the upper limit of TSH is defined by the upper limit of TSH in nonpregnant individuals minus 0.5, or a value of 4.0 mIU/L is used between 7 and 12 weeks. Prior to 7 weeks, nonpregnant range is used. **Table 4** summarizes the changes in guidelines over time for the upper limit of TSH during pregnancy.

Due to unreliability of free T4 assays during pregnancy, total T4 and total T3 levels are considered better. If population-specific and trimester-specific reference ranges for total T4 and total T3 are not available, the nonpregnant range of these hormones is multiplied by 1.5 to ascertain reference values for pregnancy.

## Hypothyroidism during Pregnancy

The prevalence of hypothyroidism in pregnant women has been reported to be high, with 0.5% women having overt hypothyroidism and 2.5% diagnosed as subclinical hypothyroidism. Thyroid hypofunction during pregnancy can increase the risk of adverse obstetric and neonatal outcomes, as summarized in **Table 5**. One of the most important concerns that have often been raised is the effect of untreated hypothyroidism on neurodevelopment health of infants. In rare cases, the transplacental transfer of TSH receptor blocking antibodies has been reported resulting in fetal goiter and neonatal hypothyroidism. Some women may demonstrate isolated hypothyroxinemia with normal TSH levels but its significance remains to be determined.

It is unclear whether all women should be universally screened for thyroid dysfunction during pregnancy. However, given the high prevalence of thyroid dysfunction and its

**TABLE 4:** Trimester-specific TSH reference ranges.

| Guidelines | TSH (mU/L) reference range |
| --- | --- |
| American Thyroid Association 2011 | • 1st trimester: 0.1–2.5<br>• 2nd trimester: 0.2–3.0<br>• 3rd trimester: 0.3–3.0 |
| American Thyroid Association 2017 | • TSH > upper limit of population and trimester-specific reference range<br>• Alternatively, reduce the upper limit of nonpregnant reference range by 0.5<br>• If not available, TSH >4.0 |

(TSH: thyroid-stimulating hormone)

**TABLE 5:** Complications associated with hypothyroidism during pregnancy.

| Maternal | Neonatal |
| --- | --- |
| • Anemia<br>• Postpartum hemorrhage<br>• Cardiac dysfunction<br>• Preeclampsia<br>• Placental abruption | • Fetal distress in labor<br>• Prematurity/low birth weight<br>• Congenital malformations<br>• Perinatal death<br>• Stillbirth<br>• Neurodevelopmental delay<br>• Congenital hypothyroidism (if autoimmune) |

**TABLE 6:** Indications for levothyroxine treatment in pregnant women with hypothyroidism.

| Absolute indication for levothyroxine | Relative indication for levothyroxine |
|---|---|
| • Overt hypothyroidism<br>• SCH under treatment prior to pregnancy<br>• TSH >10 mU/L irrespective of FT4 levels or TPO-Ab status<br>• TSH above population-based trimester-specific value and TPO-Ab positive | • TSH >2.5 mU/L but below upper reference limit with TPO-Ab positive<br>• TSH above upper reference limit but <10 mU/L with TPO-Ab negative<br>• Euthyroid with TPO-Ab positive with history of pregnancy loss |

(SCH: subclinical hypothyroidism; TPO-Ab: antithyroid peroxidase antibodies; TSH: thyroid-stimulating hormone)

relationship with adverse pregnancy outcomes, a high index of suspicion and a low threshold for testing should be maintained.

Levothyroxine replacement in both overt as well as subclinical hypothyroidism has been shown to reduce the risk of adverse outcomes. Therefore, there is a need for close vigilance of thyroid health during pregnancy, prompt diagnosis of thyroid dysfunction and its early and rapid treatment. The indications for initiation of LT4 treatment in women with subclinical hypothyroidism during pregnancy are listed in **Table 6**.

LT4 replacement therapy should be rapidly titrated to attain TSH levels of <2.5 mIU/L as early as possible. Ideally, optimization of LT4 therapy should be attained prior to conception with frequent monitoring and titration of doses during pregnancy. Most women would require an increase in the dose of LT4 during the first trimester due to increasing demand for thyroid hormones. If hypothyroidism is newly recognized during pregnancy, it should be fully treated as early as possible.

If a woman has already been on LT4 treatment prior to pregnancy, the dose should be optimized in the preconception period to maintain TSH in the lower half of reference range. As soon as pregnancy is confirmed, the dose should be increased to compensate for the increased demands of pregnancy. The usual dose increment can vary from 25 to 50 μg, based on TSH values. Monitoring of thyroid functions can be done at 4–6 weeks intervals to titrate LT4 dose and reach a target TSH of 0.5–2.5 mU/L. Thereafter, monitoring can be done once in each trimester or more often, if required. The physiological changes associated with pregnancy revert following delivery. Therefore, the dose of LT4 is reduced in most patients and TSH monitored after 6–8 weeks of delivery.

## Thyroid Autoantibodies and Pregnancy

Several studies suggest that thyroid autoantibodies, particularly TPOAbs, may have a role in subfertility and the risk of miscarriage and preterm delivery, even in women who have normal thyroid function. In a systematic review, Plowden et al. found a 3-fold increase in the odds ratio of miscarriage in women who had elevated titers of thyroid autoantibodies but were biochemically euthyroid.

The risk of the development of hypothyroidism during pregnancy is 5–10% in such women as they may be unable to increase thyroxine production appropriately during pregnancy. The risk of preterm labor in euthyroid women with AITD has been reported to be 2- to 4-fold greater. It would be prudent to monitor thyroid function closely during pregnancy in such women and if not already started on LT4 replacement in early pregnancy, a repeat testing at least once between 26 and 32 weeks of gestation is warranted.

Conception rates in women with subfertility were higher when treated early with LT4 with TSH maintained close to the lower end of normal. Similarly, rates of early pregnancy

## SECTION 2: Endocrinology

losses were also lower. A careful evaluation on history and physical examination for any features of thyroid dysfunction should be undertaken in all pregnant women. Those women who have elevated titers of thyroid autoantibodies also are at greater risk of postpartum thyroid dysfunction and postpartum depression.

## Management of Thyroid Disease in Women with Subfertility

All women who are undergoing evaluation and treatment for subfertility should be screened for thyroid dysfunction and it is considered appropriate to maintain TSH <2.5 mU/L if they have overt or subclinical hypothyroidism or thyroid autoantibodies. This may result in improved pregnancy outcomes. **Flowchart 1** depicts the algorithm to evaluation and treatment of thyroid dysfunction in women with subfertility.

## Thyrotoxicosis during Pregnancy

As discussed earlier, a dip in TSH levels with an increase in thyroid hormone secretion occurs in early pregnancy due to the thyrotropic effects of βhCG. Transient mild hyperthyroidism may occur in women with very high βhCG levels during the first half of gestation. Transient gestational thyrotoxicosis is reported in 1–3% pregnancies and is often seen in the setting of hyperemesis gravidarum, molar pregnancies or multiple pregnancies.

In most cases, gestational thyrotoxicosis is mild, resolves as pregnancy progresses and does not require pharmacological treatment. In the second trimester, free T4 levels begin to decline in parallel to reduction in βhCG. Therefore, most cases of gestational hyperthyroidism require only supportive symptomatic management. The use of antithyroid drugs is not indicated. Symptomatic treatment with short-term use of beta-blockers may be required in some cases. However, it is important to differentiate gestational thyrotoxicosis from Graves' disease. While clinical picture may be helpful,

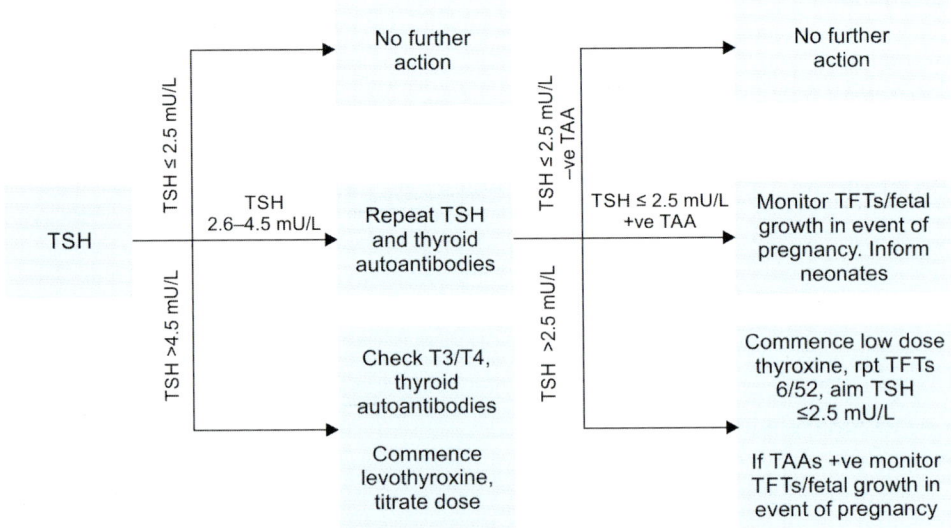

(T3: triiodothyronine; T4: thyroxine; TAA: thyroid antithyroglobulin antibody; TFT: thyroid function test; TSH: thyroid-stimulating hormone)

**FLOWCHART: 1:** Management of hypothyroidism in women undergoing evaluation for subfertility.

radionuclide scintigraphy cannot be performed during pregnancy. Hence, it is useful to assess TRAb titers to rule out Graves' disease.

Graves' disease is relatively uncommon and reported in about 0.1–0.4 pregnancies. The course of the disease is biphasic, with an exacerbation within the first trimester and an improvement thereafter, but a recurrence after delivery. Graves' disease during pregnancy poses unique challenges associated with increased risk of adverse pregnancy outcomes including preterm delivery, preeclampsia, growth restriction, heart failure, and stillbirth. The adverse effects may result from uncontrolled thyrotoxicosis, transplacental transfer of antithyroid drugs or TRAb antibodies, as summarized in **Table 7**.

Therefore, women with pre-existing Graves' disease should be advised to achieve euthyroidism before planning a pregnancy. Definitive therapy prior to pregnancy should be considered in women with large goiter, significantly high T4 levels, high titers of TRAb or high dose requirements of antithyroid drugs or inadequate response to antithyroid drugs. TRAb titers decline rapidly after thyroidectomy, while TRAb titers may rise after radioiodine therapy and remain high for 1 year. Therefore, conception should be delayed for at least 6 months after radioactive iodine therapy. For women planning pregnancy within 6 months, thyroidectomy may be the preferred definitive treatment.

Women who continue medical management with antithyroid drugs may be switched to propylthiouracil prior to conception or as soon as pregnancy is confirmed. Propylthiouracil is associated with a lower risk of teratogenicity compared to methimazole or carbimazole, which has been associated with aplasia cutis, choanal or esophageal atresia, abdominal wall defects, eye and urinary abnormalities, and congenital heart defects. Though birth defects have also been reported with propylthiouracil, they are usually milder and include face and neck defects and urinary abnormalities. However, propylthiouracil carries a greater risk of hepatotoxicity which is an idiosyncratic reaction and difficult to predict. Therefore, most guidelines recommend that women should be switched back to methimazole after 16 weeks of gestation.

Whichever agent is used, the dose of antithyroid drugs should be kept at the lowest possible level to minimize exposure to the fetus as well as to avoid overtreatment. Since antithyroid drugs freely cross the placenta, there is a risk of suppression of fetal thyroid tissue if an attempt is made to normalize maternal thyroid functions. The target is to maintain free T4 at the upper limit of normal or slightly above it and TSH between 0.1–0.4 mIU/L. TSH within the reference range should prompt reduction of antithyroid

**TABLE 7:** Risks associated with hyperthyroidism during pregnancy.

|  | Mother | Fetus | Neonate |
|---|---|---|---|
| Effect of uncontrolled thyrotoxicosis | • Congestive heart failure<br>• Pre-eclampsia<br>• Thyroid storm<br>• Miscarriage<br>• Placental abruption | • Prematurity<br>• Intrauterine growth retardation<br>• Low birth weight<br>• Still birth | • Secondary hypothyroidism |
| Effect of antithyroid drugs | • Minor reactions<br>• Agranulocytosis<br>• Hepatotoxicity | • Birth defects<br>• Fetal hypothyroidism<br>• Fetal goiter |  |
| Effect of TRAb |  | • Fetal hyperthyroidism | • Neonatal hyperthyroidism |

(GD: Graves' disease; RAI: radioiodine ablation; TRAb: TSH receptor stimulating antibodies)

drug dose and it may even be discontinued in up to 30% of women. Antithyroid drugs should be titrated regularly because of the risk of maternal or fetal hypothyroidism and subsequent risk for fetal development.

Some women with Graves' disease may enter into a phase of relative remission toward the end of pregnancy. However, following delivery, they are at risk of recurrence of Graves' disease or an exacerbation. Therefore, close monitoring for symptoms and thyroid functions after delivery is needed.

Monitoring of TRAb titers is also warranted as these antibodies may cross the placenta and result in fetal thyrotoxicosis. TRAb titers should be evaluated at the first antenatal visit and if elevated, they should be repeated at 18–22 weeks and then at 32 weeks. TRAbs may persist in fetal circulation for few weeks after delivery and may cause transient neonatal hyperthyroidism in 1–5%. In some circumstances, there may be a need for surgical treatment for hyperthyroidism during pregnancy, especially if there is severe hyperthyroidism and/ or antithyroid drugs are not being tolerated or there is a large goiter. If required, thyroidectomy is considered safe in the second trimester in an appropriately prepared woman.

## Thyroid Cancer and Pregnancy

Course of differentiated thyroid cancer is aggravated by the TSH-like effect of βhCG. Evaluation of thyroid nodules includes ultrasound and FNA. Radionuclide scans are contraindicated during pregnancy. Second trimester is the safest period for surgery and curative treatment with radioactive iodine should be deferred until after the patient has delivered.

## CONCLUSION

Hypothyroidism has a high prevalence in females at all ages and has significant effects on reproductive health, fertility, pregnancy outcomes, and neonatal health. The treatment of thyroid dysfunction in reproductive age group is known to improve reproductive health, pregnancy outcomes, and quality of life. While the benefits of LT4 replacement in hypothyroid women are well established, the benefits of treating euthyroid women with AITD both pre-conception and during pregnancy remains a gray area and further research is needed to confirm benefit of treating this population. Similarly, the management of hyperthyroidism in women of reproductive age group requires special considerations.

## SUGGESTED READING

1. Dunn D, Turner C. Hypothyroidism in Women. Nurs Women Health. 2016;20(1):93-8.
2. Lu Y, Li J, Li J. Estrogen and thyroid diseases: an update. Minerva Med. 2016;107(4):239-44.
3. Li H, Li J. Thyroid disorders in women. Minerva Med. 2015;106(2):109-14.
4. Kendle F. 1905 Case of precocious puberty in a female cretin. Br Med J. 1905;1(2301):246.
5. Jefferys A, Vanderpump M, Yasmin E. Thyroid dysfunction and reproductive health. Obstet Gynaecol. 2015;17(1):39-45.
6. Alexander EK, Pearce EN, Brent GA, Brown RS, Chen H, Dosiou C, et al. 2017 Guidelines of the American Thyroid Association for the Diagnosis and Management of Thyroid Disease During Pregnancy and the Postpartum. Thyroid. 2017;27(3):315-89.
7. Kahaly G, J, Bartalena L, Hegedüs L, Leenhardt L, Poppe K, Pearce SH. 2018 European Thyroid Association Guideline for the Management of Graves' Hyperthyroidism. Eur Thyroid J. 2018;7(4):167-86.

8. Paschou SA, Vryonidou A, Goulis DG. Thyroid nodules: A guide to assessment, treatment and follow-up. Maturitas. 2017;96:1-9.
9. Springer D, Jiskra J, Limanova Z, Zima T, Potlukova E. Thyroid in pregnancy: from physiology to screening. Crit Rev Clin Lab Sci. 2017;54(2):102-16.
10. Priya G. Subclinical hypothyroidism during pregnancy: Controversies. Journal of the Indian Medical Association. 2018;4(116):45.
11. Korevaar TIM, Medici M, Visser TJ, Peeters RP. Thyroid disease in pregnancy: new insights in diagnosis and clinical management. Nat Rev Endocrinol. 2017;13(10):610-22.
12. Nazarpour S, Tehrani FR, Simbar M, Tohidi M, AlaviMajd H, Azizi F. Comparison of universal screening with targeted high-risk case finding for diagnosis of thyroid disorders. Eur J Endocrinol. 2016;174(1):77-83.
13. Stagnaro-Green A, Abalovich M, Alexander E, Azizi F, Mestman J, Negro R, et al. Guidelines of the American Thyroid Association for the diagnosis and management of thyroid disease during pregnancy and postpartum. Thyroid. 2011;21(10):1081-125.
14. Plowden TC, Schisterman EF, Sjaarda LA, Perkins NJ, Silver R, Radin R. Thyroid-stimulating hormone, anti-thyroid antibodies, and pregnancy outcomes. Am J Obstet Gynecol. 2017;217(6):697:e1-7.
15. Chan L. Gestational transient thyrotoxicosis. Am J Emerg Med. 2003;21(6):506.
16. Cooper DS, Laurberg P. Hyperthyroidism in pregnancy. Lancet Diab Endocrinol. 2013;1(3):238-49.
17. Perros P. Thyrotoxicosis and pregnancy. PLoS Med. 2005;2(12):e370.
18. Lazarus JH. Pre-conception counselling in Graves' disease. Eur Thyroid J. 2012;1:24-9.
19. Ines B, Cesidio G, Giorgio N. Thyroid-stimulating hormone receptor antibodies in pregnancy: clinical relevance. Front Endocrinol (Lausanne). 2017;8:137.

# Polycystic Ovary Syndrome: A Multifaceted Endocrinopathy

*Savita Jain, Sarah Nadeem, Gagan Priya*

## ABSTRACT

Polycystic ovary syndrome (PCOS) is one of the most common disorders in reproductive age women, defined by a triad of chronic oligo/anovulation, hyperandrogenism, and polycystic appearance of ovaries. PCOS is a multisystem endocrinopathy associated with multiorgan involvement. While most young women present with menstrual irregularity or hyperandrogenic features such as hirsutism, acne or alopecia, it may be recognized during evaluation for subfertility. Insulin resistance is an important pathophysiological mechanism in PCOS and a significant proportion of these patients are overweight or obese. Several studies suggest that PCOS is associated with a long-term risk of diabetes mellitus, cardiovascular disease, nonalcoholic fatty liver disease (NAFLD), obstructive sleep apnea (OSA), psychological disturbances, and gynecological malignancies such as endometrial carcinoma. The management approach should take into account the predominant symptoms, lifestyle modification, and weight reduction and an assessment for cardiometabolic risk factors and their management.

## INTRODUCTION

Polycystic ovary syndrome (PCOS) is one of the most common disorders in reproductive age women, defined by a triad of chronic oligo/anovulation, hyperandrogenism, and polycystic appearance of ovaries, depicted in **Figure 1**. However, it is important to understand that PCOS is a multisystem endocrinopathy with many facets beyond reproductive health. Initially reported by American gynecologists, Irvin F Stein, and Michael L Leventhal, in 1935, in seven of their patients (earlier was known as Stein–Leventhal syndrome), PCOS was rapidly recognized to affect women of reproductive age across all ethnic groups and races. Patients have variable clinical presentation.

Classically, the endocrinopathy is recognized by hyperandrogenism, but its association with overweight/obesity and insulin resistance has shown that it is indeed a multifaceted endocrinopathy. Worldwide prevalence of PCOS is highly variable due to varied and inconsistent diagnostic criteria used. According to a meta-analysis done by Ding T et al. the prevalence is lowest in Chinese women, followed by Caucasians, middle eastern, and black women. As per WHO estimates of 2010, 116 million women worldwide are affected by PCOS (3.4% population). An Indian study reported the prevalence of 6% in south Indian girls in the age group of 18–24 years.

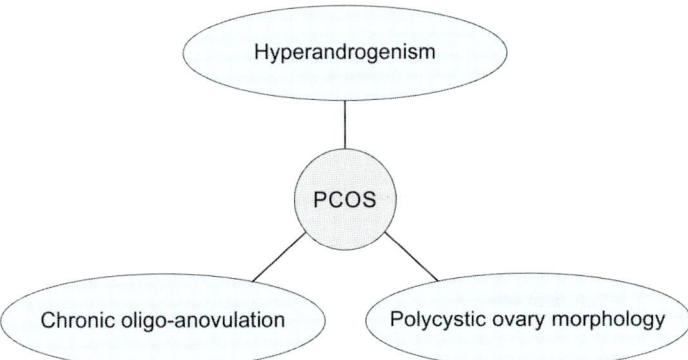

**FIG. 1:** Core components of polycystic ovary syndrome (PCOS).

## PATHOPHYSIOLOGY

The exact pathophysiology of PCOS and its manifestations remains unknown and seems to involve multiple pathways. PCOS is more prevalent among first degree relatives of patients with PCOS. Around >100 genes have been evaluated and the syndrome seems to result from the effect of environmental factors superimposed on a susceptible genetic background. An inherent ovarian dysfunction is suggested and factors such as sedentary lifestyle, access to calorie-dense foods, obesity, insulin resistance, prenatal androgen exposure during early gestation, low birth weight or macrosomia, precocious pubarche, endocrine disruptors, and stress also play a role.

Insulin resistance has been strongly associated with the pathogenesis of PCOS, even in lean women. Hyperinsulinemic-euglycemic clamp studies suggest that most women with PCOS have some degree of insulin resistance; almost 80% obese women and 30–40% of lean women with PCOS demonstrate insulin resistance. It is postulated that insulin resistance in PCOS entails a selective resistance to the metabolic effects of insulin due to altered post-receptor signaling and impaired tyrosine phosphorylation. However, serine phosphorylation and sensitivity to mitogenic effects are maintained. Therefore, unlike metabolic tissues including liver, adipose tissue, and skeletal muscle, the ovaries remain sensitive to insulin in PCOS.

Insulin resistance and resultant compensatory hyperinsulinemia play an important role in the pathogenesis of clinical manifestations of PCOS. In addition, it is associated with a chronic inflammatory state. Hyperinsulinemia can directly stimulate ovarian androgen production. This effect is further augmented by increase in gonadotropin-releasing hormone (GnRH) pulse amplitude and frequency, resulting in luteinizing hormone (LH) hypersecretion. In addition, androgen excess leads to recruitment of more primordial follicles, their premature luteinization and arrest as antral follicles. Insulin resistance is further associated with increased insulin-like growth factor-1 (IGF-1) production and decreased IGF binding protein-1 (IGFBP-1) secretion from the liver; with IGF-1 further acting similar to insulin on the ovaries. Sex hormone binding globulin (SHBG) secretion is reduced leading to more bioavailable testosterone.

Another postulated mechanism implicated in the pathogenesis of PCOS is an exaggerated GnRH pulsatility resulting in LH hypersecretion. Polycystic ovaries are overtly sensitive to LH stimulation, which leads to follicular arrest and increased androgen formation.

## CLINICAL PRESENTATION

The classic components of PCOS phenotype include ovulatory dysfunction, hyperandrogenism or metabolic dysfunction. Clinical presentation of PCOS varies across different ethnicities and evolves across various age groups. Menstrual irregularities and hyperandrogenic symptoms such as hirsutism, acne, seborrhea or alopecia are the common presentations in adolescence and young adults, followed by concerns related to subfertility. However, as women age, the concern shifts toward long-term cardiometabolic health and cancer risk. It has been suggested that ethnicity-specific guidelines for diagnosis of PCOS need to be developed as the phenotype may vary from one ethnic group to another.

### Ovulatory Dysfunction

Ovulatory dysfunction may present as delayed menarche, menstrual irregularities, amenorrhea or subfertility/infertility. Irregular menstrual cycles in the first year following menarche are considered physiological, as part of the pubertal transition. Persistent irregular cycles are suggestive of oligo-anovulation and are defined as:
- *1–3 years post-menarche:* <21 days or >45 days
- *3 years post-menarche to perimenopause:* <21 days or >35 days or <8 cycles per year
- *1 year post-menarche:* >90 days for any one cycle
- Primary amenorrhea by age 15 years or >3 years post-thelarche.

In most women, menstrual cycle history is indicative of anovulation and tests for ovulation confirmation are not generally required, but some patients may have regular cycles despite anovulation. In these women, mid-luteal serum progesterone may be used to assess ovulation. Ovulatory dysfunction may also present with primary or secondary infertility.

### Hyperandrogenism

Hyperandrogenism may be clinical or biochemical:
- Clinical hyperandrogenism presents as hirsutism (presence of excessive terminal hair in a male pattern distribution), acne, androgenic alopecia, or seborrhea. Hirsutism is generally more severe in women with central obesity and has been considered to be predictive of metabolic complications and poor response to infertility treatment. Androgenic alopecia generally occurs at a later age and is less common. Virilizing symptoms such as clitoromegaly, masculinization or voice change are rare in PCOS and should raise the suspicion of other hyperandrogenic disorders.
- Biochemical hyperandrogenism is defined as elevated serum androgen levels including total testosterone, free or bioavailable testosterone or other androgens such as dehydroepiandrosterone sulfate (DHEAS).

### Obesity

A significant proportion of adolescent girls and women with PCOS are overweight or obese with body mass index (BMI) >25 kg/m$^2$; the percentage varying from 35 to 80%. The predominant pattern is an increase in abdominal and ectopic fat. Abdominal obesity (elevated waist circumference) contributes to hyperandrogenemia. Obesity further aggravates both reproductive and metabolic dysfunction and negatively affects response to treatment.

## Metabolic Dysfunction

Insulin resistance is one of the hallmarks in many patients with PCOS. Almost 50% women have a family history of type 2 diabetes mellitus (T2DM). Women with PCOS are at increased risk of impaired glucose tolerance (IGT) and T2DM that manifests at an earlier age than non-PCOS women. The prevalence of IGT and T2DM is 30–40% and 10%, respectively in the reproductive age and rises with age. Overall risk for T2DM is increased by 2- to 3-fold; this risk rises to 3- to 5-fold with concomitant obesity. In the initial stages, postprandial hyperglycemia predominates and fasting serum glucose or glycosylated hemoglobin (HbA1c) may be unable to detect hyperglycemia. There is a more rapid rate of progression from IGT to T2DM; >50% IGT women with PCOS progress to overt diabetes within 10 years. The risk of gestational diabetes mellitus (GDM), preeclampsia, and preterm delivery is also higher in women with PCOS.

## Cardiovascular Risk

There is an almost 2-fold increase in the prevalence of metabolic syndrome. Almost 70% PCOS women have borderline or overt lipid abnormalities with a pattern of hypertriglyceridemia, elevated low-density lipoprotein cholesterol (LDL-C), and reduced high-density lipoprotein cholesterol (HDL-C). Studies have demonstrated increased levels of cardiovascular risk markers such as high-sensitivity C-reactive protein, lipoprotein A, and tumor necrosis factor $\alpha$; and higher carotid artery intima media thickness and coronary artery calcium scores. While the prevalence of cardiovascular risk markers is increased, the relationship of PCOS with cardiovascular disease has not been clearly established in prospective studies.

## Other Comorbidities

Polycystic ovary syndrome is also associated with increased prevalence of nonalcoholic fatty liver disease (NAFLD), mood disorders, and depression as well as obstructive sleep apnea (OSA).

## Endometrial Cancer

The risk for endometrial cancer was found to be 3.5-fold higher in PCOS due to prolonged exposure to unopposed estrogen. Since then, numerous studies have confirmed that relative risk is 2- to 6-fold and it generally presents before menopause. Risk factors for endometrial cancer in PCOS include nulliparity and infertility, higher hirsutism score, oligomenorrhea (<4 cycles per year), obesity, and T2DM.

## DIFFERENTIAL DIAGNOSIS OF PCOS

Although PCOS is a common endocrine disorder, it is considered a diagnosis of exclusion and other causes of ovulatory dysfunction with hyperandrogenism need to be excluded. Most common of these include hypothyroidism and hyperprolactinemia. Other less common disorders are nonclassic congenital adrenal hyperplasia (NCAH), androgen-secreting tumors of the ovaries or adrenals, and Cushing's syndrome. In women presenting with amenorrhea, it is important to rule out pregnancy, primary ovarian failure, and functional amenorrhea. In a patient presenting with rapid onset features of hyperandrogenism, particularly virilization (male pattern baldness, clitoromegaly, masculinization of voice, etc.), it is important to exclude androgen-secreting tumors.

## DIAGNOSTIC CRITERIA AND PCOS PHENOTYPES

Several expert groups have proposed varying diagnostic criteria for PCOS over the decades, often leading to confusion. The most commonly used criteria include the Rotterdam consensus criteria given by the European Society of Human Reproduction and Embryology (ESHRE), the American Society of Reproductive Medicine (ASRM), National Institute of Health (NIH), and the Androgen Excess Society (AES) criteria. In general, the prevalence of PCOS is higher when using the 2003 Rotterdam criteria than 1990 NIH criteria. These are summarized in **Table 1**. The AES recognizes the presence of clinical or biochemical hyperandrogenism as a mandatory criterion for the diagnosis of PCOS, thus excluding nonhyperandrogenic phenotypes. All diagnostic criteria require that other diseases with similar presentation be ruled out.

To minimize the confusion within clinical practice due to variable diagnostic criteria, NIH organized a PCOS workshop in 2012 with 29 experts. They recommended using the Rotterdam criteria along with a classification into four phenotypes: A, B, C, and D, as depicted in **Table 2**. Phenotypes A and B, characterized by both oligo/anovulation and hyperandrogenism, are considered more severe and have been strongly associated with cardiovascular risk. The prevalence of different phenotypes varies across ethnic groups. Ganie MA et al. from North India reported two distinct phenotypes—obese hyperinsulinemic women with dysglycemia and lean hyperandrogenic women.

## DIAGNOSTIC APPROACH TO PCOS

Evaluation of an individual should begin with clinical history, physical examination, and appropriate laboratory evaluation to rule out secondary causes.

**TABLE 1:** Diagnostic criteria for polycystic ovary syndrome.

| National Institute of Health (NIH) criteria, 1990 | Rotterdam criteria, 2003 | Androgen Excess Society (AES), 2006 |
|---|---|---|
| 1. Oligo-anovulation and<br>2. Clinical or biochemical hyperandrogenism | At least 2 out of 3:<br>1. Chronic oligo-anovulation<br>2. Clinical or biochemical hyperandrogenism<br>3. Polycystic ovaries on ultrasound | Clinical or biochemical hyperandrogenism and at least 1 out of 2:<br>1. Chronic oligo-anovulation<br>2. Polycystic ovaries on ultrasound |

All diagnostic criteria require exclusion of the secondary causes of polycystic ovary syndrome.

**TABLE 2:** Phenotypes of polycystic ovary syndrome.

| Diagnostic criteria | Phenotype A | Phenotype B | Phenotype C | Phenotype D |
|---|---|---|---|---|
| Oligo/anovulation | + | + | – | + |
| Hyperandrogenism | + | + | + | – |
| Polycystic ovaries | + | – | + | + |
| | Classic PCOS | Essential NIH criteria | Ovulatory PCOS | Nonhyper-androgenic PCOS |

(NIH: National Institute of Health; PCOS: polycystic ovary syndrome)

# CHAPTER 3: Polycystic Ovary Syndrome: A Multifaceted Endocrinopathy

## Clinical History

Clinical history should be taken with regards to age of menarche, menstrual cycle regularity and its duration, hirsutism, acne, fluctuations in weight, and other associated diseases or previous/current medications. It is also important to note the age of onset, rate of progression, and change in symptoms with treatment. Lifestyle parameters such as diet, physical activity, smoking, etc., should be assessed. Past history including symptoms of depression, medication and family history of PCOS, hirsutism, T2DM, and premature cardiovascular disease (<55 years in a male relative; <65 years in a female relative) should also be noted.

## Physical Examination

A detailed physical examination should focus on evaluation for obesity (BMI, waist circumference), insulin resistance (acanthosis nigricans, skin tags), hyperandrogenic features (acne, hirsutism score, alopecia, seborrhea), and blood pressure. Clinically, hirsutism is commonly assessed and scored by the modified Ferriman–Gallwey hirsutism scoring system as depicted in **Figure 2**. It considers the nine most androgen-sensitive areas of the body and assigns scores from 0 (no hair) to 4 (terminal hair as in males). These areas include upper lip, chin, chest, upper abdomen, thighs, back, arm, and buttocks. Total score is calculated by adding the individual nine scores. Score of 8-15 is defined as mild hirsutism, 15-26 as moderate, and 26-36 as severe hirsutism. Only terminal hair growing >5 mm if untreated and pigmented are considered. Ludwig visual score is used for assessing the degree and distribution of alopecia.

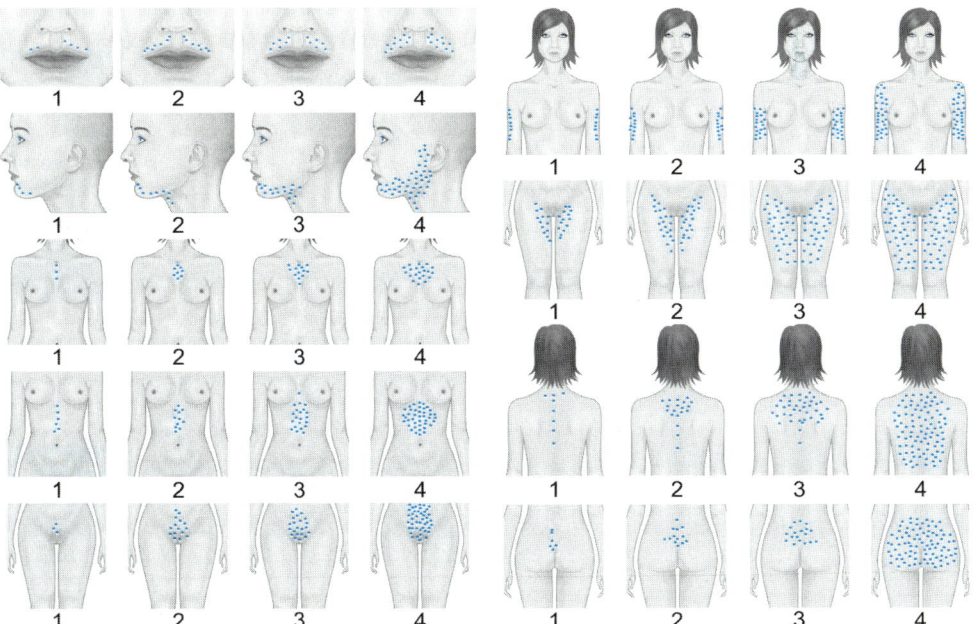

**FIG. 2:** Modified Ferriman–Gallwey scoring system for hirsutism.
Score of 8–15: Mild hirsutism, 15–26: Moderate hirsutism, and 26–36: Severe hirsutism.

In patients having history of rapid onset worsening of hyperandrogenism, features of virilization should be noted (clitoromegaly, deep voice, masculine body habitus). Clinical features raising the suspicion of Cushing's syndrome such as moon facies, prominent supraclavicular fat pad, violaceous striae, proximal muscle weakness, etc., should also be noted when present.

In **Table 3**, we summarize the relevant aspects of clinical history and physical examination.

## Radiological Evaluation

If patient has irregular cycles and hyperandrogenism, ultrasound is not necessary for diagnosis of PCOS but may be supportive in defining the phenotype. Polycystic ovaries on ultrasound demonstrate numerous ovarian follicles. Polycystic ovary morphology as per Rotterdam criteria is defined as an ovarian follicle count ≥12 follicles, of 2–9 mm in size, and/or increased ovarian volume >10 mL, in either ovary, in the absence of a dominant follicle.

**TABLE 3:** Clinical history and physical examination in women with PCOS.

| History | |
|---|---|
| Menstrual history | • Age at menarche<br>• Cycle regularity<br>• Duration |
| Cutaneous manifestations | • Acne<br>• Hirsutism |
| Lifestyle parameters | • Diet<br>• Physical activity<br>• Weight fluctuation<br>• Smoking |
| Past history | • Diabetes mellitus<br>• Hypertension/CVD<br>• Medication<br>• Depression/Anxiety |
| Family history | • PCOS/Hirsutism<br>• Metabolic diseases<br>• Premature CAD |
| **Physical examination** | |
| Obesity | • BMI<br>• Waist circumference |
| Blood pressure | • Every 6 months |
| Hirsutism | • Modified FG score |
| Alopecia | • Ludwig visual score |
| Acne | • Recurrent, refractory or severe |
| Virilization | • Clitoromegaly<br>• Deep voice<br>• Male habitus |

(BMI: body mass index; CAD: coronary artery disease; CVD: cardiovascular disease; FG: Ferriman–Gallwey; PCOS: polycystic ovary syndrome)

The American Society of Reproductive Medicine recommends that transvaginal ultrasound should be preferred in sexually active women and ultrasound should not be used in those with <1 year after menarche. If using newer endovaginal transducers with frequency bandwidth 8 MHz, follicle number per ovary of ≥25 should be considered. In women with extended periods of amenorrhea, ultrasound may be repeated to diagnose endometrial hyperplasia and cancer (not recommended routinely in all patients).

## Laboratory Evaluation

Laboratory investigations should focus on establishing biochemical hyperandrogenism (if not clinically evident), evaluating for secondary causes, and assessing for comorbid conditions such as IGT, T2DM or dyslipidemia.

For biochemical hyperandrogenism, free testosterone or bioavailable testosterone is recommended, using high quality assays such as liquid chromatography-mass spectrometry and extraction/chromatography immunoassays. However, since these assays are not readily available and the current commercial assays are highly unreliable, total testosterone is most commonly used. Simultaneous measurement of SHBG, which is often reduced in PCOS, can be helpful in calculation of free androgen index (FAI) which is calculated as the ratio of total testosterone to SHBG.

Free androgen index = total testosterone (nmol/L) × 100/SHBG (nmol/L)

Elevated total or free testosterone or FAI >5 is a key diagnostic feature of biochemical hyperandrogenism. Measurement of DHEAS and androstenedione levels may be considered if testosterone levels are not elevated.

Serum anti-Müllerian hormone (AMH) is a new biomarker that is considered a surrogate marker of antral follicle count. The levels have been found to be elevated in PCOS and its measurement may be helpful in the absence of reliable ultrasound. However, there is a lack of international standard assays and adequate normative data and it is not routinely used in the evaluation of PCOS.

Measurement of LH and follicle-stimulating hormone (FSH) is no longer considered in the diagnosis of PCOS, but may help in differentiation from primary ovarian failure. Thyroid functions, serum prolactin, and 17-hydroxyprogesterone levels should be measured to exclude hypothyroidism, hyperprolactinemia, and NCAH. In addition, other rare diseases may lead to similar symptoms and appropriate evaluation is needed if there are clinical indicators. **Table 4** summarizes specific case-specific endocrine evaluation for secondary causes when suspected.

Additional evaluation should focus on screening for comorbid conditions, as summarized in **Table 5**. Oral glucose tolerance test with 75 g glucose is recommended for all PCOS patients (including adolescents). Measurement of fasting serum glucose or HbA1c may miss a substantial number of women with IGT, which is the earliest abnormality. If normal, repeat screening should be done every 1–3 years or earlier if patient gains substantial weight or develops symptoms of diabetes. Measurement of fasting lipid profile is also recommended. Assessment of liver functions and ultrasound abdomen for evidence of NAFLD should be considered in women with metabolic risk factors. If symptoms are suggestive of OSA, polysomnography should be considered. In women with prolonged unopposed estrogen exposure, endometrial biopsy may be required to rule out endometrial hyperplasia. Data supports that women with severe oligo-ovulation are at higher risk of endometrial hyperplasia and endometrial cancer. To reduce this risk, women should have a minimum of four withdrawal bleeds per year.

## SECTION 2: Endocrinology

**TABLE 4:** Investigations to rule out diseases having similar presentation as PCOS.

| Disorders that may mimic PCOS | Laboratory evaluation |
|---|---|
| Hypothyroidism | Thyroid function |
| Hyperprolactinemia | Serum prolactin |
| Nonclassic congenital adrenal hyperplasia | Basal 17OHP (during early follicular phase)<br>If borderline—ACTH stimulated 17OHP |
| Pregnancy | Serum or urine hCG |
| Androgen secreting tumor | • Serum testosterone<br>• DHEAS<br>• USG ovaries<br>• CECT or MRI abdomen and pelvis |
| Cushing's syndrome | • Overnight dexamethasone suppression test<br>• 24-h urinary free cortisol<br>• Late night salivary cortisol |
| Primary ovarian failure | • Serum FSH<br>• Serum estradiol |
| Hypothalamic amenorrhea | • Serum FSH<br>• Serum LH<br>• Serum estradiol |

(17OHP: 17-hydroxyprogesterone; ACTH: adrenocorticotropic hormone; CECT: contrast-enhanced computed tomography; DHEAS: dehydroepiandrosterone sulfate; hCG: human chorionic gonadotropin; FSH: follicle-stimulating hormone; LH: luteinizing hormone; MRI: magnetic resonance imaging; PCOS: polycystic ovary syndrome; USG: ultrasonography)

**TABLE 5:** Investigations for associated complications in PCOS.

| Comorbidity | When to screen | How to screen |
|---|---|---|
| Type 2 diabetes mellitus | All patients | • Oral glucose tolerance test<br>• Reassess every 1–3 years |
| Cardiovascular risk | All patients | • Weight and body mass index<br>• Blood pressure<br>• Lipid profile |
| Obstructive sleep apnea | If symptomatic<br>• Snoring<br>• Waking tired from sleep<br>• Daytime sleepiness<br>• Fatigue | • Polysomnography |
| Endometrial cancer | • Prolonged amenorrhea (<4 cycles per year)<br>• Abnormal uterine bleeding | • USG endometrium<br>• Endometrial biopsy |

(PCOS: polycystic ovary syndrome; USG: ultrasonography)

## MANAGEMENT

Polycystic ovary syndrome is not a life-threatening condition, but can cause a lot of distress and psychosocial issues. As the symptoms vary over a spectrum, there is no single best treatment. Treatment should be tailored according to the presenting phenotype, troubling symptoms, and whether patient desires pregnancy or not.

## Lifestyle Modification and Weight Reduction

Since insulin resistance and obesity contribute to ovulatory dysfunction and metabolic complications, so lifestyle modification is of utmost importance. In addition to improving metabolic parameters, about 5–10% weight loss itself can decrease serum androgen levels thus improving ovulation, menstrual irregularities, and even fertility in addition to improving metabolic parameters.

Diet modification and physical activity form the cornerstone of weight management plan in women with PCOS. Obese patients should be suggested calorie-restricted diets and moderate-to-high intensity exercise to reduce weight.

- Healthy eating principles should be followed lifelong. No specific food is considered better than the other and diet advice should be individualized based on food preferences and allowing flexibility.
- Physical activity should be realistic and include activities of daily living (household chores, leisure activity, transportation such as walking or cycling, occupational work) as well as structured aerobic activity.
- Pharmacological therapy for obesity (orlistat, lorcaserin, phentermine-topiramate extended release, or liraglutide) and bariatric surgery may be used if lifestyle modification fails to achieve desired weight loss.

## Management of Menstrual Irregularity

### Hormonal Therapy

- Oral contraceptive pills (OCPs) are recommended as first choice agents to treat menstrual irregularities and hirsutism in women not desiring pregnancy. Most commonly used agents are the combination low-dose oral contraceptives. Both estrogen and progestin suppress LH secretion and reduce ovarian androgen production. In addition, estrogen increases SHBG, thus reducing bioavailable androgens. Among progestins, drospirenone, cyproterone acetate, and dienogest have anti-androgenic potential. Other progestins have androgenic potential which is variable. Norethindrone, levonorgestrel, and norgestrel are more androgenic as compared to desogestrel and norgestimate. But trials have failed to show any significant difference in testosterone levels with the use of different progestins.

    Oral contraceptive pills should be used cautiously in women >40 years (>35 years if smoker), hypertension (controlled or uncontrolled), dyslipidemia, unexplained vaginal bleeding, and women with diabetes >20 years duration or having microvascular complications.
- Progestin-only pills or intrauterine devices may be used, especially for endometrial protection against prolonged estrogen exposure, but they are associated with abnormal bleeding patterns.

## Metformin

Metformin can be used as second line therapy for menstrual irregularity in women who do not tolerate hormonal contraceptives or when they are contraindicated. However, its efficacy is limited.

## Inositol

There is limited data with myo-inositol and d-chiro inositol. The use of these agents is currently not recommended and it is still considered an experimental therapy.

There is no defined interval of time for which therapy is required; treatment is usually prolonged.

# Management of Hirsutism

- First line of treatment remains oral contraceptives. Treatment has to be continued for at least 6 months before benefits are visible and is often required long-term.
- Anti-androgens should be considered for hirsutism if there is inadequate response to oral contraceptives or they cannot be used and there is cosmetic therapy failure (tried for at least 6 months). These agents must be used with effective contraception due to potential for fetal toxicity.
    - *Spironolactone*: Aldosterone antagonist having anti-androgenic action (dose 100–200 mg/day in two divided doses).
    - *Flutamide*: Androgen receptor antagonist (Dose: 62.5–250 mg/day), potentially hepatotoxic, so not recommended over long-term.
    - *Finasteride*: 5α reductase type 2 inhibitor (Dose: 2.5–5 mg/day).
- Additional topical therapy includes use of eflornithine ointment and cosmetic treatments such as laser and intense pulse light ablation or electrolysis of hair follicles.

# Fertility Management

- Ovulation induction with letrozole, clomiphene citrate or other estrogen modulators is recommended as the first line treatment to treat anovulation in PCOS. Prolonged use should be avoided in unsuccessful cases.
- Metformin may be used as adjuvant therapy to prevent hyperstimulation in women undergoing in vitro fertilization (IVF).
- Gonadotropins are required in women who fail to conceive on ovulation induction therapy. Gonadotropins are expensive, not easily available, need intensive ultrasound monitoring, and increase the likelihood of multiple pregnancy.
- Laparoscopic ovarian surgery may be used in women with anovulatory infertility and clomiphene resistance.
- In vitro fertilization with/without intracytoplasmic sperm injection (ICSI) is considered third line therapy.

# Management of Insulin Resistance and Diabetes

Both metformin and thiazolidinediones have been studied to combat insulin resistance and glucose intolerance in PCOS patients. Metformin is recommended in patients with IGT or T2DM who fail to show improvement with lifestyle modification only. It is not recommended to treat only cutaneous manifestations of PCOS. Thiazolidinediones are best avoided in reproductive age group due to potential teratogenic effects.

## CONCLUSION

Polycystic ovary syndrome has profound medical implications in a woman in her reproductive years and even beyond. A patient of PCOS faces different issues in various phases. She may have early pubarche or menarche, menstrual irregularity, and hyperandrogenic features commencing in adolescence, infertility due to anovulation, subsequently pregnancy complications, and high-risk of miscarriage when she conceives and later metabolic diseases and endometrial cancer. Healthcare professional should be vigilant about long-term health of women with this multifaceted disorder.

## SUGGESTED READING

1. Ding T, Paul JH, Peterson I, Wang FF, Qu F, Baio G, et al. The prevalence of polycystic ovary syndrome in reproductive-aged women of different ethnicity: a systematic review and met-analysis. Oncotarget. 2017;8(56):96351-58.
2. Kabel AM. Polycystic ovarian syndrome: insights into pathogenesis, diagnosis, prognosis, pharmacological and non-pharmacological treatment. J Pharma Reports. 2016;4(1).
3. Bharathi V, Swetha S, Neerajaa J, Madhavica J, Moorthy J, Rekha SN, et al. An epidemiological survey: effect of predisposing factors for PCOS in Indian urban and rural population. MEFS. 2017;22(4):313-6.
4. Rosenfield RL, Ehrmann DA. The pathogenesis of polycystic ovary syndrome (PCOS): The hypothesis of PCOS as functional ovarian hyperandrogenism revisited. Endocr Rev. 2016;37(5):467-520.
5. Balen A. The pathophysiology of polycystic ovary syndrome: trying to understand PCOS and its endocrinology. Best Pract Res Clin Obstet Gynaecol. 2004;18(5):685-706.
6. Teede HJ, Misso ML, Costello MF, Dokras A, Laven J, Moran L, et al. Recommendations from the international evidence-based guideline for the assessment and management of polycystic ovarian syndrome. Fertil Steril. 2018;110(3):364-79.
7. Legro RS, Arslanian SA, Ehrmann DA, Hoeger KM, Murad MH, Pasquali R, et al. Diagnosis and treatment of polycystic ovary syndrome: an Endocrine Society Clinical Practice Guideline. JCEM. 2013;98(12):4565-92.
8. Wild S, Pierpoint T, Jacobs H, McKeigue P. Long-term consequences of polycystic ovary syndrome: results of a 31 year follow-up study. Hum Fertil (Camb). 2000;3(2):101-5.
9. Zawadzki JK, Dunaif A. Diagnostic criteria for polycystic ovary syndrome: Towards a rational approach. In: Dunaif A, Givens JR, Haseltine FP, Merriam GR (Eds). Polycystic ovary syndrome. Boston: Blackwell Scientific Publications;1992. pp. 377-84.
10. Rotterdam ESHRE/ASRM-Sponsored PCOS Consensus Workshop Group. Revised 2003 consensus on diagnostic criteria and long-term health risks related to polycystic ovary syndrome. Fertil Steril. 2004;81(1):19-25.
11. Azziz R, Carmina E, Dewailly D, Diamanti-Kandarakis E, Escobar-Morreale HF, Futterweit W, et al. Criteria for defining polycystic ovary syndrome as a predominantly hyperandrogenic syndrome: An Androgen Excess Society guideline. JCEM. 2006;91(11):4237-45.
12. Ganie MA, Marwaha RK, Dhingra A, Nisar S, Mani K, Masoodi S, et al. Observation of phenotypic variation among Indian women with polycystic ovary syndrome from Delhi and Srinagar. Gynaecol Endocrinol. 2016;32(7):566-70.
13. Eckland CL, Usadi RS. Endocrine and reproductive effects of polycystic ovarian syndrome. Obstet Gynecol Clin N Am. 2015;42(1):55-65.

# Contraception and Women's Health

*Arundhati Dasgupta, Faria Afsana*

## ABSTRACT

Hormonal contraceptives comprise of a very efficient method of contraception, and have been used by hundreds of millions of women around the world for decades. The formulation of contraceptives has changed over this period from high-dose estrogen to low-dose estrogen. While there remains some health concern including risk of breast cancer, cervical cancer, liver dysfunction, and thromboembolism, most of the risks decline substantially over a period of time following the withdrawal of the drug. Apart from having a big role to play in terms of prevention of pregnancy and childbirth-related complications due to its contraceptive action per se, hormonal contraceptives also provide certain other gynecological and nongynecological benefits to the user. Judicious use with individualization of therapy is the key to safe and successful use of hormonal contraception.

## INTRODUCTION

Birth control or contraception has been used since ancient times to prevent unplanned pregnancies and complications resulting from them. Several methods of female contraception have found widespread acceptance across the world as depicted in **Flowchart 1**. Oral contraception seems to be most widely used. In the early 1950s, Carl Djerassi, an Austrian-American chemist had synthesized the first oral contraceptive,

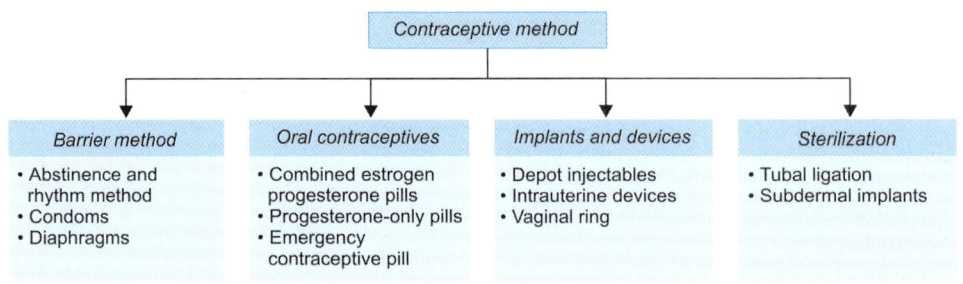

**FLOWCHART 1:** Types of contraceptives used in women.

norethindrone. For decades thereafter, combined oral contraceptives (COCs) have been an extremely effective and popular means of contraception. Data suggest that around 780 million women around the world currently use this method of contraception with the usage being to the tune of 80% in developed countries. There are over 17 different oral contraceptive formulations now available across the world. With the increasing use of COCs, it is important to understand their health implications.

While discussing the long-term health effects of oral contraceptives, it is important to recognize the changing trend in the use of contraceptives. It is important to appreciate the fact that unlike hormone replacement therapy (HRT), COCs use much higher supraphysiological doses of estrogen and progesterone and therefore the health effects of COC are much different from that seen with HRT. However, currently, much smaller doses of more active hormones (5–30 µg of ethinyl estradiol as compared to earlier used doses of 50–60 µg) are being used. In addition, there is increasing use of COCs by younger women to prevent the first pregnancy rather than to space successive pregnancies, thereby resulting in longer years of use. This makes it all the more important to understand the impact that oral contraceptives have on the health of women who use them.

# EFFECT OF ORAL CONTRACEPTIVES ON VARIOUS ORGAN SYSTEMS

## Effect on Glucose Metabolism

Estrogen-progestin combination therapy has been implicated in the development of insulin resistance. While previous data had suggested an association between COC use and glucose intolerance, recent meta-analysis has found significant heterogeneity in the association with glucose levels, fasting glucose to insulin ratios, and homeostatic model assessment-insulin resistance (HOMA-IR). The American College of Obstetricians and Gynecologists (ACOG) recommends that in women with diabetes, the use of COCs be limited to women who are otherwise healthy, do not smoke, are younger than 35 years, and show no evidence of hypertension, nephropathy, retinopathy, or other vascular disease.

## Effect on Lipid Metabolism

Estrogen, in general, has a favorable effect on lipid metabolism. The estrogen component of COCs enhances the removal of low-density lipoprotein cholesterol (LDL-C) by reducing the degradation of LDL receptors and inhibiting proprotein convertase subtilisin kinase-9 (PCSK-9) enzyme. Estrogen also increases the levels of high-density lipoprotein cholesterol (HDL-C). However, estrogen can also cause an increase in serum triglycerides. The effect of progestin component on lipid metabolism is varied and depends on the type and the dose of progestin being used. Progestins may adversely impact lipid health via their action on androgen receptors. More androgenic progestins may have a negative effect on total and LDL-C, while less androgenic progestins or those with antiandrogenic effects have minimal effects on lipids.

Serum triglyceride levels have been seen to rise with COC use and COCs need to be used cautiously in women with baseline hypertriglyceridemia. Fasting serum lipid levels need to be monitored after initiation of COC in women with dyslipidemia. Alternative forms of contraception should be considered for women with uncontrolled LDL-C (≥160 mg/dL) or multiple cardiovascular risk factors.

## Effect on Cardiovascular Health

A major concern with the use of COCs has been their association with thromboembolic risk. Estrogen increases the levels of procoagulant factors such as fibrinogen, factors VII, VIII, and X, and plasminogen while it decreases the levels of antithrombin III, protein S, and plasminogen activator inhibitor-1 (PAI-1) and mediates activated protein C resistance. The net effect of these procoagulant and anticoagulant changes is a small increase in coagulation raising the concern about increase in cardiovascular disease (CVD). The risk of vascular thromboembolism (VTE) is largely attributed to the type of progestin used—risk is higher among the third- and fourth-generation progestins desogestrel, drospirenone, gestodene, and cyproterone acetate as compared to second-generation progestin levonorgestrel.

Data suggest that women with known dyslipidemias using COC may be at increased risk for myocardial infarction (MI) and may experience a minimal increase in stroke risk. The risk profile varies between second and third-generation pills. While VTE seems to be somewhat more prevalent with third-generation pills, the risk of MI is higher among second-generation pill users. The relative risk of MI increases as estrogen dose rises, increasing by 60% with doses of 20 µg and more than doubling when doses of 50 µg or more are used. Risk of MI does not vary with the type or generation of progestin.

Before prescribing COCs, patients should be screened for other cardiovascular risk factors including hypertension, diabetes, and dyslipidemia. Appropriate management of these risk factors is required, as the combination of COC and multiple cardiovascular risk factors has been found to significantly increase cardiovascular event rates. In women with high cardiovascular risks, progesterone only pills are better than COCs.

In women who are postpartum, as the hypercoagulable condition persists for weeks after childbirth, it is advisable to defer the use of oral contraceptives containing estrogen until 4 weeks postpartum. However, as hypercoagulability is not a concern with depot medroxyprogesterone acetate (DMPA) and progestin-only pills, their use at 6 weeks postpartum in lactating women and immediately after delivery in nonlactating women is reasonable.

## Effect on Blood Pressure

The use of oral contraceptives (including newer agents) may increase blood pressure by as much as 8 mm Hg systolic and 6 mm Hg diastolic. In women who are non-smokers, have controlled hypertension and no signs of end-organ disease, a trial of COCs may be appropriate as long as the patient is otherwise healthy. If blood pressure remains controlled, COCs may be continued. Progestin-only contraceptives are, however, better options in women with hypertension.

## Effect on Brain and Neurocognitive Health

Recent data suggests that hormonal contraceptives influence neurohormones, neurotransmitters, and neuropeptides in the brain and impact emotional, cognitive, social, and sexual behavior. However, the net impact of these actions is yet to be understood. COCs have been found to be an independent risk factor for ischemic stroke in some studies. But recent studies and meta-analysis indicate that low-dose estrogen preparations (i.e., preparations containing <50 µg of estrogen) have not been associated with an increased risk of stroke in the absence of migraine. ACOG and the WHO state that in women with migraine, the use of combination estrogen-progesterone contraception may be considered for those who are healthy, <35 years, without aura, and nonsmokers. Progesterone-only contraceptives are safe for use in women who have migraine with aura, even in the presence of other risk factors for stroke.

However, it is important to understand that pregnancy likely poses a far greater cardiovascular risk to women than does the use of estrogen-containing contraception, even in the high-risk group of migraineurs with aura. Pregnancy, delivery, and more importantly the postpartum period is associated with a significantly elevated relative risk (RR) of both ischemic (RR = 8.7) and hemorrhagic (RR = 28.3) stroke.

## Effect on the Liver

Older higher-dose formulations of COCs have been associated with elevated liver enzymes. However, this effect is not commonly observed with current formulations. COCs may cause mild inhibition of bilirubin excretion, leading to jaundice in patients with inherited disorders like Dubin–Johnson syndrome. COCs may also be associated with cholestatic liver injury which appears to be related to inhibition of bilirubin and bile acid secretion and typically occurs within the first few months of therapy. The cholestasis associated with COCs is typically mild and resolves rapidly with discontinuation of the drug. Several reports of hepatic adenomas have been linked to prolonged COC use with the reported risk being around 0.5% per year. Other associations include gall bladder disease, Budd–Chiari syndrome, and peliosis hepatis.

## Effect on Bone Health

In general, HRT in hypogonadal or menopausal women is strongly associated with improvements in bone mass. However, the reports are to the contrary when progesterone only or low-dose estrogen-progesterone contraceptive pills are used in early years. The reason being that these formulations suppress the synthesis and secretion of ovarian estradiol, which is required for bone health. Data on DMPA has shown that in women who had attained peak bone mass, DMPA use was associated with reduced bone mineral density (BMD) and in those who had not yet attained peak bone mass (adolescents and young women), it impaired the acquisition of BMD. In longitudinal studies of adults and adolescents, approximately 5–7% of bone was reported to be lost. However, the rate of loss appeared to decrease over time and BMD increased after discontinuation of the drug and within a 2–3-year period, recovered to the level of a comparable non-DMPA user population. Low-dose estrogen combination COCs have also been associated with lower BMD in adolescent and young women users. A study looking at the association between COC use and fracture risk consisting of women aged between 25 and 65 years, that contributed 484,083 women-years of follow-up found that the group of ever-users of COCs were more likely to have a fracture than never-users. However, a Cochrane review concluded that with existing evidence, the effect of hormonal contraceptives on fracture risk cannot be determined.

## Effect on Mortality

A long-term follow-up of a prospective cohort in the Nurses' Health Study analyzed the association between COC use and mortality after 36 years. There was no significant difference in the rate of mortality amongst ever-users and never-users. A sub-analysis of the study proved that most of the results pertained to first-generation pills with higher hormone doses, rather than the presently used third and fourth generation lower estrogen formulations.

In the light of mortality analyses, the benefits of using oral contraceptives in drastically reducing maternal mortality by lowering the chance of pregnancy and its complications as well as reducing the risk of having an unsafe abortion should also be kept in mind. The World Health Organization (WHO) has recently estimated that over 295,000 women died during and following pregnancy and childbirth in 2017. With a worldwide estimate of 36–53 million induced abortions performed each year, between 125,000 and 170,000 women die each year because of unsafe abortions.

In **Table 1**, we summarize the WHO Medical Eligibility Criteria for the use of hormonal contraceptives in women with obesity, hypertension, dyslipidemia, diabetes, and/or high cardiovascular risk.

**TABLE 1:** WHO eligibility criteria for hormonal contraceptives.

|  | Combined oral contraceptive | Combined contraceptive patch | Combined contraceptive vaginal ring | Combined injectable contraceptives | Progesterone-only pill |
|---|---|---|---|---|---|
| *Obesity* | | | | | |
| • BMI >30 kg/m$^2$ | 2 | 2 | 2 | 2 | 1 |
| *Hypertension* | | | | | |
| • BP adequately controlled | 3 | 3 | 3 | 3 | 1 |
| • Uncontrolled or vascular disease | 4 | 4 | 4 | 4 | 2 |
| *Dyslipidemia* | | | | | |
| • With no other risk factors | 2 | 2 | 2 | 2 | 2 |
| • With other risk factors | 3/4 | 3/4 | 3/4 | 2 | 2 |
| *Diabetes* | | | | | |
| • No vascular disease | 2 | 2 | 2 | 2 | 2 |
| • Nephropathy, retinopathy, or other vascular disease or duration >20 years | 3/4 | 3/4 | 3 | 2 | 2 |
| *Cardiovascular disease* | | | | | |
| • Multiple CV risk factors | 3/4 | 3/4 | 3/4 | 3/4 | 2 |
| • Established CVD | 4 | 4 | 4 | 4 | 2 |

*Note:* Medical eligibility criteria (MEC) categories for contraceptive use include:
- Category 1: Condition for which there is no restriction for the use of the contraceptive method.
- Category 2: Condition where advantages of using the method generally outweigh theoretical or proven risks.
- Category 3: condition where theoretical or proven risks usually outweigh advantages of using the method.
- Category 4: condition which represents an unacceptable health risk if the contraceptive method is used.

(BMI: body mass index; BP: blood pressure; CVD: cardiovascular disease; WHO: World Health Organization)

## NONCONTRACEPTIVE HEALTH BENEFITS OF ORAL CONTRACEPTIVE PILL

It is becoming increasingly evident that besides being well-established contraceptives, COCs seem to have a positive role to play in many functional or organic disturbances of the female reproductive axis and also have systemic effects.

- *Gynecological benefits*:
    - *Menstrual irregularities*: Combined oral contraceptives have received Food and Drug Administration (FDA) approval for the treatment of menstrual cyclical disorders. They can also be used to reduce dysmenorrhea and excessive menstrual bleeding.
    - *Ovarian cysts*: By suppressing the hypothalamo-pituitary-ovarian axis, COC offers protection from both follicular and corpus luteum cysts.
    - *Endometriosis/adenomyosis*: Combined pills with a dominant progestogen action can effectively decrease endometriosis-related pain symptoms and have also been found to be effective in reducing the size of endometriosis lesions.
    - *Myoma:* The risk of development of myoma has been found to be significantly reduced among users of combined estrogen/progestogen preparations with constant users showing around 70% reduction and those with a history of usage for 7 years or longer, demonstrating around 50% reduction of myoma size.
    - *Endometrial hyperplasia*: Oral hormonal contraceptives have been successfully used in the prevention and/or treatment of endometrial hyperplasia.
    - *Pelvic inflammatory disease*: WHO's minimal estimate for yearly incidence of bacterial and viral STDs (excluding HIV infection) is 130 million. Oral hormonal contraceptives have been found to reduce the risk of pelvic inflammatory disease (PID) by around 50–60%.
    - *Premenstrual syndrome and premenstrual dysphoric disorder*: Hormonal contraceptives containing drospirenone, which has a strong anti-mineralocorticoid effect, have been used in alleviating premenstrual symptoms that characterize premenstrual syndrome (PMS) and premenstrual dysphoric disorder (PMDD).
    - *Symptoms of hyperandrogenism*: Combined oral contraceptives are the first-line drugs for the management of hyperandrogenic symptoms such as hirsutism, acne, seborrhea or alopecia related to polycystic ovary syndrome or nonclassic congenital adrenal hyperplasia (NCAH). COCs act through multiple mechanisms to counter hyperandrogenism as depicted in **Flowchart 2**. COCs act on the hypothalamic-pituitary axis to reduce the secretion of luteinizing hormone (LH), that in turn reduces follicular arrest and ovarian androgen secretion. Androgen secretion is also reduced by direct effect of COCs on ovarian and adrenal androgen secretion. In addition, estrogen increases levels of sex hormone-binding globulin (SHBG) resulting in reduced amount of free, biologically active androgens and their consequent action on sebaceous glands and hair follicles. Many new preparations of COCs contain progestogens with anti-androgenic activity. These progestogens including cyproterone acetate, dienogest, drospirenone, and chlormadinone acetate, also block the androgen receptor and 5α-reductase activity to inhibit the action of circulating androgens.
    - *Effect on gynecological malignancy risk*: Combined oral contraceptives have differential effect on the risk of gynecological malignancies. They may reduce the risk of ovarian and endometrial cancer, while concerns have been raised over an increased risk of breast cancer. This is discussed in a subsequent section of this chapter.

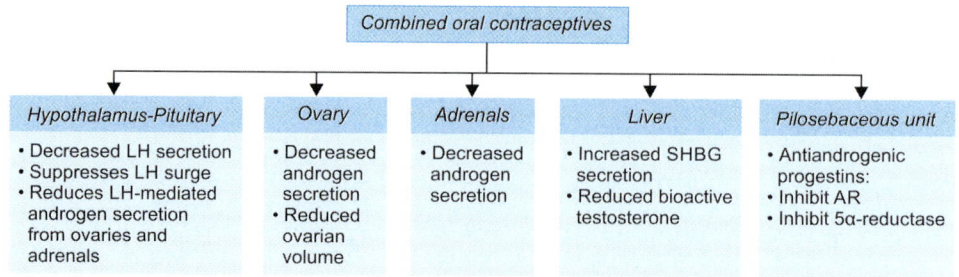

(AR: androgen receptor; LH: luteinizing hormone; SHBG: sex hormone-binding globulin).
**FLOWCHART 2:** Mechanism of action of combined oral contraceptives in hyperandrogenism.

- *Nongynecological benefits*:
  - *Rheumatoid arthritis*: The risk of rheumatoid arthritis has been found to be substantially decreased by about 30% in users of COCs. However, long-term outcome of connective tissue disorders does not seem to be influenced by COC use.
  - *Multiple sclerosis*: Recent reports suggest that the age of occurrence of first symptoms of multiple sclerosis was significantly higher among women who had oral hormonal contraceptives compared to women who did not (onset at 31 years vs. 33 years).

## ORAL CONTRACEPTIVES AND RISK OF MALIGNANCIES

### Ovarian Cancer

Oral contraceptive use has been associated with a 6% reduction in the relative risk of ovarian cancer per year, persisting beyond 15 years of exposure with no difference seen amongst different formulations of COCs. The beneficial effect is evident with even short-term use of as little as 3–6 months; however, marked risk reduction is only achieved after intake for >10 years. A collaborative analysis of 45 epidemiologic studies from worldwide data on combined oral hormonal contraceptives and ovarian cancer has demonstrated that use of COCs decreases the risk of ovarian cancer by 20% after every 5 years of use, a benefit which persisted for >30 years. This analysis calculated that combined COC usage has already prevented around 200,000 ovarian cancers and 100,000 deaths due to ovarian cancer.

The mechanisms hypothesized to cause reduction in the incidence of ovarian cancer include:
- Suppression of ovulation which decreases injury and causes subsequent regression of the ovarian surface epithelium.
- Constant low levels of FSH and LH which subsequently affect the ovarian surface epithelium.

### Endometrial Cancer

Continued use of COCs for at least 1 year has demonstrated a reduction in the risk of endometrial cancer to the tune of 50% as compared to never-users. This protective effect increases with the duration of use and has been seen to persist for >20 or more years after discontinuation.

## Breast Cancer

One major concern related to long-term use of hormonal contraceptives is an elevated risk of breast cancer. Estrogen causes proliferation of breast tissue and would be expected to increase the risk of breast cancer by stimulating growth of stem cells and intermediate cells. On the other hand, while progestin causes alveolar cell growth in the estrogen-primed breast, it also promotes cell differentiation. It is thus unclear whether the net effect would be to increase or decrease breast cancer risk. The Collaborative Group on Hormonal Factors in Breast Cancer, a collaborative reanalysis of individual data of 153,536 women, found a small but significant increase in the relative risk of breast cancer (odds ratio or OR $1.07 \pm 0.02$) but did not identify an increase in risk with increasing duration of use. In fact, after discontinuation of use for >10 years, the risk among users has been considered as equivalent to never-users.

## Cervical Cancer

The Oxford-Family Planning Association study found an elevated risk of cervical cancer among ever-users of oral contraceptives while other studies failed to identify such an association. The International Collaborative of Epidemiological Studies of Cervical Cancer undertook a collaborative patient-level reanalysis of 24 observational studies. The analysis found that there was an excess risk of cervical cancers which increases with duration of use, but this effect declined after stopping oral contraceptive use and was, similar to data about breast cancer, equivalent to the risk of nonusers after 10 years of nonuse.

## Other Cancers

Hormonal contraception has not been found to alter the risk of thyroid, lung, stomach, urinary tract, gallbladder or pancreatic cancer, or the risk of lymphoma, cutaneous melanoma, and tumors of the central nervous system.

### Are there any determinants of cancer risk with oral contraceptive use?
The patterns of cancer risk with the use of hormonal contraceptive use over a women's entire lifetime may be determined by personal factors like gravidity, parity, breastfeeding, etc. The total duration of oral contraceptive use or length of time since the use has been stopped may also modify the risk of cancers associated with oral contraceptives.

## CONCLUSION

It is evident that oral contraceptives have widespread effects on women health that extend far beyond contraception. While the risks of breast and cervical cancer needs to be kept in mind, the overall decrease in pregnancy and childbirth-related complications as well as the other beneficial aspects with the use of COC provide adequate basis for their widespread use. The impact of oral contraceptive use on the metabolism and various organ systems of the body need to be kept in mind while deciding on whether to initiate and continue COCs and to decide on which contraceptive is best suited for the individual.

## SUGGESTED READING

1. Christin-Maitre S. History of oral contraceptive drugs and their use worldwide. Best Pract Res Clin Endocrinol Metab. 2013;27(1):3-12.
2. De Leo V, Musacchio MC, Cappelli V, Piomboni P, Morgante G. Hormonal contraceptives: pharmacology tailored to women's health. Hum Reprod Update. 2016;22(5):634-46.
3. Visser J, Snel M, Van Vliet HA. Hormonal versus non-hormonal contraceptives in women with diabetes mellitus type 1 and 2. Cochrane Database Syst Rev. 2013;(3):CD003990.
4. ACOG practice bulletin No. 206: Use of hormonal contraception in women with coexisting medical conditions. Obstet Gynecol. 2019;133(2):128-50.
5. Bastianelli C, Farris M, Rosato E, Brosens I, Benagiano G. Pharmacodynamics of combined estrogen-progestin oral contraceptives: effects on metabolism. Expert Rev Clin Pharmacol. 2017;10(3):315-26.
6. Gialeraki A, Valsami S, Pittaras T, Panayiotakopoulos G, Politou M. Oral contraceptives and HRT risk of thrombosis. Clin Appl Thromb Hemost. 2018;24(2):217-25.
7. Saguil A. Risk of venous thromboembolism with use of combined oral contraceptives. Am Fam Physician. 2015;91(5):287-8.
8. Edlow AG, Bartz D. Hormonal contraceptive options for women with headache: a review of the evidence. Rev Obstet Gynecol. 2010;3(2):55-65.
9. WHO Medical eligibility criteria for contraceptive use, Fifth edition. WHO. [Online] Available at https://apps.who.int/iris/bitstream/handle/10665/181468/9789241549158_eng.pdf?sequence=9. [Last accessed January, 2020].
10. Ponnatapura J, Kielar A, Burke LMB, Lockhart ME, Abualruz AR, Tappouni R, et al. Hepatic complications of oral contraceptive pills and estrogen on MRI: controversies and update – adenoma and beyond. Magn Reson Imaging. 2019;60:110-21.
11. Lopez LM, Grimes DA, Schulz KF, Curtis KM, Chen M. Steroidal contraceptives: effect on bone fractures in women. Cochrane Database Sys Rev. 2014;(6):CD006033.
12. Charlton BM, Rich-Edwards JW, Colditz GA, Missmer SA, Rosner BA, Hankinson SE, et al. Oral contraceptive use and mortality after 36 years of follow-up in the Nurses' Health Study: prospective cohort study. BMJ. 2014;349:g6356.
13. Schindler AE. Non-contraceptive benefits of oral hormonal contraceptives. Int J Endocrinol Metab. 2013;11(1):41-7.
14. Chiaffarino F, Parazzini F, La Vecchia C, Marsico S, Surace M, Ricci E. Use of oral contraceptives and uterine fibroids: results from a case-control study. Br J Obstet Gynaecol. 1999;106(8):857-60.
15. Gierisch JM, Coeytaux RR, Urrutia RP, Havrilesky LJ, Moorman PG, Lowery WJ, et al. Oral contraceptive use and risk of breast, cervical, colorectal, and endometrial cancers: a systematic review. Cancer Epidemiol Biomarkers Prev. 2013;22(11):1931-43.
16. Amiri M, Kabir A, Nahidi F, Shekofteh M, Ramezani Tehrani F. Effects of combined oral contraceptives on the clinical and biochemical parameters of hyperandrogenism in patients with polycystic ovary syndrome: a systematic review and meta-analysis. Eur J Contracept Reprod Health Care. 2018;23(1):64-77.
17. Helvaci N, Yildiz BO. Oral contraceptives in polycystic ovary syndrome. Minerva Endocrinol. 2014;39(3):175-87.
18. Holmqvist ST, Hammar M, Lindblom AM, Brynhildsen J. Age at onset of multiple sclerosis is correlated to use of combined oral hormonal contraceptives and child birth before diagnosis. Fert Steril. 2010;94:2835-7.
19. Beral V, Doll R, Hermon C, Peto R, Reeves G. Ovarian cancer and oral contraceptives: collaborative reanalysis of data from 45 epidemiological studies including 23,257 women with ovarian cancer and 87,303 controls. Lancet. 2008;371(9609):303-14.
20. Breast cancer and hormone replacement therapy: collaborative reanalysis of data from 51 epidemiological studies of 52,705 women with breast cancer and 108,411 women without breast cancer. Collaborative Group on Hormonal Factors in Breast Cancer. Lancet. 1997;350(9084):1047-59.
21. Appleby P, Beral V, Berrington de González A, Colin D, Franceschi S, Goodhill A, et al. International Collaboration of Epidemiological Studies of Cervical Cancer. Cervical cancer and hormonal contraceptives: collaborative reanalysis of individual data for 16,573 women with cervical cancer and 35,509 women without cervical cancer from 24 epidemiological studies. Lancet. 2007;370(9599):1609-21.

# CHAPTER 5

# Health Issues during Menopausal Transition

*Tejal Lathia, Than Than Aye*

## ABSTRACT

The menopausal transition is a critical period in a woman's life that poses unique health challenges. Diabetes and menopause are irretrievably linked and the menopausal transition is a window of opportunity to screen women for diabetes and emphasize the benefits of lifestyle modification for prevention of diabetes. Women undergoing surgical menopause need special attention. Hormone therapy, if initiated, is safe from a diabetes perspective.

Osteoporosis is a major issue in menopausal women. Appropriate risk stratification based on dual-energy X-ray absorptiometry (DXA) and country specific fracture-risk assessment (FRAX) scores with timely initiation of treatment is imperative to prevent fractures. Overt hypothyroidism needs to be treated but initiation of levothyroxine in subclinical hypothyroidism (SCH) needs to be carefully considered in menopausal women due to lack of clear evidence of benefits and risk of iatrogenic thyrotoxicosis. Postmenopausal hyperandrogenism is of cosmetic importance to most women. However, it is important to exclude androgen-secreting tumors.

## INTRODUCTION

Menopause is a signal event in a woman's life that marks the end of reproductive competence. It is a retrospective diagnosis, which can only be made with certainty with absence of menses for a year or more. Menopause heralds significant cardiometabolic, neurocognitive, and skeletal changes. In this chapter, we discuss some of the key health issues that arise at the time of menopausal transition and after.

## THE MENOPAUSAL TRANSITION

Menopausal transition signals a time of reproductive aging in women that begins earlier than the actual cessation of menstruation or the final menopausal period (FMP). Reproductive aging results from a progressive decline in ovarian follicle pool, which becomes accelerated toward the end.

*The menopausal transition includes the following phases*:
- As the secretion of gonadal hormones and reproductive competence of the gonads begins to decline, there is an initial rise in follicle stimulating hormone (FSH) and

luteinizing hormone (LH) due to compensatory response of the hypothalamic-pituitary-ovarian axis. A decline in the secretion of inhibin B leads to a loss of negative feedback of FSH secretion.
- This is followed by significant variability in ovarian hormone secretion and follicle development. Typical menopausal symptoms may appear intermittently in this time.
- The final phase is characterized by low estrogen levels resulting from persistently low ovarian hormone secretion, and cessation of menstrual cycles.

## Age at Menopause

The mean menopausal age of the Indian women as interpreted from a pan-India survey conducted by the Indian Menopause Society is 46.2 ± 4.9 years. Multiple regression analysis showed a positive correlation between natural menopause age and marital status, marriage duration, socioeconomic status, education, and body mass index. A negative correlation was observed between natural menopause age and parity status.

## Other Endocrine Changes with Menopause

There are a host of physical and psychological changes that a woman undergoes at the time of menopause. Menopause is characterized by a change from gynoid pattern to android pattern of fat distribution with an increase in central adiposity rather than an increase in body weight per se. Along with an increase in visceral adiposity, menopausal women also demonstrate an increase in pro-inflammatory markers, suggesting that adiposity is associated with a chronic inflammatory state. The levels of sex hormone binding globulin (SHBG) also tend to decrease in parallel with rise in visceral fat, unfavorable adipocytokine profile, and insulin resistance. Low SHBG levels have been found to be an independent marker of insulin resistance, increased risk of diabetes mellitus, and cardiovascular disease (CVD) in postmenopausal women. However, this relationship has not been demonstrated consistently. Often, thyroid dysfunction is held responsible for the weight gain and thyroid medications may be initiated in the hope of weight loss. It is important to assess if levothyroxine replacement in subclinical hypothyroidism (SCH) would really have benefits in postmenopausal women.

On an average, a woman loses up to 5% of her bone mass in the first 5 years after menopause. It is important to recognize osteoporosis and assess women for fracture risk, while at the same time exclude secondary causes such as hyperparathyroidism. Many menopausal women experience some degree of hyperandrogenism with increase in facial hair and loss of scalp hair. While in most, this is a cosmetic concern, androgen-secreting tumors should be carefully ruled out.

## MENOPAUSE AND DIABETES

Most women struggle with weight gain during the menopausal transition. This primarily results from the altered hormonal milieu that characterizes menopause. In addition to an increase in total body fat, there occurs an increase in abdominal and visceral fat, leading to an unfavorable adipocytokine profile, chronic inflammation, and oxidative stress.

A retrospective study showed that weight increase around pregnancy and menopause correlated significantly with higher odds for the diagnosis of diabetes and/or hypertension. Midlife women are at significant diabetes risk due to the high prevalence of excess adiposity, insulin resistance, and disorders that contribute separately to diabetes risk such as sleep disorders and depression.

It is well known that there are gender differences in the burden of complications of diabetes. Several large epidemiological studies and meta-analyses have assessed the risk of coronary heart disease and stroke with diabetes in women versus men. There is compelling evidence to suggest that risk of coronary heart disease is 44% greater in women with diabetes than men with diabetes, while the risk of stroke is 27% greater. This risk remains even adjusting for other sex-specific major risk factors for CVD.

Thus, weight redistribution with increase in total body fat may predispose a woman to diabetes and the complications of diabetes tend to be more severe for women. Menopause is a golden window where early diagnosis of diabetes is feasible and this window must not be missed.

The timing of menopause, the type of menopause, and the treatment of vasomotor symptoms with hormonal therapy all impact diabetes and are important to consider.

## Timing of Menopause

In the prospective, population-based Rotterdam study that followed 3,639 postmenopausal women for 9.2 years, 348 women developed incident type 2 diabetes mellitus (T2DM). After adjustment for confounders, hazard ratios (HRs) for T2DM were 3.7 [95% confidence interval (CI) 1.8–7.5] 2.4 (95% CI 1.3–4.3), and 1.60 (95% CI 1.0–2.8) for women with premature (<40 years), early (40–45 years), and normal (>45 years) menopause, respectively, relative to those with late menopause ($p < 0.001$). In contrast, a study by Qiu et al. found no association of age at menarche or menopause with diabetes though higher menopause age was associated with decreasing CVD risk ($p = 0.020$) and earlier menopause (46 years) with significantly higher osteoporosis risk (odds ratio 1.59, 95% CI 1.07–2.36, $p = 0.023$).

Women with earlier menopause require focused screening, appropriate counseling and strategies for prevention must be in place to prevent T2DM. It is well known that early intensive glucose lowering reduces the risk of microvascular and macrovascular complications of diabetes.

## Type of Menopause: Natural versus Surgical

The NHEFS (National Health and Nutrition Examination Survey-I Epidemiological Follow-up Study) evaluated the data of 2,597 postmenopausal women. Over a period of 9.2 years, the incidence of new-onset diabetes was 7.4 cases/1,000 person-years for women with no history of surgical menopause, while it was 8.2/1,000 person-years for women who had undergone hysterectomy alone and 8.5/1,000 person-years who had undergone hysterectomy with bilateral salpingo-oophorectomy (BSO). When assessed for confounding factors, the risk of diabetes was found to be elevated only in women who had undergone hysterectomy with BSO (HR 1.57, 95% CI 1.03–2.41).

This suggests that the risk of diabetes is increased with surgical menopause in women who have both the ovaries removed as compared to those in whom ovaries were left intact. The preservation of ovaries, if feasible, mitigates the risk of diabetes to a certain extent and must be given due consideration prior to planning surgery.

## Impact of Hormonal Therapy on Diabetes

Hormone replacement therapy (HRT) is used to treat severe vasomotor symptoms that may accompany the menopause transition. It is now clear that HRT can be safely given to early menopausal women [<10 years since menopause (YSM)], <60 years of age,

> **BOX 1** **Menopause and diabetes: Summary points.**
> - Early menopause increases the risk of type 2 diabetes mellitus
> - Surgical menopause increases the risk of diabetes which is partially mitigated by the preservation of ovaries
> - There is conflicting evidence as to whether diabetes leads to early menopause
> - In women with severe vasomotor symptoms, it is safe to give hormone replacement therapy especially if they are <60 years of age within 10 years of menopause and are at low-risk of VTE, CVD, and breast cancer
> - HRT reduces the risk of diabetes in women without pre-existing diabetes
> - HRT does not worsen diabetes risk and may improve glycemia in women with pre-existing diabetes
>
> (CVD: cardiovascular disease; HRT: hormone replacement therapy, VTE: venous thromboembolism)

with low-risk of breast cancer and CVD, if they are willing to take HRT. However, the Endocrine Society guidelines for the treatment of symptoms of menopause recommend using systemic HRT with caution in women with diabetes.

- *Without pre-existing diabetes*: Salpeter et al. reviewed 107 randomized trials that compared menopausal hormone therapy (MHT) to placebo or no treatment in nondiabetic women. They reported lower fasting plasma glucose and insulin levels in MHT users, with a 13% reduction in insulin resistance, measured by Homeostatic Model Assessment of Insulin Resistance (HOMA-IR). The incidence of new-onset diabetes was reduced by 30%. It was also observed that the beneficial metabolic effects of estrogen were attenuated when simultaneous progesterone was being administered.
- *With pre-existing diabetes:* Several placebo-controlled randomized trials have evaluated the effect of oral conjugated estrogen (CE) or estradiol (E2) in postmenopausal women with diabetes. The use of estrogen was associated with reduction in insulin resistance, fasting plasma glucose, and glycosylated hemoglobin (HbA1c) but not postprandial glucose values. A decrease in HbA1c along with reduced hepatic glucose production (HGP) was also observed in another study using oral E2 in postmenopausal diabetic women. However, most of these studies have been of short duration with smaller number of subjects and evaluated the role of estrogen alone.

It has been suggested that oral estrogen, particularly CE, has a greater beneficial effect on insulin resistance compared to transdermal E2 preparation. This is possibly because oral estrogen undergoes first-pass metabolism and has a greater effect on the suppression of hepatic glucose output.

Though HRT is not recommended for the prevention of diabetes, if HRT is needed for a woman for severe vasomotor symptoms, it can be safely used without fear of worsening diabetes. There is also very little data on the effect of HRT on complications of diabetes. It may be prudent to use other nonhormonal alternatives such as selective serotonin reuptake inhibitors for the treatment of vasomotor symptoms in patients already suffering from diabetes complications. We summarize the salient points related to diabetes and menopause in **Box 1**.

## MENOPAUSE AND CARDIOVASCULAR HEALTH

Though cardiovascular health in postmenopausal women is outside the purview of this chapter, the issue of cardiovascular health comes into focus when hormone therapy is to be initiated for women in early menopause.

Menopausal hormone therapy can be considered in women who are <60 years of age and <10 years postmenopausal, if required for troublesome menopausal symptoms. However, several factors should be taken into consideration when deciding whether to use MHT in such individuals including an assessment of the baseline risk of CVD. If MHT is being considered, the type of MHT to be used, its dose, and route of administration (oral versus transdermal) should also be individualized based on cardiovascular risk. The Menopause Decision-Support Algorithm can be used for the same. It begins with the calculation of the American College of Cardiology/American Heart Association (ACC/AHA) 10-year CVD risk. Age since menopause is an additional factor that helps stratify women as those in whom MHT use is associated with low, intermediate, or high-risk.

Those women who are deemed to be at low-risk (<5%) can be prescribed MHT. In those who are at intermediate risk (5–10%), transdermal estrogen alone is preferred over oral estrogen if there is no uterus. If a woman has intact uterus, micronized progesterone is added as this has less adverse impact on carbohydrate and lipid metabolism or blood pressure. Other factors that should be considered for risk stratification include family history of CVD, coronary artery calcium score, ankle-brachial pressure index, and C-reactive protein.

Menopausal hormone therapy should be avoided in women at high-risk (>10%). In addition to ACC/AHA risk score, other factors that put a woman at high-risk include previous history of acute coronary syndrome, cerebrovascular or peripheral artery disease, aortic aneurysm, diabetes or chronic kidney disease. In all high-risk women, if there are troublesome vasomotor symptoms, nonhormonal therapies only should be considered

## MENOPAUSE AND OSTEOPOROSIS

The Food and Agriculture Organization (FAO) and World Health Organization (WHO) recommend total daily calcium intake of 1,000–1,300 mg/day. However, most Asian countries have average calcium intake below these recommended values with a mean of 450 mg/day. In addition, studies from most countries of South and South East Asia also show a high prevalence of vitamin D insufficiency and deficiency in both men and women and across all age groups. This is associated with a detrimental impact on bone health.

Menopause is an important event in a woman's life cycle that affects bone health with the prevalence of osteoporosis and osteopenia increasing with increasing years since menopause. Postmenopausal osteoporosis is a well-studied and established phenomenon. However, appropriate screening and timely intervention are still not performed.

A study by Khadilkar et al. from Pune, India to estimate prevalence of osteoporosis above 40 years of age showed that men had similar bone mineral density (BMD) values at each age group compared to premenopausal women up to the age of 50 years. Postmenopause, there was a significant sharp decline in BMD noted for women. This indicates that rapid bone loss may occur during menopausal transition. In men, a gradual decline in BMD was observed at the lumbar spine till the 55–60 years age group indicating that men also undergo bone loss but at a later age than women.

This warrants that adequate precaution should be taken during menopausal years to prevent osteoporosis during later years, as age-related bone loss is a continuous process throughout life. However, osteoporosis remains greatly underdiagnosed and undertreated in Asia, even in the most high-risk patients who have already fractured. The problem is particularly acute in rural areas where hip fractures are often treated conservatively. In addition, dual-energy X-ray absorptiometry (DXA) technology is relatively expensive and not widely available.

## Treatment of Osteoporosis in Menopausal Women

The Endocrine Society guidelines recommend that all postmenopausal women who are at high-risk of fractures should be treated, especially if they have had a recent osteoporotic fracture. The benefits of antiosteoporosis therapies in such women clearly outweigh the risks of pharmacological treatment. In addition, one must consider other patient-specific factors as well patient preferences when deciding the choice of treatment.

If there is a history of previous spine or hip fracture, or BMD T-score at the hip or spine is ≤ −2.5, or 10-year hip fracture risk is >3%, or the risk of major osteoporotic fracture on the country-specific fracture-risk assessment (FRAX) score is >20%, the individual is considered at "high-risk." If there is history of multiple spine fractures or a BMD T-score at the spine or hip is ≤ −2.5, the individual is categorized as "very high-risk".

Postmenopausal women who are at high fracture risk can be treated initially with bisphosphonates (alendronate, risedronate, zoledronic acid or ibandronate). Bisphosphonate therapy can reduce fracture risk in such individuals. However, ibandronate does not reduce nonvertebral or hip fracture risk. When a woman is on bisphosphonates, fracture risk is to be reassessed after 3–5 years of continued treatment. If the risk of fractures remains to be high, pharmacological treatment is continued. In those women where risk is reduced to low or moderate risk, a "bisphosphonate holiday" can be considered.

Another option to bisphosphonates in postmenopausal women at high-risk of osteoporotic fractures is denosumab. When denosumab is started, fracture risk should be reassessed after 5–10 years of therapy. If fracture risk remains persistently high, denosumab is continued or a switch is made to other osteoporosis therapies. If denosumab is discontinued, antiresorptive treatment (bisphosphonates, hormone therapy or selective estrogen receptor modulator) should be started to prevent a rebound increase in bone turnover that could lead to a rapid decline in BMD and a rise in fracture risk.

For postmenopausal women who have osteoporosis and are at very high-risk of fractures, initial treatment with teriparatide or abaloparatide for up to 2 years is a better approach as it reduces the risk of both vertebral and nonvertebral fractures. This is especially useful in women with history of severe or multiple vertebral fractures. After completion of teriparatide or abaloparatide, antiresorptive drug treatment is continued to ensure that bone density gains during previous treatment are maintained.

Selective estrogen receptor modulators (SERMs), HRT or tibolone are not routinely recommended for the management of postmenopausal osteoporosis. Their use is considered in women who do not tolerate bisphosphonates, denosumab or teriparatide/abaloparatide or in whom these medications are contraindicated. SERMs should not be used if a woman has high-risk of deep vein thrombosis (DVT), but will offer additional advantage in women at risk of breast cancer. HRT use is restricted to women who are younger than 60 years and <10 years postmenopausal, have low-risk of DVT, low cardiovascular risk, low-risk of breast cancer, and have bothersome vasomotor or other menopausal symptoms.

## THYROID AND MENOPAUSE

Etiology and management of thyroid disease, especially primary hypothyroidism and overt hyperthyroidism, does not differ substantially in the menopausal woman as compared with younger women. However, some dilemmas are encountered in the menopausal group—what is the thyroid-stimulating hormone (TSH) level at which treatment should be initiated for SCH and what should be the TSH target during treatment? It is imperative to avoid iatrogenic thyrotoxicosis to prevent worsening of osteoporosis in women going through the menopausal transition. Similarly, what level of low TSH warrants treatment? Does subclinical hyperthyroidism need to be treated at all in menopausal women?

## Subclinical Hypothyroidism

The weight redistribution and early physical and psychological symptoms of the menopausal transition mimic the signs and symptoms of hypothyroidism. This prompts many women to take a TSH test. Often these values are in the SCH range (normal free T4 but elevated TSH).

A recent clinical practice guideline based on a systematic review issued a strong recommendation against thyroxine replacement in adults with SCH. The reason for this was that no important differences were found in patients offered thyroxine replacement in the subclinical range for the following parameters: General quality of life, thyroid related symptoms, fatigue/tiredness or depression. No significant differences were found for cognitive function, mortality or cardiovascular events. Though there was no harm with initiation of therapy but no benefit was demonstrated either. Initiation of treatment often sets up expectation of weight loss which does not occur. On the other hand, the need for regular testing, doctor visits, and medications increase, as does the risk of overtreatment.

## Subclinical Hyperthyroidism

While the overall burden of subclinical hyperthyroidism is low, it poses specific challenges in postmenopausal women. The risks of subclinical hyperthyroidism, especially with a TSH <0.1 mIU/mL include increased risk of atrial fibrillation, overall mortality, cardiovascular mortality, and reduction in BMD in postmenopausal women. The American Thyroid Association (ATA) clinical practice guidelines recommend detailed evaluation and treatment for subclinical hyperthyroidism when TSH is persistently below 0.1 in all individuals above 65 years of age, those who have cardiovascular risk factors or CVD, osteoporosis, or postmenopausal women not on any HRT or bisphosphonates, and in individuals with symptoms.

## POSTMENOPAUSAL HYPERANDROGENISM

The menopausal transition is associated with a gradual decline in circulating androgen levels. However, with a rise in LH levels that occur in menopause, it can lead to increased secretion of androgens from the ovaries as well adrenals. In addition, peripheral conversion of androgens also contributes to the circulating pool of androgens. Therefore, in some pathological states, the serum concentrations of androgens are elevated after menopause. The most common of these is polycystic ovary syndrome and we enlist other causes of postmenopausal hyperandrogenism is **Table 1**.

Women who present with hyperandrogenic features should be evaluated clinically and with appropriate laboratory tests, including measurement of serum total, free or bioavailable testosterone and dehydroepiandrosterone sulfate (DHEAS) levels. If total testosterone is significantly elevated (>150 ng/dL), it should raise the suspicion of androgen-secreting tumors, usually of the ovaries. Similarly, if DHEAS levels are >700 µg/dL, adrenal tumor needs to be excluded. Therefore, in women who have rapid onset of symptoms or virilizing symptoms and very high levels of androgens, suitable imaging studies including transvaginal ultrasound and magnetic resonance imaging (MRI) for ovaries and adrenals should be considered. Treatment depends on the cause of the postmenopausal hyperandrogenism.

**TABLE 1:** Causes of postmenopausal hyperandrogenism.

| Nontumorous/Functional | Tumorous |
|---|---|
| • Polycystic ovary syndrome<br>• Obesity<br>• Nonclassic congenital adrenal hyperplasia<br>• Cushing's syndrome<br>• Acromegaly<br>• Ovarian hyperthecosis<br>• Drug use or abuse | • Adrenocortical cancer<br>• Adrenal benign adenomas<br>• Ovarian sex-cord stromal tumors<br>• Metastases to ovary |

## ADRENOCORTICAL AXIS AND MENOPAUSE

Some studies such as the Seattle Midlife Women's Health Study suggest that cortisol levels increase during later stage of menopausal transition. The significance of such changes in adrenocortical function and their association with vasomotor symptoms remain to be determined. DHEAS levels decline with age and DHEA supplementation has been attempted in postmenopausal women with the aim of improving metabolic and musculoskeletal health. However, most studies have demonstrated no benefits of DHEA supplementation.

## NEUROCOGNITIVE HEALTH

Neurocognitive health of perimenopausal women was assessed in the cross-sectional study of Women's Health Across the Nation (SWAN). This included a large sample of 12,425 women between 40 and 55 years age; self-reported forgetfulness was very common in this population which had a large percentage of perimenopausal women. When adjusted for factors such as ethnicity, age, socioeconomic status, education, marital status, parity, health habits, body weight, and symptoms of depression or anxiety, perimenopausal women reported forgetfulness more commonly than premenopausal women. On the other hand, interventional studies have not reported any sustained or consistent benefit of MHT on neurocognitive function. The WHIMS of Younger Women (WHIMSY) failed to demonstrate any benefit of CE-based MHT on cognitive function in postmenopausal women between the age of 50–55 years.

Depression has also been commonly reported during the menopausal transition, with studies reporting rates as high as 15–50%. These have been attributed to both direct effect of hormonal changes as well as the vasomotor symptoms. Quite often, the diagnosis of clinical depression may be overlooked as the symptoms may get attributed to menopause, per se. There is a need to be vigilant of this possibility. However, the effect of hormonal therapy on mood is not well-established and depression should be appropriately treated with psychological counseling and appropriate antidepressant pharmacological treatment, as necessary.

The Cache County Study including 1,768 postmenopausal women examined the effect of MHT on the risk of Alzheimer's disease (AD) and reported that women who took MHT within 5 years of menopause had a 30% lower risk of AD in later life, especially if they had continued MHT for 10 or more years. Similar findings were reported in the KEEPS (Kronos Early Estrogen Prevention Study), where MHT use during perimenopausal period was associated with reduced future risk of neurodegenerative diseases including mild cognitive impairment and AD. Women who took oral CE also performed better in measures of depression, anxiety or memory recall than placebo.

## CONCLUSION

Menopausal women face a host of endocrinologic changes during the transition. The approach to treatment differs in this group of often-neglected women. Focused sensitization of all healthcare personnel about common problems in menopausal women of this age range can help improve their quality of life.

## SUGGESTED READING

1. Hall JE. Endocrinology of the Menopause. Endocrinol Metab Clin N Am. 2015;44(3):485-96.
2. Ahuja M. Age of menopause and determinants of menopause age: A PAN India survey by IMS. J Midlife Health. 2016;7(3):126-31.
3. Davis SR, Castelo-Branco C, Chedraui P, Lumsden MA, Nappi RE, Shah D, et al. Understanding weight gain at menopause. Climacteric. 2012;15(5):419-29.
4. Rurik I, Móczár C, Buono N, Frese T, Kolesnyk P, Mahlmeister J, et al. Early and menopausal weight gain and its relationship with the development of diabetes and hypertension. Exp Clin Endocrinol Diabetes. 2017;125(4):241-50.
5. Kim C. Does menopause increase diabetes risk? Strategies for diabetes prevention in midlife women. Womens Health (Lond). 2012;8(2):155–67.
6. Peters SAE, Huxley RR, Woodward M. Diabetes as risk factor for incident coronary heart disease in women compared with men: a systematic review and meta-analysis of 64 cohorts including 858,507 individuals and 28,203 coronary events. Diabetologia. 2014;57(8):1542-51.
7. Peters SAE, Huxley RR, Woodward M. Diabetes as a risk factor for stroke in women compared with men: a systematic review and meta-analysis of 64 cohorts, including 775,385 individuals and 12,539 strokes. Lancet. 2014;383(9933):1973-80.
8. Muka T, Asllanaj E, Avazverdi N, Jaspers L, Stringa N, Milic J, et al. Age at natural menopause and risk of type 2 diabetes: a prospective cohort study. Diabetologia. 2017;60(10):1951-60.
9. Qiu C, Chen H, Wen J, Zhu P, Lin F, Huang B, et al. Associations between age at menarche and menopause with cardiovascular disease, diabetes, and osteoporosis in Chinese Women. J Clin Endocrinol Metab. 2013;98(4):1612-21.
10. King P, Peacock I, Donnelly R. The UK prospective diabetes study (UKPDS): clinical and therapeutic implications for type 2 diabetes. Br J Clin Pharmacol. 1999;48(5):643-8.
11. Appiah D, Winters SJ, Hornung CA. Bilateral oophorectomy and the risk of incident diabetes in postmenopausal women. Diabetes Care. 2014;37(3):725.
12. Stuenkel CA, Davis SR, Gompel A, Lumsden MA, Murad MH, Pinkerton JV, et al. Treatment of symptoms of the menopause: An Endocrine Society clinical practice guideline. J Clin Endocrinol Metab. 2015;100(11):3975-4011.
13. Salpeter SR, Walsh JME, Ormiston TM, Greyber E, Buckley NS, Salpeter EE. Meta-analysis: effect of hormone-replacement therapy on components of the metabolic syndrome in postmenopausal women. Diabetes Obes Metab. 2006;8(5):538-54.
14. Friday KE, Dong C, Fontenot RU. Conjugated equine estrogen improves glycemic control and blood lipoproteins in postmenopausal women with type 2 diabetes 1. J Clin Endocrinol Metab. 2001;86(1):48-52.
15. Brussaard HE, Leuven JAG, Frölich M, Kluft C, Krans HM. Short-term oestrogen replacement therapy improves insulin resistance, lipids and fibrinolysis in postmenopausal women with NIDDM. Diabetologia. 1997;40(7):843-9.
16. Mauvais-Jarvis F, Manson JE, Stevenson JC, Fonseca VA. Menopausal hormone therapy and type 2 diabetes prevention: Evidence, mechanisms, and clinical implications. Endocrin Rev. 2017;38(3):173-88.

17. Manson JE. Current recommendations: what is the clinician to do? Fertil Steril. 2014;101(4):916-21.
18. Mithal A, Wahl DA, Bonjour J-P, Burckhardt P, Dawson-Hughes B, Eisman JA, et al. Global vitamin D status and determinants of hypovitaminosis D. Osteoporos Int. 2009;20(11):1807-20.
19. Kadam NS, Chiplonkar SA, Khadilkar AV, Khadilkar VV. Prevalence of osteoporosis in apparently healthy adults above 40 years of age in Pune City, India. Indian J Endocr Metab. 2018;22:67-73.
20. Eastell R, Rosen CJ, Black DM, Cheung AM, Murad MH, Shoback D. Pharmacological management of osteoporosis in postmenopausal women: An Endocrine Society clinical practice guideline. J Clin Endocrinol Metab. 2019;104(5):1595-622.
21. Bekkering GE, Agoritsas T, Lytvyn L, Heen AF, Feller M, Moutzouri E, et al. Thyroid hormones treatment for subclinical hypothyroidism: a clinical practice guideline. BMJ. 2019;365:l2006.
22. Ross DS, Burch HB, Cooper DS, Greenlee MC, Laurberg P, Maia AL, et al. 2016 American Thyroid Association Guidelines for diagnosis and management of hyperthyroidism and other causes of thyrotoxicosis. Thyroid. 2016;26(10):1343-421.
23. Woods NF, Mitchell ES, Smith-Dijulio K. Cortisol levels during the menopausal transition and early postmenopause: observations from the Seattle Midlife Women's Health Study. Menopause. 2009;16(4):708-18.
24. Gold EB, Sternfeld B, Kelsey JL, Brown C, Mouton C, Reame N, et al. Relation of demographic and lifestyle factors to symptoms in a multi-racial/ethnic population of women 40-55 years of age. Am J Epidemiol. 2000;152(5):463-73.
25. Espeland MA, Shumaker SA, Leng I, Manson JE, Brown CM, LeBlanc ES, et al. Long-term effects on cognitive function of postmenopausal hormone therapy prescribed to women aged 50 to 55 years. JAMA Intern Med. 2013;173(15):1429-36.
26. Shao H, Breitner JCS, Whitmer RA, Wang J, Hayden K, Wengreen H, et al. Hormone therapy and Alzheimer disease dementia: new findings from the Cache County Study. Neurology. 2012;79(18):1846-52.
27. Wharton W, Gleason CE, Dowling NM, Carlsson CM, Brinton EA, Santoro MN, et al. The KEEPS-Cognitive and Affective Study: baseline associations between vascular risk factors and cognition. J Alzheimers Dis. 2014;40(2):331-41.

# SECTION 3

# Rheumatology

**SECTION EDITORS**
Mohanjeet Kaur, Vikas Gupta

# CHAPTER 1

# Pertinent Rheumatological Issues in Women

*Benzeeta Pinto, Ramya Janardana*

## ABSTRACT

Rheumatic diseases are common in women and occur at every age group. Autoimmune diseases are frequent in the reproductive age group and degenerative in older women. Chronic nonspecific musculoskeletal pain and fibromyalgia are responsible for significant burden in general outpatient department (OPD) patients. Evaluation requires assessment for the cause and appropriate treatment. Pregnancy and lactation are special concerns in women with rheumatic diseases as both disease and drugs may have an impact. Management of these diseases requires early diagnosis and multidisciplinary care to improve outcomes.

## INTRODUCTION

Rheumatic disorders are extremely common in the general population and affect both genders across a wide range of age groups. They encompass diseases affecting the musculoskeletal system and connective tissue due to various etiologies. They are the second leading cause of disability causing significant morbidity with resultant healthcare utilization. More than 150 clinical conditions are included in the list of rheumatic diseases. Rheumatic diseases can be divided into two major groups: Inflammatory rheumatic diseases (IRDs) and noninflammatory rheumatic diseases.

It is well recognized that rheumatic disease especially autoimmune rheumatic diseases are more common in women than in men. Although they can occur at any age, they are particularly common in the reproductive age group and have a significant impact on the quality of life. In addition, there are concerns of the impact of these diseases and treatment on pregnancy and lactation. The recent advances in the management of these diseases including the many new targeted therapies have contributed to decreasing the morbidity and mortality. However, the lack of awareness of these diseases both in the general population and medical fraternity contribute to delayed diagnosis and treatment. In this chapter, we summarize the diagnosis and treatment of common rheumatic disease in women.

# RHEUMATOID ARTHRITIS

Rheumatoid arthritis (RA) is a common disease affecting 0.5–1% of the general population. It is a chronic, multisystem, autoimmune, inflammatory arthritis that primarily affects the joints but can have extra-articular manifestations. The disease is more common in women with a M:F ratio of 1:2. The characteristic clinical feature of RA is chronic, symmetric synovitis involving large and small joints (**Fig. 1**). The axial skeleton other than the cervical spine is classically spared, as are the distal interphalangeal joints. RA is an erosive arthritis and untreated, leads to deformities. Extra-articular features include Sicca syndrome (secondary Sjögren's), ocular manifestations, anemia, Felty's syndrome, pleuritis, pericarditis, interstitial lung disease, and secondary vasculitis. Extra-articular manifestations are more common in long-standing, untreated seropositive disease.

The diagnosis of RA is clinical and supported by laboratory investigations. The American college of rheumatology (ACR)/European league against Rheumatism (EULAR) proposed updated classification criteria in 2010. However, these criteria are primarily for classification and not diagnosis. Of note, rheumatoid factor (RF) and anticyclic citrullinated peptide (anti-CCP) are not essential for diagnosis. RF occurs in 70–80% of patients with RA but they have relatively poor specificity and can occur in other disease like primary Sjögren's, systemic lupus erythematosus (SLE), cryoglobulinemia, and other chronic inflammatory diseases. Hence, the mere presence of RF does not confirm the diagnosis of RA since RF may be positive in many conditions and even normally in older individuals. Anti-CCP has similar sensitivity but much higher specificity (95–98%).

Prompt diagnosis and aggressive treatment by a specialist trained in the management of rheumatic diseases is important to improve outcomes in RA. The backbone of treatment is disease-modifying antirheumatic drugs (DMARDs) (**Table 1**). There are numerous newer treatments in RA including anticytokine therapy (biologic—bDMARDS) and targeted small molecules (ts—targeted synthetic DMARDs). All current guidelines recommend a treat to target approach with frequent assessment of disease activity and titration of DMARDs accordingly, the target being remission or low disease activity. In addition, nonpharmacological interventions, physiotherapy, and psychosocial interventions are necessary to improve quality of life.

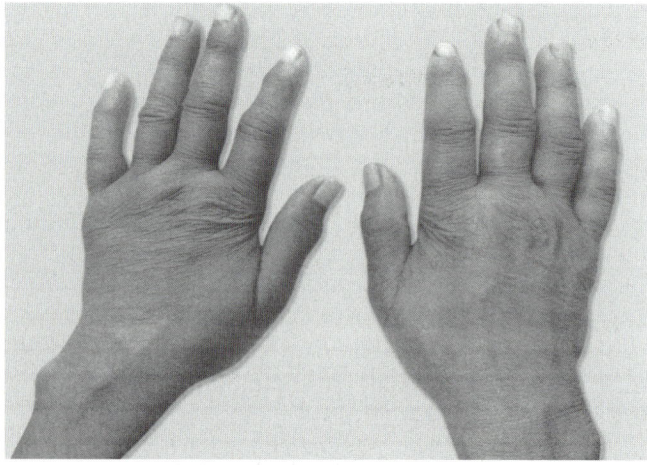

**FIG. 1:** Both hands showing swelling of proximal interphalangeal joints and wrists without deformities. *(For color version, see Plate 5)*

**TABLE 1:** Disease modifying drugs in rheumatoid arthritis.

| Drugs | Route of administration | Dose |
|---|---|---|
| • Conventional DMARDs | | |
|   ○ Methotrexate | Oral/IM or SC | 7.5–25 mg weekly once |
|   ○ Leflunomide | Oral | 20 mg OD |
|   ○ Hydroxychloroquine | Oral | 200–400 mg OD |
|   ○ Sulfasalazine | Oral | 2–3 g/day in divided doses |
| • Biological DMARDs | | |
|   ○ Anti TNFs | | |
|     – Etanercept | SC | 50 mg weekly |
|     – Infliximab | IV | 400 mg every 8 weeks |
|     – Adalimumab | SC | 40 mg every 2 weeks |
|     – Golimumab | SC | 50 mg monthly |
|   ○ Anti CD20 | IV | 1 g × 2 dose or 500 mg × 2 doses |
|     – Rituximab | | |
|   ○ Anti IL-6 | | |
|     – Tocilizumab | IV | 8 mg/kg IV monthly |
| • Targeted synthetic DMARDs | | |
|   ○ Tofacitinib | Oral | 5 mg BD |
|   ○ Baricitinib | Oral | 4 mg OD |

## OSTEOARTHRITIS

Osteoarthritis (OA) is the most important joint disease worldwide affecting 10% of the men and 18% of women above the age of 60 years. Both hand and knee OA are more common in women than men. OA ranges from an asymptomatic radiologic finding to debilitating joint disease. Knee OA is more common in India compared to western countries due to our lifestyle. OA is associated with significant morbidity and loss of function. The most important risk factor for OA is age. Other nonmodifiable risk factors include gender, genetics, and ethnicity. Modifiable risk factors include obesity, muscle strength, injury to the joint, physical activity, and occupation.

Osteoarthritis may affect a single joint or be generalized. OA has a predilection to involve the knees, hips, interphalangeal joints of hand, 1st carpometacarpal joints, 1st metatarsophalangeal joints, apophyseal (facet) joints of the lower cervical, and lower lumbar spine. Heberden's nodes (nodular swellings of DIP) and Bouchard's nodes (nodular swelling of PIP) are features of generalized OA. The symptoms of OA range from joint pain which is worse after exertion, stiffness, functional limitation, and deformity depending on the joints involved.

Management of OA requires both pharmacological and nonpharmacological measures. Exercise to improve neuromuscular balance and gait, weight reduction, lifestyle modifications, and pain relief with topical and oral treatment are important measures. Knee replacement surgery is reserved for severe symptoms not responding to conservative treatment. Several other treatments have been tried both surgical and medical including glucosamine, chondroitin supplements, hyaluronate injections, and regenerative surgical techniques. Most of these are found to have conflicting results in clinical trials and are yet to be approved by regulatory bodies.

# CHRONIC MUSCULOSKELETAL PAIN

Chronic pain is extremely common in the general population and musculoskeletal problems are the most common cause. Chronic pain affects at least 20% of the adult population and is associated with both physical and psychosocial morbidity. It is more common in women than men. Chronic musculoskeletal pain (CMP) may be regional or generalized. Regional pain may be inflammatory or mechanical depending on the cause. OA, inflammatory arthritis, and periarticular conditions are important considerations. Generalized pain may be due to inflammatory causes or fibromyalgia which is characterized by diffuse pains without any specific etiology (**Table 2**). However, many patients with a peripheral nociceptive trigger like OA and inflammatory arthritis may present with diffuse pains and require management for both components.

Fibromyalgia syndrome (FMS) is characterized by chronic widespread musculoskeletal pain and tenderness, mood, and cognitive dysfunction. It occurs in 2–4% of general population and is more common in women. The prevalence of FMS is increased in rheumatic diseases like RA, OA, and primary Sjögren's syndrome. FMS is associated with psychiatric comorbidities like depression, anxiety, and sleep disorders.

Evaluation of CMP should focus on detailed physical examination and directed investigations to identify the cause of pain. The role of vitamin D supplementation in nonspecific CMP is conflicting and most studies do not show a benefit. Non-pharmacological measures such as exercise and physiotherapy and treatment of psychiatric comorbidity are essential for better outcomes.

# OTHER RHEUMATOLOGICAL DISEASES

Spondyloarthropathies (SpA) are a group of inflammatory arthritis that include axial SpA and ankylosing spondylitis, peripheral SpA, psoriatic arthritis, inflammatory bowel diseases associated arthritis, and reactive arthritis. They are more common in men and have common clinical features of sacroiliitis, axial involvement, enthesitis, dactylitis, and asymmetric oligoarthritis. Women tend to have less radiographic damage and there is often a significant delay in diagnosis of SpA in women.

Systemic lupus erythematosus is a heterogenous autoimmune disease that affects women more commonly than men (M:F—1:9). It has multisystem manifestations including constitutional symptoms, joint pains, fatigue, cutaneous rash, hematological, renal, neuropsychiatric, and cardiac involvement. It should be suspected in women of reproductive age group presenting with unexplained multisystem manifestations.

**TABLE 2:** Causes of generalized chronic musculoskeletal pain (CMP).

| Type of CMP | Examples | Mechanism |
| --- | --- | --- |
| Peripheral nociceptive trigger | • Inflammatory arthritis—rheumatoid arthritis, primary Sjögren's syndrome<br>• Degenerative—osteoarthritis chronic low back ache | • Decreased descending analgesic input<br>• Lower pain threshold Central augmentation |
| Centralized pain | Fibromyalgia tension, headache | Disturbance in central processing of pain |

Primary Sjögren's syndrome is a common autoimmune disease with a prevalence 0.3–1/1,000 persons with a female preponderance. The hallmark of the disease is exocrine dysfunction which manifests as dryness of the mouth and eyes. Other symptoms include fatigue and joint pain. Patients may also have involvement of other organs such as interstitial nephritis presenting as distal renal tubular acidosis, palpable purpura, cryoglobulinemia, and obstructive bronchiolitis.

Systemic sclerosis is an uncommon immune-mediated rheumatic disease more common in women than men. It is characterized by thickening and fibrosis of skin and internal organs and vasculopathy. Raynaud's phenomenon is a typical symptom of the vasculopathy. The skin thickening may be diffuse or limited. Internal organ involvement includes gastrointestinal, pulmonary hypertension, interstitial lung disease, and rarely renal crisis.

Gout is an inflammatory arthritis that occurs due to deposition of the monosodium urate crystals in the joints. The prevalence in developed countries is 3–6% in men and 1–2% in women. Women with gout are likely to be older (postmenopausal) and have other etiologies for hyperuricemia like diuretic use or renal failure. Gout usually presents with acute arthritis usually of the first metatarsophalangeal joint which subsides on its own in 1–2 weeks. This is usually preceded by asymptomatic hyperuricemia. Recurrent flares can occur in untreated patients, which become increasingly frequent and prolonged and polyarticular. Advanced gout is associated with tophi or chronic gouty arthritis with structural damage or both can develop in some individuals. Diagnosis is based on typical history and demonstration of monosodium urate crystals in the synovial fluid. The presence of hyperuricemia in a patient with arthritis is not diagnostic of gout as hyperuricemia is common in the general population. This is common error encountered in clinical practice and leads to incorrect diagnosis of other inflammatory and degenerative arthritis as gout. In addition, it must be kept in mind that gout is uncommon in premenopausal women unless there is a secondary cause for hyperuricemia.

Evaluation and treatment of connective tissue diseases is complex and should involve a trained specialist. Early diagnosis and prompt treatment is the key to decreasing mortality and morbidity of these diseases. Treatment in general includes immunosuppression or immunomodulatory drugs, which are decided based on the extent and severity of the disease and organ involvement. The treatment is associated with various side effects including the risk of serious infections. Multidisciplinary care is required in most patients for the best outcomes.

## PREGNANCY AND RHEUMATOLOGICAL ILLNESS

### Fertility in Rheumatic Diseases

Mixed results have been found in various studies regarding time to pregnancy and ovarian reserve in women with rheumatological illnesses. Fertility may not be affected directly by the rheumatological illnesses, however, impaired sexual function both disease related (connective tissue diseases) and due to psychological burden of chronic disease are under recognized by health professionals. Except for cyclophosphamide (CYC), most drugs do not have any irreversible effect on fertility. The risk of CYC related premature gonadal failure increases with age and cumulative dose of the drug administered. Sustained amenorrhea is rare in women under 25 years treated with doses of 3.5–7 g. At a cumulative CYC dose >10 g, women with SLE aged >30 years are at risk of developing premature ovarian failure. NSAIDs can delay or temporarily inhibit ovulation. Prednisolone at doses of >7.5 mg/day can prolong time to pregnancy.

## Pregnancy Risks and Complications

Rheumatoid arthritis disease activity improves during pregnancy in more than half; around 40% have increase in their disease activity during 6 weeks postpartum. Majority of studies describe increased risk of preterm births in RA associated with increased HAQ (health assessment questionnaire) scores. There is no association with congenital birth defects.

The risk for severe disease during pregnancy is increased in women with active SLE in the 6 months prior to conception, in those with repeated flares in the years prior to conception, and in those who discontinue needed medications due to pregnancy. About 81% of large cohort of pregnant lupus patients with inactive or active stable lupus prior to conception had uncomplicated pregnancies. The risks include early pregnancy loss, intrauterine death, prematurity, low birth weight, hypertensive disorders of pregnancy, disease flare, and maternal death.

In addition to disease activity assessment, specific maternal antibody status such as antiphospholipid antibodies (aPL) and antibodies to Ro/La should be assessed in the preconception period; these form part of risk assessment for the future pregnancy. The risk of neonatal lupus, development of complete congenital heart block (CHB) is 2% in high titer Ro/Ro52 positive pregnancies and the recurrence risk is 16–18%. HCQS is safe in pregnancy and its use is associated with reduced risk of flare, recurrence of CHB and aPL antibody- related pregnancy losses during pregnancy.

Considering the above risks, contraceptive advise is of paramount importance in lupus patients who are not suited/ may not tolerate pregnancy during the course of follow-up. Barrier contraception, intrauterine contraceptive device, and surgical sterilization are considered safe. Of the oral contraceptive pills (OCPs), estrogen contains pills are associated with risk of thrombosis in lupus patients with moderate-to-severe disease activity, positive aPLs, and previous thrombotic events. Progesterone only pills are a safer alternative in these situations. In lupus with mild disease activity, aPL antibody negative lupus subjects combined OCPs are considered safe.

## Antiphospholipid Antibody Syndrome and Pregnancy

Antiphospholipid antibody syndrome (APS) is an autoimmune disease characterized by the presence of aPL that predispose to thrombotic and obstetric complications. The three antibodies included in the criteria are lupus anticoagulant (LA), anticardiolipin (ACLA), and beta-2 glycoprotein 1($\beta$2GP1). APS may be primary or associated with other diseases, the most common association being SLE. In addition to the criteria manifestations of recurrent first trimester pregnancy loss, intrauterine deaths due to placental insufficiency, APS is associated with pregnancy-induced hypertension, intrauterine growth restriction, and maternal thrombosis. Depending on the prepregnancy, APS-related complication in the individual patient's heparin is recommended at varying doses; therapeutic dose in patients with thrombotic disease whereas, prophylactic dose in pure obstetric APS. In addition to low-dose aspirin and hydroxychloroquine in all pregnancies. LA positivity, triple positivity (LA, ACLA, and $\beta$2GP1) is associated with increased risk.

## Systemic Sclerosis and Pregnancy

Increased risk of miscarriages and preterm births (26%) more so in long-standing diffuse disease. Overall rate of a successful live birth of 84% in limited and 77% in diffuse scleroderma is reported. Scleroderma activity does not change with pregnancy; however,

**TABLE 3:** Commonly used drugs in rheumatic diseases and safety in pregnancy.

| Preferred | Relatively safe (requires individualized approach) | Contraindicated | Inadequate data to support safety |
|---|---|---|---|
| Glucocorticoids (B) | TNF alpha inhibitors (B) | Methotrexate (X) | Anakinra (B) |
| NSAIDs (B) | Azathioprine (D) | Leflunomide (X) | Abatacept (C) |
| Hydroxychloroquine (C) | Cyclosporine (C) | Cyclophosphamide (D) | Tofacitinib (C) |
| Sulfasalazine (B) | Tacrolimus (NA) | Mycophenolate (D) | Rituximab (C) |
| Low-dose aspirin (NA) | | ERA (NA) | |
| PDE-5 inhibitors (B) | | | |

*Note:* Pregnancy FDA category in () A, B, C, D—FDA pregnancy categories, NA—FDA pregnancy categories not assigned.

it may be a relative contraindication in those with rapidly progressive diffuse disease, moderate-to-severe pulmonary hypertension, and interstitial lung disease. Risk is highest in those with moderate-to-severe pulmonary hypertension. Reflux disease does increase along the course of pregnancy. The prevalence of scleroderma renal crisis in pregnancy is controversial; if suspected, one needs to bear in mind the teratogenic potential of angiotensin-convertase enzyme (ACE) inhibitors in the first trimester.

## Drugs in Pregnancy and Lactation

An extremely important consideration is the safety of medications in pregnancy and lactation. Women should be appropriately counseled about the risk of teratogenicity of various drugs and appropriate family planning measures. Ideally disease should be inactive at the time of planning a pregnancy and the patients should be changed to safer drugs such as low-dose steroids, hydroxychloroquine, sulfasalazine, and azathioprine (**Table 3**).

## CONCLUSION

Rheumatic diseases are common in women and are responsible for significant morbidity. They require appropriate investigations and treatment. With the advent of numerous advances, women with rheumatic diseases can lead a near normal life. Early diagnosis and multidisciplinary management are essential to improve outcomes.

## SUGGESTED READING

1. Jokar M, Jokar M. Prevalence of inflammatory rheumatic diseases in a rheumatologic outpatient clinic: analysis of 12626 cases. Rheumatol Res. 2018;3:21-7.
2. Schuna AA. Autoimmune rheumatic diseases in women. J Am Pharm Assoc (Wash). 2002;42(4):612-23.
3. Smolen JS, Aletaha D, McInnes IB. Rheumatoid arthritis. Lancet. 2016;388(10055):2023-38.
4. Smolen JS, Landewé R, Bijlsma J, Burmester G, Chatzidionysiou K, Dougados M, et al. EULAR recommendations for the management of rheumatoid arthritis with synthetic and biological disease-modifying antirheumatic drugs: 2016 update. Ann Rheum Dis. 2017;76(6):960-77.
5. Johnson VL, Hunter DJ. The epidemiology of osteoarthritis. Best Pract Res Clin Rheumatol. 2014;28(1):5-15.
6. Hunter DJ, Bierma-Zeinstra S. Osteoarthritis. Lancet. 2019;393(10182):1745-59.

7. Lichtenstein A, Tiosano S, Amital H. The complexities of fibromyalgia and its comorbidities. Curr Opin Rheumatol. 2018;30:94-100.
8. Clauw DJ. Diagnosing and treating chronic musculoskeletal pain based on the underlying mechanism(s). Best Pract Res Clin Rheumatol. 2015;29:6-19.
9. Gaikwad M, Vanlint S, Mittinity M, Moseley GL, Stocks N. Does vitamin D supplementation alleviate chronic nonspecific musculoskeletal pain? A systematic review and meta-analysis. Clin Rheumatol. 2017;36(5):1201-8.
10. Tsokos GC. Mechanisms of disease: Systemic lupus erythematosus. N Engl J Med. 2011;365:2110-21.
11. Mariette X, Criswell LA. Primary Sjögren's syndrome. N Engl J Med. 2018;378:931-9.
12. Denton CP, Khanna D. Systemic sclerosis. Lancet. 2017;390:1685-99.
13. Harrold LR, Etzel CJ, Gibofsky A, Kremer JM, Pillinger MH, Saag KG, et al. Sex differences in gout characteristics: Tailoring care for women and men. BMC Musculoskelet. Disord. 2017;18(1):108.
14. Østensen, M. Sexual and reproductive health in rheumatic disease. Nat Rev Rheumatol. 2017;13: 485-93.
15. Morel N, Bachelot A, Chakhtoura Z, Ghillani-Dalbin P, Amoura Z, Galicier L, et al. Study of anti-Müllerian hormone and its relation to the subsequent probability of pregnancy in 112 patients with systemic lupus erythematosus, exposed or not to cyclophosphamide. J Clin Endocrinol Metab. 2013;98:3785-92.
16. Brouwer J, Hazes JMW, Laven JSE, Dolhain RJEM. Fertility in women with rheumatoid arthritis: Influence of disease activity and medication. Ann. Rheum. Dis. 2015;74:1836-41.
17. De Man YA, Dolhain RJEM, Van De Geijn FE, Willemsen SP, Hazes JMW. Disease activity of rheumatoid arthritis during pregnancy: Results from a nationwide prospective study. Arthritis Care Res. 2008;59:1241-8.
18. Clowse MEB, Magder LS, Witter F, Petri M. The impact of increased lupus activity on obstetric outcomes. Arthritis Rheum. 2005;52(2):514-21.
19. Clowse MEB, Magder L, Witter F, Petri M. Hydroxychloroquine in lupus pregnancy. Arthritis Rheum. 2006;54(11):3640-7.
20. Eudy AM, Siega-Riz AM, Engel SM, Franceschini N, Howard AG, Clowse MEB, et al. Effect of pregnancy on disease flares in patients with systemic lupus erythematosus. Ann Rheum Dis. 2018;77(6):855-60.
21. Andreoli L, Bertsias GK, Agmon-Levin N, Brown S, Cervera R, Costedoat-Chalumeau N, et al. EULAR recommendations for women's health and the management of family planning, assisted reproduction, pregnancy and menopause in patients with systemic lupus erythematosus and/or antiphospholipid syndrome. Ann Rheum Dis. 2017;76(3):476-85.
22. Kutteh WH, Hinote CD. Antiphospholipid antibody syndrome. Obstet Gynecol Clin North Am. 2014;41(1):113-32.
23. Steen VD. Pregnancy in women with systemic sclerosis. Obstet Gynecol. 1999;94(1):15-20.

# CHAPTER 2

# Risk of Cardiovascular Events in the Presence of Autoimmune Diseases

*Nupoor Acharya, Debasish Mishra*

## ABSTRACT

Cardiovascular diseases (CVDs) are one of the leading causes of mortality in autoimmune rheumatic diseases and the increased risk of same is associated with heightened proinflammatory state. Both traditional and specific disease-related risk factors are implicated in the increased CVD risk. Various scoring methods, imaging modalities, and biomarkers have been developed to assess the CVD risk, however, each has its own pros and cons. Management strategies aim at primary and secondary prevention of CVD. European League Against Rheumatism (EULAR) recommendations for screening and assessment of CVD risk in autoimmune rheumatic diseases have been developed. Early recognition and treatment of CVD risk factors can reduce preventable mortalities in these diseases.

## INTRODUCTION

Autoimmune diseases are caused due to aberrant immune activation and may involve a single system or more commonly have multisystemic involvement. These diseases are associated with an imbalance between proinflammatory and anti-inflammatory cytokines. This imbalance leads to a persistent inflammatory state. The heightened inflammatory state seen in autoimmune diseases is responsible for the increased cardiovascular risk. Cardiovascular diseases (CVDs) account for a major cause of morbidity and mortality in patients with autoimmune diseases. Several manifestations of CVD are seen in association with rheumatological illnesses and include hypertension, accelerated atherosclerosis, coronary artery disease, cerebrovascular accidents, and peripheral vascular involvement.

## EPIDEMIOLOGY

Autoimmune diseases are associated with increased cardiovascular risk. Rheumatoid arthritis (RA) is associated with 1.5-folds increased risk of coronary artery disease and other CVD outcomes along with mortality. The risk of CVD related mortality is also high in systemic connective tissue diseases such as systemic lupus erythematosus (SLE) and systemic sclerosis (SSc) with a high-risk of mortality (HR–1.5). Incidence of CVD is also high in spondyloarthropathy (SpA) and the risk ranges between 1.5 to 1.6 times (OR–1.6) for different SpA. Inflammatory arthritides are also associated with a slightly increased risk of stroke (HR–1.09).

## PATHOPHYSIOLOGY

- *Proinflammatory cytokines*: These play a major role in the pathogenesis of CVD. The cytokines predominantly involved are tumor necrosis factor alpha (TNF-α), interleukins 1 and 6, and C-reactive protein (CRP). This proinflammatory state leads to increased levels of low-density lipoprotein (LDL), very low-density lipoprotein (VLDL), lipoprotein (a) (LpA), hypercoagulability, and platelet dysfunction. This in turn leads to accelerated atherosclerosis, increased carotid intima medial thickness (cIMT), plaque rupture, and endothelial dysfunction.
- *Accelerated atherosclerosis*: Diseases such as RA, SLE, SpA, antiphospholipid syndrome (APS), and SSc are associated with accelerated atherosclerosis.
- *Proliferative obliteration*: Connective tissue diseases are associated with proliferative arteriopathy that may lead to obliteration of vessels, leading to coronary artery disease, pulmonary artery hypertension, and peripheral vascular disease. Few of the diseases associated with obliterative vasculopathy are SSc, mixed connective tissue disease (MCTD), SLE, and overlap syndromes.
- *Autoantibody*: Circulating autoantibodies may directly attack the antigens present on vessel wall leading to a cascade of reactions that ultimately leads to atherosclerosis, thrombosis, and coagulation abnormalities. This is seen in association with disease such as SLE, anti-phospholipid syndrome, and other autoimmune diseases.
- *Coronary arteritis*: Apart from accelerated atherosclerosis, coronary arteritis is another cause for myocardial ischemia and increased cardiovascular morbidity. Vasculitis syndromes such as Takayasu arteritis, Kawasaki disease, giant cell arteritis, polyarteritis nodosa, SLE, other primary or secondary vasculitis, are the diseases that can manifest as coronary arteritis.
- *Myocarditis*: Inflammatory processes involving the myocardium are seen in association with various systemic autoimmune diseases, such as, SLE, MCTD, Takayasu arteritis, macrophage activation syndrome, vasculitides, and other connective tissue disease. These may lead to cardiomyopathy, arrhythmias, and heart failure.

## DISEASE-SPECIFIC RISK FACTORS

There are certain traditional and nontraditional risk factors that are associated with CVD in patients with autoimmune disease. The important traditional risk factors are obesity, dyslipidemia, diabetes, hypertension, and smoking; all are associated with an increased CV risk in patients with underlying autoimmune diseases. Apart from the traditional risk factors associated with CVD, autoimmune diseases add to the risk of CVD due to nontraditional risk factors. They are listed as following.

### Rheumatoid Arthritis

There are multiple risk factors that play an important role in CVD in RA. Disease flare in RA is associated with a peculiar metabolic state known as lipid paradox. The paradoxical effect is the nonlinear relationship between cholesterol levels and cardiovascular risk. The lower total cholesterol and higher high-density lipoprotein (HDL) are associated with increased risk of CVD. High inflammatory markers, i.e., high erythrocyte sedimentation rate (ESR) and CRP suggests active inflammation and are associated with higher CVD risk. High disease activity is also associated with persistently high inflammation and increased risk of CVD. There is an increased risk of having CVD with an odds ratio (OR) of 1.61 and 2.59 for moderate and high disease activity in RA. The cytokine milieu in RA favors a proinflammatory phenotype. Proinflammatory cytokines are associated with atherogenesis leading to increased CV risk. The presence of rheumatoid factor and anti-citrullinated peptide antibodies (ACPA) have shown inconsistent association with increased cardiovascular risk, though ACPA may have a stronger correlation with CV risk. Drugs used in the treatment of RA also have an impact on the underlying CVD risk. Methotrexate, hydroxychloroquine, and TNF inhibitors reduce the CVD risk by negatively affecting the proinflammatory state. The nonsteroidal anti-inflammatory drugs (NSAIDs), steroids and other biologicals such as tocilizumab (an IL-6R inhibitor) and Jak inhibitors can cause dyslipidemia–whether this translates into an increased CVD risk is currently unknown. Caution has been advised on the use of NSAIDs and TNF inhibitors in patients with congestive heart failure Class III/IV.

## Systemic Lupus Erythematosus and Antiphospholipid Syndrome

Systemic lupus erythematosus is associated with an increased risk of myocardial ischemia. There are various risk factors that are specific to SLE which play a role in increasing CV morbidities associated with SLE. The important ones are long-standing disease, prolonged usage of steroids, cumulative dose of steroids, renal dysfunction, nephrotic syndrome, premature ovarian failure due to disease activity or as an adverse effect of therapy, presence of antiphospholipid antibodies, proinflammatory cytokines, hypertension, and oxidized LDL Proteinuria and raised serum creatinine are strongly associated with increased CV risk. Amongst the antiphospholipid antibodies, lupus anticoagulant is more strongly associated with myocardial ischemia. Also, SLE patients have been found to have higher serum levels of very low density lipoprotein, triglycerides, and homocysteine than general population in a Canadian study. Antiphospholipid antibodies may also have a direct impact on endothelial cells producing endothelial dysfunction and vascular insufficiency, in addition to thrombosis. There is insufficient evidence to suggest a direct role of antiphospholipid antibodies in atherogenesis and myocardial dysfunction.

## Spondyloarthropathy

The risk factors for CVD in SpA are similar to RA. SpA is a pro-inflammatory state with especially high levels of TNF-α that exert an atherogenic effect. Endothelial dysfunction is another factor responsible for increased CVD risk. Use of NSAIDs and disease modifying antirheumatic drugs have same effects as in RA.

## Systemic Sclerosis and Overlap Syndromes

In a population-based study in patients of SSc, increased risk of CVD was found with hazard ratios (HR ) of 1.8 and 2.61 for myocardial infarction and stroke, respectively. Another study found that male gender, older age, pulmonary artery hypertension, hypercholesterolemia, diabetes mellitus, hypertension, and duration of SSc are important predictors of CVD in SSc. Presence of antiendothelial antibodies, reactive oxygen species, and oxidized LDL are other cardiovascular risk factors. Traditional risk factors were found to be less prevalent in SSc. In MCTD, age and hypertension are the important predictors of increased CV risk and associated with increased aortic stiffness.

## Vasculitis

Small vessel, medium vessel, as well as large vessel vasculitis, are all associated with increased CV risk. In addition to direct involvement of coronary arteries by the inflammatory processes seen in vasculitis, other factors also play a role in accelerated atherogenesis. Corticosteroids use, renal dysfunction, and proinflammatory cytokines, are amongst the important risk factors.

## Gout and Hyperuricemia

Gout and hyperuricemia are known to be associated with metabolic syndrome. Hyperuricemia is an independent risk factor for hypertension, endothelial dysfunction, and vascular disease, leading to increased CV mortality. Gout is an inflammatory state and independently associated with increased cardiovascular mortality.

# CARDIOVASCULAR RISK ASSESSMENT IN AUTOIMMUNE DISEASES

Different algorithms are being used for cardiovascular risk assessment in general population. The different scores that are commonly used for CV risk assessment are, Framingham Risk Score, SCORE (Systematic Coronary Risk Evaluation) chart, QRISK1/2/3, Reynold's Risk Score, and atherosclerotic cardiovascular disease (ASCVD) score. Most of these scores assess 10 years CV risk. These scores tend to underestimate the CVD risk in autoimmune diseases. These scores can also be used for CV risk assessment in autoimmune diseases with some modifications. The EULAR has given a set of recommendations for the assessment and management of CV risk in chronic inflammatory arthritides. The recommendations are summarized in **Box 1**.

---

**BOX 1** — **Summary of EULAR recommendations for CV risk management.**

**Principles and recommendations**
- CV risk is to be managed by treating rheumatologists
- Optimal disease control to lower CV risk
- Assessment of CVD risk every 5 years or less
- Assessment of CVD risk as per national guidelines. Use SCORE model if no national guidelines are present
- Estimation of serum lipids to be performed when disease is stable
- Multiply the risk score by 1.5 for RA if it is not included in the model
- Carotid ultrasound for determining asymptomatic atherosclerosis can be used for CVD screening
- CVD risk management, antihypertensives, statins as per national guidelines
- Lifestyle recommendations should include dietary advice, exercise, and smoking cessation for everyone
- Use NSAIDs with caution in subjects with known CVD risk
- Minimize the dose of glucocorticoids and taper as soon as possible. The indications for prolonged usage should be checked regularly

(CV: cardiovascular; CVD: cardiovascular diseases; NSAIDs: nonsteroidal anti-inflammatory drugs; RA: rheumatoid arthritis)

## Assessment of Vascular Function

Different ultrasound-based imaging techniques have been studied for noninvasive assessment of vascular function in patients with autoimmune diseases. Carotid intimal media thickness (cIMT) is the most widely studied tool and a good marker for generalized atherosclerosis. Endothelial function can be assessed by using flow mediated (FMD) and nitroglycerine mediated (NMD) dilation of brachial artery by B-mode ultrasound. Arterial stiffness can be measured in the peripheral vessels pulse wave velocity (PWV). Coronary flow reserve (CFR) is an important tool for assessment of myocardial perfusion. All these modalities have been studied in inflammatory arthritis and associated with increased CV risk.

## Biomarkers for Cardiovascular risk

There are various antigens, autoantibodies, inflammatory markers, that can be used as molecular markers to predict CVD risk. Inflammatory markers such as, highly sensitive C-reactive protein (hsCRP), interleukins, TNF-α, vascular and intercellular adhesion molecules (VCAM/ICAM), and acute phase reactants such as haptoglobin, have been found to be associated with increased CVD risk. Autoantigens such as heat shock protein-60 (HSP-60), oxidized-LDL, apolipoprotein-A1, angiopoietin 2, dimethylarginine, highly atherogenic HDL, and their respective autoantibodies, serum uric acid, NT Pro-BNP, and osteoprotegerin predict high CVD risk. Proteomics is an upcoming area of research that studies the cellular expression of proteins under different conditions. Proteomics can also be used to assess CVD risk in a patient with autoimmune diseases.

## MANAGEMENT OF CARDIOVASCULAR RISK

Decreasing the CVD risk in autoimmune diseases requires prevention of both traditional and disease-specific risk factors.

*Prevention of traditional risk factors*: There are no specific guidelines for management of traditional risk factors in autoimmune diseases. General measures are used for their prevention. These include smoking cessation, deaddiction strategies for smoking, monitoring of blood pressure, antihypertensives, assessment of lipid profile at regular intervals, statins, low-dose aspirin for primary or secondary prevention (especially in prothrombotic states), weight control, dietary advice, physical therapy, counseling, treatment of diabetes, and early recognition of increased CVD risk. Patient education and periodic evaluation is very important in prevention of CVD.

*Prevention of disease-specific risk factors includes the following measures*:
- *Early and effective control of disease activity*: Since high disease activity is an important factor responsible for accelerated atherosclerosis, it is imperative to control disease activity to reduce the CVD risk.
- *Minimizing NSAIDs and corticosteroids use*: Both NSAIDs and corticosteroids use increase CVD risk. They should be minimized to lowest possible dose and shortest duration, to reduce CVD risk.
- *Drugs reducing CVD risk*: Multiple studies have found that disease-modifying anti-rheumatic drugs (DMARDs), particularly hydroxychloroquine reduces overall mortality in SLE. It shows cardioprotective effect and decreases dyslipidemia and insulin resistance when used in SLE and other diseases. Methotrexate has also been shown to reduce CV and overall mortality in RA patients. The effect of TNF inhibitors on CV morbidity and mortality is controversial. Though they reduce inflammation and suppress the effect of TNF-α, thus reducing CVD risk, they are also known to produce

cardiac failure. The effect of smaller molecules, rituximab, abatacept, and tocilizumab on CVD risk is not extensively studied yet. In SLE, mycophenolate mofetil has shown some promise in reducing CV mortality. More aggressive immunosuppression with stronger disease control seems to have better cardioprotective effect.

## CONCLUSION

Autoimmune diseases are associated with increased CVD risk as compared to general population. Early detection and management of traditional and disease-specific risk factors is the key to reduce CVD risk in such patients. Early and effective disease control is essential in reducing CV morbidity and mortality.

## SUGGESTED READING

1. England BR, Thiele GM, Anderson DR, Mikuls TR. Increased cardiovascular risk in rheumatoid arthritis: mechanisms and implications. BMJ. 2018;361:k1036.
2. Mackey RH, Kuller LH, Moreland LW. Update on cardiovascular disease risk in patients with rheumatic diseases. Rheum Dis Clin North Am. 2018;44(3):475-87.
3. Mason JC, Libby P. Cardiovascular disease in patients with chronic inflammation: mechanisms underlying premature cardiovascular events in rheumatologic conditions. Eur Heart J. 2015;36(8):482-9c.
4. Myasoedova E, Crowson CS, Kremers HM, Roger VL, Fitz-Gibbon PD, Therneau TM, et al. Lipid paradox in rheumatoid arthritis: the impact of serum lipid measures and systemic inflammation on the risk of cardiovascular disease. Ann Rheum Dis. 2011;70(3):482-7.
5. Mantel Ä, Holmqvist M, Nyberg F, Tornling G, Frisell T, Alfredsson L, et al. Risk factors for the rapid increase in risk of acute coronary events in patients with new-onset rheumatoid arthritis: a nested case-control study. Arthritis Rheumatol. 2015;67(11):2845-54.
6. Bessant R, Duncan R, Ambler G, Swanton J, Isenberg DA, Gordon C, et al. Prevalence of conventional and lupus-specific risk factors for cardiovascular disease in patients with systemic lupus erythematosus: A case–control study. Arthritis Rheum. 2006;55(6):892-9.
7. Sinicato NA, da Silva Cardoso PA, Appenzeller S. Risk factors in cardiovascular disease in systemic lupus erythematosus. Curr Cardiol Rev. 2013;9(1):15-19.
8. Bruce IN, Urowitz MB, Gladman DD, Ibañez D, Steiner G. Risk factors for coronary heart disease in women with systemic lupus erythematosus: The Toronto Risk Factor Study. Arthritis Rheum. 2003;48(11):3159-67.
9. Man A, Zhu Y, Zhang Y, Dubreuil M, Rho YH, Peloquin C, et al. The risk of cardiovascular disease in systemic sclerosis: a population-based cohort study. Ann Rheum Dis. 2013;72(7):1188-93.
10. Ngian G-S, Sahhar J, Proudman SM, Stevens W, Wicks IP, Doornum SV. Prevalence of coronary heart disease and cardiovascular risk factors in a national cross-sectional cohort study of systemic sclerosis. Ann Rheum Dis. 2012;71(12):1980-3.
11. Triantafyllias K, de Blasi M, Lütgendorf F, Cavagna L, Stortz M, Weinmann-Menke J, et al. (2019). High cardiovascular risk in mixed connective tissue disease: evaluation of macrovascular involvement and its predictors by aortic pulse wave velocity. Clin Exp Rheumatol. 2019;37(6):994-1002.
12. Feig DI, Kang D-H, Johnson RJ. Uric acid and cardiovascular risk. N Engl J Med. 2008;359(17):1811-21.
13. Kuo CF, See LC, Luo SF, Ko YS, Lin YS, Hwang JS, et al. Gout: an independent risk factor for all-cause and cardiovascular mortality. Rheumatology. 2010;49(1):141-6.
14. Cooney MT, Dudina AL, Graham IM. Value and limitations of existing scores for the assessment of cardiovascular risk: A review for clinicians. J Am Coll Cardiol. 2009;54(14):1209-27.
15. Agca R, Heslinga SC, Rollefstad S, Heslinga M, McInnes IB, Peters MJL, et al. EULAR recommendations for cardiovascular disease risk management in patients with rheumatoid arthritis and other forms of inflammatory joint disorders: 2015/2016 update. Ann Rheum Dis. 2017;76(1):17-28.
16. Soltész P, Kerekes G, Dér H, Szücs G, Szántó S, Kiss E, et al. Comparative assessment of vascular function in autoimmune rheumatic diseases: Considerations of prevention and treatment. Autoimmun Rev. 2011;10(7):416-25.
17. Teixeira PC, Ferber P, Vuilleumier N, Cutler P. Biomarkers for cardiovascular risk assessment in autoimmune diseases. Proteomics Clin Appl. 2015;9(1-2):4-57.

# SECTION 4

# Neurology

**SECTION EDITORS**
Monika Singla, Aastha Takkar Kapila

# CHAPTER 1

# Epilepsy in Women

*Anuja Patil, Sita Jayalakshmi*

## ABSTRACT

Epilepsy in women poses a challenge due to complex interactions with the sex hormones, pharmacodynamic differences with antiepileptic drugs (AEDs), and potential reproductive consequences nearly in every phase of their lives from puberty to menopause. Catamenial epilepsy with periodic seizure clustering along the menstrual cycle suggests the cyclic hormonal changes affecting seizure threshold. These bidirectional interactions also pose a chance of seizure exacerbation with the hormonal contraceptives as well as risk of contraceptive failure with the enzyme inducing AEDs. Some of the AEDs especially valproate is associated with major congenital malformations (MCMs) and needs caution against use in women in reproductive age group. Regular folate supplementation is beneficial in mitigating the risk of malformations as well as the cognitive teratogenesis. During pregnancy, management of seizures should be balanced against the likely immediate- and long-term fetal outcomes, although benefits with AEDs far outweigh the risks. The postpartum period is likely to have seizure exacerbation with maternal pharmacodynamic changes as well as altered sleep patterns and needs dose adjustment accordingly. Elderly women with new-onset seizures must be evaluated for likely immune-mediated encephalitis. Also for those on chronic AED therapy, regular bone mineral density assessments and calcium and vitamin D supplements are indicated. The probable social implications need to be considered while treating women with epilepsy with a joint effort from the social supporter and psychologist as well as the physicians.

## INTRODUCTION

The World Health Organization (WHO), 2010 Global Burden of Disease Study underlines epilepsy as the second most serious neurologic disorder. Although it affects every person in a different way, epilepsy in women merits special interest. Not only does epilepsy behave differently in women as opposed to men, but also women respond differently to the antiepileptic drugs (AEDs) used in their management and may have implications on their reproductive outcomes. These gender differences stem from the physiological, endocrine, pharmacodynamic as well as sociocultural variations among the two. The current chapter reviews the existing literature and provides an overview into various aspects of epilepsy in women.

## EPIDEMIOLOGY: EPILEPSY IN WOMEN

The overall prevalence of epilepsy is shown to be nearly same in both the sexes. However, men are likely to be more susceptible to have a seizure as well as higher likelihood of lifetime risk of developing epilepsy attributed to greater likelihood of exposure to the traumatic, toxic, and other causes likely to cause or trigger seizures. The precise rates of incidence or prevalence of epilepsy across the genders vary widely across in different studies and are influenced by geography, reporting biases, and inclusion criteria of the study. The most often reported trends include: Generalized seizures are observed more commonly in girls below 1 year of age. The prevalence of generalized seizures remains comparable among both genders till about 45 years after which it raises in men. Similarly, focal seizures are seen almost equally in both genders in childhood and early adulthood, but later the prevalence increases among men. Among the specific epileptic syndromes, primary generalized epilepsy (PGE or formerly IGE) including childhood and juvenile absence epilepsy and juvenile myoclonic epilepsy is seen more commonly among women. The difference is invariably noted in 15–50 years age group highlighting the interplay of hormonal factors in the reproductive age group. In the localization-related epilepsies (LREs), symptomatic especially those due to traumatic, alcohol related, and also structural lesions are seen more commonly in men than in women while cryptogenic LREs are more commonly seen in women. Women with mesial temporal lobe epilepsy (MTLE) are more likely to have isolated auras and lateralizing electroencephalography (EEG) than men. Men with MTLE are more likely to have secondarily generalized seizures than women. Interestingly, despite these differences, gender was not found to be a significant outcome variable in studies comparing the long-term prognosis of epilepsy. Also, rate of sudden unexpected death in epilepsy (SUDEP) is similar among both genders. In-depth review of the rationale behind these variations is beyond the scope of this chapter. However, implications of these gender differences among the epileptic syndromes are under constant scrutiny of various clinical studies.

## CATAMENIAL EPILEPSY

The pattern of seizure clustering in relation to the menstrual cycle in women is termed as catamenial epilepsy. The word is derived from Greek "katamenios" meaning monthly. Almost 70% women report exacerbation of seizures in relation to menstruation. But only one-third of all women with intractable partial epilepsy are diagnosed to be catamenial as per the criteria of "2-fold increase in the average daily seizure frequency during the specific phases" of the cycle. Three patterns of exacerbation of seizures have been described (**Fig. 1**). The C1 pattern with perimenstrual occurrence (day –3 to 3 with first day being onset of menstruation) and C2 with periovulatory (day 10–13 or –13 of the cycle with ovulation at D14) are noted in routine ovulatory cycles. While pattern C3 is seen in inadequate luteal phase irrespective of ovulation or in anovulatory cycles, seizures occur around day 10 of one cycle to third day of next. Of all types, secondarily generalized seizures are found to exacerbate in anovulatory cycles than the complex or simple partial seizures. While temporal lobe seizures, especially left sided are seen to cluster mainly around menstruation than the extratemporal or undifferentiated seizures.

The cyclic exacerbation of seizures at certain points suggests the influence of hormonal processes on occurrence of seizures correlating with the serum estradiol:progesterone ratio. Estrogen or its metabolite estradiol exerts proconvulsant effect by stimulation of the N-methyl-D-aspartate (NMDA) receptors seen especially in hippocampus. It has also been seen to interact with non-NMDA kainate receptors and quisqualate-mediated

# CHAPTER 1: Epilepsy in Women

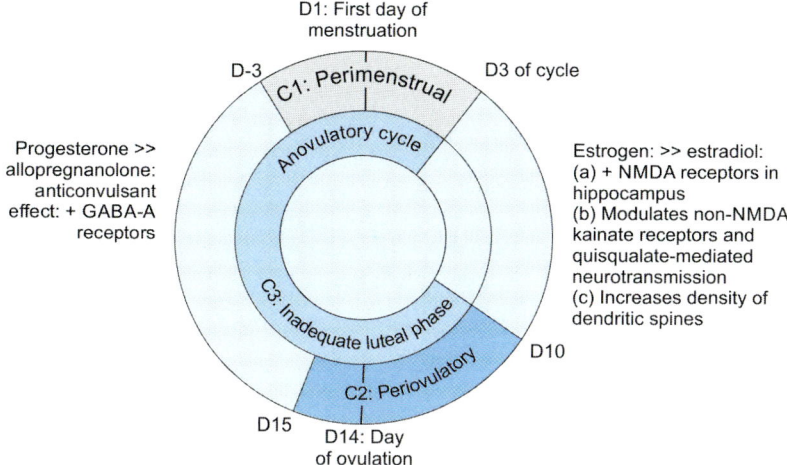

(GABA-A: gamma-aminobutyric acid type A; NMDA: N-methyl-D-aspartate)

**FIG. 1:** Patterns of catamenial epilepsy in relation to menstrual cycle.

neurotransmission and increasing the density of dendritic spines. This explains the periovulatory seizure exacerbation correlating with estrogen surge. Progesterone and its metabolite allopregnanolone on the other hand are shown to be anticonvulsant with stimulation of the gamma-aminobutyric acid type A (GABA-A) receptors. This correlates to the perimenstrual seizure clustering with progesterone withdrawal as also the C3 pattern is noted in inadequate luteal phase. Anti-Müllerian hormone a member of transforming growth factor-β (TGF-β) family is shown to be protective against the NMDA receptor-mediated neurotoxicity. Its receptors are seen in hippocampus, cortex, and hypothalamus.

Management involves documentation of the periodic seizure clustering using seizure diaries and keeping track of menstrual cycle phases with basal body temperature. Acetazolamide 250–500 mg BD or clobazam 20–30 mg/day can be given for 7–10 days starting 2 days prior to the period of seizure exacerbation. Synthetic progestins or oral natural progesterone lozenges have been shown to be beneficial, especially for C1 pattern of catamenial epilepsies. Alternative options include slight dose increment of the regularly used AEDs around the noted period with monitoring for signs of toxicity.

## REPRODUCTIVE AND SEXUAL DYSFUNCTION IN WOMEN WITH EPILEPSY

Compared to the general population, women with epilepsy tend to have higher rates of reproductive disorders including menstrual irregularities, reproductive endocrinopathies such as polycystic ovarian syndrome (PCOS), hyperandrogenism, decreased libido, infertility, premature menopause, and hyperprolactinemia. Importantly, these effects are irrespective of the use of AEDs. Amygdala and the associated limbic cortex have reciprocal connections with hypothalamus which in turn modulates the hypothalamic–pituitary–ovarian axis. Seizures arising from the mesial temporal lobe can disrupt this hormonal balance and cause reduced secretion of the gonadotropic hormones. Fertility rate in women with epilepsy was earlier reported to be 85%. Recently, an observational cohort study compared women with epilepsy without previous known infertility versus aged-matched healthy women. The study reported similar rates of achieving pregnancy in both the groups including time to pregnancy, ovulatory rate, live birth rates, and sexual activity. However, these differences may arise with the complex interplay of multiple factors including the age-related physiological and hormonal, social, and psychological nature, comorbidities as well as the seizure frequency, severity of epilepsy, and the neurocognitive status in the women under consideration.

## HORMONAL INTERACTIONS OF ANTIEPILEPTIC DRUGS

Antiepileptic drugs affect internal hormonal milieu. The effects may range from cosmetic such as acne, hirsutism to reproductive affecting fertility, pregnancy to reducing bone mineral density, and asymptomatic thyroid hormone alterations. The AEDs that induce hepatic microsomal enzymes (**Box 1**) increase metabolism of sex steroids and also tend to increase sex hormone-binding globulin (SHBG) thus reducing the circulating free hormone levels. Valproate is one of the most widely known and studied AED for its hormonal side effects. It has been associated with PCOS or hyperandrogenism in almost 90% and menstrual irregularities in 45% of women on treatment. These effects are partly reversible and are common in younger women and those gaining weight with valproate. Switching over to AEDs with least known hormonal interactions such as lamotrigine or levetiracetam for women developing these adverse effects beneficial. Estrogen either in hormonal contraceptives or during pregnancy is known to induce metabolism of some AEDs, especially lamotrigine and to some extent valproate and reduce their therapeutic efficacy.

## CONTRACEPTION IN WOMEN WITH EPILEPSY

The interactions of routinely used AEDs with the hormonal contraceptives are bidirectional and may cause contraceptive failure as well as cause decline in AED levels below therapeutic efficacy. AEDs induce metabolism of synthetic estrogen and progestins in combined contraceptive pills and progesterone only pills or depot implants. This may lead to contraceptive failure in women on enzyme-inducing AEDs. The rate of oral

| BOX 1 | Degree of microsomal enzyme induction by antiepileptic drugs (AEDs). |
|---|---|
| **Strong enzyme-inducing AEDs:**<br>• Phenobarbitone<br>• Phenytoin<br>• Primidone<br>• Carbamazepine<br>• Oxcarbazepine<br>• Perampanel<br>**Weak enzyme-inducing AEDs:**<br>• Topiramate<br>• Lamotrigine<br>• Clobazam<br>• Eslicarbazepine<br>• Felbamate<br>• Rufinamide | **Noninducer AEDs:**<br>• Ethosuximide<br>• Valproate<br>• Levetiracetam<br>• Gabapentin<br>• Clonazepam<br>• Tiagabine<br>• Zonisamide<br>• Pregabalin<br>• Vigabatrin<br>• Lacosamide<br>• Ezogabine |

contraceptive failure is up to 3–6% in women on AEDs as compared to 1% in their healthy counterparts. Knowing the potential teratogenicity of AEDs, any unintended pregnancies while on treatment may bear devastating consequences. Intrauterine devices may prove to be better option for women on these AEDs.

## TERATOGENICITY AND FETAL RISK OF ANTIEPILEPTIC DRUGS

Children born to women with epilepsy on treatment are at increased risk of congenital malformations as well as premature birth, low birth weight, and low 1 minute Apgar scores. Major congenital malformations (MCMs) are overt structural or other anomalies detected within 5 days of birth that are life-threatening or have major impact on life and/or require surgical correction. The rate of developing MCMs is higher in women with epilepsy on AEDs (6.1%) than the untreated ones (2.8%) and general population (2.2%). Also, the risk is considerably higher while on polytherapy (6.8%) than on monotherapy (4%). Furthermore, the risk is higher with first trimester (organogenesis) than later exposure. Individual risk for causing MCMs of the commonly used AEDs has been reported by the North American AED Pregnancy Registry (NAAPR) (**Table 1**). There is high-risk of intrauterine death with spontaneous abortion or a stillbirth in women exposed to polytherapy with AEDs and when either of the parent had a history of any MCM.

Other than congenital malformations, AED exposure has been known to affect cognitive and behavioral development till early childhood causing low intelligence quotient (IQ), decreased verbal intelligence, language deficits, autism, and attention deficit hyperactivity disorder. A prospective study of children exposed to AEDs observed till 6 years of age [NEAD (Neurodevelopmental Effects of Antiepileptic Drugs) study] showed that high dose of valproate (>800 mg/day) exposure was associated with significantly lower adjusted mean IQ levels by 9.7 points compared to controls. Other AEDs including carbamazepine, lamotrigine, and phenytoin were not seen to affect the IQ levels in exposed children.

**TABLE 1:** Percent frequency and the commonly observed MCMs of AEDs.

| AED name | Rate of causing MCMs (%) | Commonly observed malformations, growth, and neurobehavioral disorders |
|---|---|---|
| Valproate | 8.9 | Neural tube defects, lower IQ, verbal intelligence, and autism |
| Phenobarbital | 5.9 | Cardiac defects, oral clefts |
| Topiramate | 4.4 | Facial clefts, hypospadias |
| Carbamazepine | 3.0 | Neural tube defects (lower risk than VPA) |
| Phenytoin | 2.8 | Growth retardation, microcephaly, cardiac defects, and hypoplastic digits |
| Lamotrigine | 2.1 | Orofacial clefts, transposition of great arteries, and anencephaly |
| Levetiracetam | 2.0 | None specifically associated |
| Clonazepam | 2.3 | None specifically associated |
| Oxcarbazepine | 1.7 | None specifically associated |
| Zonisamide | 1.5 | Low birth weight |
| Gabapentin | 1.2 | None specifically associated |

(AEDs: antiepileptic drugs; IQ: intelligence quotient; MCMs: major congenital malformations; VPA: valproate)

Intranatal screening for possible malformations must be offered to gravid women. Depending on the potential risk of MCMs, invasive screening with chorionic villus sampling (CVS) in first trimester or genetic amniocentesis in second trimester may be offered for high-risk pregnancies, especially with prior gestations with MCMs or symptomatic parent. In patients with relative risk monitoring with guidance of the obstetrician with maternal serum alpha-fetoprotein, β-human chorionic gonadotropin (β-HCG), placental-associated pregnancy protein-A, and fetal malformation scans regularly as per the fetal growth must be considered.

## PRENATAL COUNSELING FOR WOMEN WITH EPILEPSY

While treating women in reproductive age group, it is important to explain the women about the likely interactions of AEDs with hormonal contraceptives, likelihood for unintended pregnancies, potential teratogenic effects of AEDs, need to control seizures especially during pregnancy, and the need for strict compliance to medication. The treating neurologist should choose AEDs with least side effect, attempt monotherapy or least interacting combinations of AEDs and include folate supplementation even prior to conception. It is important to ensure proper social and family support. Managing pregnant women with epilepsy is a teamwork involving neurophysicians, obstetricians experienced in high-risk pregnancy care and if need be, psychologists, and social support workers. Prepregnancy baseline AED levels may help to guide the management of AEDs during pregnancy.

## SEIZURE CONTROL AND ANTIEPILEPTIC DRUG MANAGEMENT DURING PREGNANCY

Seizure frequency remains largely unchanged or surprisingly may even reduce during pregnancy. As per the European Registry of AEDs and pregnancy nearly 70.5% women have seizures at similar rate as their baseline during pregnancy, 12% may have lower seizure rate while 15.8% may have an exacerbation. The reasons for seizure recurrence during pregnancy are multifactorial including the physiologic and pharmacodynamic alterations with increased volume of distribution, increased renal clearance, reduced gastric transit and absorption, increased hepatic metabolization, increased estrogen to progesterone ratio especially midterm, increased psychosocial stress, disturbed sleep pattern as well as likelihood of reducing the dosage or missing AEDs with fear of fetal well-being. Seizure control prior to pregnancy also seems to affect the seizure recurrence as 78.4% of women with active epilepsy are known to have seizures during their pregnancy as against 22.3% of those with controlled or inactive epilepsy. Also, those women with catamenial epilepsy were observed to have better seizure control during pregnancy likely due to absence of the cyclic hormonal changes and raised progesterone levels. Drop in AED blood levels by 35% or more than the preconception level may lead to seizure recurrence.

Recurrent seizures during pregnancy may lead to placental hypoperfusion causing fetal hypoxia, acidosis, even trauma due to maternal falls, or injuries during tonic-clonic seizures. Thus, women with seizures during pregnancy are at risk of preterm delivery, intrauterine growth retardation, and small for gestational weight babies. Hence, AED dose adjustment must be made considering the seizure frequency and blood AED levels, especially for women on lamotrigine but also for oxcarbazepine, carbamazepine, phenytoin, and levetiracetam. The benefits of continuing AEDs may far outweigh the

## CHAPTER 1: Epilepsy in Women

---

**Seizures during pregnancy**

Etiology: Eclampsia, PRES, RCVS, CVT, AIE, lupus, CNS vasculitis, CNS infections, breakthrough seizures due to noncompliance

↓

**Status epilepticus**

Rx: Primary care ABC, left lateral position, lorazepam/midazolam, LEV/PHT
$MgSO_4$ if s/o eclampsia, thiamine, and fetal risk assessment

↓ Persistent seizures: consider CEEG to r/o NCSE

**Refractory/super-refractory status epilepticus**

Add on AED/midazolam/propofol/pentobarbital/ketamine infusion
persistent seizures: IV methylprednisolone, if s/o AIE: IVIg/PLEX
1st or 2nd trimester: Termination if maternal high-risk state, term gestation: deliver,
if status controlled, then regular fetal monitoring and deliver at term

---

(ABC: airway, breathing and circulation; AED: antiepileptic drug; AIE: autoimmune encephalitis; CNS: central nervous system; CVT: cerebral venous thrombosis; IVIg: intravenous immunoglobulin; CEEG: continuous EEG monitoring; LEV: levetiracetam; $MgSO_4$: magnesium sulfate; NCSE: non-convulsive status epilepticus; PHT: phenytoin; PRES: posterior reversible encephalopathy syndrome; PLEX: plasmapheresis; RCVS: reversible cerebral vasoconstriction syndrome)

**FLOWCHART 1:** Management of seizures/status epilepticus during pregnancy.

likelihood of their potential harm during pregnancy. Management of seizure exacerbation with status epilepticus during pregnancy is shown in **Flowchart 1**. For women with new-onset seizures during pregnancy, levetiracetam may be the preferred choice, while for those with breakthrough seizures, loading of the prior AED must be considered if noncompliance is the cause.

## POSTNATAL CARE AND BREASTFEEDING

Postpartum period is another risk period for seizure exacerbation and needs to be monitored cautiously. Apart from the underlying primary cause of epilepsy, immune-mediated causes such as autoimmune encephalitis and lupus are known to flare postpartum and need to be considered especially in women with postpartum psychosis and seizure exacerbation. All AEDs can be transferred to baby through breast milk, although the levels are lower than transplacental in-utero exposure. The level of exposure depends on the maternal blood AED levels and rate of absorption and clearance by baby. The relative adverse effects are observed mainly with the barbiturate and benzodiazepine group with sedation, lethargy, poor sucking, and sometimes dependence in baby. Breastfeeding is associated with major benefits in baby such as reduced risk of respiratory and gastrointestinal infections, asthma, atopic dermatitis in later childhood as well as lower maternal risk of ovarian and breast cancer, postpartum hemorrhage, depression, and diabetes mellitus. Also, in the extended analysis of the NEAD study out of all the children exposed in utero to single AED those who were breastfed had relatively higher IQ levels than those who were not. Thus, the benefits far outweigh the risks associated with AED exposure during breastfeeding. The nursing mothers should therefore be educated to make an informed decision knowing the potential risks and benefits associated with breastfeeding and continuing AEDs postpartum.

## PERIMENOPAUSAL WOMEN WITH EPILEPSY

Perimenopausal period is associated with elevated estrogen and decreasing progesterone levels, thereby causing increased risk of seizures. Later as menopause sets in, with diminished secretion of pituitary gonadotropic hormones, a hypogonadal state is reached thereby stabilizing seizure frequency. Nearly two-thirds of women experiencing menopausal symptoms tend to have seizure exacerbation. This is especially seen in those with catamenial epilepsy in youth and those on hormonal replacement therapy, the frequency gradually decreases in menopausal period. Thus, AED doses need to be monitored and adjusted based on seizure frequency and comorbid conditions in this age group. For those with new-onset seizures or multifocal and changing pattern of seizure, behavioral or cognitive changes should be evaluated for immune-mediated encephalitis such as Hashimoto's encephalitis or voltage-gated potassium channel (VGKC)-associated encephalitis.

Another concern in perimenopausal women is risk of osteoporosis. With longer seizure duration and larger cumulative AED load, they are predisposed to increased bone turnover. Compared to general population, people with epilepsy are at almost two to six times increased risk of fractures due to reduced bone mineral density, increased tendency to fall during seizures, and gait disturbances with chronic AED use. The risk is especially high with enzyme-inducing AEDs especially phenytoin, phenobarbitone, and primidone, but also associated with valproate, carbamazepine, gabapentin, oxcarbazepine, zonisamide, and may be seen with levetiracetam and topiramate. Lamotrigine however, is not associated with either reduced serum calcium levels or increased bone turnover. Thus, in perimenopausal epileptic women, lamotrigine or the newer nonenzyme-inducing AEDs must be the first choice while initiating treatment. While for those on polytherapy, care should be taken to stabilize on preferable AED combination with least side effect profile, keeping in mind the likelihood of seizure exacerbation during this period. Regular dual X-ray absorptiometry (DEXA) scans and serum vitamin D levels to monitor for osteoporosis with calcium and vitamin D supplements for those at risk are recommended. Those with osteopenia or osteoporosis should be consulted with endocrinologist for need for bisphosphonates and other therapeutic measures.

## SOCIAL ISSUES IN INDIA

In developing countries such as India, epilepsy is still considered as a social stigma. In a recent hospital-based study, about 42% women concealed the history of epilepsy prior to marriage and were observed to have adverse marital outcome. This also tends to affect the compliance with AEDs, adequacy in seizure reporting, acceptance of further invasive procedures in drug-resistant epilepsies, and overall follow-up. Multiple factors including the level of education, family structure, socioeconomic background, fear of fetal risks, and occupational status of the women as well as psychosocial support systems play a role. Overcoming these social hurdles proves to be an important challenge apart from the management of epilepsy in India. Social awareness programs for families with epileptic women as well as including these topics in education programs and imparting the knowledge and recommended treatment norms of epilepsy in practitioners across the society may help in overcoming these issues.

## CONCLUSION

Treating women with epilepsy is challenging considering the complex hormonal interactions, likelihood of fetal risks, changes at every phase of their lives from puberty to adulthood to maternal and nursing phase to menopause, and the associated psychosocial implications. It is not mere seizure control, but merits keeping in mind all the long-term implications and change in AED management in accordance. An attempt should be made at monotherapy when feasible or favorable AED combinations with folate and vitamin D supplements as per need might help in mitigating likely adverse effects. Spreading the knowledge of these issues will help in better patient interactions and informed decision-making.

## SUGGESTED READING

1. Murray CJ, Vos T, Lozano R, Naghavi M, Flaxman AD, Michaud C, et al. Disability-adjusted life years (DALYs) for 291 diseases and injuries in 21 regions, 1990-2010: a systematic analysis for the Global Burden of Disease Study 2010. Lancet. 2012;380(9859):2197-223.
2. Fiest KM, Sauro KM, Wiebe S, Patten SB, Kwon CS, Dykeman J, et al. Prevalence and incidence of epilepsy: A systematic review and meta-analysis of international studies. Neurology. 2017;88(3):296-303.
3. Reddy DS. The neuroendocrine basis of sex differences in epilepsy. Pharmacol Biochem Behav. 2017;152:97-104.
4. McHugh J, Delanty N. Epidemiology and classification of epilepsy: gender comparisons. In: Bradley R, Harris R, Jenner P (Eds). International Review of Neurobiology. USA: Elsevier; 2008.
5. Hauser WA, Annegers JF, Kurland LT. Incidence of epilepsy and unprovoked seizures in Rochester, Minnesota: 1935-1984. Epilepsia. 1993;34(3):453-68.
6. Janszky J, Schulz R, Janszky I, Ebner A. Medial temporal lobe epilepsy: gender differences. J Neurol Neurosurg Psychiatry. 2004;75(5):773-5.
7. Cockerell OC, Johnson AL, Sander JW, Shorvon SD. Prognosis of epilepsy: a review and further analysis of the first nine years of the British National General Practice Study of Epilepsy, a prospective population-based study. Epilepsia. 1997;38(1):31-46.
8. Vélez-Ruiz NJ, Pennell PB. Issues for Women with Epilepsy. Neurol Clin. 2016;34(2):411-25.
9. Herzog AG, Klein P, Ransil BJ. Three patterns of catamenial epilepsy. Epilepsia. 1997;38(10):1082-8.
10. Herzog AG. Catamenial epilepsy: Update on prevalence, pathophysiology and treatment from the findings of the NIH Progesterone Treatment Trial. Seizure. 2015;28:18-25.
11. Sazgar M. Treatment of Women with Epilepsy. Continuum (Minneap Minn). 2019;25(2):408-30.
12. Webber MP, Hauser WA, Ottman R, Annegers JF. Fertility in persons with epilepsy: 1935-1974. Epilepsia. 1986;27(6):746-52.
13. Pennell PB, French JA, Harden CL, Davis A, Bagiella E, Andreopoulos E, et al. Fertility and Birth Outcomes in Women With Epilepsy Seeking Pregnancy. JAMA Neurol. 2018;75(8):962-9.
14. Reimers A, Brodtkorb E, Sabers A. Interactions between hormonal contraception and antiepileptic drugs: clinical and mechanistic considerations. Seizure. 2015;28:66-70.
15. Shorvon SD, Tomson T, Cock HR. The management of epilepsy during pregnancy—progress is painfully slow. Epilepsia. 2009;50(5):973-4.
16. North American Antiepileptic Drug Pregnancy Registry. (2016). Update on monotherapy findings: Comparative safety of 11 antiepileptic drugs used during pregnancy. [online] Available from http://www.aedpregnancyregistry.org/wp-content/uploads/2016-newsletter-Winter-2016.pdf. [Last accessed January, 2020].
17. Meador KJ, Baker GA, Browning N. Fetal antiepileptic drug exposure and cognitive outcome at age 6 years (NEAD study): a prospective observational study. Lancet Neurol. 2013;12(3):244-52.

18. de Jong J, Garne E, de Jong-van den Berg LT, Wang H. The Risk of Specific Congenital Anomalies in Relation to Newer Antiepileptic Drugs: A Literature Review. Drugs Real World Outcomes. 2016;3(2):131-43.
19. Battino D, Tomson T, Bonizzoni E, Craig J, Lindhout D, Sabers A, et al. Seizure control and treatment changes in pregnancy: observations from the EURAP epilepsy pregnancy registry. Epilepsia. 2013;54(9):1621-7.
20. Vajda FJE, O'Brien TJ, Graham JE, Hitchcock AA, Lander CM, Eadie MJ. Predicting epileptic seizure control during pregnancy. Epilepsy Behav. 2018;78:91-5.
21. Cagnetti C, Lattanzi S, Foschi N, Provinciali L, Silvestrini M. Seizure course during pregnancy in catamenial epilepsy. Neurology. 2014;83(4):339-44.
22. Meador KJ, Baker GA, Browning N, Cohen MJ, Bromley RL, Clayton-Smith J, et al. Breastfeeding in children of women taking antiepileptic drugs: cognitive outcomes at age 6 years. JAMA Pediatr. 2014;168(8):729-36.
23. Harden CL, Pulver MC, Ravdin L, Jacobs AR. The effect of menopause and perimenopause on the course of epilepsy. Epilepsia. 1999;40(10):1402-7.
24. Sharma SK, Sardana V, Maheshwari D, Bhushan B, Jain N, Shringi P, et al. Problems faced by married women with epilepsy in Indian scenario: a hospital based study. Int J Epilepsy. 2018;5(2):80-6.

# CHAPTER 2

# Specific Issues of Stroke in Women

*Sucharita Ray, MV Padma Srivastava*

## ABSTRACT

Strokes occupy the bulk of the causes of morbidity and mortality in the modern world. Women are a special population when it comes to strokes. Treating clinicians need to have knowledge about the risk factors that predispose women to have strokes. They should also be able to decide the best treating option for women. These awareness and ability to distinguish strokes in women versus men are important because the statistics including deaths from stroke are worse in women as compared to men. In addition, they constitute a special group requiring increased care and attention after a stroke for multiple reasons. In this chapter, we have a concise review of the risk factors pertaining to women regarding stroke, discuss special scenarios and conditions that have an influence on cerebrovascular disorders in women, and discuss the treatment options available for treating them.

## INTRODUCTION

Modern civilization has brought about the rise of noncommunicable diseases like strokes and other cerebrovascular diseases which are one of the most common causes of mortality and chronicity. It is especially important to know all aspects of this disease as together they present one of the largest group of diseases that are well amenable to prevention. Even after presentation, a thorough knowledge of its treatment aspects can help in improving the quality of life of the affected patients to a significant extent. It is even more worthwhile to consider the special aspects of stroke pertaining to women.

## CLINICAL PRESENTATION

Women tend to differ from men in their presentation of a stroke. It is important to keep in mind that women tend to present with completely nontraditional symptoms of stroke-like reduced consciousness instead of focal deficits as seen by their male counterparts. Secondly, they are way more likely to present late to the emergency with their symptoms and are also less likely to receive thrombolysis for stroke when indicated as compared to their male counterparts. Such glaring differences in all aspects of stroke related to women ranging from risk factors to presentation to modes of treatment options have assumed special significance leading to the status culminating in the formulation of the "sex as a biological variable" initiative by the National Institutes of Health. Hence, it becomes imperative to discuss the spectrum of stroke with reference to women as a special category of patients with distinctive/unique biological characteristics.

## EPIDEMIOLOGY AND RISK FACTORS IN WOMEN FOR STROKE

Women have significantly higher risk factors for stroke as compared to men and the relationship of risk factors for stroke is much more complicated in women than it is for men. In general, the risk for stroke is higher in men as compared to women, up to the age of 75 years, after which the risk for women is higher than that of men. Overall, women not just tend to be older than men to experience the first-ever stroke, but also have a higher lifetime risk of stroke than men (20% vs. 16.7%).

Indian women, like the rest of them from Asia, have chances of higher mortality in stroke as well as a higher risk of stroke than their male counterparts, after the age of 55 years. A significant proportion of women under 40 years of age who suffered stroke had cerebral venous thrombosis (CVT) or stroke in and around the period of pregnancy and puerperium. In contrast in the elderly, there was a strong correlation to hypertension for the occurrence of ischemic strokes.

## ROLE OF ESTROGEN IN STROKES IN WOMEN

Estrogen can change the balance between procoagulant forces and the anticoagulant and fibrinolytic drive by lowering the level of plasminogen activator inhibitor-1 (PAI-1). This factor is a serine protease inhibitor that can potentially decrease the efficacy of intravenous thrombolysis. This is evidenced by the fact that premenopausal women with high levels of circulating estrogen and postmenopausal women on hormone replacement therapy (HRT) with higher circulating levels of estrogen have lower levels of PAI-1 and hence benefit more from intravenous thrombolysis as compared to those without HRT or postmenopausal women.

## HORMONE REPLACEMENT AND STROKE RISK

Hormones, particularly the balance between estrogen and progesterone, are crucial in determining the risk of stroke in women. Both early and delayed menopause is associated with an increased risk of stroke in women. Several trials and the prospective observational cohort in the Women's Health Initiative (WHI) have proven that estrogen, alone or with a progestogen, increases a woman's risk of stroke. The risk of stroke increases by approximately one-third with standard-dose hormone therapy in healthy postmenopausal women. The risk is said to be similar for unopposed estrogen as it is for estrogen plus progestogen. However, lower doses of transdermal estrogen (<50 μg/day) or oral conjugated estrogens (0.3 mg/day) may not significantly alter the risk of stroke.

## ORAL CONTRACEPTIVES AND RISK OF STROKES

Ever since the earliest oral contraceptive pills (OCP) came about, concern has been rife regarding their role in the coagulation cascade. To date, OCPs have been associated with a rise in procoagulant factors, like fibrinogen, prothrombin and clotting factors, VII and VIII, and a reduction in the levels of antithrombin III. All these effects are compounded in patients with higher age, blood pressure, and smoking. The type of oral contraceptive use also determines the risk of stroke. Modern oral contraceptive formulations containing low doses of ethinyl estradiol or progestin-only pills do not seem to have any added risk of stroke. Similarly, parenteral methods of contraception like hormonal patches or vaginal rings also do not seem to carry any extra risk of stroke.

It is important to know that other valid risk factors of stroke add up in determining the total risk for stroke. For example, the presence of migraines irrespective of an aura has an odds ratio (OR) of 3 for increasing the risk of stroke. However, the addition of OCPs increases the OR anywhere from 5 to 17. This increase in the odds of stroke also holds for other risk factors like age and obesity. The International Headache Society does not discourage the use of combination of OCPs in patients with migraine without aura. However, recommendations for contraception in women with migraines and other focal deficits in women older than 35 years and in smokers are isolated progestin preparations like pills, intrauterine devices (IUDs), injection and implant, and nonhormonal means like use of a barrier method of contraception, surgical, or copper-containing IUDs.

## PREGNANCY AND STROKE

Pregnancy is a state of hormonal overdrive that brings a lot of factors to clash with each other. At the heart of it is the dynamic shift in the levels of the circulating reproductive hormones, estrogen and progesterone. The levels of these determine the risk of stroke in pregnancy which is considered a hypercoagulable state. While the absolute risk of stroke in a healthy nonpregnant woman is low at 21/100,000 patients, the risk increases to 34/100,000 patients in pregnant females. The postpartum state is considered to be a higher prothrombotic state than the antepartum period. Even though the risk of both ischemic as well as hemorrhagic strokes increases during pregnancy, the incidence of ischemic stroke far outweighs that of hemorrhagic stroke and accounts for almost 80% of all strokes. Preeclampsia and eclampsia are two complications that predominate during the last trimester of pregnancy and both the conditions can be accompanied by high blood pressures and can culminate in a stroke. CVT is another complication in pregnancy which occurs due to hypercoagulability and can cause both ischemic and hemorrhagic strokes.

Arterial dissections and subarachnoid hemorrhages occur less commonly in stroke and can also be a cause of ischemic and hemorrhagic strokes, respectively. It is important to look out for these causes in pregnant patients as well in order to maximize results.

## THROMBOLYSIS IN WOMEN

Thrombolysis is a critical step in the management of acute ischemic stroke. It yields the best results when done in the window period of 4.5 hours. However, gender-wise differences exist in the utilization as well as results of thrombolysis and thrombolysis is a paradox in women in that there is a significantly higher benefit with thrombolysis but the utilization rates of thrombolysis are uniformly poorer in women as compared to men. These rates of lower utilization of thrombolysis extend to women of higher age or with a history of previous stroke, diabetes, or carotid stenosis. Such situations demand a thorough analysis of factors operating for utilization of emergency care services when it concerns stroke or other cerebrovascular events.

Recanalization rates in women when thrombolysed within 6 hours of stroke onset were significantly higher in women as compared to men (94% vs. 59%; $p = 0.02$). These rates remained statistically significant even after omitting patients with occlusive internal carotid artery disease and those thrombolysed within 3 hours of stroke onset.

A meta-analysis found that women were more likely to experience a worse outcome after intravenous thrombolysis than men after intravenous thrombolysis [risk ratio (RR) 1.24, 95% confidence interval (CI) 1.11–1.36, p < 0.001]. However, no significant difference can be seen in rates of recanalization after thrombolysis or in hemorrhagic transformation after thrombolysis.

## SAFETY OF THROMBOLYSIS IN PREGNANCY AND MENSTRUATION

Pregnancy was considered to be a contraindication to thrombolysis in earlier guidelines for acute ischemic stroke but has since then been revoked. rtPA has been listed as a Category C drug which is relatively contraindicated in pregnancy. However, it does not cross the placenta and has a short half-life of about 5 minutes. The present guidelines ask to consider the use of rtPA in patients judiciously when the benefits of stroke thrombolysis outweigh the apprehended risks of uterine bleeding. Similarly, while thrombolysis is not contraindicated during menstruation, patients should be advised that thrombolysis can increase the amount of bleeding especially if they experience menorrhagia. However, caution is expressed and a consultation with a gynecologist is required if there is a history of recent or active vaginal bleeding causing significant anemia or hypotension.

## MECHANICAL THROMBECTOMY IN ISCHEMIC STROKE

Mechanical thrombectomy has one of the best numbers needed to treat for patients with ischemic stroke. However, the majority of the trials have excluded pregnant patients and hence the safety and efficacy of these two interventions in these groups are unclear. However, several case reports of successful mechanical thrombectomy have been reported in the literature. These cases highlight that pregnancy may be a special circumstance for the use of mechanical thrombectomy in women when indicated and is probably safe unless hemorrhage or preterm labor is a consideration in them.

## ANTIPLATELET USE IN WOMEN

Female sex hormones, especially estrogen, have a complicated relationship with coagulation cascade in women as outlined earlier. Hence, the relationship of antiplatelets is very different in women as compared to men. However, even if the theoretical concerns remain, the clinical effect size of the difference in responses is minimal. Certain reports suggest higher protection and efficacy of antiplatelets in secondary prevention of stroke in women as compared to myocardial infarction.

## USE OF STATINS IN PREGNANCY

There is a concern for teratogenic risk of statins in pregnancy and there exist certain reports of congenital abnormalities with the use of a statin in the antepartum period. However, a recent systematic review refutes these small case series and found no clear increase in the risk of congenital abnormalities with the use of statins in control groups or in the general population. In the recent guidelines for stroke, patients with hypercholesterolemia are advised to stop statins at least 2 months before they desire to conceive. However, if they become pregnant while they are on statins, it is advisable to stop statins as soon as possible.

## INTRACEREBRAL HEMORRHAGE AND WOMEN

Women tend to have lower rates of intracerebral hemorrhage than males in all age groups up to the age of 80 years after which the trends are reversed. One of the most important phases of women to experience intracerebral hemorrhage is during the pregnancy and postpartum period wherein the relative risk was 2.5 (CI 1.0–6.4) and 28.3 (CI 13.0–61.4), respectively. Arteriovascular malformations account for nearly 4.4% of all maternal deaths. Hypertension is a strong risk factor in most cases of nonaneurysmal intracerebral hemorrhage in women. Apart from hypertension, advanced maternal age, coagulation disorders, abuse of tobacco, and presence of other vascular disorders in the form of aneurysms or malformations should be sought after. Management of these emergencies are along the lines of the generally established guidelines of stroke and there is no difference in the rate of aggressiveness in the management of intracerebral hemorrhage in women after adjusting for the comorbidities.

## CEREBRAL VENOUS THROMBOSIS

One of the most common varieties of a stroke to affect women due to their hormonal influences is CVT. It also affects women about three times more common than men. Female sex hormones have an important role to play in the pathogenesis of CVT. However, apart from that, several other causes can cause venous strokes including anemia, infections, hematological abnormalities, and malignancies.

The occurrence of venous strokes also explains the atypical presentations for the same including headache, seizures, papilledema, cranial nerve palsies, etc. Overall, the prognosis of CVT is better than reported previously with a direct correlation to the severity of symptoms at the onset or presence of hemorrhage on admission CT scan. Similarly, the involvement of the deep cerebral venous system carries a worse prognosis than the involvement of the superficial venous system. Anticoagulation is the main line of management, although surgery has a place if there is a significant mass effect or midline shift. The duration of anticoagulants is temporary up to a period of around 6 months if the occurrence of the venous stroke was provoked due to some reversible factors. However, the anticoagulants are continued indefinitely if the occurrence of venous stroke is due to an inherent thrombophilia or hypercoagulable state.

## CONCLUSION

Women are special by virtue of their internal milieu as well as external factors. During the reproductively active age group, they have some protection against strokes but higher age predisposes them to experience a higher number of strokes and overall higher mortality. Despite this, treatment measures are found to be as effective in men as women and it is important to keep these differences in mind when treating women to achieve the best possible clinical outcome for them.

## SUGGESTED READING

1. McGregor AJ, Beauchamp GA, Wira CR, Perman SM, Safdar B. Sex as a Biological Variable in Emergency Medicine Research and Clinical Practice: A Brief Narrative Review. West J Emerg Med. 2017;18(6):1079-90.

2. Mandelzweig L, Goldbourt U, Boyko V, Tanne D. Perceptual, social, and behavioral factors associated with delays in seeking medical care in patients with symptoms of acute stroke. Stroke. 2006;37(5):1248-53.
3. Bushnell CD. Stroke and the female brain. Nat Clin Pract Neurol. 2008;4(1):22-33.
4. Yu C, An Z, Zhao W, Wang W, Gao C, Liu S, et al. Sex Differences in Stroke Subtypes, Severity, Risk Factors, and Outcomes among Elderly Patients with Acute Ischemic Stroke. Front Aging Neurosci. 2015;7:174.
5. Barker-Collo S, Bennett DA, Krishnamurthi RV, Parmar P, Feigin VL, Naghavi M, et al. Sex Differences in Stroke Incidence, Prevalence, Mortality and Disability-Adjusted Life Years: Results from the Global Burden of Disease Study 2013. Neuroepidemiology. 2015;45(3):203-14.
6. Giralt D, Domingues-Montanari S, Mendioroz M, Ortega L, Maisterra O, Perea-Gainza M, et al. The gender gap in stroke: a meta-analysis. Acta Neurol Scand. 2012;125(2):83-90.
7. Banerjee TK, Das SK. Fifty years of stroke researches in India. Ann Indian Acad Neurol. 2016;19(1):1-8.
8. Mehndiratta P, Wasay M, Mehndiratta MM. Implications of female sex on stroke risk factors, care, outcome and rehabilitation: an Asian perspective. Cerebrovasc Dis. 2015;39(5-6):302-8.
9. Liu M, Li G, Tang J, Liao Y, Li L, Zheng Y, et al. The Influence of Sex in Stroke Thrombolysis: A Systematic Review and Meta-Analysis. J Clin Neurol. 2018;14(2):141-52.
10. Yang SH, Shi J, Day AL, Simpkins JW. Estradiol exerts neuroprotective effects when administered after ischemic insult. Stroke. 2000;31(3):745-9.
11. Meyer DM, Eastwood JA, Compton MP, Gylys K, Zivin JA, Ovbiagele B. Sex differences in antiplatelet response in ischemic stroke. Womens Health (Lond). 2011;7(4):465-74.
12. Henderson VW, Lobo RA. Hormone therapy and the risk of stroke: perspectives ten years after the Women's Health Initiative trials. Climacteric J Int Menopause Soc. 2012;15(3):229-34.
13. Schierbeck LL, Rejnmark L, Tofteng CL, Stilgren L, Eiken P, Mosekilde L, et al. Effect of hormone replacement therapy on cardiovascular events in recently postmenopausal women: randomised trial. BMJ. 2012;345:e6409.
14. Carlton C, Banks M, Sundararajan S. Oral Contraceptives and Ischemic Stroke Risk. Stroke. 2018;49(4):e157-9.
15. Bushnell C, McCullough LD, Awad IA, Chireau MV, Fedder WN, Furie KL, et al. Guidelines for the Prevention of Stroke in Women: A Statement for Healthcare Professionals From the American Heart Association/American Stroke Association. Stroke. 2014;45(5):1545-88.
16. Bousser MG, Conard J, Kittner S, de Lignières B, MacGregor EA, Massiou H, et al. Recommendations on the risk of ischaemic stroke associated with use of combined oral contraceptives and hormone replacement therapy in women with migraine. The International Headache Society Task Force on Combined Oral Contraceptives & Hormone Replacement Therapy. Cephalalgia. 2000;20(3):155-6.
17. ACOG Practice Bulletin No. 110: noncontraceptive uses of hormonal contraceptives. Obstet Gynecol. 2010;115(1):206-18.
18. Tate J, Bushnell C. Pregnancy and stroke risk in women. Womens Health (Lond). 2011;7(3):363-74.
19. Grear KE, Bushnell CD. Stroke and Pregnancy: Clinical Presentation, Evaluation, Treatment and Epidemiology. Clin Obstet Gynecol. 2013;56(2):350-9.
20. Reeves MJ, Wilkins T, Lisabeth LD, Schwamm LH. Thrombolysis treatment for acute stroke: issues of efficacy and utilization in women. Womens Health (Lond). 2011;7(3):383-90.
21. Blum B, Wormack L, Holtel M, Penwell A, Lari S, Walker B, et al. Gender and thrombolysis therapy in stroke patients with incidence of dyslipidemia. BMC Womens Health. 2019;19(1):11.
22. Colello MJ, Ivey LE, Gainey J, Faulkner RV, Johnson A, Brechtel L, et al. Pharmacological thrombolysis for acute ischemic stroke treatment: Gender differences in clinical risk factors. Adv Med Sci. 2018;63(1):100-6.
23. Powers WJ, Rabinstein AA, Ackerson T, Adeoye OM, Bambakidis NC, Becker K, et al. 2018 Guidelines for the Early Management of Patients With Acute Ischemic Stroke: A Guideline for Healthcare Professionals From the American Heart Association/American Stroke Association. Stroke. 2018;49(3):e46-110.
24. Blythe R, Ismail A, Naqvi A. Mechanical Thrombectomy for Acute Ischemic Stroke in Pregnancy. J Stroke Cerebrovasc Dis. 2019;28(6):e75-6.

25. Watanabe TT, Ichijo M, Kamata T. Uneventful Pregnancy and Delivery after Thrombolysis Plus Thrombectomy for Acute Ischemic Stroke: Case Study and Literature Review. J Stroke Cerebrovasc Dis. 2019;28(1):70-5.
26. Karalis DG, Hill AN, Clifton S, Wild RA. The risks of statin use in pregnancy: A systematic review. J Clin Lipidol. 2016;10(5):1081-90.
27. Hsieh JT, Ang BT, Ng YP, Allen JC, King NK. Comparison of Gender Differences in Intracerebral Hemorrhage in a Multi-Ethnic Asian Population. PLoS One. 2016;11(4):e0152945.
28. Toossi S, Moheet AM. Intracerebral Hemorrhage in Women: A Review with Special Attention to Pregnancy and the Post-Partum Period. Neurocrit Care. 2019;31(2):390-8.
29. Guha R, Boehme A, Demel SL, Li JJ, Cai X, James ML, et al. Aggressiveness of care following intracerebral hemorrhage in women and men. Neurology. 2017;89(4):349-54.
30. Ferro JM, Canhão P, Stam J, Bousser MG, Barinagarrementeria F. Prognosis of cerebral vein and dural sinus thrombosis: results of the International Study on Cerebral Vein and Dural Sinus Thrombosis (ISCVT). Stroke. 2004;35(3):664-70.

# Movement Disorders: Gender Issues and Management Strategies

*Roopa Rajan, Asha Kishore*

## ABSTRACT

Movement disorders are neurological disorders characterized by abnormal (hyperkinetic or hypokinetic) movements of various parts of body. The dominant motor phenomenology in these disorders may include parkinsonism, tremor, dystonia, chorea, myoclonus, tics, or stereotypies. Nonmotor manifestations accompanying these disorders further contribute to much disability in these conditions. Structurally, basal ganglia and its connection and functionally dopamine metabolism are responsible for abnormal motor symptoms. Common movement disorders include Parkinson's disease, essential tremors, dystonia, chorea, etc. Gender differences exist in the epidemiology and clinical presentation of many of the abovementioned movement disorders. While therapeutic strategies remain the same, response to treatment may be different in women. Special situations such as pregnancy and breastfeeding may require slightly different management approach. We discuss about the gender differences and practical implications of these disorders in this chapter.

Understanding of these gender-specific issues may help prioritize and individualize the treatment of these disabling conditions.

## INTRODUCTION

Movement disorders encompass a wide variety of neurological disorders characterized by an excess (hyperkinetic) or paucity (hypokinetic) of movement. The dominant motor phenomenology in these disorders may include parkinsonism, tremor, dystonia, chorea, myoclonus, tics, or stereotypies. Movement disorders often result from aberrant functioning of a neuronal network subserving motor functions and the diagnostic process is complicated by similar phenotypes resulting from malfunction at a variety of nodes in the motor network. In addition to motor symptoms, nonmotor manifestations accompany many movement disorders and contribute to much disability and morbidity. Women suffering from movement disorders often face many barriers including delay in diagnosis, lack of access to treatment, and may experience symptoms differently from their male counterparts. There are also differences in the epidemiology of the common movement disorders in terms of gender and some unique movement disorders may be specific to women. As movement disorders can affect women at any stage of the life cycle, concerns regarding pregnancy and breastfeeding can affect the choice of treatment in women with movement disorders. This chapter provides an overview of the gender-specific issues and management strategies in women with movement disorders focusing on the common conditions of Parkinson's disease (PD), essential tremor (ET), and dystonia.

## PARKINSON'S DISEASE

Parkinson's disease is the second most common neurodegenerative disorder in adults older than 60 years. It is characterized by the classical motor symptoms of bradykinesia, rigidity, resting tremor, and postural instability. A multitude of nonmotor symptoms ranging from hyposmia, pain, and autonomic and sleep disturbances among others accompany the cardinal motor symptoms. Some of the nonmotor symptoms may be premotor, i.e., appear prior to onset of motor symptoms. An integrated, multidisciplinary approach is essential to effectively control the motor and nonmotor symptoms and improves the quality of life of patients living with PD.

### Epidemiology

According to the Global Burden of Disease Study (2018), the worldwide burden of PD has more than doubled over the past two decades from 2.5 million patients in 1990 to 6.1 million patients in 2016. PD is more common in men than women.

### Clinical Features

Clinical features of PD differ slightly in men and women. Women tend to be older at presentation and are more likely to have a tremor-dominant disease. Symptoms in women are milder as assessed by the UPDRS (Unified Parkinson's Disease Rating Scale) and adjusted for duration of illness. In spite of this, women report worse quality of life and higher levels of functional disability. Nonmotor symptoms vary greatly according to gender. Women report more depression, anxiety, and fatigue. Hyposmia and sexual dysfunction are less often reported by women. Risk of significant cognitive impairment is thought to be lesser in women and women often perform better on cognitive tasks. Rapid eye movement sleep behavior disorder (RBD) occurs equally in both men and women, however women often report only disturbed sleep, the classical symptoms of dream enactment may not be forthcoming.

### Management Issues

Levodopa in combination with a peripheral decarboxylase inhibitor like carbidopa is the mainstay of treatment in PD. Additional drugs used for monotherapy and as add-on include dopamine agonists (pramipexole, ropinirole), monoamine oxidase (MAO) inhibitors (rasagiline, selegiline), catechol-O-methyltransferase (COMT) inhibitor (entacapone), and the N-methyl-D-aspartate (NMDA) antagonist (amantadine). Choice of drugs to initiate treatment is decided by the severity of motor symptoms. In general, gender does not guide the choice of therapeutic agent. Nevertheless, the risk and nature of motor and nonmotor complications may be different in men and women. Pharmacological studies have identified greater bioavailability of levodopa in women.

Female gender is an established risk factor for developing earlier levodopa-induced dyskinesias. Other risk factors include young-onset PD, long disease duration, and higher cumulative levodopa dose. These factors are to be considered when initiating treatment, although gender alone does not guide the choice of treatment.

Among the nonmotor symptoms, impulse control disorders (ICDs) and related behaviors are reported in up to 13–30% of patients with PD. Dopamine agonists are among the strongest risk factors associated with development of ICD, although many other drugs, age, and genetics also play a role. Overall risk of developing ICD is similar in men and women. However, women develop compulsive shopping and compulsive eating more frequently and less frequently report hypersexuality. Women are also less likely to develop dopamine dysregulation syndrome (DDS) which is characterized by compulsive use of dopaminergic medications in excess of the doses required to control motor or nonmotor symptoms.

As the usual age of onset of PD is in the sixth to seventh decades, most women diagnosed with PD are beyond the childbearing age. Nevertheless, some patients develop symptoms of PD in the second decade (juvenile PD) or the third/fourth decade (young-onset PD). In these patients, medications choices and responses may be complicated by physiological hormonal fluctuations and during pregnancy and breastfeeding. Symptoms of PD were noted to increase when women were taking oral contraceptives. Some patients report worsening of PD symptoms during menstruation while other reports suggest that menstrual symptoms can worsen after the onset of PD. Anecdotal evidence suggests that PD symptoms remain static or may worsen during pregnancy. This may be due to withdrawal of medications or reduction of doses during pregnancy. Among the dopaminergic drugs, levodopa appears to be generally safe during pregnancy based on data from case reports and registries. Animal studies suggest teratogenic effects on the fetus on exposure to amantadine and selegiline and these should be avoided in pregnancy. There is insufficient data regarding the safety of other commonly used drugs like dopamine agonists. Obstetric and fetal complications during the perinatal period are not increased in women with PD.

Deep brain stimulation is the standard of care for control of motor fluctuations and levodopa-induced dyskinesias. As mentioned earlier, women are less likely to receive surgical treatments for PD as compared to men. They also undergo surgery after a longer delay than men with similar levels of disability. Few studies have suggested that women have better outcomes after functional neurosurgery for PD compared to men. Due to higher dyskinesias, women are more likely to be undertreated with medications and hence may benefit earlier surgery. Access to informal, unpaid caregiving is lesser for women with PD. Women are also likely to be underrepresented in clinical trials of new therapies for PD, with implications to the generalizability of results.

## ESSENTIAL TREMOR

Essential tremor is characterized by an action or postural tremor of the upper limbs, with additional findings like subtle dystonia, rest tremor, or ataxia in a subset (ET plus). Tremor usually starts in the upper limb and may spread to the head, voice, and legs. Tremor can be quite disabling functionally and may be a source of social embarrassment. Women report being more bothered and embarrassed by the tremor, after adjusting for severity. Head tremor and voice tremor are much more common in women with ET. Head tremor may be accompanied by dystonia (dystonic tremor) which is also more common in women. Medications like propranolol, primidone, and topiramate may be useful in treating the tremor symptomatically. Thalamic deep brain stimulation and stereotactic or focused ultrasound-guided thalamotomy are therapeutic options for refractory ET.

# DYSTONIA

Dystonia is an abnormal involuntary posturing of a body part, characterized by sustained or repetitive and often twisting postures. Dystonias may be focal (affecting a single body part, like blepharospasm), segmental (two contiguous body parts), multifocal (two noncontiguous or more than two sites), or generalized (trunk and at least two other body parts). Focal dystonias are common in adults whereas childhood-onset dystonias have a tendency to generalize. Focal craniocervical dystonias which are the most commonly encountered focal dystonias are more common in women with a female:male ratio of 16–33:1. On the other hand, writer's cramp, another common focal dystonia, is more common in men (male:female ratio 2:1). Some dystonias like the X-linked dystonia-parkinsonism (DYT-*TAF1*) are almost exclusively found in men. Others like dopa-responsive dystonia (DYT-*GCH1*) are more common in women. In myoclonus-dystonia (DYT-*SCGE*), the gene expression is maternally imprinted. This means that children of affected women are less likely to manifest the disease, even if they inherit the aberrant allele from their mother. This has implications for genetic counseling. Although few anecdotal reports have suggested that hormonal fluctuations can affect the severity of dystonic symptoms, larger series identify no major fluctuations in symptoms with pregnancy, menopause, or hormone replacement. Botulinum toxin is the treatment of choice for focal dystonias and is equally effective in men and women. Women with spasmodic adductor dysphonia may require larger doses for symptom control compared to men. Patients with early-onset isolated dystonias are often given a trial of levodopa to check for response (dopa-responsive dystonia). Trihexyphenidyl, baclofen, tetrabenazine, and clonazepam are medications used to treat dystonia. Patients with severe generalized dystonia benefit from deep brain stimulation of the globus pallidus interna. Gender does not modify the effects of deep brain stimulation in dystonia.

# OTHER MOVEMENT DISORDERS

Sydenham's chorea is a delayed manifestation of rheumatic fever. It is more common in girls and may appear for the first time or recur in pregnancy as chorea gravidarum. Mild forms of chorea gravidarum may be left untreated considering the benefit-risk ratio with respect to the fetus. In cases of severe chorea, high potency dopamine receptor blockers may be considered although animal studies have demonstrated occasional teratogenic potential with these drugs. Chorea can be precipitated by oral contraceptive pills. Among the genetic causes of chorea, Huntington's disease (HD) is the most common. Gender of the affected parent influences the expression of disease in offspring. Children receiving the *HD* gene from their mother usually develop later-onset chorea while those receiving it from the father manifest the disease at younger ages, often resulting in a Westphal phenotype. Advanced paternal age at the time of conception is also associated with higher gene expression and earlier and more severe phenotype in the offspring. Prenatal testing is available for HD, though often underutilized.

Tourette syndrome (TS) is characterized by multiple motor and vocal tics, beginning in early childhood with a waxing and waning course. TS is more prevalent in men than women. Neuropsychiatric symptoms like obsessive compulsive disorder and attention deficit hyperactivity disorder often accompany TS. Female patients are especially more likely to manifest obsessive compulsive disorder, depression, and anxiety. Hormonal fluctuations affect the severity of symptoms, with about one-fourth of patients reporting worsening tic severity in the premenstrual phase.

Wilson's disease is a treatable neurometabolic disorder that presents with a spectrum of movement disorders including dystonia, tremor, and ataxia. Hepatic presentations were more common in women whereas the neuropsychiatric presentation was dominated in men. Standard therapy consists of copper chelation with D-penicillamine, oral zinc, or trientine. Although none of these drugs are proven to be safe in pregnancy, considering the essentiality of copper chelation for both neurological and hepatic involvement, the drugs may need to be continued during pregnancy. Case reports have described patients with successful pregnancy outcomes while continuing chelation therapy.

## CONCLUSION

Gender differences exist in the epidemiology and clinical features of many movement disorders. Although therapeutic strategies remain the same, response to treatment and special situations such as pregnancy and breastfeeding may require slightly different approaches to treatment. Understanding of these gender-specific issues may help prioritize and individualize the treatment of these disabling conditions.

## SUGGESTED READING

1. Albaugh DL, Shih YY. Neural circuit modulation during deep brain stimulation at the subthalamic nucleus for Parkinson's disease: what have we learned from neuroimaging studies? Brain Connect. 2014;4(1):1-14.
2. Schapira AH, Chaudhuri KR, Jenner P. Non-motor features of Parkinson disease. Nat Rev Neurosci. 2017;18(7):435-50.
3. Baker JM, Hung AY. Movement Disorders in Women. Semin Neurol. 2017;37(6):653-60.
4. Rabin ML, Stevens-Haas C, Havrilla E, Devi T, Kurlan R. Movement disorders in women: a review. Mov Disord. 2014;29(2):177-83.
5. Ascherio A, Schwarzschild MA. The epidemiology of Parkinson's disease: risk factors and prevention. Lancet Neurol. 2016;15(12):1257-72.
6. Postuma RB, Berg D, Adler CH, Bloem BR, Chan P, Deuschl G, et al. The new definition and diagnostic criteria of Parkinson's disease. Lancet Neurol. 2016;15(6):546-8.
7. Postuma RB, Berg D. Advances in markers of prodromal Parkinson disease. Nat Rev Neurol. 2016;12(11):622-34.
8. Dorsey ER, Elbaz A, Nichols E, Abd-Allah F, Abdelalim A, Adsuar JC, et al. Global, regional, and national burden of Parkinson's disease, 1990–2016: a systematic analysis for the Global Burden of Disease Study 2016. Lancet Neurol. 2018;17(11):939-53.
9. Wooten GF, Currie LJ, Bovbjerg VE, Lee JK, Patrie J. Are men at greater risk for Parkinson's disease than women? J Neurol Neurosurg Psychiatry. 2004;75(4):637-9.
10. Haaxma CA, Bloem BR, Borm GF, Oyen WJG, Leenders KL, Eshuis S, et al. Gender differences in Parkinson's disease. J Neurol Neurosurg Psychiatry. 2007;78(8):819-24.
11. Nandipati S, Litvan I. Environmental Exposures and Parkinson's Disease. Int J Environ Res Public Health. 2016;13(9):E881.
12. Smith KM, Dahodwala N. Sex differences in Parkinson's disease and other movement disorders. Exp Neurol. 2014;259:44-56.
13. Rocca WA, Bower JH, Maraganore DM, Ahlskog JE, Grossardt BR, de Andrade M, et al. Increased risk of parkinsonism in women who underwent oophorectomy before menopause. Neurology. 2008;70(3):200-9.
14. Benedetti MD, Maraganore DM, Bower JH, McDonnell SK, Peterson BJ, Ahlskog JE, et al. Hysterectomy, menopause, and estrogen use preceding Parkinson's disease: an exploratory case-control study. Mov Disord. 2001;16(5):830-7.
15. Rugbjerg K, Christensen J, Tjønneland A, Olsen JH. Exposure to estrogen and women's risk for Parkinson's disease: a prospective cohort study in Denmark. Parkinsonism Relat Disord. 2013;19(4):457-60.

16. Liu R, Baird D, Park Y, Freedman ND, Huang X, Hollenbeck A, et al. Female reproductive factors, menopausal hormone use, and Parkinson's disease. Mov Disord. 2014;29(7):889-96.
17. Weisskopf MG, O'Reilly E, Chen H, Schwarzschild MA, Ascherio A. Plasma urate and risk of Parkinson's disease. Am J Epidemiol. 2007;166(5):561-7.
18. Gao X, O'Reilly ÉJ, Schwarzschild MA, Ascherio A. Prospective study of plasma urate and risk of Parkinson disease in men and women. Neurology. 2016;86(6):520-6.
19. Szewczyk-Krolikowski K, Tomlinson P, Nithi K, Wade-Martins R, Talbot K, Ben-Shlomo Y, et al. The influence of age and gender on motor and non-motor features of early Parkinson's disease: initial findings from the Oxford Parkinson Disease Center (OPDC) discovery cohort. Parkinsonism Relat Disord. 2014;20(1):99-105.
20. Perrin AJ, Nosova E, Co K, Book A, Iu O, Silva V, et al. Gender differences in Parkinson's disease depression. Parkinsonism Relat Disord. 2017;36:93-7.
21. Martinez-Martin P, Falup-Pecurariu C, Odin P, van Hilten JJ, Antonini A, Rojo-Abuin JM, et al. Gender-related differences in the burden of non-motor symptoms in Parkinson's disease. J Neurol. 2012;259(8):1639-47.
22. Pigott K, Rick J, Xie SX, Hurtig H, Chen-Plotkin A, Duda JE, et al. Longitudinal study of normal cognition in Parkinson disease. Neurology. 2015;85(15):1276–82.
23. Mahale RR, Yadav R, Pal PK. Rapid eye movement sleep behaviour disorder in women with Parkinson's disease is an underdiagnosed entity. J Clin Neurosci. 2016;28:43-6.
24. Connolly BS, Lang AE. Pharmacological treatment of Parkinson disease: a review. JAMA. 2014;311(16):1670-83.
25. Umeh CC, Pérez A, Augustine EF, Dhall R, Dewey RB, Mari Z, et al. No sex differences in use of dopaminergic medication in early Parkinson disease in the US and Canada—baseline findings of a multicenter trial. PLoS One. 2014;9(12):e112287.
26. Hassin-Baer S, Molchadski I, Cohen OS, Nitzan Z, Efrati L, Tunkel O, et al. Gender effect on time to levodopa-induced dyskinesias. J Neurol. 2011;258(11):2048-53.
27. Warren Olanow C, Kieburtz K, Rascol O, Poewe W, Schapira AH, Emre M, et al. Factors predictive of the development of Levodopa-induced dyskinesia and wearing-off in Parkinson's disease. Mov Disord. 2013;28(8):1064-71.
28. Hariz GM, Nakajima T, Limousin P, Foltynie T, Zrinzo L, Jahanshahi M, et al. Gender distribution of patients with Parkinson's disease treated with subthalamic deep brain stimulation: a review of the 2000-2009 literature. Parkinsonism Relat Disord. 2011;17(3):146-9.
29. Willis AW, Schootman M, Kung N, Wang XY, Perlmutter JS, Racette BA. Disparities in deep brain stimulation surgery among insured elders with Parkinson disease. Neurology. 2014;82(2):163-71.
30. Picillo M, Palladino R, Moccia M, Erro R, Amboni M, Vitale C, et al. Gender and non motor fluctuations in Parkinson's disease: A prospective study. Parkinsonism Relat Disord. 2016;27:89-92.
31. Weintraub D, Koester J, Potenza MN, Siderowf AD, Stacy M, Voon V, et al. Impulse control disorders in Parkinson disease: a cross-sectional study of 3090 patients. Arch Neurol. 2010;67(5):589-95.
32. Sarathchandran P, Soman S, Sarma G, Krishnan S, Kishore A. Impulse control disorders and related behaviors in Indian patients with Parkinson's disease. Mov Disord. 2013;28(13):1901-2.
33. Giovannoni G, O'Sullivan JD, Turner K, Manson AJ, Lees AJ. Hedonistic homeostatic dysregulation in patients with Parkinson's disease on dopamine replacement therapies. J Neurol Neurosurg Psychiatry. 2000;68(4):423-8.
34. Maeda T, Shimo Y, Chiu SW, Yamaguchi T, Kashihara K, Tsuboi Y, et al. Clinical manifestations of nonmotor symptoms in 1021 Japanese Parkinson's disease patients from 35 medical centers. Parkinsonism Relat Disord. 2017;38:54-60.
35. Kompoliti K, Comella CL, Jaglin JA, Leurgans S, Raman R, Goetz CG. Menstrual-related changes in motoric function in women with Parkinson's disease. Neurology. 2000;55(10):1572-5.
36. Seier M, Hiller A. Parkinson's disease and pregnancy: An updated review. Parkinsonism Relat Disord. 2017;40:11-7.
37. Anderson VC, Burchiel KJ, Hogarth P, Favre J, Hammerstad JP. Pallidal vs subthalamic nucleus deep brain stimulation in Parkinson disease. Arch Neurol. 2005;62(4):554-60.
38. Accolla E, Caputo E, Cogiamanian F, Tamma F, Mrakic-Sposta S, Marceglia S, et al. Gender differences in patients with Parkinson's disease treated with subthalamic deep brain stimulation. Mov Disord. 2007;22(8):1150-6.

39. Chandran S, Krishnan S, Rao RM, Sarma SG, Sarma PS, Kishore A. Gender influence on selection and outcome of deep brain stimulation for Parkinson's disease. Ann Indian Acad Neurol. 2014;17(1):66-70.
40. Dahodwala N, Shah K, He Y, Wu SS, Schmidt P, Cubillos F, et al. Sex disparities in access to caregiving in Parkinson disease. Neurology. 2018;90(1):e48-54.
41. Tosserams A, Araújo R, Pringsheim T, Post B, Darweesh SK, IntHout J, et al. Underrepresentation of women in Parkinson's disease trials. Mov Disord. 2018;33(11):1825-6.
42. Bhatia KP, Bain P, Bajaj N, Elble RJ, Hallett M, Louis ED, et al. Consensus Statement on the Classification of Tremors. From the Task Force on Tremor of the International Parkinson and Movement Disorder Society. Mov Disord. 2018;33(1):75-87.
43. Louis ED, Rios E. Embarrassment in essential tremor: prevalence, clinical correlates and therapeutic implications. Parkinsonism Relat Disord. 2009;15(7):535-8.
44. Louis ED, Ford B, Frucht S. Factors associated with increased risk of head tremor in essential tremor: a community-based study in northern Manhattan. Mov Disord. 2003;18(4):432-6.
45. Godeiro-Junior C, Felicio AC, Aguiar PC, Borges V, Silva S, Ferraz HB. Head tremor in patients with cervical dystonia: different outcome? Arq Neuropsiquiatr. 2008;66(4):805-8.
46. Puschmann A, Wszolek ZK. Diagnosis and treatment of common forms of tremor. Semin Neurol. 2011;31(1):65-77.
47. Albanese A, Bhatia K, Bressman SB, DeLong MR, Fahn S, Fung VS, et al. Phenomenology and classification of dystonia: A consensus update. Mov Disord. 2013;28(7):863-73.
48. Soland VL, Bhatia KP, Marsden CD. Sex prevalence of focal dystonias. J Neurol Neurosurg Psychiatry. 1996;60(2):204-5.
49. Domingo A, Westenberger A, Lee LV, Brænne I, Liu T, Vater I, et al. New insights into the genetics of X-linked dystonia-parkinsonism (XDP, DYT3). Eur J Hum Genet. 2015;23(10):1334-40.
50. Lee WW, Jeon BS. Clinical spectrum of dopa-responsive dystonia and related disorders. Curr Neurol Neurosci Rep. 2014;14(7):461.
51. Grabowski M, Zimprich A, Lorenz-Depiereux B, Kalscheuer V, Asmus F, Gasser T, et al. The epsilon-sarcoglycan gene (SGCE), mutated in myoclonus-dystonia syndrome, is maternally imprinted. Eur J Hum Genet. 2003;11(2):138-44.
52. Gwinn-Hardy KA, Adler CH, Weaver AL, Fish NM, Newman SJ. Effect of hormone variations and other factors on symptom severity in women with dystonia. Mayo Clin Proc. 2000;75(3):235-40.
53. Anderson TJ, Rivest J, Stell R, Steiger MJ, Cohen H, Thompson PD, et al. Botulinum toxin treatment of spasmodic torticollis. J Royal Soc Med. 1992;85(9):524-9.
54. Lerner MZ, Lerner BA, Patel AA, Blitzer A. Gender differences in onabotulinum toxin A dosing for adductor spasmodic dysphonia. Laryngoscope. 2017;127(5):1131-4.
55. Luc QN, Querubin J. Clinical Management of Dystonia in Childhood. Paediatr Drugs. 2017;19(5):447-61.
56. Brüggemann N, Kühn A, Schneider SA, Kamm C, Wolters A, Krause P, et al. Short- and long-term outcome of chronic pallidal neurostimulation in monogenic isolated dystonia. Neurology. 2015;84(9):895-903.
57. Maia DP, Fonseca PG, Camargos ST, Pfannes C, Cunningham MC, Cardoso F. Pregnancy in patients with Sydenham's Chorea. Parkinsonism Relat Disord. 2012;18(5):458-61.
58. Riddoch D, Jefferson M, Bickerstaff ER. Chorea and the oral contraceptives. Br Med J. 1971;4(5781):217-8.
59. Farrer LA, Cupples LA, Kiely DK, Conneally PM, Myers RH. Inverse relationship between age at onset of Huntington disease and paternal age suggests involvement of genetic imprinting. Am J Hum Genet. 1992;50(3):528-35.
60. Jankovic J. Tourette's syndrome. N Engl J Med. 2001;345(16):1184-92.
61. Lewin AB, Murphy TK, Storch EA, Conelea CA, Woods DW, Scahill LD, et al. A phenomenological investigation of women with Tourette or other chronic tic disorders. Compr Psychiatry. 2012;53(5):525-34.
62. Schwabe MJ, Konkol RJ. Menstrual cycle-related fluctuations of tics in Tourette syndrome. Pediatr Neurol. 1992;8(1):43-6.
63. Litwin T, Gromadzka G, Członkowska A. Gender differences in Wilson's disease. J Neurol Sci. 2012;312(1-2):31-5.
64. Roberts EA. Update on the Diagnosis and Management of Wilson Disease. Curr Gastroenterol Rep. 2018;20(12):56.

# CHAPTER 4

# Headache Disorders: Are They Different in Women?

*Monika Singla, Sulena, Aastha Takkar Kapila*

## ABSTRACT

Headache is one of the most common neurological symptoms of patients presenting to neurology outpatient department (OPD). Most common primary headaches are migraine, tension headache, and cluster headache. Out of various headaches, migraine is the most common type of headache. It is about two to three times more common in women as compared to men. According to the International Classification of Headache Disorders-3 (ICHD-3), headache is divided into various different types. Clinical profile, severity, triggers, and duration of migraine may vary in women. In this chapter, we would like to discuss migraine in women, its implications, and relation with hormones.

## INTRODUCTION

Headache has been a common complaint since the dawn of civilization to this present day technological world of artificial intelligence.

According to the Global Burden of Diseases 2016, neurological disorders are the leading group cause of disability-adjusted life years (DALYs) and the second leading group cause of deaths in the world. Migraine is the second largest contributor to DALYs with male-to-female ratios of <0.7.

Headache is divided into two broad categories of primary and secondary headache according to the International Classification of Headache Disorders-3 (ICHD-3).

Primary headache is the one where diagnosis is made on pattern recognition of presenting symptoms and no cause found on examination or investigation. The examples for primary headache are migraine, tension-type headache (TTH), or cluster headache, most common being migraine. Secondary headache has an identifiable cause on examination or investigation like cerebral venous thrombosis or brain tumor. Although the most common type of headache is primary type (90%), most pertinent thing is not to miss a secondary cause of headache in clinical practice. The various red flags (**Table 1**) for headache guide so that ominous causes are not missed and if any of these are present, we should consider secondary headache and patient should undergo neuroimaging.

## SECTION 4: Neurology

**TABLE 1 :** Headache 'RED FLAGS'.

- Acute or sudden onset headache
- First or worst headache
- New onset headache
- Headache onset after age of 50 years
- Headache with change in pattern
- Progressive or worsening headache
- Headache that is sudden in onset during exertion, with coughing, with sneezing, sex related or with Valsalva maneuver
- Headache with postural link
- Headache in a setting of malignancy or retroviral disease
- Headache with accompanying neurologic symptoms or signs
- Headache with systemic symptoms (fever, weight loss, cough)

## TYPES OF MIGRAINE

Migraine has mainly two main types:
1. *Migraine without aura*: Migraine without aura, i.e., common migraine is a clinical syndrome characterized by headache, lasting for 4–72 hours, usually pulsating or throbbing unilateral temporal or holocranial headache, and commonly associated with photophobia, phonophobia, nausea, and vomiting.
2. *Migraine with aura*: Other type is migraine with aura or classical migraine. It is primarily characterized by the transient focal neurological symptoms in form of visual aura like zigzag lines, flashes of light, scotomas, homonymous hemianopia, etc., auditory aura, sensory aura, or weakness of any side that usually precede the headache by few minutes or sometimes accompany the headache.

Migraine headache in children and adolescents is usually bilateral as compared to adults where it is unilateral. Few patients may complain of typical facial location of pain, which is called "facial migraine" in the literature.

## PATHOPHYSIOLOGY OF MIGRAINE

The various theories of origin of migraine are cortical spreading depression (CSD), vascular theory, and trigeminovascular system involvement. During migraine without aura, there is no evidence of CSD on regional cerebral blood flow imaging. There may be spreading oligemia seen in migraine with aura patients. Glial waves or other cortical phenomena may be involved in migraine without aura as per literature. Various messenger molecules like nitric oxide (NO), calcitonin gene-related peptide (CGRP), and 5-hydroxytryptamine (5-HT) are involved in migraine pain. The importance of sensitization of pain pathways has been proven in few studies. Triptans, the highly receptor-specific acute medications which are 5-HT1B/D receptor agonists, 5-HT1F receptor agonists, and CGRP receptor antagonists, have demonstrated high efficacy in the acute treatment of migraine attacks. Because of their high receptor specificity, their mechanism of action provides new insight into migraine mechanisms.

## CHAPTER 4: Headache Disorders: Are They Different in Women?

# PREVALENCE OF MIGRAINE

The cumulative incidence of migraine is 43% with annual incidence ranging from 0.8 to 2.38% per year. In India, the prevalence of migraine varies from 1.37 to 72%. Migraine starts with second decade of life with disability reaching its peak at 20–24 years of age—childbearing age. In this chapter, we plan to discuss migraine in women specifically related with hormones.

Migraine varies in different phases of life of female due to a cyclical alteration in hormonal level in blood. This can be understood by dividing them into as follows:
- Menstrual migraine (MM)
- Migraine in pregnant women
- Migraine in postpartum and lactation period
- Migraine in perimenopausal state

## Role of Hormones in Migraine

The cyclical changes in various hormones like hypothalamus secreted gonadotropin-releasing hormone (GnRH), pituitary secreted luteinizing hormone and follicle-stimulating hormone which stimulates the ovarian secretion of estrogen and progesterone that influence migraine. During the luteal phase of menstruation, an abrupt decrease in both estrogen and progesterone levels occurs which possibly trigger MM and prime blood vessels to other factors, such as prostaglandins (PGs).

## Menstrual Migraine

Menstrual migraine first noted in 1666 by Van der Linden is now seen in 60% of women with migraine.

As compared to migraines occurring at other times of the cycle, MM attacks are more severe, of longer duration, more disabling, and less responsive to both acute and prophylactic treatment.

The ICHD-3 defines MM as pure menstrual migraine (PMM) without aura and menstrually-related migraine without aura (MRM) (**Table 2**).

Pure menstrual migraine without aura is less common, affecting 10–14% of female migraineurs as compared to MRM which affects >50% of women with migraine.

Treatment of MM includes nonpharmacological and pharmacological measures. Nonpharmacological treatment includes avoidance of known triggers, regular exercise, sleep hygiene, good hydration, education, reassurance, and behavioral therapy. Pharmacological treatment includes acute treatment and short- and long-term prophylaxis. Women should be counseled well in advance regarding side effects of the medicines and contraception, e.g., topiramate in doses >200 mg/day can cause hormonal birth control failure due to rapid metabolism of estrogens and progestins.

For females who have headache mainly with menses, it can be managed with acute treatment. Acute treatment consists of nonsteroidal anti-inflammatory drugs (NSAIDs), triptans, or dihydroergotamine (DHE) which can be used for the duration of MM which may be 5–7 days. Women who have less frequent attacks can be managed with short-term prophylaxis for 5–7 days with NSAIDs, triptans or DHE, methergine, and magnesium.

Women who have severe MM and also headache during other days of cycle may need long-term prophylaxis with hormonal therapy with estrogens alone or combined with

**TABLE 2:** Diagnostic criteria for menstrual migraine.

**Pure menstrual migraine without aura:**
A. Attacks, in a menstruating woman,[1] fulfilling criteria for migraine without aura as per ICHD-3 classification and Criterion B given below
B. Documented and prospectively-recorded evidence over at least three consecutive cycles has confirmed that attacks occur exclusively on day 1 ± 2 (i.e., days −2 to +3)[2] of menstruation[1] in at least two out of three menstrual cycles and at no other times of the cycle

**Menstrually-related migraine without aura**
A. Attacks, in a menstruating woman,[1] fulfilling criteria for migraine without aura as per ICHD-3 classification and criterion B below
A. Documented and prospectively-recorded evidence over at least three consecutive cycles has confirmed that attacks occur on day 1 ± 2 (i.e., days −2 to +3)[2] of menstruation[1] in at least two out of three menstrual cycles, and additionally at other times of the cycle

[1]For the purposes of ICHD-3 menstruation is considered to be endometrial bleeding resulting from either the normal menstrual cycle or from the withdrawal of exogenous progestogens, as in the use of combined oral contraceptives or cyclical hormone replacement therapy.
[2]The first day of menstruation is day 1 and the preceding day is day −1; there is no day 0.

progestins, estrogens modulators and antagonists, pharmacological oophorectomy with GnRH analog with or without add-back therapy, and prolactin release inhibitors.

# Migraine During Pregnancy, Postpartum, and Lactation State

As in general population, important point is to rule out secondary cause of headache. New onset or new type of headache confers 50% chances of secondary headache. Presence of hypertension and proteinuria along with headache suggests preeclampsia.

Migraine with aura has an unpredictable course during pregnancy. Its frequency tends to increase during pregnancy and postpartum and decrease with breastfeeding.

The prognosis of migraine with aura varies according to the trimester. In first trimester, migraine tends to worsen but improves in subsequent trimesters. Migraine with onset at menarche and MM tend to improve during pregnancy.

Women with migraine are at an increased risk of developing hypertensive disorder and vascular events—cardiovascular and cerebrovascular events including venous thromboembolism. They are also at higher risk of delivering a low birth weight or a preterm child and undergoing cesarean section and placental abruption. However, migraine does not seem to increase the risk of miscarriage, congenital anomalies, and stillbirth.

The management of migraine in women begins with a preconception visit in anticipation of pregnancy to plan the treatment for acute attacks and prophylactic medication. The treatment consists of nonpharmacological treatment as discussed above. Pharmacological treatment includes acute treatment and preventive medication. All medications have uncertainty regarding their safety for use in pregnancy. The Food and Drug Administration (FDA) prescription drug labeling should be consulted before prescription in pregnancy.

In acute attacks, acetaminophen (oral or intravenous) with doses limited to 4 g/day along with prochlorperazine and metoclopramide can be used in all trimesters. NSAIDs may be used during second trimester, but avoided in first trimester due to risk of spontaneous abortion and third trimester due to risk of premature closure of fetal ductus arteriosus.

## CHAPTER 4: Headache Disorders: Are They Different in Women?

For prevention of further attacks in disabling migraine, drugs which can be used are magnesium, metoprolol, amitriptyline (doses of 10–50 mg), and lidocaine peripheral nerve block every 2–4 weeks.

Beta-blockers (metoprolol and propranolol) are not the first-line option for prophylaxis in pregnant women. The potential fetal side effects are intrauterine growth retardation, preterm birth and respiratory distress, and bradycardia. If patient already taking beta-blockers, they should be tapered 2–3 days prior to labor. Magnesium sulfate (350 mg/day) is a FDA-approved drug for prophylaxis. Other drugs considered with uncertain safety value are coenzyme Q10 (100 mg twice daily) and riboflavin. Onabotulinumtoxin-A is a FDA-approved Category C drug for chronic migraine in pregnancy. Pericranial peripheral nerve block with lidocaine has also shown positive result in migraine.

Acute and preventive medications for migraine during breastfeeding are given in **Table 3**.

## Migraine in Perimenopausal Period

There may be improvement or worsening of migraine during menopause. Natural menopause is associated with a lower prevalence of migraine compared to surgical menopause. The prevalence of migraine with aura does not improve with menopause as compared to migraine without aura.

Hormone replacement therapy (HRT) has a variable effect on migraine. Though, most women have decrease in the frequency of attacks, few report worsening of migraine.

The effect of HRT on migraine depends on regimen, type of hormonal preparation, dose, and route of delivery. Nonoral routes are better as compared to oral formulations of estrogen replacement for migraine, possibly due to more stable serum hormone levels.

## NEW MARKERS IN FEMALES WITH MIGRAINE

The pathophysiology of migraines is complex and involves multiple factors. The psychological and physical symptoms associated with migraine have been linked to abnormal cytokine production, increased proinflammatory interleukin (IL)-1β, IL-6,

**TABLE 3:** Acute and preventive medications for migraine during breastfeeding.

|  | Considered safe | Use with caution | Contraindications |
|---|---|---|---|
| Acute | • Acetaminophen<br>• Caffeine<br>• Ibuprofen<br>• Diclofenac<br>• Low dose aspirin<br>• Eletriptan<br>• Sumatriptan | • Naproxen<br>• Indomethacin<br>• Codeine<br>• Metoclopramide<br>• Prochlorperazine | • High dose aspirin<br>• Ergot derivative<br>• Ketorolac |
| Preventive | • Metoprolol<br>• Propranolol<br>• Amitriptyline<br>• Nortriptyline<br>• Onabotulinum toxin A | • Topiramate<br>• Valproic acid | • Atenolol<br>• Nadolol<br>• Ergot derivatives<br>• Riboflavin<br>• Candesartan<br>• Memantine |

tumor necrosis factor-α (TNF-α), proinflammatory chemokine IL-8, and an exaggeratedly skewed cytokine profile, in particular the TNF-α and 12p70/IL-10.

## OTHER CAUSES OF HEADACHE DURING PREGNANCY

Around 30–50% women have headache during pregnancy. Primary headaches such as migraine without aura, TTH, and migraine with aura are more common than secondary headache.

New-onset migraine without aura and migraine with aura during pregnancy are reported in 1–10% and 14% of the cases, respectively. Secondary headaches are seen in 42% of patient with common causes being cerebral venous thrombosis, ischemic and hemorrhagic stroke, arterial dissection and subarachnoid hemorrhage, hypertensive disorders including preeclampsia, common viral infections, and acute sinusitis. Magnetic resonance imaging is the preferred imaging method for evaluating these patients as it involves no exposure to ionizing radiation.

There may be various triggers for migraine in women which may act alone or in combination are stress, sun exposure, sleep deprivation, travel, hair wash or head bath, missing meals, and fasting.

## CONCLUSION

Migraine with its accompanying disability is more common in females as compared to males. Due to cyclical alteration in hormonal level, migraine varies in different phases of life of female and so treatment also varies accordingly. Thereby, a compassionate, meticulous, and open minded approach toward treatment of migraine is warranted in females.

## SUGGESTED READING

1. Critchley M. Migraine: from cappadocia to queen square. In: Smith R (Ed). Background to Migraine. London: Heinemann; 1967. pp. 28-38.
2. Feigin VL, Nichols E, Alam T, Bannick MS, Beghi E, Blake N, et al. Global, regional, and national burden of neurological disorders, 1990–2016: a systematic analysis for the Global Burden of Disease Study 2016. Lancet Neurol. 2019;18(5):459-80.
3. Olesen J, Dodick DW, Ducros A, Evers S, First MB, Goadsby PJ, et al. The International Classification of Headache Disorders, 3rd edition (ICHD-3). Cephalalgia. 2018;33(9):629-808.
4. Rasmusssen BK, Jensen R, Schroll M, Olessen J. Epidemiology of headache in a general population—a prevalence study. J Clin Epidemiol. 1991;44(11):1147-57.
5. Stewart WF, Wood C, Reed ML, Roy J, Lipton RB. Cumulative lifetime migraine incidence in women and men. Cephalalgia. 2008;28(11):1170-8.
6. Stovner LJ, Hagen K, Jensen R, Katsarava Z, Lipton RB, Scher AI, et al. The global burden of headache: a documentation of headache prevalence and disability worldwide. Cephalalgia. 2007;27(3):193-210.
7. Das SK, Sanyal K. Neuroepidemiology of major neurological disorders in rural Bengal. Neurol India. 1996;44(2):47-58.
8. Saha SP, Bhattacharya S, Das SK, Maity B, Roy T, Raut DK. Epidemiological study of neurological disorders in a rural population of Eastern India. J Indian Med Assoc. 2003;101(5):299-300.
9. Ray BK, Paul N, Hazra A, Das S, Ghosal MK, Misra AK, et al. Prevalence, burden, and risk factors of migraine: a community-based study from Eastern India. Neurol India. 2017;65(6):1280-8.
10. Abu-Arafeh I, Razak S, Sivaraman B, Graham C. Prevalence of headache and migraine in children and adolescents: a systematic review of population-based studies. Dev Med Child Neurol. 2010;52(12):1088-97.

11. Laurell K, Larsson B, Eeg-Olofsson O. Prevalence of headache in Swedish schoolchildren, with a focus on tension-type headache. Cephalalgia. 2004;24(5):380-8.
12. Lipton RB, Bigal EM. The epidemiology of migraine. Am J Med. 2005;118 (Suppl 1):3S-10.
13. Horrobin D. Prostaglandins and migraine. Headache. 1977;16(2):113-6.
14. Somerville BW. The role of estradiol withdrawal in the etiology of menstrual migraine. Neurology. 1972;22(4):355-65.
15. Van der Linden JA. De Hemicrania Menstrua Historia et Consilium. London: Bavarian State Library; 1660.
16. Allais G, Benedetto C. Update on menstrual migraine: from clinical aspects to therapeutic strategies. Neurol Sci. 2004;25 (Suppl 3):S229-31.
17. MacGregor EA. Oestrogen and attacks of migraine with and without aura. Lancet Neurol. 2004;3(6):354-61.
18. MacGregor EA, Hackshaw A. Prevalence of migraine on each day of the natural menstrual cycle. Neurology. 2004;63(2):351-3.
19. Granella F, Sances G, Allais G, Nappi R, Tirelli A, Ferraris A, et al. Characteristics of menstrual and non-menstrual attacks in women with menstrually related migraine. Cephalalgia. 2001;21(4):263-4.
20. Olesen J, Steiner TJ. The International Classification of Headache Disorders, 2nd Edn (ICDH-II). J Neurol Neurosurg Psychiatry. 2004;75(6):808-11.
21. Silberstein SD, Merriam GR. Sex hormones and headache. J Pain Symptom Manage. 1993;8(2):98-114.
22. Johannessen SI, Landmark CJ. Antiepileptic drug interactions—principles and clinical implications. Curr Neuropharmacol. 2010;8(3):254-67.
23. Wells RE, Turner DP, Lee M, Bishop L, Strauss L. Managing Migraine During Pregnancy and Lactation. Curr Neurol Neurosci Rep. 2016;16(4):40.
24. Melhado EM, Maciel JA, Guerreiro CA. Headache during gestation: evaluation of 1101 women. Can J Neurol Sci. 2007;34(2):187-92.
25. Aubé M. Migraine in pregnancy. Neurology. 1999;53 4 (Suppl 1):S26-8.
26. Sances G, Granella F, Nappi RE, Fignon A, Ghiotto N, Polatti F, et al. Course of migraine during pregnancy and postpartum: a prospective study. Cephalalgia. 2003;23(3):197-205.
27. Wabnitz A, Bushnell C. Migraine, cardiovascular disease, and stroke during pregnancy: systematic review of the literature. Cephalalgia. 2015;35(2):132-9.
28. Gassman AL, Nguyen CP, Joffe HV. FDA regulation of prescription drugs. N Engl J Med. 2017;376(7):674-82.
29. Freeman EW, Sammel MD, Lin H, Gracia CR, Kapoor S. Symptoms in the menopausal transition: hormone and behavioral correlates. Obstet Gynecol. 2008;111(1):127-36.
30. Wang SJ, Fuh JL, Lu SR, Juang KD, Wang PH. Migraine prevalence during menopausal transition. Headache. 2003;43(5):470-8.
31. Neri I, Granella F, Nappi R, Manzoni GC, Facchinetti F, Genazzani AR. Characteristics of headache at menopause: a clinico-epidemiologic study. Maturitas. 1993;17(1):31-7.
32. Mattsson P. Hormonal factors in migraine: a population-based study of women aged 40 to 74 years. Headache. 2003;43(1):27-35.
33. MacGregor A. Effects of oral and transdermal estrogen replacement on migraine. Cephalalgia. 1999;19(2):124-5.
34. MacGregor EA. Migraine, the menopause and hormone replacement therapy: a clinical review. J Fam Plann Reprod Health Care. 2007;33(4):245-9.
35. Buse DC, Loder EW, Gorman JA, Stewart WF, Reed ML, Fanning KM, et al. Sex differences in the prevalence, symptoms, and associated features of migraine, probable migraine and other severe headache: results of the American Migraine Prevalence and Prevention (AMPP) Study. Headache. 2013;53(8):1278-99.
36. Maleki N, Linnman C, Brawn J, Burstein R, Becerra L, Borsook D. Her versus his migraine: multiple sex differences in brain function and structure. Brain. 2012;135 (Pt 8):2546-59.
37. Dai Z, Zhong J, Xiao P, Zhu Y, Chen F, Pan P, et al. Gray matter correlates of migraine and gender effect: A meta-analysis of voxel-based morphometry studies. Neuroscience. 2015;299:88-96.
38. Maniyar FH, Sprenger T, Monteith T, Schankin CJ, Goadsby PJ. The premonitory phase of migraine–what can we learn from it? Headache. 2015;55(5):609-20.

39. Schulte LH, Allers A, May A. Hypothalamus as a mediator of chronic migraine: Evidence from high-resolution fMRI. Neurology. 2017;88(21):2011-6.
40. Moulton EA, Becerra L, Johnson A, Burstein R, Borsook D. Altered hypothalamic functional connectivity with autonomic circuits and the locus coeruleus in migraine. PLoS One. 2014;9(4):e95508.
41. Bahra A, Matharu MS, Buchel C, Frackowiak RS, Goadsby PJ. Brainstem activation specific to migraine headache. Lancet. 2001;357(9261):1016-7.
42. Tso AR, Trujillo A, Guo CC, Goadsby PJ, Seeley WW. The anterior insula shows heightened interictal intrinsic connectivity in migraine without aura. Neurology. 2015;84(10):1043-50.
43. Akerman S, Holland PR, Goadsby PJ. Diencephalic and brainstem mechanisms in migraine. Nat Rev Neurosci. 2011;12(10):570-84.
44. Noseda R, Burstein R. Migraine pathophysiology: anatomy of the trigeminovascular pathway and associated neurological symptoms, cortical spreading depression, sensitization, and modulation of pain. Pain. 2013;154 (Suppl 1):S44-53.
45. Boćkowski L, Śmigielska-Kuzia J, Sobaniec W, Żelazowska-Rutkowska B, Kułak W, Sendrowski K. Anti-inflammatory plasma cytokines in children and adolescents with migraine headaches. Pharmacol Rep. 2010;62(2):287-91.
46. Uzar E, Evliyaoglu O, Yucel Y, Ugur Cevik M, Acar A, Guzel I, et al. Serum cytokine and pro-brain natriuretic peptide (BNP) levels in patients with migraine. Eur Rev Med Pharmacol Sci. 2011;15(10):1111-6.
47. Kemper RH, Meijler WJ, Korf J, Ter Horst GJ. Migraine and function of the immune system: a meta-analysis of clinical literature published between 1966 and 1999. Cephalalgia. 2001;21(5):549-57.
48. Duarte H, Teixeira AL, Rocha NP, Domingues RB. Increased interictal serum levels of CXCL8/IL-8 and CCL3/MIP-1α in migraine. Neurol Sci. 2015;36(2):203-8.
49. Oliveira AB, Bachi AL, Ribeiro RT, Mello MT, Tufik S, Peres MF. Unbalanced plasma TNF-α and IL-12/IL-10 profile in women with migraine is associated with psychological and physiological outcomes. J Neuroimmunol. 2017;313:138-44.
50. Maggioni F, Alessi C, Maggino T, Zanchin G. Headache during pregnancy. Cephalalgia. 1997;17(7):765-9.
51. Raffaelli B, Siebert E, Körner J, Liman T, Reuter U, Neeb L. Characteristics and diagnoses of acute headache in pregnant women—a retrospective cross-sectional study. J Headache Pain. 2017;18(1):114.
52. Edlow JA, Caplan LR, O'Brien K, Tibbles CD. Diagnosis of acute neurological emergencies in pregnant and post-partum women. Lancet Neurol. 2013;12(2):175-85.
53. Granella F, Sances G, Pucci E, Nappi RE, Ghiotto N, Nappi G. Migraine with aura and reproductive life events: a case control study. Cephalalgia. 2000;20(8):701-7.
54. Ravishankar K. 'Hair wash' or 'head bath' triggering migraine—observations in 94 Indian patients. Cephalalgia. 2006;26(11):1330-4.
55. Turner LC, Molgaard CA, Gardner CH, Rothrock JF, Stang PE. Migraine trigger factors in a non-clinical Mexican-American population in San Diego country: implications for etiology. Cephalalgia. 1995;15(6):523-30.
56. Hauge AW, Kirchmann M, Olesen J. Trigger factors in migraine with aura. Cephalalgia. 2010;30(3):346-53.

# CHAPTER 5

# Neuroimmunology: Special Considerations in Women

*Aastha Takkar Kapila, Anu Gupta, Julie Sachdeva, Monika Singla*

## ABSTRACT

Neuroimmunology deals with disorders involving immune aberrations of the nervous system. The immunological and endocrinal differences in women make them more prone to develop these disorders underscoring the importance of understanding the special considerations of these disorders in women. For a long time, neuroinflammatory diseases like multiple sclerosis (MS) received majority of the attention by researchers worldwide. Paradigm change was witnessed in this branch when other neuroimmunological diseases like other inflammatory demyelinating diseases including neuromyelitis optica (NMO), autoimmune encephalopathies, and vasculitic disorders affecting the nervous system were recognized. Autoimmune encephalopathies represent noninfectious, immunotherapy responsive encephalopathies, specially affecting individuals of younger age group. Vasculitic disorders affecting the nervous system are characterized by vascular inflammation affecting vessels of different sizes. This chapter discusses these neuroimmunological disorders with special considerations in women.

## INTRODUCTION

The breakdown of immunological tolerance leading to immune reaction against a self-molecule leads to autoimmune disorders. Various studies suggest associations of environmental, genetic factors, and certain types of infections with autoimmune disorders. Prevalence of autoimmune disorders in the Indian subcontinent is not known, but approximately 3% of the Western populations currently suffer from autoimmune diseases. The field of neuroimmunology deals with interaction of neurosciences and immunology. Women are found to be at significantly higher risk of developing an autoimmune disease than men. The risk increases to almost 10-folds in young, postpubescent women. Although the mechanisms for this predisposition are not entirely known, but it is a known fact that females and castrated males produce much higher levels of estrogen and reduced levels of testosterone which may alter the immune response. In addition, women undergo sweeping endocrinological changes at least twice during their lifetime, i.e., puberty and menopause and these endocrinological transitions exert significant effects on the immune system due to interactions between the hormonal milieu, innate, and adaptive immune systems as well as pro- and anti-inflammatory cytokines and thereby modulate the susceptibility of women to autoimmune diseases.

SECTION 4: Neurology

## AUTOIMMUNE DISORDERS AFFECTING THE NERVOUS SYSTEM

Common autoimmune disorders affecting the central nervous system (CNS) include multiple sclerosis (MS), neuromyelitis optica spectrum disorders (NMOSDs), autoimmune encephalitis (AE), and vasculitic disorders—primary and secondary.

## SPECIFIC NEUROIMMUNOLOGICAL DISORDERS

### Multiple Sclerosis and Neuromyelitis Optica Spectrum Disorders

Multiple sclerosis is a chronic demyelinating disease of the CNS. MS typically presents as relapsing-remitting attacks of inflammation, demyelination, and axonal damage leading to various degrees of neurological symptoms and disability.

Neuromyelitis optica spectrum disorders, traditionally known as Devic disease, are inflammatory demyelinating disorders (IDDs) affecting CNS and are probably the most common IDD apart from MS. These debilitating disorders affect the optic nerves and spinal cord often with frequent relapses resulting in significant mortality and morbidity.

### Prevalence

The prevalence of MS varies from 0.5 to 1.5/100,000. However, there is a relatively wide range in the prevalence of Neuromyelitis optica (NMO) depending upon the differences in geographic and ethnicity of the cohorts which varies from 1 to 5/100,000 population.

The prevalence of MS in women has increased markedly during the last decades (2.3–3.5:1). MS primarily affects young adults between 20 and 40 years of age. NMO is up to nine times more prevalent in females compared to males and has the median age of onset in the late fourth decade. However, it is known to occur in all age groups including children and elderly.

### Pathogenesis of Multiple Sclerosis and Neuromyelitis Optica

White and gray matter tissue inflammation due to focal immune cell infiltration and associated cytokines is the cause of damage in MS. Also, studies have suggested that T-helper cell intervention and adaptive immune responses [which are initiated by interaction between antigen-presenting cells (APCs) with T lymphocytes] play an important role in the initiation and progression of MS.

In NMO, an antigenic stimulus leads to the peripheral production of circulating immunoglobulins (NMO-IgG). Through a presumed breach or deficiency in the blood–brain barrier, the antibody is able to access the extracellular domain of aquaporin-4 (AQP4) at the glia limitans resulting in its internalization and subsequent degeneration. The peripheral source of NMO-IgG may also explain the excellent response to plasma exchange in patients with NMO.

### Types of Multiple Sclerosis

- Benign MS/clinically isolated syndrome (CIS)
- Relapsing-remitting MS (RRMS)
- *Progressive MS*:
    - Secondary progressive MS (SPMS)
    - Primary progressive MS (PPMS)
    - Progressive-relapsing MS (PRMS)

### Benign Multiple Sclerosis/Clinically Isolated Syndrome (Table 1)

Clinically isolated syndrome is the first episode of neurologic symptoms caused by demyelination in the CNS. The episode, which by definition must last for at least 24 hours, is characteristic of MS but does not yet meet the criteria (clinical/radiological) for a diagnosis of MS because people who experience a CIS may or may not go on to develop MS.

### Relapsing-remitting Multiple Sclerosis (Table 1)

It is the most common type of MS, accounting for 85% of cases. It is characterized by relapses of focal neurological deficits without concomitant fever. Complete remissions/period of stability may be seen in between relapses. Radiologically, many more brain lesions than expected of the clinical condition are seen on imaging.

### Secondary Progressive Multiple Sclerosis

Relapsing-remitting multiple sclerosis can progress to SPMS which is characterized by axonal injury and atrophy in white and gray matter. Clinically, the neurological symptoms become progressive after initial relapses.

### Primary Progressive Multiple Sclerosis

It is seen in <15% of patients and is characterized by symptoms that worsen from onset of disease without relapse or remission.

### Progressive-relapsing Multiple Sclerosis

It is characterized by progressive disease from the start with intermittent flare-up and no period of remission.

## Clinical Features and Diagnostic Criteria

The clinical features of MS and NMO are shown in **Tables 1** and **2A and B**.

## Investigations

### Neuroimaging

On spinal magnetic resonance imaging (MRI), NMO is characterized by acute continuous longitudinal lesions covering three/more vertebral levels [longitudinally extensive or patchy transverse myelitis (TM)] while MS is suggested by patchy lesions that are rarely continuous over more than one vertebral segment (short segment TM). In NMO, spinal cord lesions tend to be centrally located, rarely extending to the surface of the cord, whereas in MS such lesions are located peripherally or eccentrically. Normal brain imaging is initially present in 55–84% of the patients with NMO, but cerebral white matter lesions can be expected over the course of the disease. NMO typical lesions correspond to areas with high AQP4 expression such as hypothalamus, ependymal cells, and brainstem. MS typical lesions are distributed in the periventricular, cortical, juxtacortical, and infratentorial regions of the brain.

### Cerebrospinal Fluid Analysis

Patients of NMOSD frequently have cerebrospinal fluid (CSF) pleocytosis (>50 cells/µL) while the CSF in MS rarely reveals a pleocytosis. The peripheral synthesis of NMO-IgG is consistent with the relative lack of CSF oligoclonal bands in the NMO, as NMO-IgG is not generated primarily by intrathecal synthesis, this in contrast to MS, which is characterized

**TABLE 1:** Clinical features of MS and NMO.

| Clinical features | Multiple sclerosis (MS) | Neuromyelitis optica (NMO) |
|---|---|---|
| Classical symptoms | Sensory loss—paresthesias<br>*Spinal cord symptoms:*<br>• Motor symptoms—weakness, muscle cramps secondary to spasticity<br>• Autonomic symptoms—bladder, bowel, and sexual dysfunction<br>• Symptoms associated with partial acute transverse myelitis<br>• Cerebellar symptoms—Charcot triad of dysarthria, nystagmus, and intention tremor<br>*Optic neuritis:*<br>• Trigeminal neuralgia—bilateral facial weakness or trigeminal neuralgia<br>*Facial myokymia:*<br>• Eye symptoms—diplopia, internuclear ophthalmoplegia<br>*Heat intolerance:*<br>• Constitutional symptoms—fatigability, dizziness, and lack of sleep<br>• Pain—Occurs in 30–50% of patients at some point in their illness<br>• Subjective cognitive difficulties<br>• Depression<br>• Euphoria<br>• Bipolar disorder or frank dementia | • Optic neuritis—Isolated/simultaneous/sequential<br>• Myelitis<br>• Brainstem presentation—intractable hiccups, nausea and vomiting, vertigo, ataxia, and bulbar symptoms<br>• Hypothalamic presentation—narcolepsy, syndrome of inappropriate antidiuretic hormone secretion, anorexia, or hyperphagia<br>• Cerebral presentations—posterior reversible encephalopathy syndrome, impairment of consciousness, and seizures |

by synthesis of oligoclonal immunoglobulin within the CNS by B cells recruited from the periphery.

### *Antibody Testing*
Presence of Anti-AQP4 antibody (NMO-IgG) or myelin oligodendrocyte glycoprotein (MOG) antibodies can be used as potential biomarkers of NMO (60–94% sensitivity).

## Treatment Protocol for Multiple Sclerosis and Neuromyelitis Optica
### *Acute Relapses*
Treatment with high-dose corticosteroids (high-dose methylprednisolone pulse—1 g/ day for 5 days) has been the mainstay of acute therapy of MS and NMOSD relapses. In addition, plasma exchange is recommended for the acute relapse of NMOSD. Intravenous immunoglobulin (IVIG—dose 0.4 g/kg body weight over 5 days) is a safe and well-tolerated immunotherapy that could also be used as a treatment alternative for MS and NMOSD.

## Attack Prevention
### *Disease-modifying Therapy in Multiple Sclerosis*
The available disease-modifying drugs are beneficial for controlling inflammation and have a poor effect on the degenerative component of the disease. The United States Food

# CHAPTER 5: Neuroimmunology: Special Considerations in Women

**TABLE 2:** Diagnostic criteria of MS and NMO.

**TABLE 2A:** Revised McDonald's diagnostic criteria of MS.

Requires elimination of more likely diagnoses

Requires demonstration of dissemination of lesions in the CNS in space and time. In order to meet the criteria for dissemination in time, 30 days or more are required between events of neurological disturbance

| Clinical presentation | Additional criteria to make MS diagnosis |
|---|---|
| In a person who has experienced a typical attack/CIS at onset | |
| Two or more attacks and clinical evidence of two or more lesions OR Two or more attacks and clinical evidence of one lesion with clear historical evidence of prior attack involving lesion in different location | None. DIS and DIT have been met |
| Two or more attacks and clinical evidence of one lesion | DIS shown by one of these criteria:<br>• Additional clinical attack implicating different CNS site<br>• One or more MS-typical T2 lesions in two or more areas of CNS: Periventricular, cortical, juxtacortical, infratentorial, or spinal cord |
| One attack and clinical evidence of two or more lesions | DIT shown by one of these criteria:<br>• Additional clinical attack<br>• Simultaneous presence of both enhancing and nonenhancing MS-typical MRI lesions or new T2 or enhancing MRI lesion compared to baseline scan (without regard to timing of baseline scan)<br>• CSF oligoclonal bands |
| One attack and clinical evidence of one lesion | DIS shown by one of these criteria:<br>• Additional attack implicating different CNS site<br>• One or more MS-typical T2 lesions in two or more areas of CNS: Periventricular, cortical, juxtacortical, infratentorial, or spinal cord<br>And<br>DIT shown by one of these criteria:<br>• Additional clinical attack<br>• Simultaneous presence of both enhancing and nonenhancing MS-typical MRI lesions or new T2 or enhancing MRI lesion compared to baseline scan (without regard to timing of baseline scan)<br>• CSF oligoclonal bands |
| In a person who has steady progression of disease since onset | |
| About 1 year of disease progression (retrospective or prospective) | At least two of these criteria:<br>• One or more MS-typical T2 lesions (periventricular, cortical, juxtacortical, or infratentorial)<br>• Two or more T2 spinal cord lesions<br>• CSF oligoclonal bands |

(CIS: clinically isolated syndrome; CNS: central nervous system; CSF: cerebrospinal fluid; DIS: dissemination in space; DIT: dissemination in time; MS: multiple sclerosis)

**TABLE 2B:** Diagnostic criteria of NMO.

Diagnostic criteria for NMOSD with AQP4-IgG:
- At least one core clinical characteristic
- Positive test for AQP4-IgG using best available detection method (cell-based assay is strongly recommended)
- Exclusion of alternative diagnoses

Diagnostic criteria for NMOSD without AQP4-IgG or NMOSD with unknown AQP4-IgG status:
- At least two core clinical characteristics occurring as a result of one or more clinical attacks and meeting all of the following requirements:
    - At least one core clinical characteristic must be optic neuritis, acute myelitis with LETM, or area postrema syndrome
    - Dissemination in space (two or more different core clinical characteristics)
    - Fulfillment of additional MRI requirements, as applicable
- Negative tests for AQP4-IgG using best available detection method or testing unavailable
- Exclusion of alternative diagnoses

Core clinical characteristics:
- Optic neuritis
- Acute myelitis
- Area postrema syndrome: Episode of otherwise unexplained hiccups or nausea and vomiting
- Acute brainstem syndrome
- Symptomatic narcolepsy or acute diencephalic clinical syndrome with NMOSD—typical diencephalic MRI lesions
- Symptomatic cerebral syndrome with NMOSD—typical brain lesions

(AQP4: aquaporin-4; IgG: immunoglobulin G; LETM: longitudinally extensive transverse myelitis; NMOSD: neuromyelitis optica spectrum disorder)

and Drug Administration (USFDA) approved disease-modifying drugs for MS include interferon-beta1b (IFN-beta 1b), interferon beta-1a (IFN-beta 1a), glatiramer acetate, mitoxantrone, natalizumab, fingolimod, teriflunomide, dimethyl fumarate, alemtuzumab, pegylated IFN-beta 1a, ocrelizumab, cladribine, and siponimod. The three types of interferons: (1) Glatiramer acetate, (2) Teriflunomide, and (3) Dimethyl fumarate are approved as first-line therapies for RRMS. Alemtuzumab, fingolimod, and natalizumab are recommended for patients with highly active MS. Ocrelizumab, which has anti-CD20 action, is the only drug approved for PPMS patients who are ambulatory. Siponimod has been approved by the FDA and reduces disability accrual in SPMS.

### Attack Prevention in Neuromyelitis Optica Spectrum Disorder

The prevention of future attacks in NMOSD is crucial for long-term efficacy as cumulative inflammatory damage caused by acute attacks leads to disability. The first-line immunotherapies for prevention of relapses in NMOSD include azathioprine, mycophenolate mofetil, and rituximab. Other immunosuppressants that have been used to treat NMOSD are tacrolimus, cyclosporine A, methotrexate, and cyclophosphamide.

## Effects of Pregnancy and Lactation on Multiple Sclerosis and Neuromyelitis Optica Spectrum Disorder

Pregnancy is considered to be an immune privileged state. In MS, the relapses decrease in frequency during pregnancy and increase in the immediate postpartum period.

Breastfeeding may extend the period of pregnancy—conferred protection in MS. In contrast, NMOSD may be associated with a higher risk of relapse both during pregnancy and postpartum.

## Autoimmune Encephalitis

Autoimmune encephalitis is a complex category of diseases with diverse immunologic associations, clinical phenotypes, and management outcomes. These represent major noninfectious and a major emerging causes of encephalopathies, especially in individuals of younger age group. This group of immunotherapy-responsive encephalopathies has been recognized to be mediated by various antibodies (Abs) directed against either intracellular antigens or against membrane receptors or surface ion channel-associated proteins. Broadly, these antibodies can be divided into:

- Antibodies directed against the intracellular antigens which are nuclear or cytoplasmic proteins and are usually associated with certain malignancies (**Table 3**). These are also known as onconeural antibodies and the AE associated with these antibodies is known as paraneoplastic AE. The usual course of these syndromes is monophasic, the progression is relentless, and prognosis is guarded.
- Antibodies directed against the extracellular antigens—targeting neuronal cell surface (**Table 4**). These antigens are usually the cell surface receptors or the synaptic protein complexes. The syndromes associated with these antibodies are more commonly prevalent as compared to paraneoplastic AE. They have a relapsing course, are usually not associated with malignancies, and have a better prognosis.

The clinical features common to most AE are new onset and rapidly progressive memory loss or behavioral abnormalities, changes in state of consciousness, seizures, sleep disturbances, dysautonomia, and movement disorders. In practice, the symptoms often occur in various combinations (**Tables 3** and **4**). Limbic encephalitis (LE) is a common syndrome which occurs in many of these AE. It refers to subacute onset of episodic memory loss, confusion, and agitation. It is usually associated with hallucinations, seizures, sleep disturbances, and signal changes in medial temporal lobes and hippocampi on imaging.

**TABLE 3:** Autoimmune encephalitis associated with antibodies directed against intracellular antigens.

| Antibodies | Clinical symptoms | Malignancy |
|---|---|---|
| Anti-Hu (ANNA-1) | Encephalomyelitis, cerebellar degeneration, sensory neuronopathy, and dysautonomia | Lung carcinoma (small cell) |
| Anti-Yo (PCA-1) | Cerebellar degeneration | Breast, Ovary, and other gynecological |
| Anti-Ri (ANNA-2) | Cerebellar degeneration and opsoclonus-myoclonus | Breast, gynecological, and lung (small cell) |
| Anti-Tr | Cerebellar degeneration | Hodgkin lymphoma |
| Anti-CV2/CRMP5 | Encephalomyelitis, cerebellar degeneration, peripheral neuropathy, chorea, and uveitis | Lung (small cell) |
| Anti-Ma | Limbic, diencephalic, brainstem encephalitis, and cerebellar degeneration | Germ cell tumors of testis and other solid tumors |

(ANNA-1: antineuronal nuclear antibody type 1; ANNA-2: antineuronal nuclear antibody type 2; CRMP5: collapsin response mediator protein 5; PCA-1: Purkinje cell cytoplasmic antibody type 1)

TABLE 4: Autoimmune encephalitis associated with antibodies directed against extracellular antigens.

| Antibodies | Age in years range (median) | F:M | Clinical symptoms | Malignancy associated |
|---|---|---|---|---|
| NMDA receptor | 0.6–85 (21) | 4:1 | Behavioral and psychiatric symptoms, amnesia, seizures, catatonia, and dysautonomia | Ovarian teratomas (10–50%) |
| LGI1 | 30–80 (60) | 1:2 | LE, FBDS, myoclonus, and hyponatremia | Lung and thymoma (<10%) |
| CASPR2 | 45–80 (60) | 1:2 | Encephalitis and neuromyotonia (Morvan syndrome) | Lung and thymoma (<20%) |
| AMPA | 40–90 (60) | 9:1 | LE and psychiatric symptoms | Lung, Breast, and thymoma (70%) |
| GABA (B) | 25–75 (60) | 1:1 | LE | Lung (60%) |
| Glycine | 5–68 (60) | 6:5 | Encephalomyelitis with rigidity and myoclonus, hyperplexia, and stiff person syndrome | Rare |
| mGluR5 | 46 (15) | 1:1 | LE and myoclonus | Lung, Hodgkin's lymphoma, and thymoma (usually nonparaneoplastic) |
| DPPX | 45–76 | 1:1 | LE, myoclonus, and diarrhea | – |

(AMPA: α-amino-3-hydroxy-5-methyl-4-isoxazolepropionic acid; CASPR2: contactin-associated protein 2; DPPX: dipeptidyl peptidase-like protein 6; GABA: gamma-aminobutyric acid; LGI1: Leucine-rich glioma-inactivated protein 1; LE: limbic encephalitis; mGluR5: metabotropic glutamate receptor subtype 5; NMDA: N-methyl-D-aspartate)

## Gender-specific Issues in Autoimmune Encephalitis

Women are more susceptible to autoimmune diseases. Like MS and NMO, there is a subset of AE which occurs more often in women. Also, few paraneoplastic AE is associated with the malignancies of female urogenital system. **Tables 3** and **4** depict the salient features of various AE. AE which occur in women are discussed in brief.

### N-methyl-D-aspartate Receptor-mediated Autoimmune Encephalitis

N-methyl-D-aspartate receptor (NMDA-R) antibody-mediated AE is one of the most frequently encountered AE in neurological practice. As highlighted in **Table 3**, around 80% of patients of this disorder are women. NMDA-R antibody-mediated AE can inflict females at almost any age, including infancy. The earlier descriptions of this syndrome also consisted of young women presenting with viral prodrome followed by psychiatric and cognitive disturbances, seizures, orofacial dyskinesias, dysautonomia, and central hypoventilation. Many patients are actually treated as having psychiatric disorders because of personality and behavioral changes early in the course at times associated with paranoia, agitation, catatonia, and even frank psychosis at times. Dystonia, rigidity, hyperkinetic movements like chorea, opisthotonus, and oculogyric crisis may also occur. Many patients are young girls in their teens and it is not uncommon to see these patients getting referred to psychiatrists because of the initial phenotype. Isolated psychiatric symptoms, though rare, can occur as initial presentation or relapse in a few patients.

It is important to diagnose these patients early in the course to avoid the ongoing cortical and subcortical pathological cell loss. Another important aspect is the association of ovarian teratomas in such patients. Adequate screening and the removal of tumor if found are the cornerstone of management. The tumor association is however less strong and female overrepresentation may be absent in young children.

### *Onconeural Antibody-mediated Autoimmune Encephalitis*

Paraneoplastic encephalitis may occur in women of almost any age, though postelderly, menopausal women have a higher predisposition (**Table 3**).

The phenotype of paraneoplastic AE varies, depending upon the malignancy and antibodies formed in its response. AE encephalitis may predate or postdate the malignancy. It is specifically vital to recognize the syndrome and consider the possibility of malignancy in patients where the encephalitis predates the malignancy. As elucidated in **Table 3**, anti-Yo antibodies are almost exclusively associated with breast, ovarian, and other gynecological malignancies (anti-Ri antibodies may be associated with gynecological and lung malignancy) underscoring the importance of recognizing these syndromes in women.

## Diagnosis of Autoimmune Encephalitis

Diagnosis of AE is often complicated difficult in the clinical setting due to varied clinical symptoms and overlapping laboratory and radiological findings.

While clinical suspicion guides a physician to evaluate for AE, neuroimaging if often helpful. It is essential to rule out common causes of encephalopathy like metabolic, infectious, structural, and toxic causes. Neuroimaging reliably helps in exclusion of various structural, infectious, and other inflammatory causes of encephalopathy. Bilateral symmetrical medial temporal lobe hyperintensities on T2-weighted/fluid-attenuated inversion recovery (FLAIR) images is the hallmark of AE (**Figs. 1** and **2**). However, as acknowledged by Graus and colleagues, AE may occur with nonspecific MRI changes like hyperintensities in extralimbic, cortical, and subcortical regions.

Making a diagnosis of definite AE requires the detection of suspected antibodies in serum or the CSF of patients. The antibodies are specific for the type of AE; however, the currently available techniques have limited sensitivity for their detection. The proposed diagnostic criteria for the diagnosis of AE are given in **Box 1**.

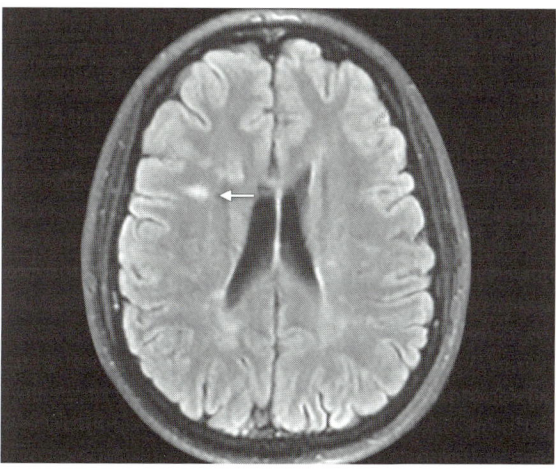

**FIG. 1:** Magnetic resonance imaging of brain: T2 fluid-attenuated inversion recovery (FLAIR) image showing a juxtacortical demyelinating plaque (arrow).

**SECTION 4:** Neurology

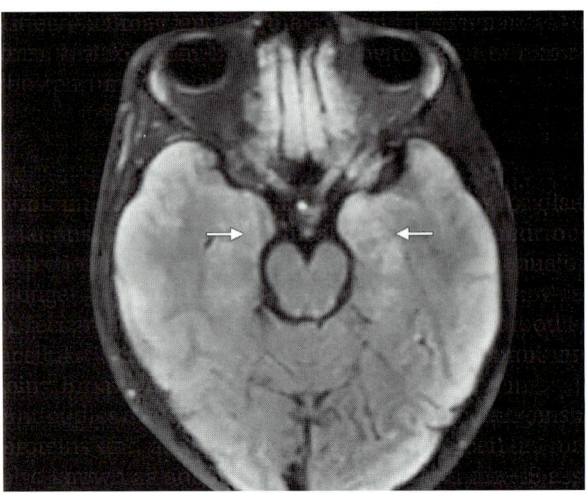

**FIG. 2:** Magnetic resonance imaging of brain: T2 fluid-attenuated inversion recovery (FLAIR) image showing bilateral medial temporal lobe hyperintensities (arrows).

> **BOX 1: Diagnostic criteria for definite autoimmune encephalitis (AE).**
>
> - Clinical phenotype: Subacute (usually within a few weeks but <3 months) onset alteration of personality or level of consciousness and symptoms suggesting involvement of the limbic system like memory deficits, psychiatric and behavioral symptoms, and seizures.
> - At least one of the following:
>   - EEG suggestive of AE
>   - CSF analysis suggestive of pleocytosis or elevated proteins
> - Typical MRI findings: Bilateral hyperintensities on T2-weighted/FLAIR sequence highly restricted to the medial temporal lobes
> - Detection of specific antibodies in serum/CSF
> - Reasonable exclusion of alternative causes
>
> (CSF: cerebrospinal fluid; EEG: electroencephalogram, FLAIR: fluid-attenuated inversion recovery)

As the deficit in AE is not essentially structural, functional and metabolic studies like 18F-fluorodeoxyglucose (18F-FDG)-positron emission tomography (PET) imaging have been reported to typically reveal changes in MRI-negative or inconclusive cases. The usual findings are hypermetabolism in medial temporal/limbic cortex (NMDA-R AE), bilateral striatal hypermetabolism (LGI1-Ab AE), and nonspecific hypometabolism in bilateral frontal/parieto-occipital cortices.

Though nonspecific, electroencephalogram (EEG) may reveal specific patterns like extreme delta brush which is seen in around 30% patients of NMDA-R encephalitis. Nonspecific patterns include diffuse or scattered slowing or occasional epileptic sharp and slow wave activity. CSF analysis may reveal lymphocytic pleocytosis and elevated proteins in a few patients. Other recommended tests to rule out associated malignancies in patients of suspected AE are given in **Box 2**.

## Treatment of Autoimmune Encephalitis

The current treatment approach involves removal of the immunological trigger and modulation or suppression of abnormal immunity. Prompt diagnosis and early removal

> **BOX 2** **Recommended screening for patients with suspected autoimmune encephalitis (AE).**
> - Women: Gynecological examination, PAPS smear, mammography, ultrasonography—for breast and ovarian screening, CT of chest and abdomen, and MRI of pelvis (to look for tiny ovarian teratoma)
> - Men: Urological examination, serum PSA levels, ultrasonography—for prostate in specific, and CT of chest and abdomen
> - More than 60 years: Whole body 18F-FDG/PET-CT
>
> (18F-FDG: 18F-fluorodeoxyglucose; PET: positron emission tomography; PSA: prostate-specific antigen)

of malignancy responsible for generation immune response are the cornerstone of management in patients with onconeural antibody syndromes.

In most patients of AE, treatment with glucocorticoids, IVIGs, and plasmapheresis is offered as the first-line treatment. In patients refractory to this therapy, rituximab or cyclophosphamide may be given. The long-term effects of this therapy in young women need a detailed risk–benefit assessment before initiation. Long-term therapy with steroid-sparing agents is often required.

# Vasculitis

Vasculitic disorders are characterized by vascular inflammation affecting vessels of different sizes. Vasculitis may be a primary vasculitis (classified as per vessel size into large vessel, medium vessel, and small vessel) or secondary to systemic collagen vascular disorders like systemic lupus erythematosus (SLE), infections, and toxins. This section is an overview of the vasculitis and related autoimmune disorders that tend to affect women more commonly.

## Primary Vasculitis

The 2012 Revised Chapel Hill Consensus Conference categorizes the diverse forms of vasculitis into large vessel—Takayasu arteritis (TAK) and giant cell arteritis (GCA), medium vessel—polyarteritis nodosa (PAN) and Kawasaki disease, and small vessel vasculitis—antineutrophil cytoplasmic antibody-associated vasculitis (granulomatosis with polyangiitis, eosinophilic granulomatosis with polyangiitis, and microscopic polyangiitis) and immune complex-associated vasculitis (Henoch–Schönlein purpura, cryoglobulinemia, and hypocomplementemic urticarial vasculitis). Vasculitis may also be limited to single organ—CNS angiitis, peripheral nerve vasculitis, and IgG4-related aortitis. Of all these, TAK and GCA are the ones which more commonly affect females.

### Takayasu Arteritis

Takayasu arteritis or pulseless disease or occlusive thromboaortopathy is the most common large vessel vasculitis seen in Asian women. It usually manifests with constitutional symptoms followed by local signs of vasculitis in young females. As per the American College of Rheumatology criteria of TAK, three or more of the following features can diagnose it with a sensitivity of 90.5% and specificity of 97.8%. Age ≤40 years, claudication of an extremity, reduced brachial artery pulse, >10 mm Hg difference in systolic blood pressure between arms, a bruit over the subclavian arteries or aorta, and arteriographic evidence of narrowing or occlusion of the entire aorta, its primary branches or large arteries in the proximal upper or lower extremities. Involvement of these vessels can manifest as limb claudication, limb ischemia, acute ischemic stroke (thromboembolism, hypoperfusion-induced brain infarction), retinopathy (peridiskal neovascularization on fundus examination), arteritic anterior ischemic optic neuropathy, central retinal artery occlusion, ocular ischemic syndrome, renal hypertension, and abdominal pain. Noninvasive disease assessment includes color Doppler sonography, contrast enhanced MRI with magnetic resonance angiography, and contrast enhanced computed tomography scan with computed tomography angiography. These may reveal vessel irregularities, stenosis, poststenotic dilatation, aneurysm formation, occlusions, and increased collateralization. Inflammation in the vessel wall can be ascertained on 18F-FDG-PET as an increased uptake in the vessel wall. Corticosteroids and alternative immunosuppressants are used in the active phase of the disease. Inactive disease with residual stenosis requires surgical intervention. Antiplatelets decrease the frequency of arterial ischemic events. Severe retinal ischemia requires panretinal photocoagulation as an adjunctive therapy.

## Giant Cell Arteritis

Giant cell arteritis or temporal arteritis is a large vessel vasculitis that peaks in the eighth decade of life (M:F—1:3). The distinguishing clinical features of GCA include new-onset localized headache after 50 years of age, temporal artery tenderness or reduced pulsation, and erythrocyte sedimentation rate (ESR) >50 mm/h. Fever, malaise, anorexia, weight loss, polymyalgia, and jaw claudication may occur. Patient may have scalp tenderness on brushing/combing hair, wearing glasses, and resting head on pillow. Diagnosis can be confirmed by demonstrating necrotizing granulomatous arteritis with multinucleated giant cells on biopsy of temporal artery, however, the result may be false negative. Noninvasive modalities include temporal artery ultrasound (dark hypoechoic circumferential halo sign—sensitivity of 68% and specificity of 91%), contrast-enhanced high-resolution MRI (bright mural enhancement of temporal artery), and whole body 18F-FDG-PET (thoracic vascular uptake). Missing the diagnosis may be catastrophic as vasculitic involvement of ophthalmic and posterior ciliary arteries can result in sudden severe irreversible vision loss (arteritic anterior ischemic optic neuropathy). Other complications include aortic aneurysm or dissection, large artery stenosis including cervical, subclavian, and brachial artery stenosis. Intracranial arteries are largely spared and peripheral nervous system (PNS) involvement is still uncommon. Early intervention with empirical high-dose corticosteroids is imperative in cases of visual loss (sequential involvement of the other eye may occur in one-third of cases and vision may improve to some extent if treatment is started on the first day of vision loss), impending vision loss (amaurosis fugax), diplopia, and jaw claudication. For low-to-moderate likelihood of GCA, a temporal artery biopsy may be done first. Elevated C-reactive protein (CRP) may be a better predictor of obtaining a diagnostic temporal artery biopsy. Symptomatic response to corticosteroids is striking and rapid. Treatment should be continued for at least 2 years. Tocilizumab has an emerging indication as an effective and safe corticosteroid-sparing therapy in the treatment of GCA.

## Secondary Vasculitis and Related Autoimmune/Inflammatory Disorders

### Systemic Lupus Erythematosus

Systemic lupus erythematosus is an autoimmune disease with an increased production of immunogenic nucleic acids/self-antigens. These trigger generation of pathogenic autoantibodies and immune complexes that deposit in tissues, trigger inflammation, and over time lead to irreversible organ damage. Women of childbearing age are most susceptible, accounting for 90% of cases. SLE can have varied central and PNS manifestations (56% prevalence over disease course) termed as neuropsychiatric SLE (NPSLE).

## CHAPTER 5: Neuroimmunology: Special Considerations in Women

The most common neuropsychiatric manifestations include headache, followed by mood disorder, cognitive dysfunction, depression, seizures, mono-/polyneuropathy, and stroke/transient ischemic attacks (TIAs). Delirium, movement disorder, aseptic meningitis, and myelopathy may occur in <5% of patients. Optic neuritis, posterior reversible encephalopathy syndrome, and hypophysitis are other rare manifestations. Recognizing the fact that the manifestations may be related to either disease flare, or side effects of therapy, or an immunosuppressed state, it remains a cornerstone in the approach to a patient with neurolupus. For example, psychosis may be due to disease per se or glucocorticoid induced. Close temporal association with starting/increasing steroid dosage, high daily steroid dose (≥40 mg prednisone or equivalent), and resolution of symptoms after tapering of glucocorticoids helps to distinguish the two.

Cognitive dysfunction may result from a diffuse involvement of the CNS or accrue after multiple/strategic infarcts. Although headaches may indicate a more sinister cause, like an underlying meningitis (infectious due to immunocompromised state or aseptic) or cerebral venous thrombosis (particularly in patients with antiphospholipid antibodies), migraine and tension headaches are still common. Looking for red flags for a primary headache disorder like features of raised intracranial pressure, transient visual obscurations, diplopia, and visual blurring, papilledema and neck stiffness are important.

Systemic lupus erythematosus predisposes to an increased risk of both arterial and venous strokes. Arterial strokes may result from hypercoagulability (in patients with antiphospholipid antibodies), vasculitis, accelerated atherosclerosis (older age, hypertension, diabetes, dyslipidemia, high disease activity, high cumulative/daily steroid dosages, and hyperhomocysteinemia), embolization (carotid plaques or Libman–Sacks endocarditis), or multiple processes occurring together.

Pregnancy and postpartum period are associated with an increased risk of SLE flares, overall mortality, thrombosis, infection, preterm labor, and preeclampsia.

The diagnosis of neurolupus is based on the presence of other characteristic clinical features and autoantibodies. Antinuclear antibodies are positive in 95% patients during the disease course, while anti-double-stranded deoxyribonucleic acid and anti-Sm antibodies are more specific for SLE.

Immunosuppressive agents added to glucocorticoids are recommended if neurologic syndrome is due to disease activity, as is done for all serious manifestations of SLE. In addition, patient will require symptomatic treatment tailored to the disease manifestation like antiepileptics, antidepressants, or antipsychotics. Cerebrovascular disease due to hypercoagulability requires long-term anticoagulation. Myelopathy is often disabling and rapid institution of high-dose steroids remains the standard of care.

### *Antiphospholipid Antibody Syndrome*

Antiphospholipid antibody syndrome (APLA) is an antibody-mediated acquired thrombophilia, seen primarily in females. It can occur alone or in association with autoimmune disorders like SLE. Recurrent arterial or venous thrombosis and/or pregnancy loss is the hallmark of this syndrome.

Neurologically, it may present with migrainous headaches, cerebral venous thrombosis (features of raised intracranial pressure with/without focal neurological deficits and seizures), and/or arterial thrombosis (TIA, amaurosis fugax, stroke, cognitive dysfunction, retinal artery occlusion, and ischemic optic neuropathy). MS like white matter lesions, dementia, transient global amnesia, Guillain–Barré syndrome (GBS), epilepsy, chorea, cerebellar ataxia, and transverse myelopathy may also occur. Ischemic encephalopathy presenting with confusion, obtundation, quadriparesis, and bipyramidal signs may occur.

Diagnosis can be made by measuring antiphospholipid antibodies (anticardiolipin antibodies, antibodies against beta-2 glycoprotein 1, and lupus anticoagulant) in serum. Patients with APLA need anticoagulation (alone or with aspirin 80 mg daily) for rest of their life (target international normalized ratio: 2.5–3.5). Pregnancy morbidity can be prevented by using low-molecular-weight heparin with aspirin 80 mg daily. IVIGs 400 mg/kg every day for 5 days may also prevent abortions.

## Sjögren's Syndrome

Sjögren's syndrome (SS) is a disease primarily of middle-aged women (M:F—1:9–20) with a bimodal distribution (peak at age 30 and 55 years). Clinically, primary SS is diagnosed if four of the following six features are present: (1) Ocular symptoms (dry eyes for >3 months), (2) Oral symptoms (dry mouth for >3 months), (3) Evidence of ocular exocrine dysfunction (positive Schirmer test or Rose Bengal stain), (4) Evidence of oral exocrine dysfunction (reduced salivary flow, abnormal parotid, or salivary scintigraphy), (5) Histopathology (lymphocytic foci in salivary glands), and (6) Serology positive for anti-Ro/SSA and/or anti-La/SSB.

Neurologically, SS affects both the CNS and PNS, PNS being affected more commonly. Peripheral neuropathy is most commonly reported. Sensory neuronopathy is one of the characteristic neurological presentations of SS. Other presentations include trigeminal neuropathy, axonal sensorimotor polyneuropathy, demyelinating polyradiculoneuropathy, autonomic neuropathy, mononeuritis multiplex, and small fiber neuropathy. In the CNS, SS can present like MS with numerous white matter lesions or with recurrent aseptic meningoencephalitis or neuropsychiatric symptoms like depression and fibromyalgia and rarely an acute on chronic myelopathy. The course of SS is likely to worsen during and after pregnancy. Obstetric outcomes are worse and the neonate may develop congenital heart block.

## Systemic Sclerosis

Systemic sclerosis (SSc) is an acquired autoimmune disorder affecting virtually every organ in the body. It is a disorder affecting predominantly females in their childbearing years (M:F—1:4–6). Inflammation and autoimmunity trigger the initial damage, which later culminates into vascular and visceral fibrosis in multiple organs. Thick and indurated skin (scleroderma) is the distinguishing feature. The disease can be classified as diffuse or localized depending on the pattern of skin involvement, natural history, and laboratory features. Since musculoskeletal complications are common, carpal tunnel syndrome may be the presenting manifestation. Deconditioning, disuse atrophy, malnutrition, inflammation, and fibrosis may all contribute to muscle weakness. The diagnosis is primarily clinical. Characteristically distributed symmetric skin induration with visceral organ involvement indicates diffuse SSc, while Raynaud's phenomenon, sclerodactyly, nailfold capillary changes, cutaneous telangiectasias, calcinosis cutis, and gastroesophageal reflux disease hint toward limited cutaneous disease. Specific autoantibodies when present increase the diagnostic certainty (anticentromere, Scl-70, and anti-RNA polymerase III). Immunosuppressive agents generally show a modest or no benefit in SSc.

## Idiopathic Inflammatory Myopathies

Idiopathic inflammatory myopathies are a group of autoimmune diseases involving the skeletal muscles and include—polymyositis (PM), dermatomyositis (DM), inclusion body myositis (IBM), and necrotizing autoimmune myositis. Women are three times more likely to suffer from DM and PM, while IBM is more common in males. Both DM and PM manifest as progressive symmetric proximal muscle weakness. Myalgias, arthralgias, dysphagia, and dysarthria may also occur. DM has characteristic skin manifestations like heliotrope rash (erythematous discoloration of eyelids with periorbital edema), Gottron's papules (raised erythematous rash over knuckles), Gottron's sign (erythematous rash over extensor surfaces), V sign (rash on sun-exposed anterior neck and chest), shawl sign (rash over back of neck and shoulders), nail bed telangiectasias, and subcutaneous calcium deposits. The key histopathological feature of DM is perimysial inflammation and perifascicular atrophy, whereas in PM muscle biopsy typically demonstrates endomysial inflammation. Common associated conditions with both include interstitial lung disease, myocarditis, and other connective tissue disorders. DM also bears an increased risk of malignancy in 15% cases. Serum creatine kinase levels are elevated (up to 50X normal or higher) in 70–80% of patients of DM and nearly all uncontrolled PM. Electromyography (EMG) of weak muscles reveals increased insertional and abnormal spontaneous activity, along with myopathic potentials. Skeletal muscle MRI reveals edema in affected muscles. A muscle biopsy is required for definitive diagnosis, particularly in suspected PM to exclude IBM. If characteristic rash of DM is present along with myositis-specific antibodies (anti-MDA5, anti-TIF1, anti-Mi2, and anti-NXP2), muscle biopsy may be deferred. DM and PM are treated initially with corticosteroids. A steroid-sparing agent like azathioprine or mycophenolate mofetil may be added if the disease is severely disabling at onset or if prolonged therapy is required. When DM or PM is associated with another well-defined connective tissue disorder such as scleroderma, rheumatoid arthritis (RA), or SS, term overlap syndrome is used.

## CONCLUSION

Women are particularly more prone to develop neuro-immunological diseases given the major endocrine and immunity transitions, which occur in a woman's life. Multiple sclerosis and Neuro-myeltis optica are two major demyelinating diseases, which present with specific focal neurological deficits. In young women, autoimmune encephalitis is an important reversible and treatable cause of rapidly progressive dementia/behavioral disturbances. Other systemic vasculitis may present with neurological symptoms as well, underscoring the need of keeping a high index of suspicion and adequately ruling them out.

## SUGGESTED READING

1. Cooper GS, Bynum MLK, Somers EC. Recent insights in the epidemiology of autoimmune diseases: improved prevalence estimates and understanding of clustering of diseases. J Autoimmun. 2009;33(3-4):197-207.
2. Desai MK, Brinton RD. Autoimmune Disease in Women: Endocrine Transition and Risk Across the Lifespan. Front Endocrinol (Lausanne). 2019;10:265.
3. Harbo HF, Gold R, Tintoré M. Sex and gender issues in multiple sclerosis. Ther Adv Neurol Disord. 2013;6(4):237-48.
4. Pandit L, Asgari N, Apiwattanakul M, Palace J, Paul F, Leite MI, et al. Demographic and clinical features of neuromyelitis optica: A review. Mult Scler. 2015;21(7):845-53.
5. Trebst C, Jarius S, Berthele A, Paul F, Schippling S, Wildemann B, et al. Update on the diagnosis and treatment of neuromyelitis optica: recommendations of the Neuromyelitis Optica Study Group (NEMOS). J Neurol. 2014;261(1):1-16.
6. Gajofatto A, Benedetti MD. Treatment strategies for multiple sclerosis: When to start, when to change, when to stop? World J Clin Cases. 2015;3(7):545-55.
7. Dalmau J, Graus F. Antibody-Mediated Encephalitis. N Engl J Med. 2018;378(9):840-51.
8. Leypoldt F, Wandinger KP, Bien CG, Dalmau J. Autoimmune Encephalitis. Eur Neurol Rev. 2013;8(1):31-7.

9. Kayser MS, Titulaer MJ, Gresa-Arribas N, Dalmau J. Frequency and characteristics of isolated psychiatric episodes in anti-N-methyl-D-aspartate receptor encephalitis. JAMA Neurol. 2013;70(9):1133-9.
10. Ramanathan S, Mohammad SS, Brilot F, Dale RC. Autoimmune encephalitis: recent updates and emerging challenges. J Clin Neurosci. 2014;21(5):722-30.
11. Probasco JC, Solnes L, Nalluri A, Cohen J, Jones KM, Zan E, et al. Abnormal brain metabolism on FDG-PET/CT is a common early finding in autoimmune encephalitis. Neurol Neuroimmunol Neuroinflamm. 2017;4(4):e352.
12. Takkar A, Choudhary A, Ram Mittal B, Lal V. Reversible Bilateral Striatal Hypermetabolism in a Patient with Leucine-Rich Glioma Inactivated-1 Encephalitis. J Clin Neurol. 2016;12(4):519-20.
13. Shi Y. Serial EEG Monitoring in a Patient With Anti-NMDA Receptor Encephalitis. Clin EEG Neurosci. 2017;48(4):301-3.
14. Jennette JC. Overview of the 2012 Revised International Chapel Hill Consensus Conference Nomenclature of Vasculitides. Clin Exp Nephrol. 2013;17(5):603-6.
15. Arend WP, Michel BA, Bloch DA, Hunder GG, Calabrese LH, Edworthy SM, et al. The American College of Rheumatology 1990 criteria for the classification of Takayasu arteritis. Arthritis Rheum. 1990;33(8):1129-34.
16. Petri H, Nevitt A, Sarsour K, Napalkov P, Collinson N. Incidence of giant cell arteritis and characteristics of patients: data-driven analysis of comorbidities. Arthritis Care Res. 2015;67(3):390-5.
17. Younger DS. Epidemiology of the Vasculitides. Neurol Clin. 2019;37(2):201-17.
18. Unterman A, Nolte JES, Boaz M, Abady M, Shoenfeld Y, Zandman-Goddard G. Neuropsychiatric syndromes in systemic lupus erythematosus: a meta-analysis. Semin Arthritis Rheum. 2011;41(1):1-11.
19. Ryan SL, Bhattacharyya S. Connective Tissue Disorders in Pregnancy. Neurol Clin. 2019;37(1):121-9.
20. Bhattacharyya S, Helfgott SM. Neurologic complications of systemic lupus erythematosus, sjögren syndrome, and rheumatoid arthritis. Semin Neurol. 2014;34(4):425-36.
21. Allanore Y, Simms R, Distler O, Trojanowska M, Pope J, Denton CP, et al. Systemic sclerosis. Nat Rev Dis Primers. 2015;1:15002.
22. Goyal NA. Immune-Mediated Myopathies. Contin Minneap Minn. 2019;25(6):1564-85.

# SECTION 5

# Gastroenterology

SECTION EDITOR
Vandana Midha

# CHAPTER 1

# Gender Divide: Common Gastrointestinal Disorders in Women

*Shobna Bhatia, Sridhar Sundaram*

## ABSTRACT

Gastrointestinal disorders are among the most common disorders for which women seek medical attention. Most gastrointestinal diseases in women are not inherently different from those that occur in men. Nevertheless, some gastrointestinal disorders occur more frequently or present differently in women. This article reviews common gastrointestinal disorders affecting women. The pathophysiology, clinical manifestations, management, and gender-specific issues of gastroesophageal reflux disease (GERD), peptic ulcer disease, irritable bowel syndrome (IBS), and inflammatory bowel disease (IBD) are discussed.

## INTRODUCTION

Women, with their distinct physiologic variability, starting with menarche, pregnancy, and eventually menopause, constitute a large volume of patients visiting clinics for gastrointestinal (GI) complaints. The physiological hormonal fluctuations lead to changes in GI function and thus contribute to their variety of complaints, both organic and functional. In this review, we look at gender-specific issues in commonly encountered disorders in luminal gastroenterology. The focus is on alternations in physiology, including changes in pregnancy and management of these disorders in women.

## GASTROINTESTINAL PHYSIOLOGY

The gastric acid output during fasting and after a meal is higher in men than in women; in contrast, the basal- and meal-stimulated serum gastrin concentration is higher in women. Stool weight in women varies during the menstrual cycle in women consuming a low-fiber diet and is lower during the luteal phase of the menstrual cycle, when the levels of progesterone peak. GI motility is slower in women and colonic transit time is longer.

## GASTROESOPHAGEAL REFLUX DISEASE AND ESOPHAGEAL DYSMOTILITY

Gastroesophageal reflux disease (GERD) includes a vast spectrum of reflux diseases of the gastroesophageal junction. It is categorized according to endoscopy as reflux esophagitis and nonerosive reflux disease (NERD). GERD complications include reflux esophagitis and Barrett's esophagus (BE). Both functional heartburn which is retrosternal burning discomfort or pain refractory to therapy in absence of GERD and NERD are more common in women than in men. However, men suffer pathological changes more frequently through the spectrum of reflux esophagitis, BE, and esophageal adenocarcinoma (EAC). Prevalence of GERD as per population-based studies conducted in India as well as in other parts of the world does not show any difference between both genders.

Ineffective or reflux-related esophageal motility disorder is more common in men (34% vs. 23%, $p = 0.01$) as per a previous study. Nutcracker esophagus was more common in women, however, no differences were found in achalasia, distal esophageal spasm. Men had higher incidence of nonspecific motility disorders.

There are various hypotheses for the differences in GERD and esophageal motility between males and females which include:

- *Estrogen and immune response*: Estrogen has anti-inflammatory activity which protects the distal esophageal mucosa from acid-induced damage. There is an increase in reflux esophagitis after menopause in women, likely secondary to loss of protection by estrogen. Estrogen can also suppress tissue macrophage inhibitory factor leading to wound healing.
- *Esophageal epithelial barrier function*: 17β-estradiol increases expression of occludin and leads to better expression of tight junction protein leading to increased adhesion between cells. This protection is not present in men.
- *Esophageal nociception*: Transient receptor potential vanilloid 1 (TRPV1) receptors drive nociception in the esophagus. A previous study showed that levels of TRPV1 were highest in patients with reflux esophagitis, followed by NERD and controls. These differences are pronounced in females where NERD is more commonly encountered. There is no sex-related difference in thermal pain threshold. Women tend to have higher chemical pain thresholds with larger referred pain areas compared to men.
- *Esophageal acid exposure*: Women tend to have fewer reflux episodes and percentage of time with pH <4 as compared to men in a study of subjects without reflux symptoms or GERD.

## Effect of Pregnancy on Gastroesophageal Reflux Disease

As pregnancy progresses, there is an increase in incidence of GERD from 8% in first trimester, 40% in second trimester to 52% in the third trimester. GERD is multifactorial in pregnancy. With increase in estrogen and progesterone, there is reduction in lower esophageal sphincter pressure and also effective esophageal body peristalsis, leading to poor clearance of esophageal refluxate. The enlarging uterus leads to compression of the stomach and increased intragastric pressure, leading to increasing incidence of GERD.

## Effect of Hormonal Stages on Esophageal Motility

There is a small reduction in lower esophageal sphincter pressure during the luteal phase; however, the menstrual cycle otherwise has no effect on esophageal motility. During pregnancy, there is reduction in lower esophageal sphincter pressure, reduced amplitude of distal esophageal contraction, and reduced percentage transmitted contractions. Although these effects are seen during pregnancy, symptomatic dysmotility is uncommon during pregnancy.

## Psychological Factors

Depression and anxiety are more common in women. NERD and GERD are associated with higher sleep dysfunction and anxiety with poor quality of life. These psychological factors also drive extraesophageal symptoms which are more commonly seen in women than in men.

Women do not respond to proton pump inhibitor (PPI) as well as men do [relative risk (RR): 3.66, $p < 0.001$]. Women are more likely to require dose escalation for PPI, while heartburn is less responsive in women to PPI. PPIs and histamine-2 receptor antagonists (H2RAs) are safe in pregnancy; domperidone and metoclopramide can be used as antiemetics during pregnancy.

For postmenopausal women, estrogen as an anti-inflammatory agent may be protective against esophageal mucosal injury. A previous case–control study showed significantly lowered risk of EAC with hormone replacement therapy (HRT) in postmenopausal women. By lowering the lower esophageal sphincter pressure, female hormones can increase risk of symptoms of GERD. Estrogen replacement acts as an effect modifier for reflux symptoms in obese individuals.

## FUNCTIONAL GASTROINTESTINAL DISORDERS INCLUDING IRRITABLE BOWEL SYNDROME

Functional GI disorders are challenging for both physician and the patient. Considering the nature of disease and relatively healthier patient profile, physicians tend to be biased against these patients. Considering the impact on quality of life, patients must be communicated well about the nature of disease, potential therapeutic options, and expected outcomes. Communication remains the key in management of most of these disorders. Considering that a larger proportion of these are bowel disorders, most studies have focused on irritable bowel syndrome (IBS).

Almost all functional GI disorders are more common in women. Functional esophageal disorders such as rumination and globus sensation are common in women, while functional chest pain shows equal prevalence in men and women. Functional constipation and IBS are more common in women, while functional diarrhea is more common in men. In fact, the female-to-male ratio for IBS is close to 2:1. Anorectal disorders are also more common in women especially so in postpartum ones, considering the altered physiology.

Abdominal pain, pelvic cramping, nausea, and diarrhea are more in patients with IBS during the perimenstrual period suggesting impact on visceral sensitivity. Women with IBS also report higher levels of perimenstrual symptoms. In a retrospective series, IBS was three times more common in women with dysmenorrhea than those without.

Physiologic alterations associated with differences in males and females with respect to functional GI disorders include:
- *Visceral nociception*: Greater response to visceral pain is seen in women as compared to men. Stress, especially factors in early life, produces visceral hyperalgesia, more commonly in females than in males. There is an increased response to sigmoid distension in women than men with IBS.
- *Somatic nociception*: Healthy women show an increased sensitivity to somatic pain stimuli. Multiple genetic polymorphisms are also associated with gender-specific differences in somatic sensitivity to pain.
- *Motility*: Estrogen and progesterone lead to significantly decreased colonic transit. Estrogen also helps in maintaining intestinal barrier function by influence on tight

## SECTION 5: Gastroenterology

junctions and also on inflammatory response. Stress is also known to decrease upper GI motility and augment lower GI motility more in women. Gastric emptying seems to be slower for both solids and liquids in females, while fundic relaxation prolonged and perception scores also increased in females. Estrogen also helps maintain intestinal barrier function through tight junctions and influences motility and inflammatory activity.

- *Autonomic tone*: Women have higher cardiovagal tone and lower sympathetic balance. There is also significant blunting of sympathetic activity in patients with IBS in response to stress, leading to altered pathophysiology among males and females.
- *Central processing of visceral stimuli*: Significant difference in central processing is seen between men and women, with increased responsiveness in sensory and affective regions, i.e., prefrontal cortex, insula cortex, and cingulate cortex. Females also show more resource allocation to interoceptive awareness, while males rely on cognitive processes mainly. These differences with structural differences are integral to the pathophysiology of IBS in different genders.
- *Microgenderome and immune alterations*: Gender-specific differences in microbiome largely driven by sex hormones contribute to differential sensitivity to pain and also to inflammation in the bowel. Female gender is proposed to be risk factor for postinfectious IBS and the major driver for this is the microbiome, intestinal permeability, and immune alterations.
- *Psychological factors*: As described above in GERD, there is a close association between anxiety, depression, and somatization with IBS.

Clinical assessment in women requires evaluation for other pelvic floor syndromes and gynecologic pain syndromes. Extracolonic manifestations of IBS are seen in both men and women equally. Although IBS is associated with poor sleep, there is no difference in both genders. Sexual dysfunction with lowered sexual drive is reported by both men and women (36% vs. 28%) with IBS. Dyspareunia is more commonly seen in women (16% vs. 4%). Response to psychotherapy does not vary significantly in men and women in upper GI syndromes with similar response to both psychotherapy and also selective serotonin reuptake inhibitors (SSRIs) in men and women. On the other hand, hypnotherapy was more effective in women with IBS (80% vs. 62%, $p < 0.05$) in a retrospective study. These findings however, could not be replicated in a randomized control trial which showed equal efficacy in males and females for hypnotherapy. Although drug pharmacokinetics dictated by cytochrome P450 can be affected by female hormones, there is no difference in response to pharmacotherapy for functional GI disorders between both genders.

## INFLAMMATORY BOWEL DISEASE

The prevalence of inflammatory bowel disease (IBD) in both males and females is similar. Women tend to have lower rates of Crohn's disease (CD) until 10–14 years of age, while there is an increased incidence in women thereafter. Ulcerative colitis (UC) on the other hand as equal incidence till 45 years of age, with increased incidence in males thereafter. Women pose a unique challenge to gastroenterologists managing IBD considering the inherent hormonal fluctuations.

- *Menstruation*: IBD is known to impact normal menstruation and hormonal fluctuations in women also tend to impact disease activity in IBD. Patients with IBD may have delayed menarche and menstrual cycle may be irregular. In addition, they occasionally have a cyclical pattern to their complaints correlating closely with the menstrual cycle. These could be diarrhea, loose stools, constipation, abdominal cramping, and pain.

In a bid to regularize cycles, hormonal contraception is an option in these patients but larger studies needed to clearly define its role. A previous survey attempted to address this question, wherein 129 patients with IBD of whom 88% received contraceptive pills, only 5% reported worsening of cyclical symptoms. About 19% of those on estrogen pills and 47% of those on levonorgestrel reported improvement in symptoms with medications.

- *Sexuality and body image*: Women experience more body image disturbances as compared to men (81% vs. 51%) with IBD. Sexuality was more impaired in women than in men with IBD (66% vs. 41%), more so in operated patients (69% vs. 50%). While psychosocial factors were largely contributory to decreased sexuality, women also avoided intercourse for worry of abdominal pain, diarrhea, and incontinence. In a survey, <20% women interviewed felt that their issues related to sexuality or body image were addressed by their gastroenterologist. Hence, psychosocial support is important in these patients, especially women.
- *Fertility*: IBD may impact fertility in women, although the rates of infertility are similar to that in the general population (5–14%). In nonsurgically treated patients with IBD, the decreased fertility is largely due to voluntary childlessness driven by misconceptions about IBD. Studies on anti-Müllerian hormone suggest accelerated loss of fertility in patient with CD, with those having colonic disease at higher risk. Medications such as sulfasalazine, methotrexate, and corticosteroids all reduce fertility in men, however, have no effect in women. Methotrexate is known to be teratogenic in pregnant women and hence avoided. Azathioprine, 6-mercaptopurine (6-MP), and biologics have no impact on fertility. Surgery may adversely impact fertility in both males and females, with rates increasing to 26% after ileal pouch-anal anastomosis (IPAA) for UC. These may be related to pelvic adhesions and obstruction of fallopian tubes. An increase in dyspareunia and sexual dysfunction is noted after surgery. Some patients report overall improved sexual satisfaction due to overall improved general health. Pregnancy after IPAA entails need for cesarean section for delivery to avoid injury to anal sphincters and pouch.
- *Pregnancy*: Pregnancy entails a unique challenge during management of patients with IBD. Flares of UC and CD are reported in 30–35% of pregnancies. Active disease is associated with 2-fold increased risk of preterm birth. In addition, there is a higher risk of spontaneous abortion, preterm birth, low birth weight, and complications of labor and delivery. Perineal disease is a risk factor for fourth-degree perineal laceration and it is best to personalize mode of delivery based on activity of patients. Disease activity assessment involves standard blood investigations and fecal calprotectin. Flexible sigmoidoscopy is preferred over a full colonoscopy as it is easy to perform, unprepared, and in any trimester with minimal risk.
- *Medication safety*: Medications including aminosalicylates, immunomodulators, and biologics are continued throughout pregnancy without any risk of adverse pregnancy outcomes. Steroids are used primarily to manage flares and not for maintenance. Antimicrobials are used in patients with perianal disease, pouchitis, and initial management of disease flares. Thiopurines are not started in first trimester due to risk of pancreatitis, leukopenia, and also risk of infections. However, if already ongoing, thiopurines are continued in these patients as monotherapy. Stopping thiopurines is done on case-by-case basis. Surgery is done in acute flares for disease-related indications such as perforation, abscess, severe flare, obstruction, or refractory bleeding. However, need for surgery indicates a poorer prognosis during pregnancy. Newer biologics such as tofacitinib and immunomodulators like methotrexate are avoided during pregnancy due to risk of teratogenicity or limited data on the same.

Anticoagulant prophylaxis is a must in those pregnant IBD patients admitted with flare. There is no contraindication to lactation postpartum for patients on any medical management. Vaccines can be given to the newborn as per routine schedule. However, if the mother was exposed to biologics during pregnancy, it is best to avoid liver attenuated vaccines for the first 6 months of life.
- *Menopause*: Menopause in women with IBD happens at the same age as historical controls based on a small retrospective series. However, CD can be associated with premature menopause. Although no difference in disease activity was seen in patients premenopause and postmenopause, HRT seems to have a protective effect on disease activity in IBD. Those on HRT were 80% less likely to have a flare than those not on HRT.
- *Bone health*: Women with IBD are at increased risk of osteoporosis, especially those who are postmenopausal and also on significant doses of steroids. Dual-energy X-ray absorptiometry (DEXA) screening for patients with IBD for osteoporosis is a must and treatment based on fracture risk assessment using calcium supplements, vitamin D supplementation, and also bisphosphonates are recommended.

## CONCLUSION

Women form a distinct cohort of patients needing special care in certain situations such as menstruation, pregnancy, and menopause. There are significant sex-specific differences in common luminal disorders of the GI tract. As clinicians, we must be cognizant of these differences and consider individualizing management decisions for patients. Also, these differences offer plenty of avenues for research into epidemiology, pathophysiology, clinical characteristics, and management of patients with these diseases.

At least for some GI diseases, it appears that men are indeed from Mars and women are from Venus.

## SUGGESTED READING

1. Freire AC, Basit AW, Choudhary R, Piong CW, Merchant HA. Does sex matter? The influence of gender on gastrointestinal physiology and drug delivery. Int J Pharm. 2011;415(1-2):15-28.
2. Bhatia SJ, Reddy DN, Ghoshal UC, Jayanthi V, Abraham P, Choudhuri G, et al. Epidemiology and symptom profile of gastroesophageal reflux in the Indian population: report of the Indian Society of Gastroenterology Task Force. Indian J Gastroenterol. 2011;30(3):118-27.
3. Kim YS, Kim N, Kim GH. Sex and gender differences in gastroesophageal reflux disease. J Neurogastroenterol Motil. 2016;22(4):575-88.
4. Zia JK, Heitkemper MM. Upper Gastrointestinal Tract Motility Disorders in Women, Gastroparesis, and Gastroesophageal Reflux Disease. Gastroenterol Clin North Am. 2016;45(2):239-51.
5. El-Serag H, Becher A, Jones R. Systematic review: persistent reflux symptoms on proton pump inhibitor therapy in primary care and community studies. Aliment Pharmacol Ther. 2010;32(6):720-37.
6. Houghton LA, Heitkemper M, Crowell M, Emmanuel A, Halpert A, McRoberts JA, et al. Age, Gender and Women's Health and the Patient. Gastroenterology. 2016. pii: S0016-5085(16)00183-9.
7. Nilsson M, Johnsen R, Ye W, Hveem K, Lagergren J. Obesity and estrogen as risk factors for gastroesophageal reflux symptoms. JAMA. 2003;290(1):66-72.
8. Mayer EA, Naliboff B, Lee O, Munakata J, Chang L. Review article: gender-related differences in functional gastrointestinal disorders. Aliment Pharmacol Ther. 1999;13 (Suppl 2):65-9.
9. Chang L, Heitkemper MM. Gender differences in irritable bowel syndrome. Gastroenterology. 2002;123(5):1686-701.
10. Kim YS, Kim N. Sex-Gender Differences in Irritable Bowel Syndrome. J Neurogastroenterol Motil. 2018;24(4):544-58.

11. Flak MB, Neves JF, Blumberg RS. Immunology. Welcome to the microgenderome. Science. 2013;339(6123):1044-5.
12. Rosenblatt E, Kane S. Sex-Specific Issues in Inflammatory Bowel Disease. Gastroenterol Hepatol (N Y). 2015;11(9):592-601.
13. Gawron LM, Goldberger A, Gawron AJ, Hammond C, Keefer L. The impact of hormonal contraception on disease-related cyclical symptoms in women with inflammatory bowel diseases. Inflamm Bowel Dis. 2014;20(10):1729-33.
14. Fréour T, Miossec C, Bach-Ngohou K, Dejoie T, Flamant M, Maillard O, et al. Ovarian reserve in young women of reproductive age with Crohn's disease. Inflamm Bowel Dis. 2012;18(8):1515-22.
15. Cornish JA, Tan E, Teare J, Teoh TG, Rai R, Darzi AW, et al. The effect of restorative proctocolectomy on sexual function, urinary function, fertility, pregnancy and delivery: a systematic review. Dis Colon Rectum. 2007;50(8):1128-38.

# Gut Microbiome and Obesity: Ladies Corner

*Usha Dutta, Shubra Mishra*

## ABSTRACT

There is a worldwide increase in patients living with obesity. This can be attributed to the change in our lifestyle, with an increase in sedentary jobs and activities and ever-increasing availability of processed food. However, lifestyle change does not seem to be the only factor responsible for this rampant increase in obesity. Our gastrointestinal tract plays host to a number of microorganisms which together constitute the gut microbiome. It has become clear in the past decade that the gut microbiome plays an active role in the energy metabolism, interacts and modulates the immune system and also has an effect on our hormonal and inflammatory milieu. Changes in diet can change the pattern of microbiome which inhabits the duct and a different gut microbiome can change the system digestion and energy harvest from food products. Gut microbiome can be modulated by multiple external factors, including a change in quality and quantity of food intake, use of prebiotics, probiotics and antibiotics, fecal microbiota transplant and bariatric surgeries. These interventions have a direct effect on the composition of the gut microbiota and an indirect effect on energy metabolism with consequential changes in the incidence of obesity, diabetes and other diseases. Men and women are colonized by a slightly different set of microbiota and subsequently demonstrate variable responses when exposed to an unhealthy diet and lifestyle. This review aims at explaining the structure of gut microbiota and how it plays a role in development of obesity. It also highlights various interventions which may modulate the gut microbiome and have an impact on the increasing burden on lifestyle disorders.

## INTRODUCTION

Obesity is one of the most prevalent and fastest growing diseases presently in the world today. It is a major risk factor for the development of dyslipidemia, insulin resistance, and nonalcoholic fatty liver disease (NAFLD). According to the Global Burden of Disease Study, 8% of the deaths in 2017 amounting to a total of 4.7 million were attributed to obesity. In India, 3.9% adults were found to be obese and 19.3% were overweight. However, a higher percentage of women are found to be obese across the globe as well as in the Indian population.

There are multiple factors responsible for this change in phenotype over the years. It is the environmental factors, including the change in lifestyle and dietary habits which were thought to be primarily responsible. However, with time, it was realized that it was not just the increase in calorie intake which was leading to obesity. The change in quality of food products consumed has an impact on the body's metabolism. High carbohydrate and high fat food consumption leads to a spike in insulin levels which promotes lipogenesis and predisposes to obesity. It is unlikely that the human genome has evolved so rapidly so as to be the main cause for this change.

The World Obesity Federation has defined obesity as a chronic relapsing disease process. It has recognized that obese individuals are in a constant state of low-degree inflammation which leads to insulin resistance. Insulin resistance leads to development of type 2 diabetes mellitus (T2DM) and visceral fat deposition, now known as "adipogenicity" or the "bad adipose tissue" which is further causative in development of NAFLD, coronary artery disease (CAD), chronic kidney disease (CKD), and other chronic diseases. Obesity is linked with an increased risk for development of metabolic disorders including diabetes, NAFLD, and atherosclerosis; osteoarthritis and malignancies including, but not limited to, CA breast, CA uterus, and CA gallbladder. Turnbaugh et al. studied the fecal microbiota composition in twin pairs, both monozygotic and dizygotic and also studied the microbiota composition in the mother. They observed that while there was a congruity in the composition of the gut microbiome isolated from members of one family, yet each member had a distinct gut microbiome signature, differing in the specific bacterial lineages. Heterogeneity at the level of the phylum led to differences in phenotype. It was observed that a change in composition at the phylum was associated with variability in the degree of leanness and obesity. This landmark trial unraveled the potential of gut microbiome. It has since then been studied extensively in both human and mice models.

## GUT MICROBIOTA AND METABOLISM

The composition of gut microbiota is affected by multiple factors, starting from early life. It was initially thought that the gut of a neonate is sterile and is implanted with microbiota at the time of delivery. Hence, the gut microbiota composition of a neonate depends on the mode of delivery. It has now been found that some amount of low level transfer of microbiome occurs during the intrauterine period as well. The composition of gut microbiota of an infant is intricately linked to that of his mother. Further changes occur in the composition depending on whether the baby is formula fed or breastfed, food products used for weaning, and surrounding environment's hygiene. Gut microbiome of a baby changes till up to 3 years of age, after which it becomes relatively stable in its core composition. The human gut microbiome is composed of 3,000–5,000 species. These collectively form a genome comprising of 5 million genes. These microbes have a symbiotic relationship with the human host and participate in development of innate immunity, bile acid metabolism, synthesis of micronutrients as well as metabolism of food substances.

The gastrointestinal (GI) tract is colonized by microbial organism throughout its extent, starting from the oral cavity up to the anal canal. As the luminal pH, motility, and oxygen content changes from the stomach to the intestine, a change in the microbiota composition is seen. Five phyla are most commonly isolated from the intestines. These are *Acinetobacter*, Bacteroidetes, Firmicutes, Proteobacteria, and Verrucomicrobia. Firmicutes, *Lactobacilli*, and Proteobacteria are isolated mostly from the proximal GI tract.

**TABLE 1:** Increased and decreased risk of obesity.

| Increased risk of obesity | Decreased risk of obesity |
|---|---|
| Female gender | High-fiber diet |
| High-fat and high-carbohydrate diet | Intermittent fasting |
| Sedentary lifestyle | Use of symbiotics |
| Maternal obesity | Low-fat Mediterranean diet |
| Use antibiotics: Dysbiosis | Eubiosis |

Bacteroidetes, Firmicutes, and *Akkermansia muciniphila* are present more distally. This diversity in microbial composition is vital for a healthy gut.

## MICROBIOTA-DERIVED METABOLITES

Dietary fibers are digested by the gut microbiome in the large intestine. Short-chain fatty acids (SCFAs) are the end products of the process, which includes propionate, acetate, and butyrate. Butyrate is the source of energy for the intestinal cells. Propionate and acetate are absorbed and reach the liver via the portal circulation. Propionate activates adenosine monophosphate (AMP)-activated protein kinases in the liver and muscle. This leads to activation of peroxisome proliferator-activated receptor (PPAR)-gamma coactivator and other PPAR receptor family, culminating in stimulation of glucose uptake and oxidation of fatty acids. This process has been shown to be beneficial in glycemic control, at least in murine models. Role of acetate is still uncertain. Although high blood acetate levels were associated with decreased risk of obesity in murine models, they were associated with a higher risk of obesity in human studies (**Table 1**).

Other metabolites produced by the gut microbiota include carbon dioxide, hydrogen disulfide, ammonia, sulfides, phenols, choline, and carnitine. These are crucial nutrients both for the commensal gut bacteria and the host. High levels of choline may play a role in development of NAFLD. Trimethylamine N-oxide (TMAO) levels in the liver have been found to have a positive correlation with the development of CAD.

Gut microbiota is also responsible for deconjugation of secondary bile acids in the intestine and dihydroxylation. Thus, the products formed have a higher affinity for farnesoid X receptor (FXR) and Takeda G-protein receptor 5 (TGR5) receptors and play a role in modulating the immunity as well as energy metabolism by binding to the receptors on hepatocytes, L-cells, and macrophages.

## REGULATION OF ENERGY HARVEST AND BACTERIAL TRANSLOCATION

Gut microbiota also modulates the gene expression of the intestinal mucosal cells. Thereby it has an impact on the process of fatty acid absorption, metabolism, and storage. Angiopoietin-related protein 4 (Angptl4) is a potent lipoprotein lipase inhibitor. Its activity in white adipose tissue leads to a reduction in fat percentage. Role of gut microbiota was deduced from a study that demonstrated that normal mice exhibit a decreased expression of Angptl4 as compared to germ-free mice. This promotes adipose tissue development.

# CHAPTER 2: Gut Microbiome and Obesity: Ladies Corner

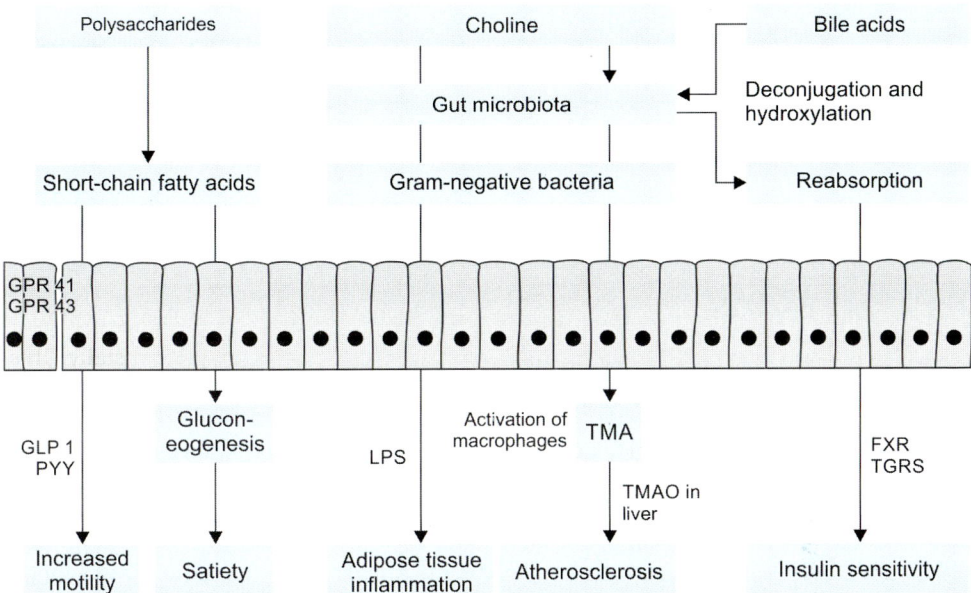

(FXR: farnesoid X receptor; GLP-1: glucagon-like peptide-1; LPS: lipopolysaccharides; PYY: peptide YY; TGR5: Takeda G-protein receptor 5; TMA: thrombotic microangiopathy; TMAO: trimethylamine N-oxide)

**FLOWCHART 1:** Characteristics of gut microbiota.

Intestinal endocannabinoid system is found to be more active in obese mice than the others. It has also been noted that the activity of the endocannabinoid system is different in germ free as compared to normal mice. This difference is of importance because activation of endocannabinoid system leads to an increased appetite by stimulation of release of glucagon-like peptide-1 (GLP-1), increased gut permeability, and systemic inflammation.

Cani et al. had observed that mice fed on a high-fat diet existed in state of low-level endotoxemia. They further linked this state to development of obesity, insulin resistance, and diabetes. They hypothesized that the changes in gut microbiome which took place in the milieu of a high-fat diet led to activation of the innate and adaptive immunity. Continuous exposure to this altered microbiota perpetuated a state of low-grade inflammation. Dietary changes in gut microbiota happen because different bacteria thrive on different substrate (**Flowchart 1**). A high-fat diet increases systemic endotoxemia. It improves the energy harvesting capacity of the gut microbiome. A positive energy balance increases the tendency for development of insulin resistance and obesity.

## CHANGES IN OBESITY

Earliest evidence of relationship between gut microbiota and body weight came from studies by Gordon et al. and Backhed et al. Germ-free mice had 40% less body weight than conventional mice, even when both were given same feed. After microbial colonization of the germ-free mice, their weight increased by 57%. Similarly, there is a difference in microbiota composition observed between lean and obese patients. Overall change in diversity of fecal microbiome is found in obese patients with an altered ratio of Firmicutes to *Bacteroides*. Firmicutes (mollicutes) are in abundance in obese patients. This change in microbial composition has been consistently observed in obese pregnant females, children with early-onset obesity, rate fed on a high-fat diet, and genetically obese rat (ob/ob). However, all studies did not show a similar pattern. Turnbaugh et al. and Faugh et al. proposed an overall greater proportion of Actinobacteria, decrease in Bacteroidetes, *Bifidobacterium*, and *Ruminococcus* with no apparent differences in Firmicutes.

## OBESITY IN WOMEN

Obesity has been observed in both males and females. There is a difference in the pattern of fat storage, mobilization, and utilization between the two groups. Women tend to store fat more in the subcutaneous tissue, especially of the gluteofemoral region. Men tend to store fat more in the abdomen, especially as visceral adipose tissue. This stems from the difference in hormonal composition and probably has an evolutionary origin. Estradiol acts both on the adipose tissue and the centers for hunger and satiety in the brain, to temper energy expenditure, and food intake. Androgens block proliferation and differentiation of preadipocytes whereas estradiol enhances it. Estradiol's action on preadipocytes is greater in females than males. It favors storage of fat in the subcutaneous tissue. Lack of estrogen in women can lead to an overall weight gain with an increased proportion of visceral fat stores. These changes have been observed in postmenopausal women as well. Treatment with estradiol in postmenopausal women has been shown to be associated with lower lipoprotein lipase activity and a healthier body fat composition. Estradiol also acts on subcutaneous adipose tissue, through alpha-2A adrenergic receptors, to decrease lipolysis. This action does not seem to occur in the visceral body fat. Adipose tissue expresses both androgen and estrogen receptors. This holds true for both men in women. The differences in hormonal concentration may be responsible for the difference in body composition and metabolic activity between the two genders.

## INTERVENTION

Dietary strategies are the primary tool for preventing and treating metabolic disorders. A study by Santos Marca et al. analyzed the fecal samples of men and women, with or without metabolic syndrome. They further studied the effect of a low-fat diet on the metabolic parameters of the cohort in 3 years and the associated change in fecal microbiome. Women with metabolic syndrome had a higher abundance of *Collinsella*, *Anaerotruncus*, and *Alistipes* whereas *Faecalibacterium* and *Prevotella* genera were more prevalent in men with metabolic syndrome. With consumption of low-fat diet for 3 years, there was a change in gut microbiota composition. Men had higher levels of *Desulfovibrio*, *Roseburia*, and *Holdemania* genera. In another Chinese cohort study, it was demonstrated that there was no significant difference in the overall gut microbiota composition (beta diversity) between men and women, but there was higher alpha diversity in female samples. An abundance of Fusobacteria was demonstrated in the fecal microbiota of obese males, while obese females had microbiota enriched with Actinobacteria. These differences in gut microbiota may be responsible for the varied efficacy of interventions in losing weight. How these differences can be utilized to tailor the weight loss plan for each and every individual should be evaluated in future projects.

## DIETARY CHANGES

The Mediterranean diet has been promoted as one of the most effective diets for fat loss. It consists of a diet full of legumes, unrefined cereals, olive oil, fruits and vegetables, moderate amount of dairy, moderate consumption of lean meat, and moderate amount of wine consumption. Such diets which are rich in plant fibers change the gut microbiota composition by increasing the diversity and restore the phyla ratio. A greater bacterial abundance of Lactobacilli and *Bifidobacterium* with a reduction in pathogens such as Enterobacteriaceae, Streptococcaceae, and Desulfovibrionaceae was observed.

## INTERMITTENT FASTING

The practice of "diet and exercise" as the main secret to control of body weight is more easily said than done. Most people find it hard to stick to such resolutions and a regaining of body weight is invariably seen in most cases. There has been a renewed interest in using intermittent fasting as a method for weight loss. It was seen that people who follow this principle had an improved metabolism and higher insulin sensitivity. However, the mechanism is not very clear. Initially, it was thought that an overall decrease in calorie intake was responsible for the changes. A study conducted by Hatori et al. on mice (Cell Metab, 2012) demonstrated an improvement in metabolism in mice who were on a time-restricted diet as compared to those on an ad libitum diet even though mice in both groups consumed equivalent calories. It was then noted that there was an increased induction of white adipose tissue into brown adipose tissue (beiging) in mice on an every other day fasting (EODF) regimen. This conversion of white adipose tissue into brown adipose tissue increases nonshivering thermogenesis, thereby increasing futile energy expenditure.

Every other day fasting regimen was associated with beiging of white adipose tissue in conventionally raised mice with intact microbiota, but not in germ-free mice. On genetic profiling of cecal microbiota of mice on EODF versus ad libitum diet, it was seen that EODF regimen increased the operational taxonomic unit (OTU) abundance of Firmicutes and decreased most other phyla. The ratio of Firmicutes/Bacteroidetes increased from 3.4 in ad libitum mice to 8.9 in EODF mice (Li G et al. 2017, Cell Metab). It is to be noted that this is in contrast to the microbiota composition seen when obese and lean mice were compared. Hence, more studies are needed to understand the relationship between gut microbiota and energy metabolism.

## PREBIOTICS

The term prebiotic was first described by Marcel Roberfroid in 1995 as "a selectively fermented ingredient that allows specific changes, both in the composition and/or activity in the GI microflora that confers benefits upon host well-being and health." Prebiotics are complex carbohydrates which are broken down by gut microbiota into SCFA. There are multiple studies available, which have assessed the changes in the gut microbiota and its milieu with the use of prebiotics. Changes in the relative abundance of gram-negative bacilli, level of gut peptides, decrease in degree of systemic inflammation, and an improvement in glucose tolerance have been noted. When RCTs (Randomized Controlled Trials) were done with prediabetic, diabetic, and obese patients, the results were equivocal with no major effect on metabolic parameters such as body weight, body mass index (BMI), insulin level, glycosylated hemoglobin (HbA1c), and homeostatic model assessment of insulin resistance (HOMA-IR). Along similar lines, variable results were seen on changes in lipid profile and there was actually no significant benefit to be found. There is a definite subclinical reduction in subclinical inflammatory markers in most studies. A systemic review by Baserra et al. (published in Clinical Nutrition, 2015) had included 13 trials of participants with BMI >25 kg/m². Use of prebiotics was associated with a reduction in total cholesterol levels as well as low-density lipoprotein (LDL) levels. In trials which included diabetic patients, there was a reduction in triglycerides and an increase in high-density lipoprotein (HDL). The effect size was small so the systematic review did not recommend the use of prebiotics in routine clinical practice.

Raw foods which are rich in prebiotics include chicory root, barley, garlic, onion, globe artichoke, rye bran, wheat bran, and banana. There are no published guidelines which recommend daily prebiotic consumption. However, a daily consumption of 4–10 g has been suggested as beneficial. Increased sensation of bloating and increase in number of bowel movements have been noted with an increase in prebiotic use. This may be a direct effect of greater fermentation and SCFA production.

## PROBIOTICS

Probiotics were described by the World Health Organization (WHO) as "live microorganisms which, when administered in adequate amounts, confer a health benefit on the host". The microorganism must be well-defined, up to the species and strain levels. The administered dose also must be predefined. Probiotics consist of the healthy microorganisms found in the gut and are expected to modulate the immune system and reduce systemic inflammation. Studies done on cell lines and animal models proposed a possible use of probiotics in the management of dyslipidemia, glycemic control, and weight loss. Preclinical studies done on animal models showed some benefit in regulation of energy metabolism. Most RCTs done have been of a small size and duration. Probiotics were administered either as yogurt or in the form of capsules. Here was small, clinically insignificant changes noted in body weight, blood pressure, HbA1c, visceral fat percentage, weight circumference, lipid profile, and the degree of inflammation. A meta-analysis of four clinical trials did not show any significant impact on body weight or BMI. Another meta-analysis of 11 RCTs, which included 614 patients with T2DM, showed a decrease in HbA1c with no impact on HOMA-IR or insulin level. A significant beneficial effect on the lipid profile was noted when fermented milk or yogurt was used instead of probiotic capsules for duration of 8 weeks. Consuming multiple strains had a greater impact than single strain. *Lactobacillus gasseri* was associated with weight loss, while *Lactobacillus acidophilus* (*L. acidophilus*) was associated with a reduction in LDL. However, there is no consensus on the strains, dosage, treatment duration, and the targeted patient profile.

Probiotics include fermented food products such as fermented milk, pickled vegetables, fermented bean paste, etc. They contain multiple lactobacilli species including *L. acidophilus*, *L. rhamnosus*, *L. plantarum*, and *L. paracasei*. Yogurt products must contain $10^8$ colony-forming units (CFUs) per gram at the time of manufacturing, to be labeled as "probiotic." Fermented plants appear to be an attractive alternative as they contain both prebiotics and probiotics.

## ANTIBIOTICS

Antibiotics use has been associated with gut dysbiosis which results in an alteration of metabolic functions with increased energy harvest from the food products and subsequent increase in obesity. Knoop et al. demonstrated in 2016 that use of oral antibiotics was associated with an increased translocation of gut commensal bacteria, further implying their role in inflammatory disorders. The effect of antibiotics on an individual depends on the baseline nutritional status, microbiota composition, and the antibiotic used. Modulation of gut microbiota in 20 male obese patients was attempted by Vrieze et al. (JOH, 2014). He randomized cases to either arm. In the first arm, patients were given amoxicillin 500 mg TID for 7 days. In the second arm, tablet vancomycin 500 mg TDS was given for 7 days. Cases in the vancomycin arm showed a reduction in fecal diversity with a decrease in gram-positive bacilli such as Firmicutes and an increase in gram-negative bacilli such as Proteobacteria. It was associated with an increase in insulin resistance. Patients in the amoxicillin arm did not show any significant changes. It has been demonstrated in mural models that administration of vancomycin may reduce the risk of type 1 diabetes mellitus and the administration of a combination of norfloxacin and ampicillin in obese mice models improved glucose tolerance. However, the same is yet to be replicated in human studies.

## OTHER DRUGS

Effect of metformin in controlling blood sugar in diabetics has been attributed partially to its impact on gut microbiota. This change in gut microbiota has also been hypothesized to be responsible for the side effects of metformin, including lactic acidosis and vitamin B12 deficiency.

Proton pump inhibitors (PPIs) are prescribed widely in both gastroenterology and internal medicine outpatient departments (OPDs). However, they have been known to change the composition of intestinal flora by increasing the intestinal pH. PPI administration has been associated with a change in microbiota composition in the terminal ileum. There is an increase in Firmicutes and a reduction in Bacteroidetes species. Hence, adverse effects of PPI including increased risk of enteric infections should not be overlooked.

## FECAL MICROBIOTA TRANSPLANT

Fecal microbiota transplant (FMT) has been firmly established as a treatment option in patients with recurrent *Clostridium difficile* (*C. difficile*) infection. It is also being explored as a treatment for other diseases linked with dysbiosis. Vrieze et al. (Gastroenterology, 2012) performed FMT obese male subjects with either autogenic fecal capsules or with feces from lean donors. When obese patients underwent FMT with feces from a lean donor, there was an improvement in insulin sensitivity at 6 weeks, but the same did not persist at 12 weeks. On the contrary, a single case was reported in 2015, where a woman developed new-onset obesity after undergoing FMT for *C. difficile* infection. The donor had been a healthy but overweight candidate. This heterogeneity in the success of FMT underlines the importance of the recipient's baseline microbiota and its resilience to any change. Nonbacterial components of gut microbiome may also play a role in energy harvest and development of obesity.

## BARIATRIC SURGERY

Bariatric surgery has been used for the treatment of obesity in patients with morbid obesity and resultant life-threatening medical conditions. Mechanism by which these operation lead to decrease in weight is 2-fold. Surgeries such as sleeve gastroplasty and adjustable gastric banding decrease the capacity of the stomach leading to early satiety. Roux-en-Y gastric bypass (RYGB) operations, with or without duodenal switch, lead to a decrease in the absorptive surface. However, these surgeries also lead to a change in the secretion of appetite and GI motility-regulating peptides such as GLP-1 and ghrelin, which cannot be completely explained by the physical change made. Microbiota changes may have a role in weight loss postbariatric surgery. Fecal microbiome analysis in patients who underwent RYGB, there was an increase in Proteobacteria and decrease in Firmicutes microbiota content. Laparoscopic sleeve gastroplasty did not lead to any drastic changes in microbiome, but an increase in abundance of anti-inflammatory bacteria *Faecalibacterium prausnitzii*. Other studies show an increase in gamma bacteria and decrease in abundance of Clostridia genus after surgery. Liou et al. had demonstrated an association between changes in gut microbiome which occurred post-RYGB and postoperative reductions in fat percentage as well as overall total body weight. Furthermore, when the fecal microbiota was transferred from a patient who underwent RYGB to germ-free mice, it led to weight loss in the murine models. A study by Aron-Wisnewsky et al. (Gut, 2019) on severely obese subjects confirmed the presence of low microbial gene richness (MGR) in such patients. Patients were then assigned either adjustable gastric balloon or RYGB. Despite major weight loss and metabolic improvements postbariatric surgery, low MGR was not fully rescued. MGR significantly increased after both surgery types, but most patients remained with low MGR at 1 year. Hence, attempts to modulate the gut microbiome could further increase postsurgical benefits.

## CONCLUSION

There is a pandemic of obesity with a steady rise in the number of people affected. Although the focus has largely been on a change in diet and lifestyle for the control of this disease, it has proven to be an incomplete, insufficient measure. Gut microbiota plays a key role in the energy harvest from ingested food substances. Gut microbiota can be modulated with changes in diet, antibiotics, prebiotics, probiotics, FMT, and even bariatric surgery. It seems to be a promising step in our fight. It is crucial to catch early-onset obese and to restore the metabolism early rather than let it worsen with time. This can prevent need for drastic procedures such as bariatric surgery.

## SUGGESTED READING

1. Turnbaugh PJ, Hamady M, Yatsunenko T, Cantarel BL, Duncan A, Ley RE, et al. A core gut microbiome in obese and lean twins. Nature. 2009;457(7228):480-4.
2. Patterson E, Ryan PM, Cryan JF, Dinan TG, Ross RP, Fitzgerald GF, et al. Gut microbiota, obesity and diabetes. Postgrad Med J. 2016;92(1087):286-300.
3. Nieuwdorp M, Gilijamse PW, Pai N, Kaplan LM. Role of the microbiome in energy regulation and metabolism. Gastroenterology. 2014;146(6):1525-33.
4. Delzenne NM, Neyrinck AM, Bäckhed F, Cani PD. Targeting gut microbiota in obesity: effects of prebiotics and probiotics. Nat Rev Endocrinol. 2011;7(11):639-46.
5. Cani PD, Bibiloni R, Knauf C, Waget A, Neyrinck AM, Delzenne NM, et al. Changes in gut microbiota control metabolic endotoxemia-induced inflammation in high-fat diet-induced obesity and diabetes in mice. Diabetes. 2008;57(6):1470-81.
6. Bäckhed F, Ding H, Wang T, Hooper LV, Koh GY, Nagy A, et al. The gut microbiota as an environmental factor that regulates fat storage. Proc Natl Acad Sci U S A. 2004;101(44):15718-23.
7. Turnbaugh PJ, Ley RE, Mahowald MA, Magrini V, Mardis ER, Gordon JI. An obesity-associated gut microbiome with increased capacity for energy harvest. Nature. 2006;444(7122):1027-31.

8. Santos-Marcos JA, Haro C, Vega-Rojas A, Alcala-Diaz JF, Molina-Abril H, Leon-Acuña A, et al. Sex Differences in the Gut Microbiota as Potential Determinants of Gender Predisposition to Disease. Mol Nutr Food Res. 2019;63(7):e1800870.
9. Griffin LE, Djuric Z, Angiletta CJ, Mitchell CM, Baugh ME, Davy KP, et al. A Mediterranean diet does not alter plasma trimethylamine N-oxide concentrations in healthy adults at risk for colon cancer. Food Funct. 2019;10(4):2138-47.
10. Hatori M, Vollmers C, Zarrinpar A, DiTacchio L, Bushong EA, Gill S, et al. Time-Restricted Feeding without Reducing Caloric Intake Prevents Metabolic Diseases in Mice Fed a High-Fat Diet. Cell Metab. 2012;15(6):848-60.
11. Li G, Xie C, Lu S, Nichols RG, Tian Y, Li L, et al. Intermittent Fasting Promotes White Adipose Browning and Decreases Obesity by Shaping the Gut Microbiota. Cell Metab. 2017;26(4):672-685.e4.
12. Beserra BTS, Fernandes R, do Rosario VA, Mocellin MC, Kuntz MGF, Trindade EBSM. A systematic review and meta-analysis of the prebiotics and synbiotics effects on glycaemia, insulin concentrations and lipid parameters in adult patients with overweight or obesity. Clin Nutr Edinb Scotl. 2015;34(5):845-58.
13. John GK, Wang L, Nanavati J, Twose C, Singh R, Mullin G. Dietary Alteration of the Gut Microbiome and Its Impact on Weight and Fat Mass: A Systematic Review and Meta-Analysis. Genes. 2018;9(3).
14. Vrieze A, Out C, Fuentes S, Jonker L, Reuling I, Kootte RS, et al. Impact of oral vancomycin on gut microbiota, bile acid metabolism, and insulin sensitivity. J Hepatol. 2014;60(4):824-31.
15. Wu H, Esteve E, Tremaroli V, Khan MT, Caesar R, Manneräs-Holm L, et al. Metformin alters the gut microbiome of individuals with treatment-naive type 2 diabetes, contributing to the therapeutic effects of the drug. Nat Med. 2017;23(7):850-8.
16. Bruno G, Zaccari P, Rocco G, Scalese G, Panetta C, Porowska B, et al. Proton pump inhibitors and dysbiosis: Current knowledge and aspects to be clarified. World J Gastroenterol. 2019;25(22):2706-19.
17. Vrieze A, de Groot PF, Kootte RS, Knaapen M, van Nood E, Nieuwdorp M. Fecal transplant: a safe and sustainable clinical therapy for restoring intestinal microbial balance in human disease? Best Pract Res Clin Gastroenterol. 2013;27(1):127-37.
18. Aron-Wisnewsky J, Prifti E, Belda E, Ichou F, Kayser BD, Dao MC, et al. Major microbiota dysbiosis in severe obesity: fate after bariatric surgery. Gut. 2019;68(1):70-82.

# CHAPTER 3

# Gastrointestinal and Liver Disorders in Pregnancy

*Vandana Midha, Harmeet Kaur*

## ABSTRACT

Liver disease occurring during pregnancy can present a challenge for both clinicians and gynecologists. Certain liver diseases are uniquely associated with pregnancy, whereas others are unrelated. This review discusses liver diseases unique to pregnancy such as hyperemesis gravidarum, acute fatty liver of pregnancy (AFLP), intrahepatic cholestasis of pregnancy (ICP), and hemolysis and elevated liver enzymes and low platelets (HELLP) syndrome.

## INTRODUCTION

Pregnancy is a special state that leads to physiological changes in multiple organs of the body including liver. Abnormal liver function tests (LFTs) can be encountered in 3–5% of pregnancies. Some of these abnormalities may be "normal" in pregnant women. However, all pregnant women with abnormal LFTs need detailed and extensive evaluation as it is important to identify underlying liver diseases that may manifest for the first time during pregnancy as well as specific diseases related to pregnancy (**Table 1**). Therefore, a pregnant woman with abnormal LFTs should undergo standard evaluation similar to a nonpregnant individual.

In this review, we discuss the physiological changes occurring in liver in pregnancy and then focus on liver diseases unique to pregnancy. A detailed description of pre-existing liver diseases is beyond the scope of this review.

## PHYSIOLOGICAL CHANGES IN LIVER IN PREGNANCY

Plasma volume increases by 50% in pregnancy. However, despite this increase and concomitant increase in cardiac output, the blood flow to liver remains unchanged and so does the liver size. The contractility of gallbladder decreases secondary to hormonal changes and there is an increase in cholesterol saturation index that makes the bile more lithogenic.

Knowledge of physiological changes in LFTs during pregnancy is important to identify pathological alterations. Serum bilirubin and albumin are decreased throughout pregnancy, the decline becoming more prominent as the pregnancy advances. This can be

**TABLE 1:** Hepatic disorders in pregnancy.

| Pregnancy related | Pre-existing or coincidental with pregnancy |
|---|---|
| • Hyperemesis gravidarum<br>• Intrahepatic cholestasis of pregnancy<br>• Acute fatty liver of pregnancy<br>• Preeclampsia and eclampsia<br>• Hemolysis and elevated liver enzymes and low platelets (HELLP) syndrome | • Hepatitis B, C<br>• Acute viral hepatitis (hepatitis A/E)<br>• Nonalcoholic fatty liver disease<br>• Cirrhosis and portal hypertension<br>• Biliary diseases (e.g., cholelithiasis, primary sclerosing cholangitis)<br>• Autoimmune liver disease<br>• Vascular alterations (Budd–Chiari syndrome)<br>• Wilson's disease<br>• Metabolic diseases<br>• Drug-induced hepatotoxicity<br>• Post liver transplantation state<br>• Liver tumors |

(HELLP: hemolysis and elevated liver enzymes and low platelets)

explained by hemodilution as the intravascular mass of albumin is normal in pregnancy. Serum aminotransferases remain within normal limits throughout the pregnancy. Only in labor, mild increase in aspartate aminotransferase (AST) can be seen due to uterine muscle contractions. Therefore, any increase in aminotransferases before labor is pathological. Serum alkaline phosphatase (ALP) increases in third trimester of pregnancy, mainly due to increased production of placental isoenzyme. The elevated levels persist for 6–8 weeks postpartum, implying that increase in serum ALP may also be partly contributed by bone isoenzyme. It also implies that measuring ALP in late pregnancy is not a sensitive marker of cholestatic liver disease. Gamma-glutamyltransferase (GGT), 5'-nucleotidase, and prothrombin time are not affected by pregnancy.

## LIVER DISEASES UNIQUE TO PREGNANCY

The liver disorders specific to pregnancy can be classified as those related to early pregnancy [hyperemesis gravidarum (HG)] and those of late pregnancy [intrahepatic cholestasis of pregnancy (ICP), hypertension-related liver diseases (preeclampsia/eclampsia, hemolysis and elevated liver enzymes and low platelets (HELLP) syndrome, liver infarction/liver rupture), and acute fatty liver of pregnancy (AFLP)].

## Hyperemesis Gravidarum

Hyperemesis gravidarum is not a true liver disease, but is associated with abnormal LFTs. Multiple gestations, molar pregnancy, history of HG in previous pregnancy, obesity, and pre-existing diabetes are risk factors for HG. HG remains a poorly understood condition and involves a combination of hormonal, immunologic, and genetic factors. Increased levels of human chorionic gonadotropin (HCG) are noted in HG that stimulates gastrointestinal secretions as well as hypothalamic-pituitary adrenal axis, increases estrogen levels, and decreases serum prolactin. Hepatic involvement is seen in 50% cases of HG and is hypothesized to result from impaired maternal or fetal mitochondrial fatty acid oxidation leading to accumulation of fatty acids.

Symptoms usually start by 8–9th weeks of gestation and disappear by late second trimester. It is characterized by intractable vomiting that result in dehydration, metabolic alkalosis, dyselectrolytemia, ketosis, and weight loss. Rise in aminotransferases [up to five times upper limit of normal (ULN)] is the most common abnormality noted in LFTs, although increases in ALP and bilirubin are also reported. The severity of nausea and vomiting in patients with HG and liver disease correlates with the degree of elevation of aminotransferases. Liver biopsy does not show distinct histopathology; normal tissue or hepatocyte necrosis, bile plugs, and steatosis may be seen. The maternofetal effects of HG have been studied in detail. It is associated with a predominance of female fetuses, lower birth weight, and shorter gestational age at birth. However, no definitive association with Apgar scores, congenital anomalies, or perinatal death has been documented.

The treatment of HG is mainly supportive and includes intravenous fluids for rehydration, correction of dyselectrolytemia, and antiemetics (vitamin B6 or vitamin B6 plus doxylamine). Patients refractory to supportive first-line therapies may need ondansetron or glucocorticoids. The prognosis of HG is good as it is a reversible condition with no permanent hepatic damage. Fulminant hepatic failure is not seen with HG. Failure to achieve clinical/biochemical improvement implies evaluation for other etiologies.

## Intrahepatic Cholestasis of Pregnancy

Intrahepatic cholestasis of pregnancy is the most common pregnancy related, reversible, and cholestatic liver disorder occurring in third trimester. Advanced maternal age, multiparous women, history of cholestasis with oral contraceptive use, history of treatment for infertility, or a family history of ICP predicts development of ICP. The current understanding of ICP is that the elevated levels of reproductive hormones unmask genetic susceptibility in some women, resulting in cholestasis and elevated serum bile acids. Molecular studies have identified increased frequency of homozygous mutations in hepatobiliary transporters in patients with ICP. Apart from these, genes encoding extracanalicular proteins such as human leukocyte antigen (HLA), cytochrome P450, estrogen receptors (alpha, beta), and receptors for advanced glycation have also been reported to influence biliary transport and hence contribute to development of ICP. The maternal serum levels of estrogen and progesterone are highest in third trimester, when ICP presents clinically. The fact that cholestasis, in women using oral contraceptives with high estrogen content, is also similar to ICP. Therefore, role of maternal reproductive hormones in ICP cannot be underestimated. Both estrogen and progesterone have been postulated to impact hepatocellular bile acid influx via inhibition of farnesoid X receptor (FXR) pathway or bile salt export pump.

Pruritus, affecting the palms and soles without associated skin changes, is the most common presenting complaint. Jaundice is uncommon and occurs 2–4 weeks after the onset of pruritus. Clay-colored stools and dark urine might also be described. Occasionally, the cholestasis is complicated by diarrhea, steatorrhea, malabsorption, and weight loss. The most common and sometimes the only biochemical abnormality is elevated serum bile acid concentration. Serum bile acids levels also correlate with the outcome of pregnancy. Perinatal complications increase if nonfasting serum bile acid levels are >40 µmol/L. Levels >100 µmol/L are associated with adverse pregnancy outcomes including stillbirth and may need premature termination of pregnancy. LFTs show elevated aminotransferases, normal or moderately elevated GGT, and mildly increased bilirubin. ALP is also elevated, but this increase is nonspecific due to placental production of the enzyme. Unlike serum bile acids, LFTs do not correlate with outcome.

Intrahepatic cholestasis of pregnancy has a benign prognosis for mothers, with no serious short-term or long-term complications. Recovery is usually complete following delivery and bile acids/LFTs normalize within few days. Liver tests and bile acid concentrations are repeated 6–8 weeks after delivery and persistent impairment for >3 months postpartum suggest underlying coexisting liver diseases requiring additional clinical investigations. ICP may also be associated with an abnormal metabolic profile, especially higher prevalence of dyslipidemia, impaired glucose tolerance, and gestational diabetes. High maternal serum bile acids may cause fetal death by cardiac arrest after entering cardiomyocytes. Fortunately, the risk of sudden intrauterine fetal death (IUFD) is currently <1% and is rarely seen before 37 weeks.

*Treatment strategy of ICP is 2-fold*: Relief of maternal symptoms and close fetal surveillance for adverse outcomes. Ursodeoxycholic acid in doses of 10–15 mg/kg/day is the treatment of choice for ICP as it provides symptomatic relief, improves LFTs, and is considered safe (Category B) during pregnancy. Cholestyramine (bile acid binder) may also relieve symptoms, however, it may lead to worsening of steatorrhea and fat-soluble vitamin deficiency. Antihistaminics and topical menthol have also been used for management of pruritus. Dexamethasone may be used, if needed, to promote fetal lung maturity before delivery. Close fetal monitoring and early delivery remain the cornerstone of obstetric management.

## Acute Fatty Liver of Pregnancy

Acute fatty liver of pregnancy is a rare, but catastrophic disorder of third trimester that carries high maternal and fetal morbidity and mortality. The basic defect lays in the fatty acid oxidation that results in microvesicular infiltration of fat into the liver parenchyma (microvesicular steatosis) and subsequent hepatocellular dysfunction. The defective fatty acid oxidation is secondary to mutations in mitochondrial trifunctional protein (TFP) and its alpha subunit long-chain 3-hydroxyacyl-CoA-dehydrogenase (LCHAD). Medium chain dehydrogenase and carnitine palmitoyltransferase 1 deficiency also exacerbate this situation. LCHAD-deficient patients accumulate 3-hydroxy fatty acids and developmental retardation, developmental disabilities, ocular abnormalities, and sudden infant death. Different risk factors for AFLP have been identified, including nulliparity, male offspring, and twin pregnancies.

Acute fatty liver of pregnancy usually present in the third trimester between the 30th and 38th weeks of gestation. Nonspecific symptoms such as nausea, vomiting, headache, right upper quadrant pain, and fatigue are common initial presentations. Jaundice at presentation is a marker of severe disease. Hypoglycemia, encephalopathy, coagulopathy, ascites, and renal failure suggest hepatocellular failure. Pancreatitis has been reported. Approximately 50% of these patients also have signs of preeclampsia, although hypertension is generally not severe. LFTs reveal hyperbilirubinemia, elevated aminotransferases, prolonged prothrombin time, and decreased fibrinogen levels. Other typical abnormalities noted in severe disease include are normochromic, normocytic anemia, high white blood cell count, metabolic acidosis, renal dysfunction, hypoglycemia, and biochemical pancreatitis. Microvesicular steatosis on liver biopsy is diagnostic, but coagulopathy precludes liver biopsy in most of the situations. Microvesicular fatty infiltration of the liver is most prominent in hepatocytes surrounding the central veins (Zone 3) and spares those surrounding portal areas. To obviate the need of liver biopsy, the diagnosis of AFLP is usually made clinically based on compatible presentation and laboratory results. The "Swansea criteria" (**Table 2**) which combine symptoms and

TABLE 2: Swansea criteria for diagnosis of AFLP.

| Clinical features | Laboratory derangements | Histology |
|---|---|---|
| • Vomiting<br>• Abdominal pain<br>• Polydipsia/polyuria<br>• Encephalopathy | • High bilirubin (>14 mmol/L)<br>• High AST/ALT (>42 IU/L)<br>• Coagulopathy (PT >14 s or aPTT >34 s)<br>• High ammonia (>47 mmol/L)<br>• Leukocytosis (>11 × 10$^6$/L)<br>• Hypoglycemia (<4 mmol/L)<br>• Serum creatinine >150 mmol/L<br>• High uric acid (>340 mmol/L)<br>• Ascites or bright liver on ultrasound | • Microvesicular steatosis on liver biopsy |

*Note:* Six or more of the clinical and laboratory features in the absence of another explanation diagnose AFLP.
(AFLP: acute fatty liver of pregnancy; ALT: alanine aminotransferase; aPTT: activated partial thromboplastin time; AST: aspartate aminotransferase; PT: prothrombin time)

laboratory derangements have been validated in large cohorts with 85% positive predictive value and 100% negative predictive value for hepatic microvesicular steatosis.

Hypertension, proteinuria, and other clinical and laboratory features have been observed to overlap between AFLP and HELLP syndrome. However, compared with HELLP syndrome, patients with AFLP are more likely to have hepatic failure with coagulopathy, hypoglycemia, encephalopathy, and renal failure.

Maternal and fetal demises in AFLP are predicted to be 18–23%, respectively. Prompt delivery with intensive care monitoring is the cornerstone of treatment. Delivery is effected immediately after initial stabilization, usually by cesarean section. Vaginal delivery is attempted only if it seems possible in <24 hours with an international normalized ratio of <1.5 and a platelet count of >50,000 cells/mm$^3$. As infections and bleeding remain the most life-threatening complications, transfusions of blood and blood products are usually required along with prophylactic antibiotics to prevent uterine infections. Most patients recover within 4 weeks postdelivery. Plasmapheresis has been used in few series in severe cases with limited success. Liver transplantation is reserved for patients who fail to recover after recovery. Monitoring subsequent pregnancies is recommended since a risk of recurrence exists particularly in cases with defects of fatty acid oxidation. The offspring of mothers affected by AFLP should be monitored carefully for manifestations of deficiency of LCHAD (including defects of heart, liver, and skeletal muscle, fatty liver, infantile cholestasis, and hypocalcemia). The international recommendation suggests that all women with AFLP and their children should have molecular testing for LCHAD/TFP.

## Preeclampsia/Eclampsia

Preeclampsia is defined as hypertension (>140/90 mm Hg) and proteinuria after 20 weeks of pregnancy and within 48 hours of delivery or one of the following features when hypertension appears: Thrombocytopenia, renal insufficiency, impaired liver function, pulmonary edema, or cerebral or visual symptoms. Liver is involved in up to one-fourth of preeclampsia patients. Liver involvement is secondary to vasospasm of the hepatic vascular bed, fibrin precipitation within the portal, and periportal areas of the liver lobule that may result in lobular ischemia and hepatocyte necrosis. Hepatic involvement is an indicator of severity of preeclampsia. Elevated aminotransferases is the most common abnormality in LFTs though mild elevations in serum bilirubin levels can also be seen. Management of precipitating factors and treatment of hypertension, associated symptoms, and seizures (in eclampsia) are needed and no specific therapy for liver involvement is required.

## Hemolysis and Elevated Liver Enzymes and Low Platelets Syndrome

Hemolysis and elevated liver enzymes and low platelets syndrome is a severe variant of preeclampsia and is characterized by hemolysis (H), elevated liver enzymes (EL), and low platelet count (LP). The pathogenesis of HELLP involves endothelial injury and fibrin deposition in blood vessels, secondary to small molecules released from the placental tissue, such as nitric oxide, prostaglandins, and endothelin, causing sinusoidal obstruction and hepatic ischemia. This leads to microangiopathic hemolytic anemia. Platelet activation, aggregation, and consumption culminate in small to diffuse areas of hemorrhage, and necrosis dissecting from zone 1 to involve the whole lobule, leading to large hematomas, capsular tears, and intraperitoneal bleeding.

The majority of patients present in the third trimester (28–36 weeks of gestation), however, nearly one-third of cases occur in the postpartum period. The presenting features are nonspecific and include upper abdominal pain and discomfort, nausea, vomiting, malaise, and headache. Jaundice is present in approximately 5% of cases. The laboratory findings are significant for intravascular hemolysis, schistocytes on peripheral smear, elevated LFTs (usually ALT), and a low platelet count. Tennessee or Mississippi classifications are used for diagnosis of HELLP syndrome (**Table 3**).

The treatment for HELLP syndrome is prompt delivery. However, complications including liver parenchymal bleed or hematoma must be confirmed radiologically if clinical suspicion is high. Cross-sectional imaging including magnetic resonance or computed tomography may be needed as ultrasonography may miss subtle findings. Adequate control of hypertension is necessary. "The Mississippi Protocol" develops as treatment includes corticosteroids, magnesium sulfate, and systolic blood pressure control. After initial optimization, delivery must immediately be effected if pregnancy is beyond 34 weeks of gestation or there is evidence of multi-organ dysfunction,

**TABLE 3:** Diagnostic criteria of HELLP syndrome.

| Tennessee classification | Mississippi classification | |
|---|---|---|
| • Platelet count ≤100 × $10^9$/L<br>• AST ≥70 IU/L and LDH ≥600 IU/L<br>• Hemolysis on peripheral blood smear<br>Two out of three criteria: Partial HELLP<br>All three criteria: Full HELLP | HELLP Class 1 | • Platelet count ≤ 50 × $10^9$/L<br>• AST ≥70 IU/L<br>• LDH ≥ 600 IU/L |
| | HELLP Class 2 | • Platelet count ≥50 × $10^9$/L, ≤100 × $10^9$/L<br>• AST ≥70 IU/L<br>• LDH ≥600 IU/L |
| | HELLP Class 3 | • Platelet count ≥100 × $10^9$/L<br>• AST ≥40 IU/L<br>• LDH ≥600 IU/L |

(AST: aspartate aminotransferase; HELLP: hemolysis and elevated liver enzymes and low platelets; LDH: lactate dehydrogenase)

disseminated intravascular coagulation (DIC), abruptio placentae, or fetal distress. In case the pregnancy is <34 weeks of gestation, management is controversial. Use of corticosteroids (betamethasone 12 mg intramuscularly every 24 h twice or four doses of intramuscular dexamethasone 6 mg every 12 h) for maturity of fetal lungs followed by delivery and intensive care of neonate has been reported. A conservative approach in cases distant from term is associated with high maternal mortality and fetal loss. Most patients have rapid and early resolution of HELLP after delivery with normalization of platelets by 5 days. Persistence of thrombocytopenia or hemolysis for >72 hours, worsening hepatic or renal failure, or life-threatening complications may need plasmapheresis, plasma volume expansion, antithrombotic agents, steroids, plasma exchange with fresh frozen plasma, or hemodialysis as specific therapies.

Complications of HELLP syndrome include intraparenchymal hemorrhage, liver infarction, subcapsular hematoma, hepatic rupture, and hepatic failure. These need aggressive correction of coagulopathy and anemia. Intensive hemodynamic monitoring should be done and exogenous trauma such as abdominal palpation and unnecessary transportation must be avoided. Surgical evacuation of hematoma and hepatic artery ligation may be lifesaving in cases of refractory shock and hepatic rupture.

## CONCLUSION

Hepatic disorders related to pregnancy are often a challenge to diagnose and treat. The timing of the condition in relation toward which trimester it starts at is the key to successful management. Accurate diagnosis can be made using specific clinical findings and blood tests. Some entities have well-defined criteria that help not only in making the diagnosis, but also in prognosticating the course of illness. Management includes supportive care, specific pharmacological therapies, and immediate termination of the pregnancy in critical illnesses.

## SUGGESTED READING

1. Ch'ng CL, Morgan M, Hainsworth I, Kingham JG. Prospective study of liver dysfunction in pregnancy in Southwest Wales. Gut. 2002;51:876-80.
2. Rodger M, Sheppard D, Gandara E, Tinmouth A. Hematological problems in obstetrics. Best Pract Res Clin Obstet Gynaecol. 2015;29:671-84.
3. Munnell EW, Taylor HC. Liver blood flow in pregnancy. Hepatic vein catheterization. J Clin Invest. 1947;26:952-6.
4. Kern F, Everson GT, DeMark B, et al. Biliary lipids, bile acids, and gallbladder function in the human female. Effects of pregnancy and the ovulatory cycle. J Clin Invest. 1981;68:1229-42.
5. Bacq Y, Zarka O, Brechot JF, et al. Liver function tests in normal pregnancy: A prospective study of 103 pregnant women and 103 matched controls. Hepatology. 1996;23:1030-4.
6. Seitanidis B, Moss DW. Serum alkaline phosphatase and 5'-nucleotidase levels during normal pregnancy. Clin Chim Acta. 1969;25:183-4.
7. Koch KL, Frissora CL. Nausea and vomiting during pregnancy. Gastroenterol Clin North Am. 2003;32:201-34.
8. Goodwin TM, Hershman JM, Cole L. Increased concentration of the free beta-subunit of human chorionic gonadotropin in hyperemesis gravidarum. Acta Obstet Gynecol Scand. 1994;73:770-2.
9. Outlaw WM, Ibdah JA. Impaired fatty acid oxidation as a cause of liver disease associated with hyperemesis gravidarum. Med Hypotheses. 2005;65:1150-3.
10. Veenendaal MV, van Abeelen AF, Painter RC, van der Post JA, Roseboom TJ. Consequences of hyperemesis gravidarum for offspring: a systematic review and meta-analysis. BJOG. 2011;118:1302-13.

11. Dixon PH, Williamson C. The pathophysiology of intrahepatic cholestasis of pregnancy. Clin Res Hepatol Gastroenterol. 2016;40:141-53.
12. Song X, Vasilenko A, Chen Y, Valanejad L, Verma R, Yan B, et al. Transcriptional dynamics of bile salt export pump during pregnancy: mechanisms and implications in intrahepatic cholestasis of pregnancy. Hepatology. 2014;60:1993-2000.
13. Geenes V, Chappell LC, Seed PT, Steer PJ, Knight M, Williamson C. Association of severe intrahepatic cholestasis of pregnancy with adverse pregnancy outcomes: a prospective population-based case-control study. Hepatology. 2014;59:1482-91.
14. Wilkström Shemer E, Marschall HU, Ludvigsson JF, Stephansson O. Intrahepatic cholestasis of pregnancy and associated adverse pregnancy and fetal outcomes: a 12-year population-based cohort study. BJOG. 2013;120:717-23.
15. Gorelik J, Patel P, Ng'andwe C, Vodyanoy I, Diakonov I, Lab M, et al. Genes encoding bile acid, phospholipid and anion transporters are expressed in a human fetal cardiomyocyte culture. BJOG. 2006;113:552-8.
16. Ylitalo K, Vanttinen T, Halmesmaki E, Tyni T. Serious pregnancy complications in a patient with previously undiagnosed carnitine palmitoyltransferase 1 deficiency. Am J Obstet Gynecol. 2005;192:2060-2.
17. Ibdah JA. Acute fatty liver of pregnancy: an update on pathogenesis and clinical implications. World J Gastroenterol. 2006;46:7397-404.
18. Goel A, Ramakrishna B, Zachariah U, Ramachandran J, Eapen CE, Kurian G, et al. How accurate are the Swansea criteria to diagnose acute fatty liver of pregnancy in predicting hepatic microvesicular steatosis? Gut. 2011;60:138-9.
19. Tran TT, Ahn J, Reau NS. ACG Clinical Guideline: liver disease and pregnancy. Am J Gastroenterol. 2016;111:176-94.
20. Gomes CF, Sousa M, Lourenço I, Martins D, Torres J. Gastrointestinal diseases during pregnancy: what does the gastroenterologist need to know? Ann Gastroenterol. 2018;31:385-94.
21. Armaly Z, Jadaon JE, Jabbour A, Abassi ZA. Preeclampsia: novel mechanisms and potential therapeutic approaches. Front Physiol. 2018;9:973.
22. Martin JN, Owens MY, Keiser SD, Parrish MR, Tam Tam KB, Brewer JM, et al. Standardized Mississippi Protocol treatment of 190 patients with HELLP syndrome: slowing disease progression and preventing new major maternal morbidity. Hypertens Pregnancy. 2012;31:79-90.

# Hepatobiliary Disorders in Females

*Shivani Mehta, Neha Berry, Praneet Wander*

## ABSTRACT

The aim of this chapter is to highlight the different hepatobiliary diseases affecting women. It focuses on the underlying hormonal and pathological differences in females in comparison to males. Women experience more severe and rapid progression of alcoholic- and drug-mediated liver injury. Females in their reproductive years are less prone to nonalcoholic fatty liver disease (NAFLD) which is one of the causes of liver transplant in women. Immune-mediated liver diseases are much more prevalent in them due to immunomodulatory effects of estrogens. They have lower predilection for fibrosis after viral hepatitis. Benign liver tumors are more common in women than malignant tumors such as hepatocellular carcinoma (HCC). The clinical manifestations of hemochromatosis present late in females. Gallstones typically present in fertile females. Acute liver failure of pregnancy and intrahepatic cholestasis of pregnancy are rare fatal hepatic disorders in pregnancy.

## INTRODUCTION

In the era of evidence-based individualized medicine, it is very important to understand the influence of gender difference on different aspects of disease process. Differences in risk factors, sexual hormones, and other physiological factors affect disease presentation, progression, treatment, and health outcomes. The patriarchal outlook of the society has affected the health-seeking behavior of females. Gaps in knowledge of women's health have led to increased focus on gender-specific medicine. The chapter elucidates the epidemiological and pathophysiological basis of the hepatobiliary disorders in females. It will cover the following diseases (**Table 1**):

- Alcoholic liver diseases
- Nonalcoholic fatty liver disease (NAFLD)
- Immune-mediated liver diseases
- Viral hepatitis
- Drug-induced liver disease
- Mass lesions
- Genetic hemochromatosis (GH)
- Acute fatty liver of pregnancy

## CHAPTER 4: Hepatobiliary Disorders in Females

**TABLE 1:** The incidence and outcome of common liver diseases: Women versus men.

| Disease | Relative incidence F:M | Outcome in women |
|---|---|---|
| **Increased incidence** | | |
| Autoimmune hepatitis | 4:1 | No survival difference |
| Benign liver lesions (most common cavernous hemangioma—1.4% prevalence) | 5–6:1 | |
| Drug-induced liver injury | 2:1 | No survival difference |
| Primary biliary cirrhosis | 10:1 | No survival difference |
| **Decreased incidence** | | |
| Alcohol-related liver disease | 2:1 | More severe |
| Hepatocellular carcinoma | 1:3 | No survival difference |
| Primary sclerosing cholangitis | 1:2.3 | No survival difference |
| **Similar incidence or conflicting data** | | |
| Hepatitis B and C infection | | Less severe |
| Hemochromatosis | | Less severe |
| Nonalcoholic fatty liver disease | | More likely to have diabetes and metabolic syndrome |

- Gallstones
- Cholestasis of pregnancy

## ALCOHOLIC LIVER DISEASE

The trend of alcohol intake has been increasing in young Indian men and women. Alcoholic liver disease is proportional to the level of alcohol consumption. Higher consumption leads to steatosis, hepatitis, and ultimately, end-stage liver disease or cirrhosis. Females are more prone to alcohol-related liver damage. Women reach higher blood alcohol concentration than men with equal doses under the same conditions. A large 12-year prospective study has shown that among the persons consuming four or more drinks per day, the relative risk of developing alcohol-induced cirrhosis was 7.0 [95% confidence interval (CI) 3.8–12.8] in men versus 17.0 (95% CI 6.8–40.8) in women. These gender differences are mainly due to differences in body structures and enzymatic activity of alcohol dehydrogenase (ADH), mainly gastric isoform and hormones. Gastric ADH is responsible for the first-pass metabolism of alcohol. The amount of alcohol not metabolized by the first-pass metabolism reaches the liver where it is metabolized by hepatic ADH. With decreased expression of the gastric enzyme in females, the alcohol reaches the liver directly and hence exacerbating the hepatic damage. The reduced content of body water compared to men increases the female susceptibility to the toxic effects of alcohol due to low distribution volume. Females have higher endotoxin levels along with increased permeability of gut to these endotoxins. In addition to this, women have more estrogen receptor concentrations in the liver causing enhanced estrogen-mediated activation of liver Kupffer cells. All these events lead to increased inflammation and necrosis. Hence, alcoholic liver disease progresses rapidly to fibrosis in women as compared to men.

## NONALCOHOLIC FATTY LIVER DISEASE

Infiltration of fatty acids in >5% of hepatocytes, in the absence of excessive alcohol intake [two standard drinks (20 g ethanol) daily for men and one standard drink (10 g ethanol) daily for women], viral, congenital, and autoimmune disorders. It ranges from simple steatosis to nonalcoholic steatohepatitis (NASH), fibrosis, and then to cirrhosis. NASH is usually seen as the hepatic manifestation of the metabolic syndrome (hypertension, diabetes mellitus, dyslipidemia, and obesity). Insulin resistance is the main disturbance leading to hepatic fat infiltration. Age and hormones influence visceral adipose tissue accumulation. Postmenopausal females accumulate visceral adipose tissue rapidly than younger females due to the protective role of endogenous estrogens against NAFLD in premenopausal women and postmenopausal women on hormone replacement therapy. The prevalence of NAFLD among women is rising due to the epidemic of metabolic diseases, particularly diabetes and obesity, with a recent study showing a prevalence of up to 24.4%. NASH is also the leading cause of liver transplant in women.

## IMMUNE-MEDIATED LIVER DISEASES

Immune-mediated liver diseases in women mainly include primary biliary cirrhosis (PBC) and autoimmune hepatitis (AIH). Immunomodulatory effects of estrogen lead to higher number of CD4+ T lymphocytes and a higher CD4+/CD8+ ratio in women. This further increases the secretion of interferon-$\gamma$ (IFN-$\gamma$) and interleukin (IL)-10. Sex steroids alter the immune system on many levels: they can regulate gene expression through steroid-responsive elements, alter antigen presentation through effects on human leukocyte antigen genes, and alter the cytokine environment. Additionally, X chromosome monosomy and fetal microchimerism (the presence of fetal cells in maternal circulation) may play a role in the pathogenesis of PBC.

Primary biliary cirrhosis is characterized by immune-mediated inflammatory destruction of the small intrahepatic bile ducts. It is a chronic cholestatic liver disease which can progress to cirrhosis and liver failure. It is 10 times more common in women than men, with an average age of onset around 50 years. Women experience more abdominal pain, constitutional (malaise, anorexia, weight loss, and fatigue) and autonomic symptoms than men. Women with PBC present at a younger age with increased rates of pruritus and slower rates of fibrosis than men.

Autoimmune hepatitis is a progressive inflammatory destruction of the liver parenchyma with female to male ratio of 4:1. There is a circulation of autoantibodies and hypergammaglobulinemia. High levels of estrogen during second trimester of pregnancy decrease the disease severity due to its anti-inflammatory effects at higher concentration. However, the rates of progression to cirrhosis, treatment failure, and death from liver failure are equivalent in men and women.

Primary sclerosing cholangitis (PSC) is a chronic inflammatory disease which causes progressive fibrosis of both the intra- and extrahepatic bile ducts and untreated results in secondary biliary cirrhosis and portal hypertension. Women are less likely to have PSC, with M:F ratio of 2–3:1.

## VIRAL HEPATITIS

Hepatitis A virus (HAV), hepatitis B virus (HBV), hepatitis C virus (HCV), and hepatitis E virus (HEV) mainly cause viral hepatitis. They have similar clinical presentations ranging from asymptomatic to acute liver failure and from subclinical infection to chronic liver disease with cirrhosis and hepatocellular carcinoma (HCC) in HBV, HCV, and hepatitis D virus (HDV). Women clear acute HCV infection at a higher rate than men do. Estrogens inhibit fibrogenesis causing stellate cells in the liver. Thus, women have less altered liver function tests and lower progression to fibrosis in viral hepatitis. In one study on long-term follow-up in women with viral hepatitis, only 27% showed progression of liver fibrosis, and cirrhosis developed in only four (2.1%) women after almost three decades. HBV affects men and women similarly. However, male sex is a risk factor for reactivation of HBV infection after seroconversion from hepatitis B e antigen (HBeAg)—positive to negative—and for the development of cirrhosis and HCC. The high levels of proinflammatory cytokines in chronic hepatitis B (CHB) can lead to complications during pregnancy, such as gestational diabetes, predelivery hemorrhages, and preterm delivery.

## DRUG-INDUCED LIVER DISEASE

Drug-induced liver injury is the major cause of the patients presenting with acute liver failure. Hepatotoxic drugs can injure the hepatocyte directly (e.g., via a free-radical or metabolic intermediate that causes peroxidation of membrane lipids) or block biochemical pathways or cellular integrity. There are gender-based differences in drug bioavailability, metabolism, and excretion. Women are more likely to express CYP3A4, an important enzyme of drug metabolism. Thus, females are more commonly affected by the toxin-mediated liver disease with a high prevalence of acute liver failure. Prospective data from the Acute Liver Failure Study Group showed that 67% of the 1,147 patients were women, and women accounted for over 70% patients hospitalized with acute liver injury due to acetaminophen or idiosyncratic drug reactions.

## MASS LESIONS IN LIVER

The incidence of benign and malignant liver tumors is different in both the genders. Benign liver tumors are more common in women, whereas malignant tumors are prevalent in men. Benign liver lesions in women include cavernous hemangioma, focal nodular hyperplasia (FNH), and hepatic adenoma. Biliary cystadenoma and adenocarcinoma are rare (1% of cystic liver lesions), and women account for 96% of cystadenomas and 66% of cystadenocarcinomas. Oral contraceptive pills are one of the main underlying causes of benign liver lesions; around 80% of women with benign liver tumors reported its use. The molecular pathogenesis of benign liver lesions suggests that women have an inactivating mutation of a gene involved in estrogen metabolism (CYP1B1), which results in an increased risk of the HNF1A (hepatocyte nuclear factor 1-a tumor suppression gene) subtype of adenomas. HCC affects men three to four times more frequently than women. It is the fifth most common malignancy in men and the ninth most common in women, with an annual incidence rate of 2.0/100,000 years for women. HCC is an androgen-sensitive tumor. Also, estrogen decreases the production of IL-6 from liver Kupffer cells leading to low occurrence of HCC in females.

## METABOLIC DISEASES: GENETIC HEMOCHROMATOSIS AND WILSON'S DISEASE

The liver plays a major role in the storage and metabolic regulation of iron. The liver produces hepcidin, which is an important mediator in the pathogenesis of GH. The manifestations of GH begin earlier in men than women, most probably due to the physiological loss of blood in women during menstruation. The clinical presentation of GH is different between women and men. Both liver disease and diabetes are less common in women. Women are less likely to be affected by Wilson's disease (WD) overall than men (47% vs. 53%); however, they are more likely to present with the hepatic form than the neuropsychiatric form.

## GALLSTONES

Gallstones are four times more prevalent in women of reproductive age than men of the same age. Estrogens stimulate hepatic lipoprotein receptors, increases biliary cholesterol secretion, and uptake of dietary cholesterol, along with decreased bile salt secretion. There is increased risk of gallstones during pregnancy. The gallbladder volume increases during the second and third trimesters with decreased gallbladder motility due to elevated progesterone levels. Steroid-induced cholesterol secretion during pregnancy causes a 50% increase in bile acid pool. All these factors contribute to the increased risk of biliary stones in pregnancy.

## GALLBLADDER MALIGNANCY

Gallbladder malignancy is one of the most common tumors of biliary tract. Its prevalence is more in females, especially those from Indian origin, than men. The risk in multiparous women is even more. The presence of estrogen and progesterone receptors on malignant as well as benign lesions plays an important role in the disease pathogenesis. But, there is not much data available related to prognostic value of presence of estrogen and progesterone receptors.

## SUGGESTED READING

1. Frezza M, di Padova C, Pozzato G, Terpin M, Baraona E, Lieber CS. High blood alcohol levels in women. The role of decreased gastric alcohol dehydrogenase activity and first-pass metabolism. N Engl J Med. 1990;322(2):95-9.
2. Ikejima K, Enomoto N, Iimuro Y, Ikejima A, Fang D, Xu J, et al. Estrogen increases sensitivity of hepatic Kupffer cells to endotoxin. Am J Physiol. 1998;274(4 pt 1):G669-76.
3. Colantoni A, Emanuele MA, Kovacs EJ, Villa E, Van Thiel DH. Hepatic estrogen receptors and alcohol intake. Mol Cell Endocrinol. 2002;193(1-2):101-104.
4. Pares A, Caballeria J, Bruguera M, Torres M, Rodes J. Histological course of alcoholic hepatitis. Influence of abstinence, sex and extent of hepatic damage. J Hepatol. 1986;2(1):33-42.
5. Völzke H, Schwarz S, Baumeister SE, Wallaschofski H, Schwahn C, Grabe HJ, et al. Menopausal status and hepatic steatosis in a general female population. Gut. 2007;56:594-5.
6. Noureddin M, Vipani A, Bresee C, Todo T, Kim IK, Alkhouri N, et al. NASH leading cause of liver transplant in women: updated analysis of indications for liver transplant and ethnic and gender variances. Am J Gastroenterol. 2018;113:1649-59.
7. Amadori A, Zamarchi R, De Silvestro G, Forza G, Cavatton G, Danieli GA, et al. Genetic control of the CD4/CD8 T-cell ratio in humans. Nat Med. 1995; 1:1279-83.
8. Gilmore W, Weiner LP, Correale J. Effect of estradiol on cytokine secretion by proteolipid protein-specific T cell clones isolated from multiple sclerosis patients and normal control subjects. J Immunol. 1997;158(1):446-51.
9. Durazzo M, Belci P, Collo A, Prandi V, Pistone E, Martorana M, et al. Gender specific medicine in liver diseases: A point of view. World J Gastroenterol. 2014;20(9):2127-35.

10. Buchel E, Van Steenbergen W, Nevens F, Fevery J. Improvement of autoimmune hepatitis during pregnancy followed by flare-up after delivery. Am J Gastroenterol. 2002;97(12):3160-5.
11. Kenny-Walsh E. Clinical outcomes after hepatitis C infection from contaminated anti-D immune globulin. Irish Hepatology Research Group. N Engl J Med. 1999;340(16):1228-33.
12. Bissell DM. Sex and hepatic fibrosis. Hepatology. 1999;29(3):988-9.
13. Bozkaya H, Bozdayi M, Türkyilmaz R, Sarioglu M, Cetinkaya H, Cinar K, et al. Circulating IL-2, IL-10 and TNF-alpha in chronic hepatitis B: their relations to HBeAg status and the activity of liver disease. Hepatogastroenterology. 2000;47(36):1675-9.
14. Luppi P, Haluszczak C, Trucco M, Deloia JA. Normal pregnancy is associated with peripheral leukocyte activation. Am J Reprod Immunol. 2002;47(2):72-81.
15. Waxman DJ, Holloway MG. Sex differences in the expression of hepatic drug metabolizing enzymes. Mol Pharmacol. 2009;76(2):215-28.
16. Wolbold R, Klein K, Burk O, Nüssler AK, Neuhaus P, Eichelbaum M, et al. Sex is a major determinant of CYP3A4 expression in human liver. Hepatology. 2003;38(4):978-88.
17. Reuben A, Koch DG, Lee WM. Drug-induced acute liver failure: results of a U.S. multicenter, prospective study. Hepatology. 2010;52(6):2065-76.
18. Balabaud C, Al-Rabih WR, Chen PJ, Evason K, Ferrell L, Hernandez-Prera JC, et al. Focal nodular hyperplasia and hepatocellular adenoma around the world viewed through the scope of the immunopathological classification. Int J Hepatol. 2013;2013:268625.
19. Rebouissou S, Bioulac-Sage P, Zucman-Rossi J. Molecular pathogenesis of focal nodular hyperplasia and hepatocellular adenoma. J Hepatol. 2008;48(1):163-70.
20. Naugler WE, Sakurai T, Kim S, Maeda S, Kim K, Elsharkawy AM, et al. Gender disparity in liver cancer due to sex differences in MyD88-dependent IL-6 production. Science. 2007;317(5834):121-4.
21. Adams PC, Deugnier Y, Moirand R, Brissot P. The relationship between iron overload, clinical symptoms, and age in 410 patients with genetic hemochromatosis. Hepatology. 1997;25(1):162-6.
22. Glenn F, McSherry CK. Gallstones and pregnancy among 300 young women treated with cholecystectomy. Surg Gynecol Obstct. 1968;127(5):1067-72.
23. Braverman DZ, Johnson ML, Kern F Jr. Effects of pregnancy and contraception steroids on gallbladder function. N Engl J Med. 1980;302(7):362-4.
24. Gupta P, Aggarwal A, Gupta V, Singh PK, Pantola C, Amit S, et al. Expression and clinicopathological significance of estrogen and progesterone receptors in gallbladder cancer. Gastrointest Cancer Res. 2012;5(2):41-7.
25. Guy J, Peters MG Liver Disease in Women: The Influence of Gender on Epidemiology, Natural History, and Patient Outcomes Gastroenterol Hepatol (N Y). 2013;9(10):633-9.

# CHAPTER 5

# Does Gender Matter in Liver Transplantation?

*Mayank Jain, Chandan Kumar Kedarisetty,
Tamarai Selvan, Senthil Kumar, Jayanthi Venkataraman*

## ABSTRACT

There are major differences in liver transplant-related outcomes between men and women. Even in countries like USA, there are fewer women who are waitlisted and are even less likely considered for a liver transplantation (LT). There are major differences in organ allocation in a woman and post-transplant outcome including graft survival. This may be influenced by differences in etiology between men and women, the smaller body build, and hormonal changes that extend across a woman's life. Postmenopausal women are at greater risk of metabolic syndrome than their counterparts in the premenopausal phase of reproductive life. The small body muscle mass in women results in lowering of serum creatinine and thereby a lowering of MELD (Model for End-stage Liver Disease), despite having a severe liver disease. The small body build also prevents woman getting an organ allocated which shifts toward the pediatric population. Till date, none of the algorithms addresses the issues of indications, pre- and post-transplant outcomes in woman that in fact can affect the clinical practice in these patients. This review highlights some of these issues with special reference to gender differences in etiology, problems related to allocation of organ, and outcomes after transplant.

## INTRODUCTION

Liver transplantation (LT) is the only recommended long-term definitive option for patients with end-stage chronic liver disease with progressive decompensation, acute-on-chronic liver failure, acute liver failure, and hepatocellular carcinoma (HCC). With improvements in surgical techniques and postoperative care, the outcomes of LT have improved considerably. Recent research has shed light on gender disparity in terms of organ donation per se, response to liver transplant, and post-transplant issues that now exist in the LT process world over.

Other reasons for gender disparity include issues related to discrepancy in body and organ size, differences in the etiology of liver disease, and limitations related to MELD (Model for End-stage Liver Disease) score.

The present review highlights some of these issues and includes discussion on factors contributing to disparity such as referral patterns, an imperfect organ allocation system that is based on the MELD score, donor-recipient liver size matching, etiology of underlying liver disease, and gender-based hormonal changes. Apart from these factors, other issues include a gender disparity in liver donation and lack of women workforce representation in this specialized field is also highlighted.

## ACCESS TO LIVER TRANSPLANTATION

### Demographic Profile and Access to Liver Transplantation

Data suggests that access to LT is considerably poor for ethnic minorities, women, and patients belonging to low socioeconomic status or inadequate insurance coverage. Over a 3-year period, 678 patients were registered for LT at Gleneagles Global Health City, Chennai. Of these, only 26.2% (178) were women that included 79 girl children. This gender disparity may be partly related because alcohol-related liver disease is relatively rare in women and it was the most common etiology of liver disease in our population. Secondly, as mentioned previously, due to poor socioeconomic conditions and lack of family support, fewer women seek further medical attention including LT, hence highlighting the gender bias when it comes to such expensive yet curative options.

### Etiology and Gender Differences: Impact on Access to Liver Transplantation

- Data from US suggests that over a 15-year period, significantly more women than men underwent LT for Wilson disease, primary biliary cirrhosis, drug-induced acute hepatic necrosis, Budd–Chiari syndrome, autoimmune-linked cirrhosis, cryptogenic cirrhosis, and nonalcoholic steatohepatitis (NASH).

  An analysis of data from our previous study from Gleneagles Global Health City, Chennai had shown that the etiology of 99 women patients listed for LT included NASH (26, 26%) to be most common followed by viral hepatitis (18, 18%), cryptogenic cirrhosis (16, 16%), autoimmune hepatitis (12, 12%), primary biliary cirrhosis (10, 10%), HCC (8, 8%), alcohol (3, 3%), and Budd–Chiari syndrome and Wilson disease (2, 2% each). A similar scenario is reported from other centers in India.
- Drug-induced liver injury is also frequent among women. They have a 1.5- to 1.7-fold greater risk of developing adverse drug reactions than men. The potential reasons for this include differences in pharmacokinetics, hormonal effects, and differences in aberrant immune response that target the liver following drug exposure. Common drugs responsible for hepatic failure among women include analgesics, antiepileptics, anti-inflammatory and antirheumatic agents, antidiabetics, and antibacterials (systemic); in men, there is a significant overrepresentation with antivirals.
- *MELD-related issues, and non-MELD as determinants of access to LT*: Other issue pertaining to organ allocation for LT includes those related to MELD score and non-MELD determinants. In women with low body weight and muscle mass, when compared to men, they are likely to have lower MELD because of lower serum creatinine levels. There is also a likelihood of an underestimation of renal dysfunction. Thus, women folk despite having a severe disease are at a distinct disadvantage when it comes to an organ allocation based on MELD score.
- *HCC and gender disparity at cross roads*: MELD exception rule for LT is usually followed for HCC that is common in men. This has resulted in increasing disparity of access to LT for new women.

More recently, estrogens seem to have a significant role to play in liver carcinogenesis. Wild-type versus variant estrogen receptors in the liver has been shown to accurately predict survival in patients with HCC. Despite this variations in estrogen receptors between the two genders, there is a striking preponderance of HCC among men. Introducing demonstration of the specific estrogen receptors in women could help reallocate organs for women with HCC with a favorable outcome.

## TECHNICAL ISSUES PERTAINING TO FEMALE GENDER

- *Size of graft*: The differences in body build result in limited access to the pool of available organs. The grafts available are either too small or too large. Due to the small build, women patients may have to wait longer for organs of an appropriate size. Livers from pediatric donors are preferentially allocated to children awaiting LT.
- *Surgery related*: It is well-established that sex mismatch is an established risk factor for chronic rejection of liver allografts. Experimental studies have shown that a female liver is more sensitive to a reperfusion injury than a male liver. Studies in male and female rats have shown an increase in oxidative stress with an increase in malondialdehyde and lactic dehydrogenase with values being significantly more in female rats. Thus, a poor outcome of a female organ after LT suggests a greater susceptibility to reperfusion injury.

  On the flip side, Eckhoff et al. in an experimental study in a rat model, had shown that injection of 17 beta-estradiol pre- and postclamping of medial lobe reduced levels of transaminases, i.e., a cytoprotective effect. It also reduced tumor necrosis factor (TNF)-alpha and increased nitric oxide levels, indicating estrogen via a receptor-mediated action may reduce ischemic-reperfusion injury. Liver biopsy had shown reduction in liver necrosis and neutrophilic infiltration.
- *Post-transplant recovery*: Post-transplant recovery in pediatric patients is better if mother is the prospective donor as explored in a Japanese study wherein they reported that maternal antigens may have an important clinical impact on graft tolerance in living donor liver transplantation (LDLT). Exposure to maternal antigens may have tolerogenic effects on offspring, resulting in acceptance or rejection of allografts expressing the maternal antigens.

  Overall outcomes after LT, especially in the long-term, are reportedly better in women as compared to men. Outcome is better in premenopausal phase wherein metabolic syndrome components such as hyperglycemia and hypertriglyceridemia are less common while poorer outcome in the menopausal phase wherein there is an increase in weight due to an increase in central adiposity, both constituting a risk factor for developing NASH and metabolic syndrome. Postmenopausal women are also at a greater risk for developing osteoporosis compared to women in the fertile age, as a consequence of decreased serum estrogen levels.

  Renal dysfunction as a complication of immunosuppression is more frequent in women than their male counterpart. Development of de novo tumors is also significantly high; specifically these include carcinoma of tongue, other tumors of the oral cavity, and head/neck cancers.
- *Post-transplant sex hormone regularization and pregnancy*: In general post-LT, there is partial or complete normalization of sex hormones and regularization of sexual function over a period of few months. Successful LT restores menstrual function in

97% and childbearing potential. However, sexual activity remains an important issue. There is decreased libido and failure to reach orgasm in 26%. The optimal timing of conception is still a matter of debate, but waiting for at least a year after LT is generally recommended.

Pregnancy outcomes after LT are acceptable in terms of the health of the mother and of the newborn and comparatively better than those following kidney transplantation. Immunosuppression, calcineurin inhibitors, and steroids are considered fairly safe during pregnancy while azathioprine and mycophenolate mofetil are associated with enhanced toxic effects during pregnancy.

## WOMEN AS LIVER DONORS

Over the past decade and a half, India has emerged as a hub for living donor organ transplants in South and Southeast Asia. Interestingly, the majority of living donors in India are women. Data from five centers across India have shown that women constitute 60.5% of the donor pool. This discrepancy probably stems from the belief that women are constant givers, increase in societal pressure, men not forthcoming for donation (as a son and breadwinner of the family), and deep set cultural prejudices. Reassessment of traditional gender roles and a woman's role in her family may help to set right these biases.

At Gleneagles Global Health City, Chennai, 55% of women of 783 donors were living donors. This data further highlights that women are the preferred and more forthcoming donors for adult as well as for pediatric LT.

## WOMEN IN THE FIELD OF LIVER TRANSPLANTATION

In the US, up to 10% of liver transplant surgeons are women and they put on an average of 70 hours per week for their work. In India, the statistics are skewed with only a handful of female LT surgeons. On the other hand, our observation has been that women are doing well as hepatologists, transplant physicians, and liver intensivists. This discrepancy is likely to be multifactorial and includes sociocultural factors, harsh working hours, a male dominant field with insufficient support from employers, further contributed by the family, and lack of advanced LT training program in India.

## CONCLUSION

This article highligts sex-based disparities in LT outcome, the differences in etiology, severity of disease, indications for LT, and transplant outcome. Most differences are subtle, but others quite distinct and marked and several still remain poorly understood. Allocation of liver is still imperfect and is based on MELD score or a bias against women, reason is still not clear. Hardcore data is needed across high volume centers so as to reduce the gender disparity in LT-related events. Efforts must be made to enhance interventions so that optimal management can be provided to women in both pre- and post-transplant period, keeping in mind that the management of women varies across the different periods of her life.

## SUGGESTED READING

1. Mindikogluy AL, Regev A, Seliger SL, Magder LS. Gender disparity in liver transplant waiting—list mortality: the importance of kidney function. Liver Transpl. 2010;16:1147-57.
2. Nephew LD, Goldberg DS, Lewis JD, Abt P, Bryan M, Forde KA. Exception Points and Body Size Contribute to Gender Disparity in Liver Transplantation. Clin Gastroenterol Hepatol. 2017;15: 1286-93.
3. Oloruntoba OO, Moylan CA. Gender-based disparities in access to and outcomes of liver transplantation. World J Hepatol. 2015;7:460-7.
4. Bryce CL, Angus DC, Arnold RM, Chang CC, Farrell MH, Manzarbeitia C, et al. Sociodemographic differences in early access to liver transplantation services. Am J Transplant. 2009;9:2092-101.
5. Guy J, Peters MG. Liver disease in women: the influence of gender in epidemiology, natural history and patient outcome. Gastroenterol Hepatol. 2013;9:633-9.
6. Sarin SK, Chari ST, Sundaram KR, Ahuja RK, Anand BS, Broor SL. Young versus adult cirrhotics: a prospective, comparative analysis of the clinical profile, natural course and survival. Gut. 1988;29:101-7.
7. Ray G, Ghoshal UC, Banerjee PK, Pal BB, Dhar K, Pal AK, et al. Aetiological spectrum of chronic liver disease in eastern India. Trop Gastroenterol. 2000;21:60-2.
8. Trimukhe R, Rai R, Narayankar SM, Shewale S, Jagtap N, Rai S, et al. Epidemiological spectrum of chronic liver disease in eastern Madhya Pradesh, India. J Assoc Physicians India. 2011;59:48.
9. Rademaker M. Do women have more adverse drug reactions? Am J Clin Dermatol. 2001;2:349-51.
10. Zopf Y, Rabe C, Neubert A, Gassmann KG, Rascher W, Hahn EG, et al. Women encounter ADRs more often than do men. Eur J Clin Pharmacol. 2008;64:999-1004.
11. Amacher DE. Female gender as a susceptibility factor for drug-induced liver injury. Hum Exp Toxicol. 2013;33:928-39.
12. Petronijevic M, Ilic K. Associations of gender and age with the reporting of drug-induced hepatic failure: data from the VigiBase™. J Clin Pharmacol. 2013;53:435-43.
13. Axelrod DA, Pomfret EA. Race and sex disparities in liver transplantation: progress toward achieving equal access? JAMA. 2008;300:2425-6.
14. Moylan CA, Brady CW, Johnson JL, Smith AD, Tuttle-Newhall JE, Muir AJ. Disparities in liver transplantation before and after introduction of the MELD score. JAMA. 2008;300:2371-8.
15. Mathur AK, Schaubel DE, Gong Q, Guidinger MK, Merion RM. Sex-based disparities in liver transplant rates in the United States. Am J Transplant. 2011;11:1435-43.
16. Villa E. Role of estrogen in liver cancer. Womens Health (Lond). 2008;4:41-50.
17. Villa E, Moles A, Ferretti I, Buttafoco P, Grottola A, Del Buono M, et al. Natural history of inoperable hepatocellular carcinoma: estrogen receptors' status in the tumor is the strongest prognostic factor for survival. Hepatology. 2000;32:233-8.
18. Gasbarrini A, Addolorato G, Di Campli C, Simoncini M, Montemagno S, Castagneto M, et al. Gender affects reperfusion injury in rat liver. Dig Dis Sci. 2001;46:1305-12.
19. Eckhoff DE, Bilbao G, Frenette L, Thompson JA, Contreras JL. 17-Beta-estradiol protects the liver against warm ischemia/reperfusion injury and is associated with increased serum nitric oxide and decreased tumor necrosis factor-alpha. Surgery. 2002;132:302-9.
20. Sanada Y, Kawano Y, Miki A, Aida J, Nakamura K, Shimomura N, et al. Maternal grafts protect daughter recipients from acute cellular rejection after pediatric living donor liver transplantation for biliary atresia. Transpl Int. 2014;27:383-90.
21. US Organ Procurement and Transplant Network Data (USOPTN). (2013). Liver transplantation between 1988 and 2013 in the United States. [online] Available from http://optn.transplan.hrsa.gov/latestData/rptData.asp. [Last accessed January, 2020].
22. Melton LJ. How many women have osteoporosis now? J Bone Miner Res. 1995;10:175-7.
23. Burra P, Senzolo M, Masier A, Prestele H, Jones R, Samuel D, et al. Factors influencing renal function after liver transplantation. Results from the MOST, an international observational study. Dig Liver Dis. 2009;41:350-6.
24. Ettorre GM, Piselli P, Galatioto L, Rendina M, Nudo F, Sforza D, et al. De novo malignancies following liver transplantation: results from a multicentric study in central and southern Italy, 1990-2008. Transplant Proc. 2013;45:2729-32.

25. Parolin MB, Rabinovitch I, Urbanetz AA, Scheidemantel C, Cat ML, Coelho JC. Impact of successful liver transplantation on reproductive function and sexuality in women with advanced liver disease. Transplant Proc. 2004;36:943-4.
26. Ho JK, Ko HH, Schaeffer DF, Erb SR, Wong C, Buczkowski AK, et al. Sexual health after orthotopic liver transplantation. Liver Transpl. 2006;12:1478-84.
27. Cundy TF, O'Grady JG, Williams R. Recovery of menstruation and pregnancy after liver transplantation. Gut. 1990;31:337-8.
28. Mass K, Quint EH, Punch MR, Merion RM. Gynecological and reproductive function after liver transplantation. Transplantation. 1996;62:476-9.
29. Jabiry-Zieniewicz Z, Cyganek A, Luterek K, Bobrowska K, Kamiński P, Ziółkowski J, et al. Pregnancy and delivery after liver transplantation. Transplant Proc. 2005;37:1197-200.
30. Burra P. Sexual dysfunction after liver transplantation. Liver Transpl. 2009;15:S50-6.
31. Murthy SK, Heathcote EJ, Nguyen GC. Impact of cirrhosis and liver transplant on maternal health during labor and delivery. Clin Gastroenterol Hepatol. 2009;7:1367-72.e1.
32. Kim HW, Seok HJ, Kim TH, Han DJ, Yang WS, Park SK. The experience of pregnancy after renal transplantation: pregnancies even within postoperative 1 year may be tolerable. Transplantation. 2008;85:1412-9.
33. Gerlei Z, Wettstein D, Rigó J, Asztalos L, Langer RM. Childbirth after organ transplantation in Hungary. Transplant Proc. 2011;43:1223-4.
34. Chattopadhyay S. (2018). Sum of her parts: Why are the vast majority of Indian organ donors women? [online] Available from https://www.thehindu.com/society/sum-of-her-parts-why-are-the-vast-majority-of-indian-organ-donors-women/article25271956.ece. [Last accessed January, 2020].
35. Florence LS, Feng S, Foster CE, Fryer JP, Olthoff KM, Pomfret E, et al. Academic careers and lifestyle characteristics of 171 transplant surgeons in ASTS. Am J Transplant. 2011;11:261-71.

# SECTION 6

# Oncology

SECTION EDITORS
Shibba Takkar Chhabra, Mohanjeet Kaur

**CHAPTER 1**

# Breast and Gynecological Cancers: An Overview

*Jaya Gosh, Davinder Paul*

## ABSTRACT

Cancer is still a major social as well as medical challenge among women. Women in low- and middle-income countries (LMICs) have higher mortality associated with female carcinoma as compared to high-income countries (HICs), in spite of their reduced overall incidence rates. This is primarily due to the inadequate access to early detection and treatment among these countries. Breast, cervix, ovary, and uterine cancer constitute >60% of the entire cancer burden among women worldwide. In this chapter, the risk factors, current burden, trends, early detection and treatment, and prevention of these cancers are outlined. In both HICs and LMICs, the burden of cancer in women could be substantially decreased through wide-ranging and impartial implementation of effective treatments, which comprise of screening of breast and cervix, and vaccination

## INTRODUCTION

Women may be affected by any of the multitude of cancers; however, breast and gynecological cancers are unique to them and affect them both physically, emotionally and are associated with a perceived loss of their very identity. With advances in the understanding of cancer, treatment, and multidisciplinary care, it is today possible to preserve organ function and achieve cure in a significant proportion of these patients. In some of these patients, it is possible to preserve fertility and they can even have successful pregnancy outcome something which was not imaginable before and after a diagnosis of cancer. In advanced or recurrent disease even if cure is not achieved, it is possible to live with cancer and lead meaningful lives like any other chronic disease and it is a constant endeavor to prolong this period. Some patients do also succumb to the disease and it is important to be able to take care of them and to be able to give them a pain free and dignified end of life care in their homes and communities and it can be done by any medical professional in the community in collaboration with the oncology team. There is thus an entire spectrum of disease and the art and science of oncology is to be striven for survivorship and also accepts palliative care with equipoise.

# BREAST CANCER

Breast cancer incidence is around 30/100,000 in India and is today the most common cancer affecting women though in rural registries cervical cancer still dominates. The median age is around 50 years which is a decade younger than the west. This rising urban incidence is attributed to several factors related to late age of first childbirth, inadequate breastfeeding, obesity, and sedentary lifestyle. Of all breast cancers only around 10–15% are hereditary. This is more likely if there is a strong family history of breast or ovarian cancer or occurs in younger women and such patients should be referred for genetic counseling and testing.

## Screening

Screening for breast cancer with mammography, though has shown mortality reduction, is associated with over diagnosis and many premalignant lesions, which may not have manifested in a woman's life time, are detected leading to unnecessary treatment and psychological stress. Thus, today the value of screening mammography for asymptomatic women over and above clinical breast examination is being put to question and even if it is done should be after the age of 50 years. Most of the data on screening is from the west (though there is an ongoing Indian study) where the incidence of breast cancer is around 100/100,000, thus in India where the incidence is less, i.e., 30/100,000 the likelihood of over diagnosis is much higher. Also, there is a paucity of dedicated multidisciplinary cancer center compared to the need and difficulty in access to care. Thus, over diagnosis would lead to more harm. In India we do not have a national breast cancer screening program and may be rightly so for the present. We await for the results of the screening study in India which tests clinical breast examination versus only health education and which would be more feasible option with less over diagnosis.

## Diagnosis and Evaluation

The diagnosis of breast cancer in a woman presenting with breast lump is based on clinical examination, mammogram, and a core needle biopsy. In very young women where the mass is freely mobile and there is a classical clinical diagnosis of a fibroadenoma which may be an exception to the above. However, it is also important to remember that some of the breast cancer occurring in young women may not have the classical signs and mammographic appearance, and their diagnosis may be delayed. Hence, it is important to keep the differential diagnosis of breast cancer even in young women.

## Treatment

Breast cancer treatment is multidisciplinary teamwork with surgical, medical, radiation oncologists, radiodiagnosis, pathologists, and also palliative care. This team effort with multidisciplinary tumor board/joint clinics is the heart of treatment and has shown improved outcomes.

## Surgery

Surgery in breast cancer has evolved from radical mastectomy and Halsteads idea of locoregional disease to Fishers concept of it being a systemic disease and thus a conservative approach. Patients with early stage disease (small <5 cm tumor confined to breast) may undergo upfront surgery. These patients may undergo either a breast conservative surgery (removal of part of breast and lymph node) or modified radical mastectomy (removal of the entire breast tissue while sparing of pectoralis major muscle along with lymph nodes). There is no difference in overall survival even after 20 years of follow-up. Thus, eligible women (i.e., those with adequate breast tumor ratio and no multicentricity) should be offered breast conservative surgery (BCS). It is, however, important to remember that all patients with BCS would need adjuvant radiotherapy. Hence, if there is no radiotherapy facility available in a center and the patient cannot travel to a tertiary center, she would best be treated with modified radical mastectomy.

Patients with locally advanced disease (i.e., larger tumors >5 cm or skin/chest wall involvement or with lymph node involvement) usually first undergo chemotherapy (neoadjuvant) followed by surgery.

In those with metastatic disease (disease at distant sites), surgery has not shown to improve survival and if anything has led to more distant relapses. Thus, the role of surgery in metastatic breast cancer is limited to achieving palliation in those with bleeding or fungation. Oligometastatic disease with up to three sites of metastasis may be considered for treatment with potential curative treatment.

## Radiotherapy

Radiotherapy to breast or chest wall with/without supraclavicular area (depending on axillary lymph node involvement) is indicated in patients with tumors >5 cm or any lymph node involvement and all patients undergoing BCS. Advances in radiotherapy techniques with computed tomography (CT) guided image-based planning have reduced local and organ toxicity. In metastatic disease, radiotherapy may be given for symptom control to affected sites and to prevent fractures in asymptomatic weight-bearing bones.

## Systemic Therapy

Breast cancer is a systemic disease and would require some form of systemic therapy in the form of either chemotherapy, hormone therapy or targeted therapy or combination of the above and now emerging role of immunotherapy. It is important to understand that today breast cancer is not a single disease but there are several subtypes each of which is treated differently. The three main subtypes are the hormone positive [estrogen receptor (ER) and/or progesterone receptor (PR) positive and human epidermal growth factor receptor 2 (HER2) negative], triple negative (i.e., ER, PR, and HER2 negative), and the HER2 positive irrespective of the hormone status. Accordingly, systemic therapy can be hormone therapy, chemotherapy, and targeted therapy, and today there is also an emerging role of immunotherapy.

*Early stage disease*: Some early stage cancers, which are hormone positive and HER2 negative, can be treated with hormone therapy alone. The decision for the same is based on clinical and histological features and, if available, feasible gene expression profiling. Most of the other hormone positive, HER2 negative cancers, all HER2 positive cancers, and all triple negative cancers need adjuvant chemotherapy.

*Locally advanced disease*: All locally advanced cancers need chemotherapy. This is usually given before surgery to downsize the tumor (neoadjuvant chemotherapy). This is followed by surgery and adjuvant chemotherapy. Anthracyclines and taxanes form the backbone of chemotherapy. In addition to common chemotherapy side effects such as alopecia, nausea, vomiting, and myelosuppression leading to low blood counts, mucositis anthracyclines are associated potential cardiotoxicity, the incidence of which increases with cumulative dose and is irreversible. Taxanes, especially, Paclitaxel are associated with hypersensitivity reactions and neuropathy. In addition, HER2 positive patients would need adjuvant HER2 targeted therapy (trastuzumab) in addition to chemotherapy for a year though there are some regimens with a shorter duration. Trastuzumab is monoclonal antibody against HER2 receptors which prevents its dimerization and activation. Its main side effect is cardiac toxicity which though reversible needs to be monitored. Those who are hormone receptor positive need adjuvant hormone therapy for 5–10 years after chemotherapy. In premenopausal women, the hormone therapy is tamoxifen (selective ER modulator) while in postmenopausal women it is an aromatase inhibitor. Both of these are oral tablets and may be associated with hot flushes, tamoxifen rarely with thromboembolic phenomenon and endometrial cancer with long-term use. The main side effect of aromatase inhibitors is osteoporosis.

*Metastatic disease*: The intent of treatment is palliative. This may be achieved with chemotherapy. In HER2 positive tumors, HER2 targeted therapy is given in addition. In those who are hormone receptor positive, palliation may be achieved with hormone therapy alone if there is no extensive visceral disease. There are several chemotherapy drugs, HER2 targeted therapy, and hormone therapy available. Other targeted therapy like CDK4/6 inhibitors may be added to hormone therapy. Bisphosphonates (e.g., zoledronic acid) or receptor activator of nuclear factor kappa-B ligand (RANKL) inhibitor denosumab is used for metastatic bone disease. Palliative care to be given to all metastatic patients for symptom control and improving quality of life.

Thus, as breast cancer today is no longer a single disease, its management depends on the subtype and involves multidisciplinary care. It also involves looking at not only the disease status but also the overall performance status and socioeconomic background, and assessing the magnitude of clinical benefit for each of the treatments planned.

## CERVICAL CANCER

Worldwide, cervical cancer is considered to be the second most common cancer among women. Annually, about 77,300 new cases are diagnosed with 37,800 deaths in India, which shows a massive case fatality rate of 49%. It contrasts sharply with data from developed countries that have an effective screening program, as a result of which the case fatality rates are substantially reduced in developed countries.

### Etiology

Among all gynecological cancers, the most preventable one is cervical cancer. It is a cancer that is caused due to unfavorable behaviors that comprise of multiple sexual partners, smoking, as well as unprotected sexual activity. All cervical cancers are caused practically by infection through human papillomavirus (HPV). Through microtraumas, which usually takes place at the time of intercourse, the oncogenic HPV gets access to the basal layer of epithelium. In susceptible patients, persistent infection results in precancerous and cancerous lesions development.

### Screening

In the western world, 74% reduction in the incidence of cervical cancer has been associated with the Papanicolaou test (Pap smear) introduction into clinical practice as well as the increase in access to and adherence with screening guidelines of cervical cancer. It is recommended to start screening for cervical cancer nearly 3 years following the onset of vaginal intercourse, but it should be not later than the age of 21 years. Screening includes a Pap smear and pelvic examination to be performed annually. According to the recent updates to the American Congress of Obstetrics and Gynecology (ACOG) screening guidelines, in case of a woman in age group 21–30 years without any known risk factors for cervical cancer and having normal findings for three or more consecutive annual examinations, it is recommended that the Pap smear can be done less often, i.e., once every 2 years, and that too based on her gynecologist's discretion. But, in women who had one or more high-risk factors, cervical cancer screening should include a Pap smear and pelvic examination to be performed annually. In the women >30 years age, it is recommended to perform HPV testing once, and it should be repeated when there is an abnormal Pap smear or periodically among women with multiple sexual partners.

## Diagnosis

Follow-up is recommended, when there is an abnormal Pap smear. A repeat follow-up Pap smear within 6 months is recommended in the presence of early signs such as mild dysplasia or atypical cells. However, the recommended follow-up in case of high-grade lesions consists of colposcopy examination along with endocervical curettage and biopsies. On the confirmation of cervical cancer in biopsy samples, additional diagnostic tests are required [such as blood tests; imaging by CT, magnetic resonance imaging (MRI), or positron emission tomography (PET)] for evaluating the extent of disease. Biopsy samples are used for determining histology. Majority of carcinomas are squamous cell carcinomas, followed by adenocarcinomas. Neuroendocrine or small cell carcinomas are found rarely.

## Treatment

Surgery at appropriate time can cure early-stage cervical cancer. Recurrent as well as metastatic cervical cancer does not respond properly to chemotherapy. The primary aim of treatment is palliation of symptoms as well as control of growth and progression of tumor. For any type of recurrent gynecologic cancer, stable disease is usually a reasonable therapeutic goal.

## Surgery and Radiation Therapy

Surgery is performed only in early-stage cervical cancer, that is, either FIGO stage IA or IB1 disease, when complete excision of the tumor with negative margins is not possible. Surgery comprise of a simple or radical hysterectomy along with dissection of pelvic and/or para-aortic lymph node. Commonly, radiation therapy is used along with chemotherapy. In the case of locally advanced cervical cancer stages IIB, IIIA, IIIB, and IVA, the standard of care is particularly radiation plus weekly cisplatin. Generally, the chemoradiation regimen consists of cisplatin 40 mg/m$^2$/week (maximum six doses) alongside receiving external beam pelvic radiation [45 Gray (Gy)]. Internal radiation (brachytherapy) follows this. Brachytherapy is most frequently administered via high-dose intracavitary brachytherapy.

## Chemotherapy

In cervical cancer, cisplatin is more effective as compared to carboplatin. Due to this, as opposed to other type of gynecologic cancers, it is not well accepted or recommended

## SECTION 6: Oncology

to substitute carboplatin for cisplatin for decreasing toxicity. Chemotherapy alone is considered only in the cases of recurrences within the radiation field or in the cases in which the desired outcome is the symptoms relief.

## Prevention

It is possible to prevent cervical cancer nearly completely. Abstinence from any type of sexual activity is the most successful prevention approach. But, to continue this for entire life is not realistic. In prevention of cervical cancer, mutual monogamy as well as condoms are not much effective. For prevention of HPV infection and reduction of the risk of development of cervical cancer, both the HPV quadrivalent vaccine (against types 6, 11, 16, and 18) as well as the bivalent HPV vaccine (against types 16 and 18) are indicated. To be effective, it is recommended to administer the HPV vaccine prior to any potential exposure to the virus (prior to any type of sexual activity). It is also effective in sexually active as well as those who are test negative for HPV. Both of these vaccines are not effective in treating HPV infections or cervical cancer.

## EPITHELIAL OVARIAN CANCER

Epithelial ovarian cancer usually presents with advanced disease in nearly 70% cases. This is because the symptoms such as dyspepsia, bloating, constipation are nonspecific and most often caused by benign conditions. There are also no effective screening tests. The incidence of ovarian cancer is around 5/100,000 women. The median age at presentation is around 60 years.

## Etiology

Ovarian cancer is a sporadic cancer; there are <10% of all cases that are attributed to hereditary risk. But, this risk increases to >50% when more than one first-degree relative, such as a mother and sister, is affected with ovarian carcinoma. It is demonstrated that the tumor suppressor genes, i.e., *BRCA1* and *BRCA2*, are involved in one or more pathways of DNA damage, which comprise both the recognition as well as the repair of genes associated with ovarian cancer development. Among these two genes, *BRCA1* is more prevalent. It is reported to be associated with 90% of the inherited cases and 10% of the sporadic cases of ovarian carcinoma. Hereditary breast or ovarian cancer syndrome and hereditary nonpolyposis colorectal cancer (HNPCC) are the two most common genetic abnormalities of familial ovarian cancer. There is an association of hereditary breast/ovarian cancer syndrome with germ-line mutations in *BRCA1* and *BRCA2* as well as with early onset of cancer and often multiple cancers in the same patient. It has also been reported that the HNPCC syndrome is associated with nearly 12% of the hereditary cases of ovarian carcinoma. Contrasting to cervical cancer, ovarian cancer has no known preinvasive component or premalignant process. Therefore, screening of the patients is difficult for detecting early disease. Large-scale clinical studies in the general population have failed to validate an advantage for routine screening using concentrations of cancer antigen (CA)-125 or transvaginal ultrasonography (TVUS).

## Diagnosis

Early stage cancer is generally asymptomatic. On the progression of disease, nonspecific symptoms are generally experienced by patients, which are usually confused with the symptoms related to common benign gastrointestinal (GI) disorders. This usually leads to delay to look for gynecologic examination as well as diagnosis. At the time of gynecological examination, signs indicating the requirement for further testing comprise of solid features, presence of an adnexal mass or any irregularity, and nodularity of the ovary. In patients with advanced disease, signs of abdominal distension may be present due to ascites and enhanced tumor burden, or cough or dyspnea due to pleural effusions. Currently, the CA-125 marker (which is a nonspecific antigen) is considered to be the best tumor marker for epithelial ovarian carcinoma. If it is increased at diagnosis, alterations in concentrations of CA-125 correlate with response as well as progression. The CA-125 concentrations can also be found to be increased in benign conditions such as during menses and/or ovulation, endometriosis, and diverticulitis. Other diagnostic tests for further evaluating the extent of disease and confirming the diagnosis may consist of abdominal ultrasonography or TVUS, GI evaluations, chest X-ray, CT, MRI, or PET.

## Treatment

In patients with early-stage ovarian cancer, timely and aggressive treatment can cure the disease; the treatment includes surgery, chemotherapy, and/or radiation. Complete response to initial surgery and chemotherapy can be achieved in several women who have advanced ovarian cancer; however, in >75% of cancers, recurrence can occur within the first 2 years. The primary goal of treatment in case of recurrent or metastatic ovarian cancer is palliation of symptoms as well as to control growth and progression of tumor. Generally, for recurrent ovarian cancer, stable disease is considered to be a reasonable therapeutic goal.

## Surgery and Radiation Therapy

For ovarian cancer, primary intervention of treatment is surgery. Diagnosis and staging is also confirmed by surgery. In case of patients who have stage IA disease, surgery is usually curative, with long-term survival >90%. For ovarian carcinoma, the surgical treatment comprises a total abdominal hysterectomy along with bilateral salpingo-oophorectomy, omentectomy, as well as lymph node dissection. Optimally debulking the tumor to <1 cm of detectable residual disease is the primary objective of surgery. Optimal cytoreduction is found to be associated with increased complete response rates to chemotherapy as well as long duration of overall survival. After the completion of chemotherapy, performing additional surgery is called secondary cytoreduction or interval debulking, if followed by more cycles of chemotherapy. In the patients with recurrent disease, further surgical interventions are considered among patients who have recurrent disease for improving quality of life by providing relief from symptoms that are associated with complications such as small bowel obstruction.

Radiotherapy plays a primary role in the palliation of symptoms among patients having recurrent pelvic disease, usually associated with small bowel obstruction. In the management of ovarian cancer, for alleviating symptoms, intraperitoneal isotopes such as 32P or external beam whole-abdominal irradiation with 35–45 Gy can be utilized. These contribute to an improvement in the quality of life of a woman.

## Systemic Treatment

There is controversy about standard post-surgery chemotherapy for ovarian cancer in the FIGO stage IA and the IB. Due to the high-risk of recurrence, several clinicians provide treatment with 3-6 cycles of paclitaxel and carboplatin. In case of patients having FIGO stage IC–IV disease or incomplete staging, the standard treatment is 6-8 cycles of a taxane plus platinum agent, which is usually carboplatin and paclitaxel.

Neoadjuvant chemotherapy is known as chemotherapy that is given prior to primary surgical intervention. In case of a patient presenting with metastatic ovarian cancer and/or not being a surgical candidate, an alternative to primary debulking surgery is neoadjuvant chemotherapy is with the aim of reducing size/volume of tumor and finally improving the chance of maximal tumor resection if surgery is feasible.

If after completion of primary treatment, the patient has no or minimal disease, an appropriate management strategy is to evaluate the patient every 3-4 months. Surveillance comprises of physical examination, CA-125 levels, as well as radiologic imaging, as indicated. While under observation, supportive care should be given during the observation period till there is progression of the disease and reinitiation of chemotherapy.

For recurrent ovarian cancer, the option of primary treatment is considered to be chemotherapy. In recurrent ovarian cancer, an important prognostic factor for any chemotherapy is platinum sensitivity. If >6 months after the last platinum therapy, cancer recurs, tumors are believed to be a platinum-sensitive disease, and in such case may respond to a second course of platinum-based treatment with 20-70% response rates. On the contrary, among patients having platinum-resistant disease, that is, those with relapse <6 months following platinum therapy, treatment options consist of agents with an optional mechanism of action (such as antiestrogens, anthracyclines, aromatase inhibitors, cytidine analogs, luteinizing hormone–releasing hormone agonists, taxanes, topoisomerase I inhibitors) or targeted agents. For all the chemotherapy agents, which are presently being used for the recurrent ovarian cancer treatment, the response rates are comparable. No guidelines exist that specify what should be the sequence or number of cycles. Decision of treatment is on the basis of preference of physician, factors related to patient (e.g., age), comorbidities, and residual toxicities from previous treatments.

Over the past 10 years, for the treatment of all gynecological malignancies, clinical research has focused on evaluating and incorporating targeted agents [such as monoclonal antibodies (bevacizumab, cetuximab)] and small-molecule tyrosine inhibitors. Most of the advancement in the treatment of recurrent ovarian cancer has been reported with bevacizumab as a single agent as well as in combination regimens. The findings of two multicenter phase III trials presented clinical data for supporting the bevacizumab to be incorporated into first-line as well as maintenance regimens for improving progression-free survival in ovarian cancer. The effect on the overall survival is still not known.

## Prevention

The risk of ovarian cancer is decreased by nearly 30% by the use of oral contraceptives. The risk continues to decline by nearly 5% every year, to a total of nearly 50% with ≥10 years of use. After discontinuing the oral contraceptive agent, protection continue for up to 20 years., For preventing sporadic (i.e., nonhereditary) ovarian cancer in the general population, it is reasonable to recommend oral contraceptives. Prophylactic surgery is considered to be an alternative among women who have known familial or genetic risk of developing ovarian carcinoma. It is usually taken into consideration following completion of childbearing. Bilateral salpingo-oophorectomy and tubal ligation with/without hysterectomy are the prophylactic procedures.

# ENDOMETRIAL CANCER

Endometrial cancer is the most common gynecological malignancy in the West, but in India, the incidence rates are low. Most of these cancers present at an early stage and are associated with a good prognosis. The treatment comprises surgical staging and adjuvant radiotherapy and/or chemotherapy depending on the final surgicopathological stage.

## Etiology

The etiology of endometrial cancer has not been fully determined. The risk of endometrial cancer is associated with either family history or factors that contribute to increased exposure to estrogen and its metabolites. Obesity is considered a major risk factor for endometrial cancer. Other conditions associated with an increased risk are polycystic ovarian syndrome, a hyper estrogenic state; and HNPCC syndrome, which is associated with a 40-60% increased risk of developing endometrial cancer. Although primarily an antiestrogen, tamoxifen use has also been associated with an increased risk of endometrial cancer because of its mixed estrogenic effects on the endometrial lining.

## Diagnosis

Although the diagnosis of endometrial cancer can be confirmed from biopsy, staging for endometrial cancer is based on a combination of diagnostic tests and surgical examination. When women present with irregular vaginal bleeding and there is a suspicion of endometrial cancer, an endometrial biopsy is usually performed during an office visit. If the biopsy is negative, then a dilation and curettage is completed to gather better sampling and confirm clinical findings. A positive biopsy is often followed up by a TVUS to determine endometrial thickness; if it is >4–5 mm, it requires further evaluation. Once a diagnosis is reached, the extent of disease in other pelvic organs and beyond the pelvic cavity is determined by diagnostic modalities such as cystoscopy, proctoscopy, CT, and MRI as appropriate.

## Treatment

Early stage endometrial cancer can be cured with timely and aggressive treatment involving surgery, chemotherapy, and/or radiation. Therapeutic goals in recurrent and metastatic cancer are to alleviate symptoms and decrease disease progression. The achievement of stable disease is often considered a reasonable therapeutic goal for recurrent gynecologic cancers.

## Surgery and Radiation

Surgery is the primary treatment for early stage endometrial cancer. This should include a thorough pathologic assessment of the depth of myometrial invasion in relation to the overall myometrial thickness, tumor size and location within the uterus, histology and grade, and extent of any lymphatic invasion. After complete resection of all disease (including a vaginal or total hysterectomy and bilateral salpingo-oophorectomy), pelvic washings are necessary to complete surgical staging. Although associated with some controversy, pelvic and/or para-aortic lymphadenectomy is a precise method for identifying nodal metastases and has been associated with improved survival rates in endometrial cancer.

Radiation alone is a treatment option to consider in patients who are medically inoperable because operative risk is high. More often, radiation is an adjuvant to either surgery or chemotherapy. After surgery, patients may receive internal radiation therapy (brachytherapy) in combination with external beam radiotherapy when there is lymph node involvement or other features that place the patient at high-risk of recurrence. Adjuvant radiation therapy is also warranted in patients with high-grade tumor and increased depth of tumor invasion in the myometrium, lymphovascular space invasion, large tumor volume, and involvement of the lower uterine segment or cervix.

## Systemic Treatment

Until recently, chemotherapy has not played a role in the primary treatment of endometrial cancer. Although clinical trials have demonstrated improved rates of complete response and progression-free survival and new regimens are beginning to emerge, most of the current regimens have been established through clinical practice experience.

For the treatment of endometrial cancer, hormonal agents (such as medroxyprogesterone or megestrol acetate) are generally used. These hormonal agents are typically selected on the basis of the hormone receptor expression of the tumor, i.e., ER or PR. In patients who have estrogen or progesterone positive tumors, hormonal agents are considered to be beneficial in recurrent disease management as they are given orally and usually are well-tolerated.

## Prevention

A protective mechanism is provided by some of the lifestyle choices and these reduce the risk of development of the endometrial cancer. Firstly, timely and proper medical treatment should be required for precursor disorders related to the endometrium for reducing the opportunity for progressing to the endometrial cancer. In the presence of an intact uterus, the use of unopposed estrogen should be avoided by women. Long-term hormone therapy should also be avoided by all women. To conclude, for decreasing the risk of obesity, it is important to take adequate diet as well as exercise interventions.

## CONCLUSION

Breast and gynecological cancers have seen significant advancements over the last 50 years in terms of detection, treatment, and prevention. Nonetheless, major challenges remain in the management of these cancers. Although cervical cancer mortality has dropped significantly in developed countries, primarily due to effective HPV vaccination program, it is still a huge cause of cancer-related mortality in India. Apart from screening for breast and cervical cancers, women education is also very essential. Women should be aware of the common symptoms related to these cancers, so that they can get themselves evaluated at an early stage.

## SUGGESTED READING

1. Gotzsche PC, Jorgensen KJ. Screening for breast cancer with mammography. Cochrane Database of Syst Rev. 2013;(6):CD001877.
2. Efiel PJ, Winter K, Morris M, Levenback C, Grigsby PW, Cooper J, et al. Pelvic irradiation with concurrent chemotherapy versus pelvic and para-aortic irradiation for high-risk cervical cancer: an update of radiation therapy oncology group trial (RTOG) 90-01. J Clin Oncol. 2004;22:872-80.

3. Villa LL, Costa RL, Petta CA, Andrade RP, Paavonen J, Iverson OE, et al. High sustained efficacy of pro- phylactic quadrivalent human papillomavirus types 6/11/16/18 L1 virus-like particle vaccine through 5 years of follow-up. Br J Cancer. 2006;95:1459-66.
4. Ford D, Easton DF, Stratton M, Narod S, Goldgar D, Devilee P, et al. Genetic heterogeneity and penetrance analysis of the BRCA1 and BRCA2 genes in breast cancer families. The Breast Cancer Linkage Consortium. Am J Hum Genet. 1998;62(3):676-89.
5. Tewari KS, Java JJ, Eskander RN, Monk BJ, Burger RA. Early initiation of chemotherapy following complete resection of advanced ovarian cancer associated with improved survival: NRG Oncology/Gynecologic Oncology Group study. Ann Oncol. 2016;27(1):114-21.
6. Lu KH, Dinh M, Kohlmann W, Watson P, Green J, Syngal S, et al. Gynecologic cancer as a "sentinel cancer" for women with hereditary nonpolyposis colorectal cancer syndrome. Obstet Gynecol. 2005;105:569-74.
7. Keys HM, Roberts JA, Brunetto VL, Zaino RJ, Spirtos NM, Bloss JD, et al. A phase III trial of surgery with or without adjunctive external pelvic radiation therapy in intermediate risk endometrial adenocarcinoma: a Gynecologic Oncology Group study. Gynecol Oncol. 2004;92(3):744-51.

# Pertinent Hemato-oncological Issues in Women

*Shruti Kakkar*

## ABSTRACT

There is an increasing risk of developing cancer during a lifetime of a woman as per the global trends. With the advances in the medical therapy, the survival for various hematological malignancies has improved significantly but these therapies are themselves associated with potential health issues. The management of the hematological malignancies involves various modalities like surgery, chemotherapy, radiotherapy, and hematopoietic stem cell (HCT) transplant. The long-term morbidities associated with these therapies may be pertaining to fertility, abnormal uterine bleeding, contraception, genital graft versus host disease (GVHD), and general health issues like osteoporosis or sexual health. This chapter deals with these complications and their available management.

## INTRODUCTION

As per the Global Burden Disease Study, there were 17.2 million (16.7–17.8 million) new cancer cases worldwide in 2016. During the same period, there were 467,000 new cases of leukemia and 461,000 cases of non-Hodgkin lymphoma. The risk of developing a cancer during a lifetime is 1 in 3 for men and 1 in 5 for women. With the advances in the medical therapy, the survival for various hematological malignancies has improved significantly over the years. There are nearly $1 \times 10^6$ survivors of hematological malignancies [acute leukemia, Hodgkin's and non-Hodgkin's lymphoma (NHL)] in United States and the expected number of hematopoietic stem cell (HCT) survivors by 2020 is $2.42 \times 10^5$.

The management of the hematological malignancies involves various modalities like chemotherapy, radiotherapy, and hematopoietic stem cell transplant. These treatment modalities, however, have serious long-term effects. The pertinent health issues in women undergoing treatment for hematological malignancies differ from those in men and have been discussed below. The long-term toxicities may affect the quality of life, thus making it necessary to recognize and manage these at the earliest.

## FERTILITY

Cancer therapy has been shown to affect both male and female fertility by various prospective and retrospective trials. Various malignancies and their treatment have effects on fertility. Oocytes begin to form in female embryos at 15 weeks of gestation and nearly 6 million oocytes can be found in the ovary by 20 weeks of gestation. Secondary follicles that depend on hormonal stimulation for development form around the ovum. Loss of follicles begins in utero and at birth, ovary contains about 1–2 million oocytes. Females of all age constantly lose follicles and menopause signifies depletion of follicles. Chemotherapy affects both mature and primordial follicles thus decreasing the ovarian reserve. The effect of treatment on fertility depends on the chemotherapeutic regimens used and patient's condition. The chemotherapeutic agents used in low and intermediate-risk acute myeloid leukemia (AML), acute lymphoblastic leukemia (ALL), and Hodgkin's lymphoma (HL) carry about 20% risk of permanent amenorrhea. Also, a significant number of females suffer from subfertility and premature menopause. Various fertility preservation methods such as hormonal therapy, oocyte preservation, and embryo cryopreservation are available. However, fertility preservation should not surpass the medical management of the cancer and should not affect the prognosis or delay initiation of chemotherapy in a woman with malignancy. Acute leukemia and NHL are aggressive tumors and it is not feasible to postpone treatment in these by even 10 days, the time period usually required for ovarian stimulation and oocyte retrieval. The poor general condition of the patient due to anemia, thrombocytopenia, active infection, and hemodynamic instability may preclude the use of fertility preservation methods. The various options currently available are.

## Hormonal Therapy

Lesser effect of chemotherapy on the fertility of prepubertal girls lead to the hypothesis that treatment with gonadotropin-releasing hormone (GnRH) analogs or combined oral contraceptive may induce a hypogonadotropic state and preserve fertility. Recent trials, however, have failed to show the benefit of hormonal therapy in preserving fertility. Prolonged use of GnRH analogs may result in low bone mineral density and increase risk the risk of fractures. The role of hormonal therapy currently is probably limited to management of abnormal uterine bleeding.

## Embryo Cryopreservation

Embryo cryopreservation involves freezing and storing the fertilized embryos. This is done via in vitro fertilization (IVF) or in vitro maturation (IVM).

Embryo cryopreservation with IVF involves many ethical and legal implications regarding parenthood. No matter how secure a relationship might appear, it is not possible to predict the same. Even though a donor sperm can be used, this process is largely for women with a partner. Thus, it is necessary to provide information regarding the preservation of patient's own fertility in addition to this process. There is an overall 19% pregnancy rate in IVF and 34% in women under the age of 35 years. The entire process of IVF requires 2–5 weeks, a delay that is again not feasible for hemato-oncological patients as stopping chemotherapy for such a prolonged period of time can alter the prognosis. There are concerns regarding the quality of embryos received via emergency IVF especially after 1–2 courses of chemotherapy. A lower risk of ovarian hyperstimulation syndrome (OHSS) is found while using GnRH antagonists and thus they should be favored.

In vitro maturation involves collection of immature oocytes after HCG administration. One of the most important benefits of this procedure is the time frame, i.e., 2–10 days during the luteal phase. This reduced time frame brings along with it many added benefits such as maintaining estrogen levels and eliminating the risk of OHSS. One caution of this process is that the pregnancy rates are lower than that of IVF.

## Oocyte Cryopreservation

Oocytes can be obtained by IVF, IVM, and cryopreserved by slow freezing. Although this process began in 1986, the birth rate after all these years has been noted to be only 2% per oocyte. Although no increase in congenital anomalies in a series of >1,000 infants was found, there are concerns of toxicity of high concentration of cryoprotectants. There is need to more published studies and experiences for this technique to move forward.

## Ovarian Tissue Cryopreservation and Reimplantation

The cryopreservation and reimplantation has one great benefit. It can be performed on prepubertal girls and has a pregnancy rate of 30%. Cryopreservation can be done at any age and there is no need to postpone chemotherapy. Majority of the studies are based on women achieving pregnancy by cryopreserving their ovarian tissue before the age of 30 years. The quantity of the tissue removed is calculated by assessing the patient and predicting the expected rate of premature ovarian failure. Once the sample has been taken, it is necessary to histologically study the sample and remove cancer cells to confirm the presence of follicles. Slow freezing is considered the best on cryopreservation. One important part of the process that needs a lot of attention is that cryopreservation and reimplantation is performed under general anesthesia, which includes a lot of risks especially in patients with mediastinal masses.

It takes about 3.5–6.5 months for the ovarian functions to restore which last for about 7 years. No congenital anomalies have been found; however, there is a risk of the possibility of the ovarian tissue to harbor malignant cells. Thus, it is vital that all required tests must be performed to reduce the risk of transmission of malignant cells.

## Ovarian Transposition

This involves placing the ovaries away from the radiation field. In craniospinal irradiation, the ovaries need to be as far from the spine as possible and can be fixed laterally. In patients receiving pelvic irradiation, a section of the utero-ovarian ligament and fallopian tube may be removed and the ovary is usually moved outside the pelvis and is anchored as high as possible to the anterior wall and two titanium clips are placed on the opposite borders of the ovary for proper identification prior to radiotherapy. Cryopreservation can be performed at the same time of transposition. A second procedure is performed to relocate the ovaries back to the pelvis as spontaneous pregnancy is not possible when the ovaries are transposed to an abdominal position. The percentage of the success of ovarian function is between 16 and 90%. These success rates depend upon patient age, radiation dose, the degree of scatter radiation, vascular compromise, and using/not using concomitant chemotherapy.

## CONTRACEPTION IN WOMEN UNDERGOING CHEMOTHERAPY

Pregnancy is undesirable in a patient diagnosed with a hematological malignancy as it interferes with the treatment plan and poses risk to the life of both the mother and fetus. Cancer survivors are more likely to terminate pregnancy as demonstrated by various studies. Advice regarding contraception should be a regular part of counseling in the diagnosis, management and follow-up phase. Contraception can be classified into four tiers depending on their efficacy.

# CHAPTER 2: Pertinent Hemato-oncological Issues in Women

Combined oral contraceptives increase the risk of venous thromboembolism in a patient with cancer and should be used with caution. These are contraindicated in patients with past history of thromboembolism, coronary artery disease, hormone sensitive tumors, liver disease, and pregnancy. History of smoking and myeloablative conditioning are relative contraindications for use of estrogen-containing contraceptives. These should also be avoided in patients who have received chest wall irradiation as it can increase the risk of subsequent breast cancer. Estrogen-containing contraception, however, is beneficial in patients with osteopenia/osteoporosis during the follow-up period. Progestin only contraceptive, e.g., norethindrone acetate, may cause irregular vaginal bleeding. An increased incidence of sinusoidal obstruction syndrome was observed in patients undergoing hematopoietic stem cell transplant on high doses of progestin. These are best avoided in patients with osteopenia.

Intrauterine contraception devices (IUCDs) may increase the risk of pelvic infections and should not be inserted just prior to high-dose chemotherapy. IUCDs have been found to be safe in patients with human immunodeficiency viruses (HIV) infection, systemic lupus erythematosus (SLE), and some solid transplants but further studies are needed regarding their use in hematological malignancies and patients undergoing stem cell transplant. Male condoms, although less effective, can be useful in prevention of sexually transmitted diseases as well as unwanted pregnancies, if used properly and consistently.

## MANAGEMENT OF ABNORMAL UTERINE BLEEDING

Therapy-induced thrombocytopenia in patients undergoing chemotherapy and HCT may lead to excessive menstrual bleed, often leading to severe anemia requiring packed red blood cell transfusions. Patients can present with different forms of abnormal vaginal bleeding, e.g., menorrhagia, metrorrhagia, or menometrorrhagia. Distinguishing between various types is essential for understanding the potential impact as well as to decide the appropriate management. The management can be classified as prophylactic or emergent.

Prophylactic treatment is used to suppress the onset of menstruation whereas emergent treatment focuses on halting the ongoing bleed. Various patient- and treatment-related factors impact the choice of treatment such as inability to take oral medications in patients with mucositis, risk of thromboembolism with estrogen containing preparations, contraindication to intramuscular injections, and intrauterine devices in patients with thrombocytopenia and neutropenia respectively. In case of severe life-threatening bleed surgical intervention like dilatation and curettage, tamponade using Foley's balloon and uterine artery embolization may be used. Uterine artery embolization must be used selectively as it leads to infertility.

## MANAGEMENT OF GENITAL GRAFT VERSUS HOST DISEASE

Genital graft versus host disease (GVHD) was first described in five women presenting with hematocolpos in 1982. Genital GVHD involves the mucosal surfaces of vulva and vagina in patients who underwent HCT and have other clinical features of GVHD. However, it could be the first manifestation of GVHD in up to a quarter of patients. Genital GVHD has been reported in 25–50% patients undergoing HCT. Vulva is the most commonly affected site followed by both vulva and vagina together. The median time of presentation of genital GVHD is about 9 months post-transplant. This gives the physicians, the opportunity to prevent GVHD by regular vaginal self-examination and early implementation of topical therapy with estrogen and other immunosuppressive agents.

The common symptoms of genital GVHD include dryness, itching, pain with urination, and dyspareunia. Patients with severe GVHD may present with amenorrhea and hematocolpos. Examination may show erythema, mucosal erosions, and leukokeratosis. Thin web like vaginal synechiae may be seen. Lichen planus, vaginal scarring, and stenosis are features of severe GVHD. Genital GVHD may be associated with herpes simplex virus (HSV) infection or human papilloma virus (HPV) reactivation.

Early recognition and management are of utmost importance in prevention of vaginal stenosis. Topical steroid therapy with clobetasol propionate 0.05% applied daily at bedtime demonstrates efficacy in 2–4 weeks. Topical cyclosporine or tacrolimus ointment may be beneficial in patients not responding to steroid therapy. Management of vaginal scarring involves lysing synechiae manually followed by insertion of estrogen containing vaginal ring or dilators. Surgical intervention may be needed in patients with extensive labial fusion and dense fibrotic vaginal scars.

## OSTEOPOROSIS

Premature menopause has been associated with low mineral density and increased risk of fractures. Bone loss is further exacerbated by prolonged immobilization, vitamin D deficiency, endocrine dysfunction such as hypothyroidism, and use of high dose corticosteroids in patients with hematological malignancies. Regular assessment of bone density by dual energy X-ray absorptiometry is recommended during follow-up. Weight-bearing exercises, regular calcium and vitamin D intake should be encouraged. Osteoporosis, if present, can be managed with bisphosphonates along with hormonal replacement therapy.

## SEXUAL HEALTH ASSESSMENT POSTCHEMOTHERAPY

Sexual function assessment in female who are long-term survivors undergoing HCT, experience sexual dysfunction. Lack of desire for sexual activity may occur due to gonadal failure, psychological issues during and post-transplant, and effect of drugs. Primary ovarian failure and chronic genital GVHD may lead to painful intercourse, noncoital pain, and vaginismus. This can affect the quality of life. A standard questionnaire can be used to assess the sexual dysfunction in the recipients by one of the team members.

## CONCLUSION

The advances in medical therapy have witnessed an increased survival for various hematological malignancies over recent years. Owing to the natural endocrine changes, the health issues in women undergoing treatment for hematological malignancies differ from those in men. Cancer treatment has a significant potential of affecting female fertility. While hormonal therapy is used to avoid abnormal uterine bleeding in these patients, embryo cryopreservation via IVF and IVM, oocyte cryopreservation, ovarian tissue cryopreservation/reimplantation, and ovarian transposition are the options available for preservation of fertility.

Pregnancy is undesirable in a patient diagnosed with a hematological malignancy but due to risks of venous thromboembolism, the use of oral contraceptive agents should be judicious. Risks of abnormal uterine bleeding, GVHD, general health concerns such as osteoporosis and sexual health concerns should always be borne into mind in order to provide holistic management in these women.

## SUGGESTED READING

1. Fitzmaurice C, Akinyemiju TF, Al Lami FH, Alam T, Alizadeh-Navaei R, Allen C, et al. Global, Regional, and National Cancer Incidence, Mortality, Years of Life Lost, Years Lived With Disability, and Disability-Adjusted Life-Years for 29 Cancer Groups, 1990 to 2016: A Systematic Analysis for the Global Burden of Disease Study. JAMA Oncol. 2018;4(11):1553-68.
2. Pulte D, Redaniel MT, Jansen L, Brenner H, Jeffreys M. Recent trends in survival of adult patients with acute leukemia: overall improvements, but persistent and partly increasing disparity in survival of patients from minority groups. Haematologica. 2013;98(2):222-9.
3. DeSantis CE, Lin CC, Mariotto AB, Siegel RL, Stein KD, Kramer JL, et al. Cancer treatment and survivorship statistics, 2014. CA Cancer J Clin. 2014;64(4):252-71.
4. Majhail NS, Tao L, Bredeson C, Davies S, Dehn J, Gajewski JL, et al. Prevalence of hematopoietic cell transplant survivors in the United States. Biol Blood Marrow Transplant. 2013;19(10):1498-501.
5. Cheng MJ, Hourigan CS, Smith TJ. Adult acute myeloid leukemia long-term survivors. J Leuk (Los Angel). 2014;2(2):26855.
6. Baker KS, Ness KK, Weisdorf D, Francisco L, Sun CL, Forman S, et al. Late effects in survivors of acute leukemia treated with hematopoietic cell transplantation: a report from the Bone Marrow Transplant Survivor Study. Leukemia. 2010;24(12):2039-47.
7. Shanis D, Merideth M, Pulanic TK, Savani BN, Battiwalla M, Stratton P. Female long-term survivors after allogeneic hematopoietic stem cell transplantation: evaluation and management. Semin Hematol. 2012;49(1):83-93.
8. Torrealday S, Kodaman P, Pal L. Premature Ovarian Insufficiency-an update on recent advances in understanding and management. F1000Res. 2017;6:2069.
9. Blumenfeld Z. Chemotherapy and fertility. Best Pract Res Clin Obstet Gynaecol. 2012; 26(3):379-90.
10. Murphy J, McKenna M, Abdelazim S, Battiwalla M, Stratton P. A practical guide to gynecologic and reproductive health in women undergoing hematopoietic stem cell transplant. Biol Blood Marrow Transplant. 2019;25(11):e331-43.
11. Poorvu PD, Frazier AL, Feraco AM, Manley PE, Ginsburg ES, Laufer MR, et al. Cancer treatment-related infertility: A critical review of the evidence. JNCI Cancer Spectr. 2019;3(1):pkz008.
12. Loren AW. Fertility issues in patients with hematologic malignancies. Hematology Am Soc Hematol Educ Program. 2015;2015(1):138-45.
13. Oktay K, Harvey BE, Partridge AH, Quinn GP, Reinecke J, Taylor HS, et al. Fertility preservation in patients with cancer: ASCO clinical practice guideline update. J Clin Oncol. 2018;36:1994-2001.
14. Donnez J, Dolmans MM. Fertility preservation in women. N Engl J Med. 2017;377:1657-65.
15. Salama M, Isachenko V, Isachenko E, Rahimi G, Mallmann P. Advances in fertility preservation of female patients with hematological malignancies. Expert Review of Hematology. 2017;10(11):951-60.
16. Patel A, Schwarz EB; Society of Family Planning. Cancer and contraception. Contraception. 2012;86:191-8.
17. Curtis KM, Jatlaoui TC, Tepper NK, Zapata LB, Horton LG, Jamieson DJ, et al. U.S. selected practice recommendations for contraceptive use, 2016. MMWR Recomm Rep. 2016;65:1-66.
18. American College of Obstetricians and Gynecologists. Committee opinion no. 606: options for prevention and management of heavy menstrual bleeding in adolescent patients undergoing cancer treatment. Obstet Gynecol. 2014;124:397-402.
19. Bates JS, Buie LW, Woodis CB. Management of menorrhagia associated with chemotherapy-induced thrombocytopenia in women with hematologic malignancy. Pharmacotherapy. 2011;31:1092-110.
20. Adegite EA, Goyal RK, Murray PJ, Marshal M, Sucato GS. The management of menstrual suppression and uterine bleeding: a survey of current practices in the Pediatric Blood and Marrow Transplant Consortium. Pediatr Blood Cancer. 2012;59:553-7.

# SECTION 7

# Nephrology

**SECTION EDITORS**
Simran Kaur, Suman Sethi

# CHAPTER 1

# Hypertensive Disorders in Pregnancy

*Suman Sethi, Nitin Sethi*

## ABSTRACT

Hypertension is responsible for complicating nearly 8–9% of maternal deaths in India and 15–20% of maternal deaths in western world. Overall, complicating about 5–10% of pregnancies in India. Recent breakthroughs in the research pertaining to its etiology have been reviewed in brief. Topics such as classification of the different forms of hypertension during pregnancy, and status of the tests available to predict preeclampsia, and strategies to prevent preeclampsia and to manage this serious disease have been included. Sadly, there is a comparative paucity of distinct randomized studies in the area of hypertension in pregnancy in contrast to trials in essential hypertension in non-pregnant cases. Subsequently, the nature of proof for the recommendations in this chapter is not graded even if corresponding references and discussions are given for every recommendation. The chapter will act as a contemporary guideline, and we intend to be capable of ranking recommendations eventually. Nevertheless, it is proposed that this chapter should be revised as and when required as more study is developed to impact the clinical practice positively. Guidelines and proposals for treating hypertension in pregnant women are customarily written for application and execution in an ideal clinical set up. It is understood that it is impossible to implement all the protocols in the guidelines across the globe; hence, choices for treatment in less-resourced clinical set up are described independently with regards to diagnosis, assessment and management.

## INTRODUCTION

Hypertension, complicating 5–7% of all pregnancies, is a leading cause of maternal and fetal morbidity, particularly when the elevated blood pressure (BP) is due to preeclampsia, either alone or "superimposed" on chronic vascular disease, and is accountable for about 8–9% and 15–20% of maternal deaths in India and in the western world, respectively. On the whole, they complicate 5–10% of pregnancies in India.

Hypertension in pregnancy is defined as BP reading ≥140/90 mm Hg on two or more occasions at least 6 hours apart or an increase in mean arterial pressure of 20 mm Hg taken at least 6 hours apart or a single reading of diastolic BP >105 mm Hg. Women with a systolic BP of 140 mm Hg must be closely followed for development of diastolic hypertension.

## CLASSIFICATION OF HYPERTENSION IN PREGNANCY

The International Society for the Study of Hypertension in Pregnancy (ISSHP) Working Group classification of hypertensive disorders complicating pregnancy is shown below in **Box 1**.

## DIAGNOSIS OF THE HYPERTENSIVE DISORDERS OF PREGNANCY

Points to be considered for ensuring the diagnosis of hypertension during pregnancy are as follows: Two readings, presenting a systolic BP of ≥140 mm Hg and/or a diastolic BP of ≥90 mm Hg, marked over a period of 4–6 hours following 20 weeks gestation, in a woman who has been normotensive before becoming pregnant. In comparison with the findings earlier, the Korotkov phase V (disappearance of the blood flow murmur) is the correct way to estimate diastolic BP during pregnancy.

Use of an automatic instrument is the most preferred choice in comparison to use of an aneroid device if it has proved reliability in both pregnancy and preeclampsia particularly; few devices may be precise for pregnant women who experience chronic or gestational hypertension but not for women with preeclampsia.

### Proteinuria

- The benchmark for evaluating abnormal proteinuria in pregnancy is a 24-hour urinary protein ≥300 mg/day; however this is regarded as a time tested value than a value with correct scientific evidence.
- If the value is positive (≥1+, 30 mg/dL), then spot urine protein/creatinine (PCr) ratio estimation is done.
- Nephrotic syndrome and its consequences like thromboprophylaxis can be identified and established by performing a 24-hour urine collection for proteinuria.
- Dipstick test may not be accurate as few proteinuria cases may be ignored by a negative dipstick test. False negative report may be possible sometimes if urine PCr is <30 mg/mmol for abnormal 24-hour proteinuria, however, in such cases, the total protein excretion is commonly <400 mg/day.
- When both 24 hour urine and PCr values are unavailable to evaluate for proteinuria, dipstick test offers a fairly good estimation of true proteinuria, especially when ranges are >1 g/L.

---

**BOX 1**   **Classification of hypertension in pregnancy.**

- Hypertension known before pregnancy or present in the first 20 weeks
- Chronic hypertension
- Essential
- Secondary
- White-coat hypertension
- Masked hypertension
- Hypertension arising de novo at or after 20 weeks
- Transient gestational hypertension
- Gestational hypertension
- Preeclampsia* de novo or superimposed on chronic hypertension

*The term severe preeclampsia should not be used in clinical practice.

## Chronic Hypertension

Chronic hypertension is increased BP that may occur either before pregnancy, become established within the initial 20 weeks of pregnancy, or may not settle by 12-week after child birth follow up. It can present as mild (up to 179 mm Hg systolic and 109 mm Hg diastolic pressure) or severe (≥180 systolic or 110 diastolic pressure) based on severity. Chronic hypertension causes complications to almost 5% of all pregnancies, and the frequency of occurrence is growing day by day because of delayed child bearing.

The ISSHP advocates the below mentioned evaluations to be done at the initial diagnostic visit for all pregnant women with chronic hypertension.
- Complete blood count (hemoglobin and platelet count).
- Liver enzymes values (aspartate aminotransferase, alanine aminotransferase, and lactate dehydrogenase) and liver functions tests (international normalized ratio, serum bilirubin, and serum albumin).
- Serum creatinine, electrolytes, and uric acid (though serum uric acid is not a diagnostic marker for preeclampsia, increased gestation-corrected serum uric acid values are connected with very bad maternal and fetal consequences and gives an alert for a complete evaluation of fetal growth, even in women with gestational hypertension. Nevertheless, uric acid value cannot be a proper guide to estimate the time of delivery).
- Urinalysis and microscopy PCr or albumin: Creatinine ratio.

## Transient Gestational Hypertension

Transient gestational hypertension cannot be considered a harmless condition; it is related to approximately 20% risk of occurrence of preeclampsia and another 20% risk of occurrence of gestational hypertension. Hence, pregnant women with transient gestational hypertension have to take more precautions and consider being more watchful along their course of pregnancy, preferably inclusive of routine BP estimation at home.

## Gestational Hypertension

The clinical diagnosis of gestational hypertension can be established by the latest development of hypertension (defined as systolic BP ≥140 mm Hg and/or diastolic BP ≥90 mm Hg) at ≥20 weeks of gestation without proteinuria or recently developed signs of end-organ dysfunction.

The primary objectives of the preliminary assessment of pregnant women with recently developed hypertension are to differentiate between gestational hypertension and preeclampsia. The later presents a distinct progress of the condition and prognosis, and to ascertain the severity of hypertension, which influences the treatment and consequence. The assessments to be done are as follows:
- *Estimation of protein excretion:* The excretion of protein through urine or proteinuria is the major clinical parameter that establishes the diagnosis of gestational hypertension or preeclampsia in a pregnant woman. As false negative and false positive results are frequent with a urine dipstick test, a negative value to trace amounts cannot be excluded as definitely proteinuria is absent. Such false negative values may be due to low specific gravity (<1.010), increased salt concentration, extremely acidic urine, or nonalbumin proteinuria. A positive urine dipstick value, especially if only +1, also requires confirmation since false positives occur. Urine protein content can be estimated by evaluating the urine protein-to-creatinine ratio; ≥0.26 mg protein/mg creatinine (30 mg/mmol) in a random urine sample or with a 24-hour urine collection.

## SECTION 7: Nephrology

> **BOX 2** **Features of severe disease in a woman with a pregnancy-related hypertensive disorder.**
>
> Systolic blood pressure ≥160 mm Hg or diastolic blood pressure ≥110 mm Hg, or both (on two separate occasions)
>
> **Symptoms of dysfunction in the central nervous system**
>
> New-onset cerebral or visual disturbance, for instance:
> - Photopsia, scotomata, cortical blindness, retinal vasospasm
> - Severe headache (described such as, "the worst headache I've ever had") or headache that persists and progresses despite analgesic therapy
>
> **Hepatic abnormality**
>
> Severe persistent right upper quadrant or epigastric pain unyielding to medication and not accounted for by an alternative diagnosis or serum transaminase concentration ≥2 times the upper limit of the normal range, or both
>
> **Thrombocytopenia**
>
> Platelet count of <100,000/μL
>
> **Renal abnormality**
>
> Progressive renal insufficiency [serum creatinine >1.1 mg/dL (97.2 μmol/L) or doubling of serum creatinine concentration in the absence of other renal disease]

- *Assessment of parameters which indicate acute disease*: A thorough history should be obtained from the patients regarding the occurrence of acute features of preeclampsia, such as recent development of cerebral or visual disturbances, epigastric or right upper quadrant pain (**Box 2**). Pulmonary edema should be determined by chest auscultation. Detection of the above mentioned features establishes the diagnosis as preeclampsia with acute features.
- *Performance of laboratory evaluation*: Analysis done in the laboratory may lead to identification of the involvement of end organ that is possible in patients with preeclampsia and not gestational hypertension. Patients with preeclampsia with severe features may indicate alterations like thrombocytopenia, elevated creatinine concentration to >1.1 mg/dL, and doubling of hepatic transaminases (**Box 2**).

## Preeclampsia

Beyond the typical definition, preeclampsia can also be described as gestational hypertension in combination with one or more of the following newly developed conditions at or after 20 weeks' gestation (**Box 3**).

*Points to remember*
- There are numerous causes of headaches during pregnancy. Nevertheless, it is a safe way to ascertain a recently developed headache in a hypertensive pregnant patient as related to preeclampsia unless it is proved to occur due to some other valid reason.
- In the presence of resources, all asymptomatic pregnant women with beginning hypertension and absence of proteinuria in dipstick test are recommended to undergo the below mentioned laboratory investigations so as to assess maternal organ dysfunction. Excluding preeclampsia is not possible if these tests are not performed. In few countries, this protocol will demand sending patients (few may not have preeclampsia) from smaller units to bigger clinical set ups where same-day laboratory facilities are present. Independent decision-making approaches become essential in such cases.

> **BOX 3** **Preeclampsia conditions in combination with gestational hypertension.**
>
> **Preeclampsia**
> - Proteinuria
> - Other maternal organ dysfunction, including
> - AKI (creatinine ≥90 µmol/L; 1 mg/dL)
> - Liver involvement (elevated transaminases, e.g., alanine aminotransferase or aspartate aminotransferase >40 IU/L) with or without right upper quadrant or epigastric abdominal pain
> - Neurological complications (examples include eclampsia, altered mental status, blindness, stroke, clonus, severe headaches, and persistent visual scotomata)
> - Hematological complications (thrombocytopenia: platelet count <150,000/µL, disseminated intravascular coagulation, hemolysis)
> - Uteroplacental dysfunction [such as fetal growth restriction, abnormal umbilical artery (UA) Doppler waveform analysis, or stillbirth]

- Hemoglobin, platelet count (and if decreased, tests of coagulation)
- Serum creatinine
- Liver enzymes
- Serum uric acid

The combination of hemolysis, increased liver enzymes and decreased platelets or any two of these conditions is described as the HELLP syndrome. Women with symptoms of HELLP syndrome should be contemplated to have preeclampsia thereby assessing for other features of preeclampsia and treating the same.

## Preeclampsia Superimposed on Chronic Hypertension

The diagnosis of this condition is arrived at when a pregnant woman with chronic essential hypertension develops any of the formerly mentioned maternal organ dysfunction in agreement with preeclampsia. This condition is expected to occur in about 25% of women with chronic hypertension.

## Prediction and Prevention of Preeclampsia

### Prediction

There are no standard test regimes like the first or second trimester test that can indicate the confirmed occurrence of preeclampsia in all cases. But a combination of maternal risk factors, BP, placental growth factor (PlGF), and uterine artery Doppler can predict women who may have specific advantages by taking 150 mg/day of aspirin in preventing preterm; however not term preeclampsia.

With the outcomes of randomized controlled trials, ISSHP guidelines specify that it is perfect to manage pregnant women who present with well determined strong clinical risk factors for preeclampsia before 16 weeks but certainly before 20 weeks, with aspirin at a dosage of 75–162 mg/day. The strong clinical risk factors include previous history of preeclampsia, chronic hypertension, pregestational diabetes mellitus, maternal body mass index >30 kg/m$^2$, antiphospholipid syndrome, and history of receiving assisted reproduction.

Maternal characteristics and history provide strong clues to which women are more at risk of developing preeclampsia than others, particularly:
- Prior preeclampsia
- Chronic hypertension
- Multiple gestation

- Pregestational diabetes mellitus
- Maternal body mass index >30
- Antiphospholipid syndrome/systemic lupus erythematosus (SLE)
- Assisted reproduction therapies

## Prevention

Use low-dose aspirin (preferably 150 mg/day) started before 16 weeks of pregnancy for women at increased risk for preeclampsia, particularly if any of the following conditions exist (**Box 4**).

# MANAGEMENT PRINCIPLES FOR THE HYPERTENSIVE DISORDERS OF PREGNANCY

The antihypertensives medications are prescribed to optimize BP within the range 110 to 140/80 to 85 mm Hg. Primarily admissible antihypertensive drugs are labetalol, oxprenolol, methyldopa, nifedipine, and diltiazem. Prazosin and hydralazine are frequently administered as second- or third-line of treatment.

Majorly chronic hypertensive women participated in the CHIPS trial (Control of Hypertension in Pregnancy Study) where a diastolic BP of 85 mm Hg was the aim; this was accompanied by decreased chances of occurrence of accelerated maternal hypertension and absence of considerable adverse events for newborn in contrast to targeting increased values of diastolic BP.

## Chronic Hypertension Because of Renal Disease

Patients suffering from progressive renal disease during pregnancy are recommended to undergo early aggressive dialysis of approximately 36 hours per week which probably gives favorable results in such cases.

## White-coat Hypertension

In case of established white-coat hypertension, pregnant women are easily maintained at home with consistent BP estimation and avoidance of antihypertensive medicines, to the minimum of about office BP levels of 160/110 mm Hg.

---

**BOX 4** | **Conditions causing increased risk for preeclampsia.**

- Previous preeclampsia
- Pre-existing medical conditions (including chronic HTN, any underlying disease of the kidneys, or pre-gestational diabetes mellitus)
- Antiphospholipid antibody syndrome
- Multiple pregnancy
- Obesity
- Assisted reproduction pregnancy
- In case of low calcium intake (<600 mg/day), use calcium 1.2–2.5 g/day in women with higher risk of HTN
- Exercise recommendation for pregnant women is thrice a week for an average 50 min, using a combination of aerobic exercise, strength, and flexibility training; which is linked to less weight gain and reduced risk of hypertensive disorders in pregnancy; there are no significant adverse effects of exercise in pregnancy

# CHAPTER 1: Hypertensive Disorders in Pregnancy

## Gestational Hypertension

- By definition, gestational hypertension is not a benign condition because approximately 25% of these patients shall develop preeclampsia eventually.
- No particular test or group of tests can indicate which particular women with gestational hypertension may eventually develop preeclampsia, the susceptibility is maximum in those women who encounter gestational hypertension at <34 weeks.
- Those women who have gestational hypertension need evaluation in a proper clinical set up if they develop preeclampsia or severe hypertension ≥160/110 mm Hg.

The precise time for delivery is still doubtful in women with gestational hypertension and no symptoms of preeclampsia. A substantial retrospective study showed outcomes that 38–39 weeks could probably be the precise time; however, the outcome needs further evidence with randomized trials eventually.

## Preeclampsia: Antenatal

- Independent of the hypertensive disorder during pregnancy, increased BP of ≥160/110 mm Hg necessitates immediate attention in a vigilant clinical set up. The value of BP increase alone cannot be taken as an authentic method to grade immediate risk of preeclampsia as acute organ dysfunction such as renal disorder or neurological consequences may occur in some women at quite moderate ranges of hypertension itself.
- In the CHIPS trial, the follow-up of pregnant patients with severe hypertension was accompanied with considerably increased chances of adverse events for both the new born (i.e., low birth weight, prematurity, fatality, and morbidity requiring neonatal unit care) and the mother (i.e., thrombocytopenia, abnormal liver enzymes with symptoms, and prolonged hospital stay). In women who were treated for an increased BP target range (of less tight control), acute hypertension was also accompanied with considerably higher acute maternal comorbidities. All women who are diagnosed with preeclampsia should undergo evaluation in a hospital set up; following which few of them can probably be treated as outpatients as their conditions is confirmed as stable and it can be recommended that they report their problems promptly and are able to gauge their BP independently.

### Intrapartum

- Oral antihypertensive agent should be administered at the initiation of labor. Decreased gastrointestinal motility possibly reduces absorption of antihypertensive drug following oral intake. Hence, intravenous antihypertensive agent would be required to optimize BP, especially if it is very acute.
- The objective of fluid balance is to attain euvolemia as always. Preeclamptic women experience capillary leak, however may possibly present lower or higher cardiac output. To achieve euvolemia, unwanted losses has to be replenished (30 mL/h) combined with expected urinary losses (0.5–1 mL/kg/h). ISSHP recommends taking 60–80 mL/h to avert susceptibility of pulmonary edema. There is no guideline to "run dry" a patient with preeclampsia as she is as such prone to acute kidney injury (AKI).

### Postpartum

Estimate BP at least every 4–6 hours in the course of the day for a minimum of 3 days postpartum. Antihypertensive medication has to be reinitiated following delivery and gradually decreased after days 3–6 postpartum unless BP is decreased (<110/70 mm Hg) or the woman encounters any further symptoms during this period.

### Short-term and Long-term Follow-up

The follow up of women with preeclampsia has to be done in a week in case the need for antihypertensive medication continues while getting discharged from the hospital. The review has to be consistent for about 3 months till such time the BP values are in optimal range. Further, women who have experienced chronic hypertension, gestational hypertension, or preeclampsia have the need for continuous follow-up throughout their life period due to higher susceptibility of cardiovascular comorbidities. Current clinical trial researches may offer precise management strategies in treating women with history of preeclampsia.

## CONCLUSION

In a conclusion, hypertensive disorders associated with pregnancy could be prevented by close antenatal follow-up and timely prediction of risk factors and reasonable management strategies.

## SUGGESTED READING

1. Ness RB, Roberts JM. Epidemiology of hypertension. In: Lindheimer MD, Roberts JM, Cunningham FG, (Eds). Chesley's Hypertensive Disorders in Pregnancy, 2nd edition. Stamford, Connecticut: Appleton & Lange; 1999. pp. 43-65.
2. Villar J, Say L, Gulmezoglu AM, Meraldi M, Lindheimer MD, Betran AP, et al. Pre-eclampsia eclampsia: a health problem for 2000 years. In: Critchly H, MacLean A, Poston L, Walker J, (Eds). Pre-eclampsia. London: RCOG Press; 2003. pp. 189-207.
3. Subramaniam V. Seasonal variation in the incidence of preeclampsia and eclampsia in tropical climatic conditions. BMC Womens Health. 2007;7:18.
4. Report of the National High Blood Pressure Education Program Working Group on high blood pressure in pregnancy. Am J Obstet Gynecol. 2000;183(1):S1-22.
5. Brown MA, Magee LA, Kenny LC, Karumanchi SA, McCarthy FP, Saito S, et al. Hypertensive disorders of pregnancy ISSHP classification, diagnosis, and management recommendations for international practice. Hypertension. 2018;72:24-43.
6. Rath W, Fischer T. The diagnosis and treatment of hypertensive disorders of pregnancy: new findings for antenatal and inpatient care. Dtsch Arztebl Int. 2009;106(45):733-8.
7. Brown MA, Roberts L, Davis G, Mangos G. Can we use the Omron T9P automated blood pressure monitor in pregnancy? Hypertens Pregnancy. 2011;30:188-93.
8. Côté AM, Firoz T, Mattman A, Lam EM, von Dadelszen P, et al. The 24-hour urine collection: gold standard or historical practice? Am J Obstet Gynecol. 2008;199:625.e1-6.
9. Mammaro A, Carrara S, Cavaliere A, Ermito S, Dinatale A, Pappalardo EM, et al. Hypertensive disorders of pregnancy. J Prenat Med. 2009;3(1):1-5.
10. Livingston JR, Payne B, Brown MA, Roberts JM, Côté AM, Magee LA, et al. Uric acid as a predictor of adverse maternal and perinatal outcomes in women hospitalized with preeclampsia. J Obstet Gynaecol Can. 2014;36:870-7.
11. Hawkins TL, Roberts JM, Mangos GJ, et al. Plasma uric acid remains a marker of poor outcome in hypertensive pregnancy: a retrospective cohort study. BJOG. 2012;119:484-92.
12. Melvin LM, Funai EF. Gestational hypertension. [online] Available from https://www.uptodate.com/contents/gestational-hypertension. [Last accessed February 2020].
13. Rumbold A DL, Crowther CA, Haslam RR. Antioxidants for preventing pre-eclampsia. Cochrane Database Syst Rev. 2008;(1):CD004227.

14. Magee LA, von Dadelszen P, Singer J, Lee T, Rey E, Ross S, et al. The CHIPS Randomized Controlled Trial (Control of Hypertension in Pregnancy Study): is severe hypertension just an elevated blood pressure? Hypertension. 2016;68(5):1153-9.
15. Saudan P, Brown MA, Buddle ML, Jones M. Does gestational hypertension become pre-eclampsia? Br J Obstet Gynaecol. 1998;105(11):1177-84.
16. Davis GK, Mackenzie C, Brown MA, Homer CS, Holt J, McHugh L, et al. Predicting transformation from gestational hypertension to preeclampsia in clinical practice: a possible role for 24 hour ambulatory blood pressure monitoring. Hypertens Pregnancy. 2007;26:77-87.
17. Cruz MO, Gao W, Hibbard JU. What is the optimal time for delivery in women with gestational hypertension? Am J Obstet Gynecol. 2012;207:214.e1-6.

# Lupus Nephritis: What's New?

*Simran Kaur, Vikas Makkar*

## ABSTRACT

The renal involvement is systemic lupus erythematosus (SLE), known as lupus nephritis (LN), affects almost half of these patients during the natural course of their disease, with almost further half of them having LN at the time of first diagnosis of SLE. The etiopathogenesis, diagnosis, and management of LN have evolved significantly in the last two decades. The diagnostic criteria of SLE have been improvised from the American College of Rheumatology (ACR) 1997 to Systemic Lupus International Collaborating Clinics (SLICC) 2012 with huge importance given to LN. The diagnosis and prognostication of LN is done by renal biopsy and classified as per the International Society of Nephrology/Renal Pathology Society (ISN/RPS) classification. In the last two decades, the treatment of LN has also evolved from steroid alone to additional immunosuppression, starting with azathioprine, then cyclophosphamide therapy (high to low dose), and mycophenolate and now rituximab and belatacept. Recently, there are efforts to analyze the role of novel biologicals in SLE and LN.

## INTRODUCTION

Lupus nephritis (LN) is the involvement of kidney in systemic lupus erythematosus (SLE). Renal involvement impacts the overall prognosis of the disease significantly. Approximately, 25–50% will have renal involvement at the time SLE is diagnosed and as many as 60% are likely to develop clinically relevant nephritis at some time in the course of their disease. The varied incidence of LN in SLE is not only affected by race and geography, but also by the diagnostic criteria used in individual studies and whether involvement is defined by renal biopsy or clinical findings.

## DIAGNOSIS OF SYSTEMIC LUPUS ERYTHEMATOSUS AND LUPUS NEPHRITIS

Patients with active lupus often have a multitude of extrarenal symptoms. Every patient may not present with prototypic signs and symptoms and serological parameters at one time, the organ involvements may unmask gradually during the natural course of the disease.

The diagnostic criteria for SLE have evolved over the past half century. The American College of Rheumatology (ACR) criteria, first published in 1971, originally proposed to diagnose SLE for research studies, and later revised twice in 1982 and 1997, were since inception used by rheumatologists to diagnose SLE if 4 or more of the 11 criteria were present in a patient. However, due to several pitfalls of ACR criteria, the Systemic Lupus International Collaborating Clinics (SLICC) criteria were proposed, by an international group focused on SLE clinical research (**Table 1**). The derivation and validations steps were published in 2012.

Based on SLICC criteria, patients are diagnosed as SLE if at least 4 of 17 criteria, including at least 1 of the 11 clinical criteria and one of the six immunologic criteria are met during evaluation. A patient with biopsy-proven LN in the presence of positivity of at least one immunological marker, such as antinuclear antibodies (ANAs), anti-double-stranded deoxyribonucleic acid (anti-dsDNA) antibodies, or low complements, can also diagnose SLE. Thus, LN being one of the strongest predictors of an unfavorable outcome of SLE has been given a huge importance in SLICC. However, validation studies for these criteria are ongoing to determine whether they perform better than the ACR criteria or not.

**TABLE 1:** Systemic lupus erythematosus: Diagnostic criteria [Systemic Lupus International Collaborating Clinics (SLICC) 2012].

| | |
|---|---|
| Cutaneous manifestations—four items | Acute cutaneous lupus erythematosus/subacute cutaneous lupus erythematosus |
| | Chronic cutaneous lupus erythematosus |
| | Oral ulcers |
| | Nonscarring alopecia |
| Joints—one item | Synovitis >2 peripheral joints (pain, tenderness, swelling, or morning stiffness >30 min) |
| Serositis—one item | Pleuritis, typical pleurisy ≥1 day, history, rub, evidence of pleural effusion, pericarditis, typical pericardial pain ≥1 day, and EKG evidence of pericardial fusion |
| Renal disorder—one item | Urine protein/creatinine ratio or urinary protein concentration of 0.5 g of protein/24 h and red blood cell casts |
| Hematological disorder—three items | Hemolytic anemia |
| | Leukopenia (<4,000 cells/mm$^3$) or lymphopenia (<1,000 cells/mm$^3$) separately at least once |
| | Thrombocytopenia (<100,000 cells/mm$^3$) at least once |
| Immunologic abnormal—six items | Positive ANA |
| | Positive anti-dsDNA (except ELISA) on ≥2 occasions |
| | Anti-Sm |
| | Antiphospholipid antibody (including lupus anticoagulant, false-positive RPR, anticardiolipin, and anti-beta-2 glycoprotein 1) |
| | Low complement (C3, C4, or CH50) |
| | Direct Coombs test in the absence of hemolytic anemia |
| Diagnosis | Fulfill four items (at least one clinical and one immunologic item) |

(ANA: antinuclear antibody; dsDNA: double-stranded deoxyribonucleic acid; EKG: electrocardiogram; ELISA: enzyme-linked immunosorbent assay; RPR: rapid plasma reagin)

## ETIOPATHOGENESIS OF LUPUS NEPHRITIS

Renal involvement occurs due to deposition of the immune complexes (ICs) in the glomerulus, which may also go on to involve the renal interstitium and vascular compartment if unchecked. Although glomerular infiltration and inflammation are the major determinant of the renal course and prognosis, vascular involvement like thrombotic microangiopathic changes portent worse prognosis. The ICs deposited in LN in the renal compartments may be derived from the circulating ICs or can form in situ from the direct cytotoxicity of a subset of pathogenic autoantibodies for glomerular cells. The autoantibodies appear against multiple circulating autoantigens and multiple epitopes in the kidney. One of the most important includes pathogenic role of DNA—anti-DNA ICs, targeting polynucleotides, ribonucleotides, and phospholipids. Besides these other ICs involved in LN include anti-smith, anti-Ro, anti-La, anti-RNP [extractable nuclear antigen (ENA)], anti-ribosomal P, or antiphospholipid antibodies. Anti-smith is most specific for LN although the incidence of positivity is 25–30% in various studies. The ICs deposits occur in the mesangium, subepithelial, or subendothelial regions of the glomerulus and generate release of proinflammatory cytokines and cell adhesion molecules causing inflammation, resulting in chemotaxis of mononuclear and polymorphonuclear cells. Proteases thus released lead to endothelial injury and mesangial proliferation.

Recently, it has been postulated that the autoantibody production and systemic interferon responses are modulated by the activation of Toll-like receptors. Also, upcoming is the role of neutrophils in pathogenesis of SLE and LN. Neutrophil cells while undergoing a novel form of cell death (NETosis) release a meshwork of chromatin, which cannot be degraded properly in patients with LN and prove to be a source of autoantigens.

## DIAGNOSIS OF LUPUS NEPHRITIS

Lupus nephritis can have a wide spectrum on presentation varying from asymptomatic urinary findings of proteinuria and microscopic hematuria to overt nephritic, nephrotic, or nephritic-nephrotic syndrome picture clinically, with varying degree of hypertension and renal dysfunction. Urinary finding includes subnephrotic to nephrotic proteinuria and presence of active sediment—microscopic to rarely gross hematuria, granular casts, red blood cell casts, white blood cell casts, waxy casts, white blood cells, and oval fat bodies. Urine with all these components is called telescopic urine. Urine and biochemical evaluation may reveal normal investigations in Class I, subnephrotic isolated proteinuria in Class II, subnephrotic proteinuria with mild microscopic hematuria/active sediment without renal dysfunction or with mild renal dysfunction in Class III, subnephrotic to nephrotic proteinuria with hematuria mostly microscopic (occasionally gross)/active sediment with renal dysfunction of varying severity suggests Class IV lesion, and often presence of overt nephrotic syndrome is seen in Class V or combination lesions (V + II, V + III, and V + IV). There is fair degree of correlation between the clinical presentation, urinary findings, and renal dysfunction with pathological diagnosis, but discordance is not uncommon. The renal manifestations can vary from acute kidney injury to rapidly progressive renal failure to chronic progressive renal insufficiency. Presence of a multisystem extrarenal involvement may or may not indicate the presence or severity of LN.

Systemic lupus erythematosus and LN involve the activation of classical as well as alternate complement pathways, hence the serum levels of C3, C4, and C1q are often decreased in active disease. The serial measurement of their levels on follow-up can also guide regarding the remission and relapse of the disease activity while on treatment.

Kidney biopsy is the mainstay of diagnosis of LN and also guides regarding the need for treatment and disease prognosis with respect to the activity and chronicity of LN. In the recent SLICC criteria, the LN is a major determinant of diagnosis of SLE, with only one immunological parameter positivity along with LN sufficient to label patient as SLE.

Kidney biopsy analysis for diagnosis of LN ideally needs two cores, one for light microscopy (LM) and second one for immunofluorescence microscopy (IF) following optimal preservation. Also, upcoming is the role of electron microscopy in kidney biopsy analysis, although not widely available and not always feasible due to cost implications.

The renal lesions in LN have a wide spectrum, the classification of which was first proposed by pathologists under the patronage of the World Health Organization in 1974. It was later modified and revised in 1982 as well as in 1995. In view of considerable advances in knowledge of clinicopathological mechanisms of LN since 1974 and inconsistencies and ambiguities of 1982 and 1995 classification schemas, a revised classification of LN was proposed by the ISN/RPS (International Society of Nephrology/Renal Pathology Society) International Society of Nephrology/Renal Pathology Society (ISN/RPS) in 2004. Like the previous classification schemas, ISN/RPS classification system is also based on glomerular pathology and more precisely defines all classes of glomerulonephritis and clearly delineates disease activity and chronicity.

The main objective ISN-RPS was to standardize the definitions of the pathologic lesions. This helped in better distinctions between classes, emphasized clinically relevant findings, and led to a uniform reporting of renal biopsy findings for appropriate treatment and prognostication of the disease. It also facilitated better reproducibility of the findings among pathologists. This classification is largely based upon the degree of glomerular involvement. The other involved substructures of the nephron, interstitial, and vascular compartments, which can severely impact the renal and overall prognosis have not been given due emphasis in ISN-RPS. Vascular compartment of the nephron can be involved in LN in varying histopathological types and intensities, sometimes presenting with distinct clinical syndromes, such as vascular IC deposition, noninflammatory necrotizing vasculopathy, thrombotic microangiopathy, and true renal vasculitis. The clinical syndromes of thrombotic thrombocytopenic purpura (TTP), anticardiolipin syndrome, and renal vein thrombosis (RVT) are also well-documented vascular complications of SLE. The pathogenesis of many of these vascular entities is not fully defined. Because glomerular pathology is of primary importance in the classification of LN, the presence and significance of these renal vascular lesions are often overlooked. However, their occurrence can have a profound effect on the clinical course and choice of therapy.

The interstitium can have varying degree of T and B lymphocytes aggregates and lymphoid granulomas. It has been found to correlate with renal dysfunction and severity of hypertension. The immune deposits can be seen along the tubular structures like the basement membrane and the luminal invasion and infiltration can also occur leading to tubulitis. The interstitial and tubular involvement can lead to chronicity changes in the form of interstitial fibrosis and tubular atrophy (IFTA), impairing long-term prognosis of LN. Rarely, tubulointerstitial nephritis can be present alone without glomerular disease resulting in acute kidney injury or renal tubular acidosis as presentations.

## TREATMENT OF LUPUS NEPHRITIS

Lupus nephritis is amenable to treatment, but if left untreated can lead to acute kidney injury, chronic kidney disease, and ultimately end-stage renal disease. The treatment of patients with active proliferative LN is divided into two phases. The initial high-dose immunosuppression is given in the induction phase and followed by a low-dose maintenance phase. The induction phase deals with acute life- or organ-threatening disease. The maintenance phase focuses on the long-term management of chronic, more indolent disease, protection from the side effects of therapy, prevention of flares, and slowing or preventing progressive renal failure.

The ISN/RPS biopsy classification should guide initial therapy. The immunosuppression for renal involvement is indicated only in severe LN, which includes Class III, IV, or V or a combination of prior two with the later. Classes I and II LN do not need immunosuppression from renal point of view, as the long-term outcome is benign in them and giving immunosuppression may be detrimental due to worse side effect profiles if risk-benefit ratio is considered. However, close surveillance is advocated as there can be change in class in the natural course of LN to the severe form. Extrarenal manifestations should be treated with immunosuppression if indicated. An exception is the group of lupus patients with lupus podocyte injury, who often respond to a short course of high-dose corticosteroids similar to patients with minimal change disease (MCD) or focal segmental glomerulosclerosis (FSGS).

In patients with active focal proliferative LN (ISN classes IIIA and IIIA/C), active diffuse proliferative LN (ISN classes IVA and IVA/C) and membranous lupus (ISN class V) immunosuppressant are given as induction therapy to abate ongoing damage to nephrons by active disease and as long-term maintenance to prevent disease flares.

Besides the immunosuppressive treatment, management of LN includes supportive treatment such as close surveillance for prevention of complications, use of angiotensin-converting enzyme inhibitors or angiotensin receptor blockers, and optimization of blood pressure control. Role of hydroxychloroquine has been proved in multiple trials to reduce the renal damage and decrease renal and extrarenal flares and also to improve patient survival.

The first-line treatment includes combination of corticosteroids and immunosuppressive medications. The role of "only steroid" based regimens and azathioprine as induction immunosuppression has now gone into oblivion. Two immunosuppressive drugs mycophenolate mofetil and cyclophosphamide have been most widely studies in past few decades. The landmark trial by the National Institutes of Health study in 2001 had demonstrated that cyclophosphamide therapy is superior to corticosteroid therapy alone. Low dose of cyclophosphamide was shown to work as well in a multicenter, prospective Euro-Lupus Nephritis Trial. Similarly role of plasmapheresis initially widely advocated is now being restricted to fewer indications like resistant SLE, central nervous system (CNS) lupus, and thrombotic microangiopathy in SLE.

In the last few years, clinical trials have shown that less toxic immunosuppressants are as effective for treating LN as their contemporary toxic counterparts.

There are numerous other newer emerging therapies for treatment of SLE and LN.

## B-cell Targeted Therapies

Anti-CD20 monoclonal antibody, rituximab, is being widely used in treatment of LN and SLE. Two open-label studies have confirmed its effectiveness and safety in refractory SLE. However, another two large multicenter randomized placebo-controlled trials in moderately-to-severely active SLE (EXPLORER) and in proliferative LN patients (LUNAR) have questioned its benefit compared to placebo. This drug is still being used in refractory cases with up to 89% response reported.

A new recombinant humanized monoclonal anti-CD20 antibody, ocrelizumab, being studied in extrarenal SLE (BEGIN study) and LN (BELONG study).

## Anti-CD22 Antibodies

A fully humanized antibody against CD22, epratuzumab, was evaluated in randomized controlled trials in patients with moderate-to-severe SLE flares. The trial was interrupted due to problems in the biologic supply. Few more studies are underway.

## B-lymphocyte Tolerogens

B-cell tolerogen consists of four dsDNA epitopes on a polyethylene glycol platform. Human trials of abetimus, the first B-cell tolerogen, for effectiveness in SLE, nonrenal lupus, and LN, are underway. However, phase III ASPEN trial in LN was terminated after interim efficacy analysis, since it not prove its benefit.

Edratide (TV-4710), another tolerogen, testing is also in progress.

## B-lymphocyte Stimulator Blockers

Belimumab has been recently approved by the Food and Drug Administration (FDA) for treatment of SLE.

Atacicept [transmembrane activator and calcium modulator and cyclophilin ligand interactor-immunoglobulin (TACI-Ig)], a soluble TACI receptor, which binds both B-cell activating factor (BAFF) and a proliferation-inducing ligand (APRIL), has been through the phase I trial in SLE.

## T-cell Target and Costimulatory Blockers

Abatacept, soluble receptor or fusion protein encoded by fusion of cytotoxic T-lymphocyte antigen-4 (CTLA-4) with the Fc portion of immunoglobulin G1 (IgG1), blocks CD28-B7 interaction and subsequent T-cell-dependent B-cell function, is undergoing testing for treatment of SLE in I–III trials.

Anti-CD40L monoclonal antibody (mAb), based on blocking CD40-CD40 ligand (CD40L), has given conflicting results.

Monoclonal antibody directed against CD11a, efalizumab, and fully humanized anti-B7RP1 antibody (AMG557) is currently being investigated as therapies for SLE.

Mammalian target of rapamycin (mTOR) inhibitors such as rapamycin (sirolimus) have proved safe and effective in refractory SLE in small studies.

## Novel Therapies Based on Cytokine Inhibition

- *Antitumor necrosis factor-α (TNF-α) inhibitors*: Infliximab, adalimumab, golimumab, certolizumab pegol, and a fusion protein that act as a "decoy receptor" for TNF-α (etanercept).
- *Anti-interferon (IFN)-α/-γ*: Sifalimumab (MEDI-545), rontalizumab, and AMG 811.
- *Anti-interleukin-1 (IL-1)*: Anakinra, a nonglycolysated version of the human IL-1Ra (IL-1 receptor antagonist).
- *Anti-IL-6 therapy*: Tocilizumab

Anti-IL-10, anti-IL-15 and anti-IL-18, and two complement inhibitors, soluble complement receptor 1 (TP10), and a monoclonal anti-C5 antibody (eculizumab) are other evolving therapies.

Last two decades have seen marked improvement in the prognosis of the disease and its complications due to early diagnosis and effective treatment options. The 5-year

## SECTION 7: Nephrology

survival of SLE is >90%. However, morbidity due to LN and mortality due to cardiovascular events still pose a significant challenge.

## CONCLUSION

There has been a considerable evolution in the criteria for diagnosis, postulated etiopathogenesis, and treatment of LN in the past decade. Their impact on the outcomes and prognosis of the disease is going to unveil in the decade to follow.

## SUGGESTED READING

1. Appel GB, Radhakrishnan J, D'Agati V. Secondary glomerular disease. In: Brenner BM (Ed). The Kidney, 8th edition. Philadelphia: Saunders; 2012. pp. 1192-277.
2. Appel GB, Jayne D, Rovin BH. Lupus nephritis. In: Johnson RJ, Feehally J, Floege J (Eds). Comprehensive Clinical Nephrology, 5th edition. Philadelphia: Saunders; 2015. pp. 303-16.
3. Hochberg MC. Updating the American College of Rheumatology revised criteria for the classification of systemic lupus erythematosus. Arthritis Rheum. 1997;40(9):1725.
4. Petri M, Orbai AM, Alarcón GS, Gordon C, Merrill JT, Fortin PR, et al. Derivation and validation of the Systemic Lupus International Collaborating Clinics classification criteria for systemic lupus erythematosus. Arthritis Rheum. 2012;64(8):2677-86.
5. KDIGO Clinical Practice Guideline for Glomerulonephritis. Lupus Nephritis. Kidney Int Suppl. 2012;2(2):221-32.
6. Davis JC, Tassiulas IO, Boumpas DT. Lupus nephritis. Curr Opin Rheumatol. 1996;8(3):415-23.
7. Salgado AZ, Herrera-Diaz C. Lupus Nephritis: An Overview of Recent Findings. Autoimmune Dis. 2012;2012:849684.
8. Bagavant H, Fu SM. Pathogenesis of kidney disease in systemic lupus erythematosus. Curr Opin Rheumatol. 2009;21(5):489-94.
9. Ourania D, Ioana R, Andreea B, Anca B, Paulina C. Immunological Profile in Patients with Lupus Nephritis and Correlations with the Histological Pattern. Curr Health Sci J. 2011;37:161-64.
10. Seshan SV, Jennette JC. Renal Disease in Systemic Lupus Erythematosus With Emphasis on Classification of Lupus Glomerulonephritis: Advances and Implications. Arch Pathol Lab Med. 2009;133(2):233-48.
11. Saxena R, Mahajan T, Mohan C. Lupus nephritis: current update. Arthritis Res Ther. 2011;13(5):240.
12. Weening JJ, D'Agate V, Schwartw MM, Seshan SV, Alpers CE, Appel GB, et al. The classification of glomerulonephritis in Systemic Lupus Erythematosus revisited. Kidney Int. 2004;65:521-30.
13. Barber C, Herzenberg A, Aghdassi E, Su J, Lou W, Qian G, et al. Evaluation of Clinical Outcomes and Renal Vascular Pathology among Patients with Lupus. Clin J Am Soc Nephrol. 2012;7(5):757-64.
14. Appel GB. New and future therapies for lupus nephritis. Cleve Clin J Med. 2012;79(2):134-40.
15. Illei GG, Austin HA, Crane M, Collins L, Gourley MF, Yarboro CH, et al. Combination therapy with pulse cyclophosphamide plus pulse methylprednisolone improves long-term renal outcome without adding toxicity in patients with lupus nephritis. Ann Intern Med. 2001;135(4):248-57.
16. Houssiau FA, Vasconcelos C, D'Cruz D, Sebastiani GD, Garrido Ed ER, Danieli MG, et al. Immunosuppressive therapy in lupus nephritis: the Euro-Lupus Nephritis Trial, a randomized trial of low-dose versus high-dose intravenous cyclophosphamide. Arthritis Rheum. 2002;46:2121-31.
17. Roccatello D, Sciascia S, Rossi D, Alpna M, Naretto C, Baldovino S, et al. Intensive short-term treatment with rituximab, cyclophosphamide and methylprednisolone pulses induces remission in severe cases of SLE with nephritis and avoids further immunosuppressive maintenance therapy. Nephrol Dial Transplant. 2011;26(12):3987-92.
18. Food and Drug Administration (FDA) Consortium. (2007). Rituxan Warning. [online] Available from https://www.accessdata.fda.gov/drugsatfda_docs/label/2012/103705s5367s5388lbl.pdf. [Last accessed January, 2020].
19. Abud-Mendoza C, Moreno-Valdés R, Cuevas-Orta E, Borjas A, Aranda F, Irazoque F, et al. Treating severe systemic lupus erythematosus with rituximab. An open study. Reumatol Clin. 2009;5(4):147-52.

20. Leandro MJ, Edwards JC, Cambridge G, Ehrenstein MR, Isenberg DA. An open study of B lymphocyte depletion in systemic lupus erythematosus. Arthritis Rheum. 2002;46(10):2673-7.
21. Merrill JT, Neuwelt CM, Wallace DJ, Shanahan JC, Latinis KM, Oates JC, et al. Efficacy and safety of rituximab in moderately-to-severely active systemic lupus erythematosus: the randomized, double-blind, phase II/III systemic lupus erythematosus evaluation of rituximab trial. Arthritis Rheum. 2010;62(1):222-33.
22. National Institutes of Health (NIH). (2011). A Study to Evaluate the Efficacy and Safety of Rituximab in Subjects With International Society of Nephrology/Renal Pathology Society (ISN/RPS) 2003 Class III or IV Lupus Nephritis (LUNAR). [online] Available from https://clinicaltrials.gov/ct2/show/NCT00282347. [Last accessed January, 2020].
23. Pinto LF, Velásquez CJ, Prieto C, Mestra L, Forero E, Márquez JD. Rituximab induces a rapid and sustained remission in Colombian patients with severe and refractory systemic lupus erythematosus. Lupus. 2011;20(11):1219-26.
24. Terrier B, Amoura Z, Ravaud P, Hachulla E, Jouenne R, Combe B, et al. Safety and efficacy of rituximab in systemic lupus erythematosus: results from 136 patients from the French autoimmunity and rituximab registry. Arthritis Rheum. 2010;62(8):2458-66.
25. Reynolds JA, Toescu V, Yee CS, Prabu A, Situnayake D, Gordon C. Effects of rituximab on resistant SLE disease including lung involvement. Lupus. 2009;18(1):67-73.
26. Turner-Stokes T, Lu TY, Ehrenstein MR, Giles I, Rahman A, Isenberg DA. The efficacy of repeated treatment with B-cell depletion therapy in systemic lupus erythematosus: an evaluation. Rheumatology (Oxford). 2011;50(8):1401-8.
27. Anolik JH, Aringer M. New treatments for SLE: cell-depleting and anti-cytokine therapies. Best Pract Res Clin Rheumatol. 2005;19(5):859-78.
28. National Institutes of Health (NIH). (2008). A Study to Evaluate Two Doses of Ocrelizumab in Patients With Active Systemic Lupus Erythematosus (BEGIN). [online] Available from https://clinicaltrials.gov/ct2/show/NCT00539838. [Last accessed January, 2020].
29. National Institutes of Health (NIH). (2008). A Study to Evaluate Ocrelizumab in Patients With Nephritis Due to Systemic Lupus Erythematosus (BELONG). [online] Available from https://clinicaltrials.gov/ct2/show/NCT00626197. [Last accessed January, 2020].
30. Petri MA, Hobbs K, Gordon C. Randomized controlled trials of epratuzumab (anti-CD-22MAB targeting B cells) reveal clinically meaningful improvements in patients with moderate and severe SLE flares. Ann Rheum Dis. 2008;67 (Suppl 2):53.
31. Fernandez D, Bonilla E, Mirza N, Niland B, Perl A. Rapamycin reduces disease activity and normalizes T cell activation-induced calcium fluxing in patients with systemic lupus erythematosus. Arthritis Rheum. 2006;54(9):2983-8.
32. Cardiel MH, Tumlin JA, Furie RA, Wallace DJ, Joh T, Linnik MD, et al. Abetimus sodium for renal flare in systemic lupus erythematosus: results of a randomized, controlled phase III trial. Arthritis Rheum. 2008;58(8):2470-80.
33. National Institutes of Health (NIH). (2004). Study of LJP 394 in Lupus Patients with History of Renal Disease (ASPEN). [online] Available from https://clinicaltrials.gov/ct2/show/NCT00089804. [Last accessed January, 2020].
34. National Institutes of Health (NIH). (2005). A Study to Evaluate the Tolerability, Safety and Effectiveness of Edratide in the Treatment of Lupus (PRELUDE). [online] Available from https://clinicaltrials.gov/ct2/show/NCT00203151. [Last accessed January, 2020].
35. Human Genome Sciences. (2010). GlaxoSmithKline and Human Genome Sciences announce FDA priority review designation for Benlysta® (belimumab) as a potential treatment for systemic lupus erythematosus. [online] Available from https://www.gsk.com/en-gb/media/press-releases/glaxosmithkline-and-human-genome-sciences-announce-fda-priority-review-designation-for-benlysta-belimumab-as-a-potential-treatment-for-systemic-lupus-erythematosus/. [Last accessed January, 2020].
36. Dall'Era M, Chakravarty E, Wallace D, Genovese M, Weisman M, Kavanaugh A, et al. Reduced B lymphocyte and immunoglobulin levels after atacicept treatment in patients with systemic lupus erythematosus: results of a multicenter, phase Ib, double-blind, placebo-controlled, dose-escalating trial. Arthritis Rheum. 2007;56(12):4142-50.
37. National Institutes of Health (NIH). (2008). Abatacept and Cyclophosphamide Combination Therapy for Lupus Nephritis (ACCESS). [online] Available from https://clinicaltrials.gov/ct2/show/NCT00774852. [Last accessed January, 2020].

38. National Institutes of Health (NIH). (2007). Efficacy and Safety Study of Abatacept to Treat Lupus Nephritis. [online] Available from https://clinicaltrials.gov/ct2/show/NCT00430677. [Last accessed January, 2020].
39. Kalunian KC, Davis JC, Merrill JT, Totoritis MC, Wofsy D. Treatment of Systemic Lupus Erythematosus by inhibition of T cell costimulation with anti-CD154: a randomized, double-blind, placebo-controlled trial. Arthritis Rheum. 2002;46(12):3251-8.
40. Wang X, Huang W, Schiffer LE, Mihara M, Akkerman A, Hiromatsu K, et al. Effects of anti-CD154 treatment on B cells in murine systemic lupus erythematosus. Arthritis Rheum. 2003;48(2):495-506.
41. Boumpas DT, Furie R, Manzi S, Illei GG, Wallace DJ, Balow JE, et al. A short course of BG9588 (anti-CD40 ligand antibody) improves serologic activity and decreases hematuria in patients with proliferative lupus glomerulonephritis. Arthritis Rheum. 2003;48(3):719-27.
42. Usmani N, Goodfield M. Efalizumab in the treatment of discoid lupus erythematosus. Arch Dermatol. 2007;143(7):873-7.
43. National Institutes of Health (NIH). (2008). A Study of AMG 557 in Adults With Systemic Lupus Erythematosus. [online] Available from https://clinicaltrials.gov/ct2/show/NCT00774943. [Last accessed January, 2020].
44. Postal M, Costallat LT, Appenzeller S. Biological therapy in systemic lupus erythematosus. Int J Rheumatol. 2012;2012:578641.
45. Haubitz M. New and emerging treatment approaches to lupus. Biologics. 2010;4:263-71.
46. Trager J, Ward MM. Mortality and causes of death in systemic lupus erythematosus. Curr Opin Rheumatol. 2001;13(5):345-51.

# CHAPTER 3

# Acute Kidney Injury in Pregnancy

*Jasmine Das*

## ABSTRACT

Pregnancy-related acute kidney injury (Pr-AKI) is a major cause of maternal and fetal morbidity and mortality worldwide. Though the incidence of Pr-AKI has decreased in developing countries due to improved prenatal care and decrease in rates of sepsis due to abortions or childbirth in last few decades, 5–20% of all AKI cases are still due to Pr-AKI. Recent data from developed countries show a rising trend in Pr-AKI due to factors like advancing age of women becoming pregnant due to assisted reproductive technology and increasing rates of hypertensive pregnancy disorders. Around 75% cases of Pr-AKI occur during the late third trimester and in the early postpartum. The hypertensive complications of pregnancy, particularly preeclampsia (PE) and/or hemolysis and elevated liver enzymes and low platelets (HELLP) syndrome, are major causes of Pr-AKI in most parts of the world. Around 1.5–2.5% cases of Pr-AKI progress to end-stage renal disease.

## INTRODUCTION

Acute kidney injury (AKI) is defined as the abrupt loss of kidney function, resulting in the retention of urea and other nitrogenous waste products and in the dysregulation of extracellular volume and electrolytes. The loss of kidney function is less as compared to acute renal failure (ARF) where overt organ failure is seen. But still, it is clinically relevant and responsible for increased morbidity and mortality.

Factors causing AKI in pregnancy are almost same as those leading to AKI in general population. Moreover, pregnancy-related complications in each trimester can also be associated with acute injury.

## EPIDEMIOLOGY

The proportion of pregnancy-related acute kidney injury (Pr-AKI) in hospitalized patients has been on declining trend in developing nations from 15% in the 1980s to 1.5% in the 2010s. In India, the associated maternal mortality rate has reduced from 20% during 1980s to 5.8% in recent studies. This is largely due to better management of postpartum hemorrhage and placental abruption and decline in sepsis rates associated with abortion and childbirth.

This situation is in contrast to developed nations where the incidence of Pr-AKI is on rise. In Canada, incidence was 1.66 per 10,000 pregnancies in 2003 and in 2010, it was 2.68 in Canada. Similarly, in United States, it increased from 2.4 in 1999–2001 to 6.3 in 2010–2011 per 10,000 deliveries. Factors responsible for this include late motherhood, pregnancies with hypertensive disorders, and underlying chronic kidney disease.

Pregnancy-related acute kidney injury is also associated with high fetal mortality and morbidity. Rates of perinatal mortality reported in several studies from India are as high as 20–45% due to intrauterine death, stillbirth, and prematurity.

Around 1.5–2.5%cases of Pr-AKI progress to end-stage renal disease. Around 40–75% of less severe Pr-AKI, in the short term, shows favorable recovery of kidney function. However, 4–9% of women with severe Pr-AKI remain dialysis dependent at 4–6 months postpartum.

## ANATOMICAL AND PHYSIOLOGICAL CHANGES IN PREGNANCY

- Increase in size of the kidneys by 1–1.5 cm due to expansion of renal vascular volume.
- Physiologic hydronephrosis resulting from compression of ureter by gravid uterus and due to the hormonal effects of progesterone.
- Increase in plasma volume by 30–50% above baseline.
- Increase in glomerular filtration rate by 40–50% of the baseline resulting in low levels of serum creatinine (Scr) usually to 0.4–0.5 mg%.
- Decrease in plasma osmolality and sodium levels by 4–5 mEq/L due to stimulation of antidiuretic hormone secondary to systemic vasodilatation.
- Chronic respiratory alkalosis due to progesterone-induced stimulation of central respiratory center in the brain.

## DIAGNOSIS

The diagnosis of AKI in pregnancy has not been standardized. The RIFLE (Risk, Injury, Failure, Loss, and End-stage) and the AKIN (Acute Kidney Injury Network) criteria used for the general population have not been well-validated in pregnancy. It has been observed in recent studies done using the RIFLE and AKIN criteria that majority of cases of Pr-AKI fall in AKIN stage 1. Also, as the RIFLE category goes up, outcome of Pr-AKI worsens.

## ETIOLOGY

The etiology behind Pr-AKI can be prerenal, intrarenal, or postrenal. Also, the timing during pregnancy suggests the underlying etiology. Important causes have been discussed in this chapter.

## HYPEREMESIS GRAVIDARUM

Its incidence varies from 3/1,000 to 1/100 pregnancies. It is the most common cause of AKI in first trimester of pregnancy. It is defined as severe and persistent nausea and vomiting, resulting in weight loss of >5% of the prepregnancy weight and ketonuria. Laboratory tests reveal deranged renal functions, hypokalemic metabolic alkalosis, increased hematocrit, mildly elevated aminotransferases, and mild hyperthyroidism due to thyroid-stimulating activity of human chorionic gonadotropin (hCG). Treatment includes antiemetics and intravenous fluids.

## ATYPICAL HEMOLYTIC UREMIC SYNDROME

Atypical hemolytic uremic syndrome (aHUS) is characterized by microangiopathic hemolytic anemia (MAHA), thrombocytopenia, and decreased kidney function. aHUS is either sporadic, which is more common (~80%) or familial, due to genetic mutations in the complement regulatory proteins, such as complement factor H, complement factor I, C3, membrane cofactor protein, or a combination resulting in an inactivation of alternative complement pathway. Pregnancy is a classic example of a condition that can trigger aHUS.

Recently, a European study explained a case of women who developed pregnancy-associated HUS has been described in a European study. The need for dialysis was more frequent at the time of presentation in those with complement gene variants. They progressed to end-stage renal disease more frequently and also increased rates of fetal loss and preeclampsia (PE) were seen.

### Treatment

- *Plasma exchange*: This is effective in about 50% of the adults. Autoantibodies to alternative complement pathway are removed and deficient gene products are replaced with plasma.
- Eculizumab, a humanized monoclonal anti-C5 antibody, inhibits the C5 cleavage by binding with it and generates membrane attack complex. The recommended regimen is 4 weekly 900 mg infusions followed by 1,200 mg every fortnight. Normalization of platelet counts, lactate dehydrogenase (LDH) levels, and decrease in Scr by 25% indicate response to therapy. In spite of it showing a good response in recent studies, it is rarely used because of its high cost.

## PREECLAMPSIA

In 2–8% of pregnancies, PE most commonly occurs in the second and third trimester period and up to 5% of cases in the postpartum period. It is characterized by new onset of hypertension and proteinuria that occurs after 20 weeks of gestation.

### Diagnostic Criteria of Preeclampsia

- Systolic blood pressure ≥140 mm Hg or diastolic blood pressure ≥90 mm Hg (measured on two occasions at least 4 h apart) and
- Proteinuria ≥300 mg/day or urine protein-to-creatinine ratio (UPCR) ≥0.3 g/g
- If no proteinuria is present, new onset of any of the following:
  - Platelets <100 × $10^3$ cells/μL
  - Scr >1.1 mg/dL or doubling of Scr concentration in the absence of other kidney disease
  - Liver transaminases 2 × Upper limits of normal
  - Pulmonary edema
  - Cerebral or visual symptoms (new onset and persistent headache, blurred vision, and flashing lights).

Around 30–40% reduction in renal blood flow and glomerular filtration rate is seen in PE as compared with a normal pregnancy. Though AKI occurs in only 1% of cases of PE, but when associated with hemolysis and elevated liver enzymes and low platelets (HELLP) syndrome, it occurs in 7–15% of cases. AKI most often develops in the setting of complication of PE such as placental abruption, disseminated intravascular coagulation (DIC), sepsis, postpartum bleeding, or intrauterine fetal death.

Placental defects and maternal susceptibility play a key role in the development of PE in the following ways:
- There is imbalance between the placental production of proangiogenic factors, e.g., vascular endothelial growth factor (VEGF) and placental growth factor (PlGF) and antiangiogenic factors like soluble fms-like tyrosine kinase-1 (sFlt-1) and soluble endoglin (sEng).
- There is excess placental production of sFlt-1, a truncated splice variant of VEGF receptor Flt-1.
- Soluble fms-like tyrosine kinase-1 antagonizes VEGF and PlGF by binding them in the circulation and preventing interaction with their endogenous receptors resulting in vasoconstriction and endothelial dysfunction evidenced by obliterative arteriolopathy and placental infarcts.
- *Complement system dysregulation:* Susceptibility to severe PE is modified with single nucleotide polymorphisms in complement gene C3. This has both predisposing and protective effects based on the allele combination.

## Treatment

- *Infusions of magnesium sulfate*: To prevent eclamptic seizures and lower blood pressure.
- *Delivery:* Severe PE in second trimester is associated with high rate of maternal complications that are common and perinatal and neonatal mortality as well. So, prompt delivery is indicated. On the other hand, women presenting between 24 and 34 weeks of gestation, expectant management results in decreased neonatal and maternal complications.
- *Dextran sulfate apheresis:* The sFlt-1 removal decreases proteinuria and prolongs the pregnancy.
- *Eculizumab:* A complement inhibitor results in favorable maternal and fetal outcomes.

# HEMOLYSIS AND ELEVATED LIVER ENZYMES AND LOW PLATELETS SYNDROME

Hemolysis and elevated liver enzymes and low platelets syndrome is reported to occur in 1–2/10,000 pregnancies. Usually, it occurs in the third trimester but may be diagnosed in the second trimester or in the postpartum period. It is considered a variant of PE. It complicates approximately 20% of women with severe PE. Increased levels of antiangiogenic factors (sFlt-1 and sEng) and decrease in the concentration of proangiogenic mediators (PlGF) have been proposed in the pathogenesis of HELLP syndrome similar to PE. It resolves with delivery and is frequently but not always associated with hypertension and proteinuria. The most common symptoms are epigastric/right upper quadrant pain, nausea, vomiting, and headache.

The diagnosis of HELLP syndrome is based on the following laboratory criteria:
- *Microangiopathic hemolytic anemia:* Schistocytes in blood smear, serum bilirubin ≥1.2 mg/dL, and LDH >600 U/L.
- Increased liver transaminases (alanine aminotransferase >70 U/L).
- Platelet count <100 × $10^3$ cells/mm$^3$.

Acute kidney injury has been reported in 3–15% cases of HELLP syndrome and overall reached up to 40% of all cases of Pr-AKI and it may increase up to 60% of cases in severe form. Dialysis is needed in approximately 10–46% of patients.

## ACUTE FATTY LIVER OF PREGNANCY

Acute fatty liver of pregnancy (AFLP) occurs in ~1 in 10,000 deliveries. Its pathogenesis is attributed to fetal deficiency of long-chain 3-hydroxyacyl-coenzyme A dehydrogenase (LCHAD). The resulting increased fetal free fatty acids cross the placenta and are hepatotoxic to the mother. The mother, mostly in her third trimester, presents with fatigue, vomiting, headache, hypoglycemia, and lactic acidosis. Around 50–75% of such patients have associated Pr-AKI of varying degrees. Treatment requires expedient delivery, supportive care, and intensive monitoring.

## THROMBOTIC THROMBOCYTOPENIC PURPURA

This is mostly caused due to deficiency of ADAMTS-13, a von Willebrand factor-cleaving protease and commonly found in the second and third trimesters of pregnancy. As pregnancy is a procoagulant state, occurrence of thrombotic thrombocytopenic purpura (TTP) is favored especially in the setting of ADAMTS-13 deficiency. Plasma exchanges or fresh frozen plasma infusions for clearance of autoantibodies and restoration of enzymatic activity are the preferred treatment choices. Platelet transfusions should be avoided as far as possible as it increases the risk of vascular thrombosis.

## LUPUS NEPHRITIS

Systemic lupus erythematosus (SLE) is mostly seen in women of childbearing age. Diagnosis of lupus nephritis for the first time in pregnancy is difficult but the presence of extrarenal manifestations of lupus such as active urinary sediments, serological markers like low complement levels, and positive antinuclear antibodies especially anti-double-stranded deoxyribonucleic acid (anti-dsDNA) antibody and anti-Smith antibody helps in making the diagnosis. Lupus during pregnancy is associated with both maternal complications such as lupus flare, PE, thrombotic events, and fetal complications like spontaneous abortions, preterm delivery, intrauterine growth retardation, and neonatal lupus. Presence of anti-Ro/anti-La antibodies is associated with neonatal lupus presenting with complete congenital heart block.

The PROMISSE (Predictors of Pregnancy Outcome: Biomarkers in Antiphospholipid Antibody Syndrome and Systemic Lupus Erythematosus) study observed that the high levels of sFlt-1 or ratio of sFlt-1:PlGF in the late first trimester/second trimester were associated with increased risk of an adverse outcome.

Pregnant women with lupus should be started on low-dose aspirin prior to 16 weeks of gestation and those having coexisting antiphospholipid syndrome (APLS). Anticoagulation with unfractionated heparin or low-molecular-weight heparin (LMWH) in addition to low-dose aspirin is recommended for those with a history of thrombotic event for APLS like three or more pregnancy losses or a late pregnancy loss. For prevention of lupus flare, hydroxychloroquine should be continued throughout the pregnancy.

## ACUTE CORTICAL NECROSIS

By 2005, the incidence of acute cortical necrosis (ACN) decreased to 0.5%. Severe hypotension usually secondary to massive antepartum or postpartum hemorrhage results in ACN and pregnancy being a hypercoagulable state predisposes to it. Histopathologically, there is patchy or diffuse cortical necrosis with sparing of medulla and intravascular thrombosis in intralobular and afferent arterioles. It usually results in permanent renal impairment.

## POSTRENAL ACUTE KIDNEY INJURY

Postrenal causes of AKI are not so common in pregnancy. They include the following:
- *Renal calculi*: Bilateral renal calculi rarely cause Pr-AKI. Urinary stasis and lithogenic factors such as increased urinary excretion of calcium, oxalate, and uric acid seen in pregnancy are responsible for calculi formation.
- *Obstructive uropathy:* It results from the uterine compression of the ureters. The risk factors are twin pregnancies, polyhydramnios, solitary kidney, and nephrolithiasis.
- *Iatrogenic injuries to the bladder and ureters:* Incidence is as low as 0.0016–0.94% and mostly occurs due to emergent C-sections, especially in women with ectopic kidney or duplication of ureter.

*Treatment depends on the underlying etiology and gestational age*:
- *At term or near-term pregnancy:* Spontaneous or induced delivery
- Preterm or too early for delivery.
  For polyhydramnios, amniotomy should be performed.
  For nephrolithiasis, placement of ureteral stents or nephrostomies is done and hemodialysis is required for severe renal failure.

## Management of Acute Kidney Injury in Pregnancy
- Treating the underlying cause of AKI.
- Maintenance of renal and uteroplacental perfusion by intravenous fluids.
- Management of associated complications such as hyperkalemia, metabolic acidosis, and anemia.
- Methyldopa and labetalol are preferred antihypertensives as angiotensin-converting enzyme (ACE) inhibitors and angiotensin receptor blockers are contraindicated in pregnancy and diuretics can result in volume depletion.
- Dialysis should be started early when estimated glomerular filtration rate (eGFR) <20 mL/min/1.73 m$^2$ with weekly increased dose of 20 hours to prevent prematurity and polyhydramnios.
- Renal biopsy is contraindicated in third trimester. It is indicated only when the biopsy diagnosis is likely to have an effect on the treatment plan.

## CONCLUSION

In the last few decades, the incidence of AKI in pregnancy has been showing a downward trend especially in developing countries. It is mainly due to improved prenatal care and decrease in the rate of septic abortions. The incidence of AKI in pregnancy in developed countries has shown increasing trend though the absolute numbers are less as compared to developing countries. Diagnosis of aHUS, TTP, AFLP, and lupus nephritis in pregnancy is challenging due to overlapping clinical features. The timing of AKI, serological markers, and newer angiogenic markers help in making the precise diagnosis. Treatment is generally supportive with expedient delivery in most of the cases. Plasmapheresis is indicated in TTP and eculizumab in aHUS.

## SUGGESTED READING

1. Mahesh E, Puri S, Varma V, Madhyastha PR, Bande S, Gurudev KC. Pregnancy-related acute kidney injury: an analysis of 165 cases. Indian J Nephrol. 2017;27:113-7.
2. Prakash J, Pant P, Prakash S, Sivasankar M, Vohra R, Doley PK, et al. Changing picture of acute kidney injury in pregnancy: study of 259 cases over a period of 33 years. Indian J Nephrol. 2016;26:262-7.
3. Mehrabadi A, Liu S, Bartholomew S, Hutcheon JA, Magee LA, Kramer MS, et al. Hypertensive disorders of pregnancy and the recent increase in obstetric acute renal failure in Canada: population based retrospective cohort study. BMJ. 2014;349:g4731.
4. Mehrabadi A, Dahhou M, Joseph KS, Kramer MS. Investigation of a rise in obstetric acute renal failure in the United States, 1999–2011. Obstet Gynecol. 2016;127:899-906.
5. Arrayhani M, El Youbi R, Sqalli T. Pregnancy-related acute kidney injury: experience of the nephrology unit at the University Hospital of Fez, Morocco. ISRN Nephrol. 2012;2013:109034.
6. Gurrieri C, Garovic VD, Gullo A, Bojanić K, Sprung J, Narr BJ, et al. Kidney injury during pregnancy: associated comorbid conditions and outcomes. Arch Gynecol Obstet. 2012;286:567-73.
7. Goodwin TM. Hyperemesis gravidarum. Clin Obstet Gynecol. 1998;41:597-605.
8. Fakhouri F, Roumenina L, Provot F, Sallée M, Caillard S, Couzi L, et al. Pregnancy-associated hemolytic uremic syndrome revisited in the era of complement gene mutations. J Am Soc Nephrol. 2010;21:859-67.
9. Bruel A, Kavanagh D, Noris M, Delmas Y, Wong EK, Bresin E, et al. Hemolytic uremic syndrome in pregnancy and postpartum. Clin J Am Soc Nephrol. 2017;12:1237-47.
10. Duley L. The global impact of preeclampsia and eclampsia. Semin Perinatol. 2009;33:130-7.
11. Suarez ML, Kattah A, Grande JP, Garovic V. Renal Disorders in Pregnancy: Core Curriculum 2019. Am J Kidney Dis. 2019;73:119-30.
12. Prakash J, Ganiger VC. Acute Kidney Injury in Pregnancy-specific Disorders. Indian J Nephrol. 2017;27:258-70.
13. Gul A, Aslan H, Cebeci A, Polat I, Ulusoy S, Ceylan Y. Maternal and fetal outcomes in HELLP syndrome complicated with acute renal failure. Ren Fail. 2004;26:557-62.
14. Silasi M, Cohen B, Karumanchi SA, Rana S. Abnormal placentation, angiogenic factors, and the pathogenesis of preeclampsia. Obstet Gynecol Clin North Am. 2010;37:239-53.
15. Lynch AM, Salmon JE. Dysregulated complement activation as a common pathway of injury in preeclampsia and other pregnancy complications. Placenta. 2010;31:561-7.
16. Thadhani R, Hagmann H, Schaarschmidt W, Roth B, Cingoez T, Karumanchi SA, et al. Removal of soluble Fms-like tyrosine kinase-1 by dextran sulfate apheresis in preeclampsia. J Am Soc Nephrol. 2016;27:903-13.
17. Jim B, Garovic VD. Acute Kidney Injury in Pregnancy. Semin Nephrol. 2017;37:378-85.
18. Kim MY, Buyon JP, Guerra MM, Zhang D, Laskin CA, Petri M, et al. Angiogenic factor imbalance early in pregnancy predicts adverse outcomes in patients with lupus and antiphospholipid antibodies: results of the PROMISSE study. Am J Obstet Gynecol. 2016;214:108.e1-14.
19. Rao S, Jim B. Acute Kidney Injury in Pregnancy: The Changing Landscape for the 21st Century. Kidney Int Rep. 2018;3:247-57.

# Challenges of Urinary Tract Infections in Females

*Harmeet Riyait*

## ABSTRACT

Between 1 and 50 years of age, urinary tract infection (UTI) and recurrent UTI are predominantly diseases of the females. The prevalence of asymptomatic bacteriuria is 5% among women between ages 20–40 years and may be as high as 40–50% among elderly women and men. As a nephrologist, I hardly ever come across the uncomplicated UTI in women as these mostly get treated empirically by over-the-counter antibiotics routinely available in our country. So, the majority of cases that reach the tertiary care center are recurrent UTI. This chapter presents the approach toward a patient with recurrent or difficult to treat UTI. It emphasizes the proper workup of the lower urinary tract and stresses on the timely referral and at least once opinion of the urologist in cases where both the doctor and the patient feel frustrated by the repeated and often failed course of antibiotics. Principles of therapy and nonpharmacological measures are briefly mentioned in the end of the chapter.

## INTRODUCTION

Between 1 and 50 years of age, urinary tract infection (UTI) and recurrent UTI are predominantly diseases of the females. The prevalence of asymptomatic bacteriuria is 5% among women between ages 20–40 years and may be as high as 40–50% among elderly women. Because of the obvious difference in the anatomy of the lower urinary tract, the risk factors and the approach to management differ between men and women (**Fig. 1**). The commonly cited reasons for higher incidence of UTI in women include the shorter length of urethra, proximity to anogenital area, and urethral trauma during sexual activity.

As a nephrologist, I hardly ever come across the uncomplicated UTI in women as most get treated by over-the-counter antibiotics, as these are routinely available in our country and self-treated empirically. So, the majority of cases that reach the tertiary care center are recurrent UTI or complicated ones.

The infection occurs due to the interplay between the host, organism, and the environment. Symptomatic UTI occurs when local defense mechanisms are overcome by virulence of invading bacteria. The exact reason why a certain colonizing bacteria will become infectious is not known. There is a possibility of genetic predisposition by the mechanism of receptors on the cell surface which act as adhering factors for the bacteria.

# CHAPTER 4: Challenges of Urinary Tract Infections in Females

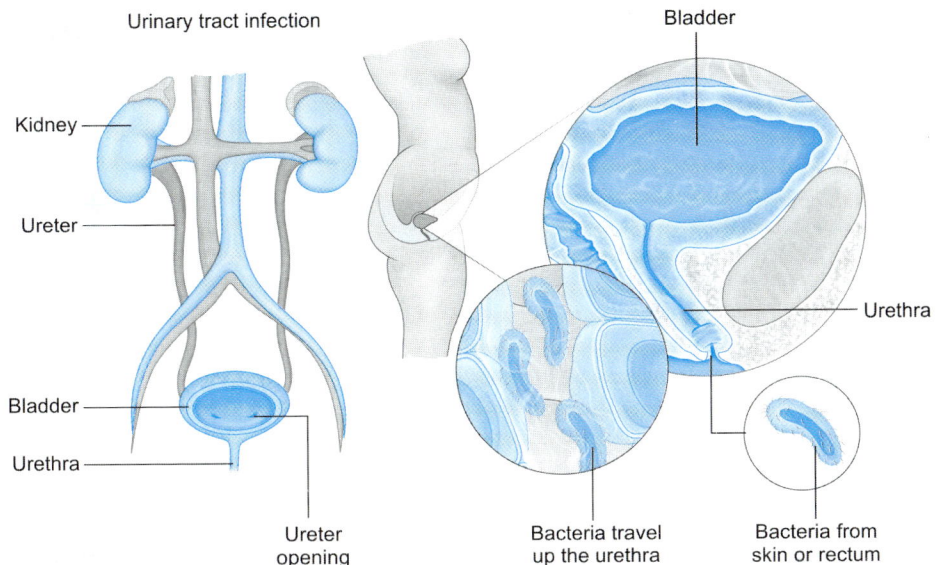

**FIG. 1:** Urinary tract anatomy.

Host immunity is also a very variable factor, difficult to quantitate. It may be influenced by nutrition, neurohormonal factors, stress, drugs, glycemic control, etc.

*Etiologic agents*: Uncomplicated lower and upper UTI is most often caused by *Escherichia coli*, present in 70–95% and *Staphylococcus saprophyticus*, present in 5% to >20%. A broader range of bacteria can cause complicated UTI and many are resistant to broad-spectrum antimicrobial agents.

## APPROACH TO A FEMALE PATIENT WITH URINARY TRACT INFECTION

### Thorough History Taking

Meticulous history is important to pinpoint the etiology and mechanism.

### Age

Elderly females have altered vaginal flora and often vaginitis due to postmenopausal hormonal changes, which may predispose to the recurrent UTI. Often some symptoms of vaginitis may be overlapping with UTI.

### Marital Status

Honeymoon cystitis is common among many women. Many times, the female may be hesitant to discuss especially when the treating doctor is a male. History of multiple partners predispose to sexually transmitted diseases (STDs).

In case of previous multiple episodes, it is usually advisable to ask the patient to make a record in calendar to exactly know the frequency of UTIs and the precipitating factors, along with the note of the antibiotics and the duration of the antibiotic use, as recurrence is common due to inadequate duration of the antibiotic treatment. Inadequate antibiotic use also increases the incidence of antibiotic resistance.

## SECTION 7: Nephrology

# Evaluation of the Voiding Symptoms

The lower urinary tract stores the urine and voids in a systematic way, so beautifully that we often take it for granted till a lapse occurs in some component.

The symptoms which indicate UTI include fever, burning micturition, increased frequency, urgency, suprapubic discomfort, and flank pain. Other causes of lower urinary tract symptoms apart from UTI are described in **Figure 2**.

A very commonly encountered problem is a patient who does not have clinical symptoms, but carrying a report of urine routine examination with pyuria and often culture positive.

Obstructive voiding symptoms include hesitancy, poor flow of urine, intermittent flow of urine, sense of incomplete evacuation, straining while micturition, prolonged voiding, etc. Storage symptoms include urgency, stress incontinence, frequency, etc. Patients are often more distressed by storage symptoms as it often lead to the soiling of the undergarments and difficulty in maintaining general hygiene.

Use of contraceptive jellies and diaphragms are not common in our country. Still, the use of type of contraception method should be asked. Many times, genital infections exist simultaneously in a couple, e.g., candidiasis especially when one of the partners is diabetic.

Diabetic status and glycemic status should be evaluated. Poor glycemic control and recurrent UTI often have cause and effect relationship. So to achieve the control, both need to be addressed simultaneously. Worsening of glycemic control in a patient with good medication and dietary compliance with otherwise asymptomatic bacteriuria may need treatment.

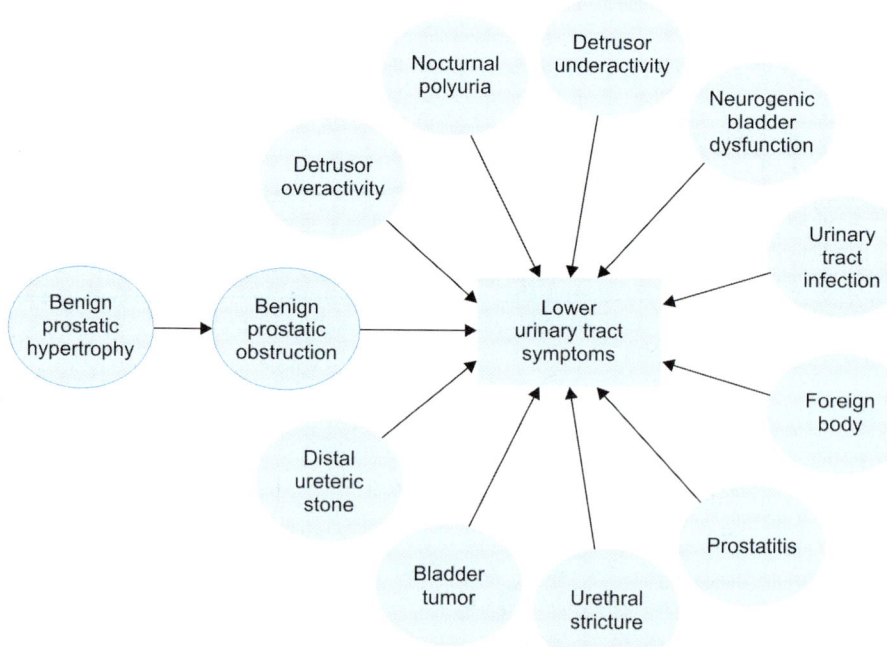

**FIG. 2:** Causes of lower urinary tract symptoms.

Past history of per urethral catheterization may predispose to urethral stricture and hence obstructive voiding. The development of obstruction is so gradual that often the patients do not realize the difference in voiding. Even after documented abnormal voiding on uroflowmetry, the patients may deny the poor stream and subsequently realize only after the flow improves after dilatation.

## EXAMINATION OF THE PATIENT WITH URINARY TRACT INFECTION

Vitals may indicate the severity of UTI and presence of sepsis. Diabetic patients may have evidence of neuropathy, which may also affect bladder autonomic functions. Clinical examination of external genitalia and the urethral orifice should be done which may reveal any evidence of vaginitis, urethral meatal stenosis, prolapse, etc., especially in the elderly multiparous women. Help of a gynecologist may be sought if history is suggestive of prolapse or there are other coexisting gynecological problems. Pruritus due to vaginitis may lead to some superficial urethral injury which may cause some dysuria. Per speculum examination will reveal the health of the vaginal mucosa, presence and nature of discharge, etc. Renal angle tenderness should be looked for if there are other systemic symptoms of UTI such as pain in abdomen, vomiting, encephalopathy, and respiratory distress indicating severe sepsis. In patients with spinal cord injuries or with other causes of spinal cord involvement, perineal sensation and anal tone should be checked.

## INVESTIGATIONS IN A PATIENT WITH URINARY TRACT INFECTION

### Hematology and Biochemistry

Complete blood count may reveal leukocytosis with neutrophilic predominance, especially if there is concomitant involvement of upper urinary tract. Renal function tests (RFTs) may be deranged. The underlying etiology of abnormal RFTs may be multifactorial, acute kidney injury due to sepsis, hypotension, dehydration (from vomiting), obstructive uropathy due to stones, papillary necrosis, and underlying chronic kidney disease (CKD) due to diabetes mellitus (DM), hypertension (HT), and chronic pyelonephritis resulting from repeated previous UTI. In case RFTs are deranged, the test should be repeated on follow-up till the level stabilizes.

Urine routine examination is the most informative investigation, easily available, and affordable. Clear instructions should be regarding midstream clean catch urine sample for culture and sensitivity. In females, the perineal area should be washed with normal water. Labia separated by fingers, initial part of urine to be discarded, and the sample be collected from the flowing part of urine (midstream). In males, the prepuce should be retracted, the glans and tip of urethra cleaned with water, and initial part of urine to be discarded and the flowing part of urine collected.

Dipstick examination should be done with 10 parameter dipstick, which will give estimate about nitrite, leukocyte esterase, hematuria, proteinuria, pH, specific gravity, etc. (**Fig. 3**).

Microscopic examination will reveal the presence of pus cells, red blood cells (RBCs) (in case there is cystitis, papillary necrosis, acute pyelonephritis, etc.), bacteria, yeast cells, and crystals.

Not all cases of pyuria are due to UTI. The differentials of sterile pyuria include tuberculosis, previously/partially treated UTI, interstitial nephritis, glomerulonephritis (usually there is associated microscopic hematuria), STDs, fungal infections, inflammation

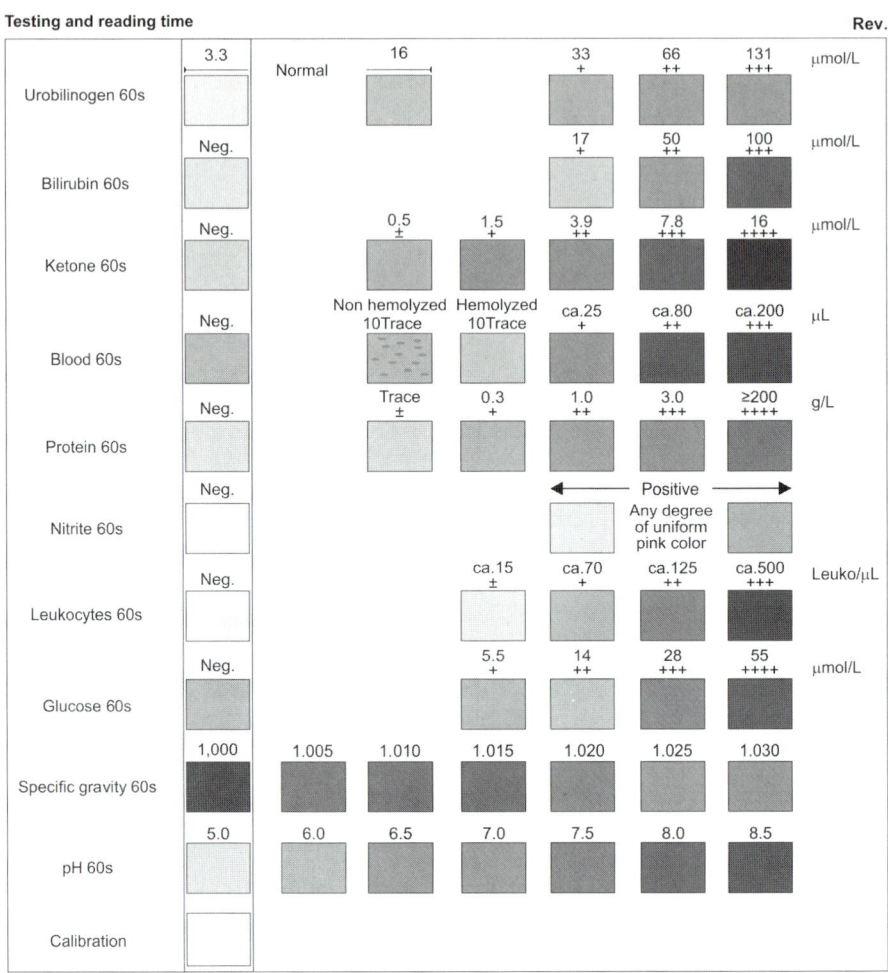

**FIG. 3:** Total 10 parameter urine dipstick. *(For color version, see Plate 5)*

in surrounding pelvic organs such as appendicitis, diverticulitis, balanitis, prostatitis, vaginitis, renal calculi, interstitial cystitis, rejection in cases of transplant, etc.

Usually a through history and physical examination help to point toward an underlying cause.

Radiological examination should include ultrasonography (USG) of kidney, ureter, and bladder (KUB), preferably whole abdomen with full bladder and postvoid residual urine (PVRU). PVRU is often missed. So, it should always be requested separately, especially if there are any obstructive voiding symptoms and history of incomplete voiding.

Uroflowmetry is a very useful investigation for the objective assessment of voiding pattern and it also has a role in documenting the improvement after initiation of treatment.

Postvoid residual urine should be done immediately after uroflowmetry. The urine flow curve is a bell-shaped graph and easy to interpret (**Figs. 4A to D**). It is noninvasive modality and usually available at centers with urology facility.

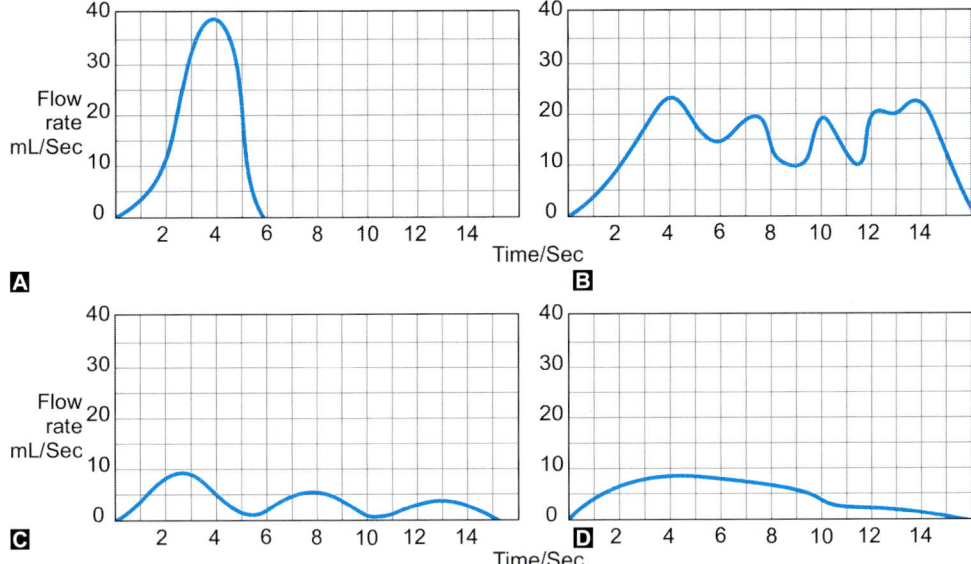

**FIGS. 4A TO D:** Graphic representation of various uroflow patterns. (A) Superflow commonly seen with poor urethral resistance. (B) Intermittent multiple peak pattern. (C) Intermittent interrupted pattern. (D) Abnormal flow rate characteristic of detrusor outlet obstruction.

Urodynamic studies help in detailed evaluation of bladder function and define the functional and structural abnormalities of the bladder (**Fig. 5**). However, it is invasive, not easily available, and costly. It should be performed after the adequate treatment of UTI otherwise during UTI it carries risk of bacteremia.

## PRINCIPLES OF MANAGEMENT

Antibiotics are the cornerstone of therapy but not the only thing in the treatment of UTI. Additional measures may include early voiding after sexual intercourse in females, adequate hydration, especially during travelling, etc., as women often drink less water to avoid urination at public places due to poor maintenance of toilets at many public places, especially in India. Maintenance of perineal hygiene and use of cotton undergarments are other suggested means, though there is no hard evidence. But these are easy to implement without any additional cost and therefore there is no harm in recommending these. Local ointments containing antibacterial, antifungal, and steroids may be used if there is local itching. The duration of the use may be restricted to 3 days as long-term and regular use may lead to atrophy of skin due to steroids and risk of emergence of resistance. Counseling for good glycemic control is very important, as it also helps to reduce the risk of further recurrences of UTI.

Bladder relaxant agents (e.g., darifenacin, solifenacin) may be required in case of storage voiding symptoms and there is often significant improvement in the quality of life. The side effects specially retention of urine and anticholinergic symptoms such as dryness of mouth may occur. Dryness of mouth may respond to reduction of the dose. Many patients may be able to discontinue these agents and may have symptom-free interval. In patients who had achieved good control, it may restart if symptoms recur. Expert urological

## SECTION 7: Nephrology

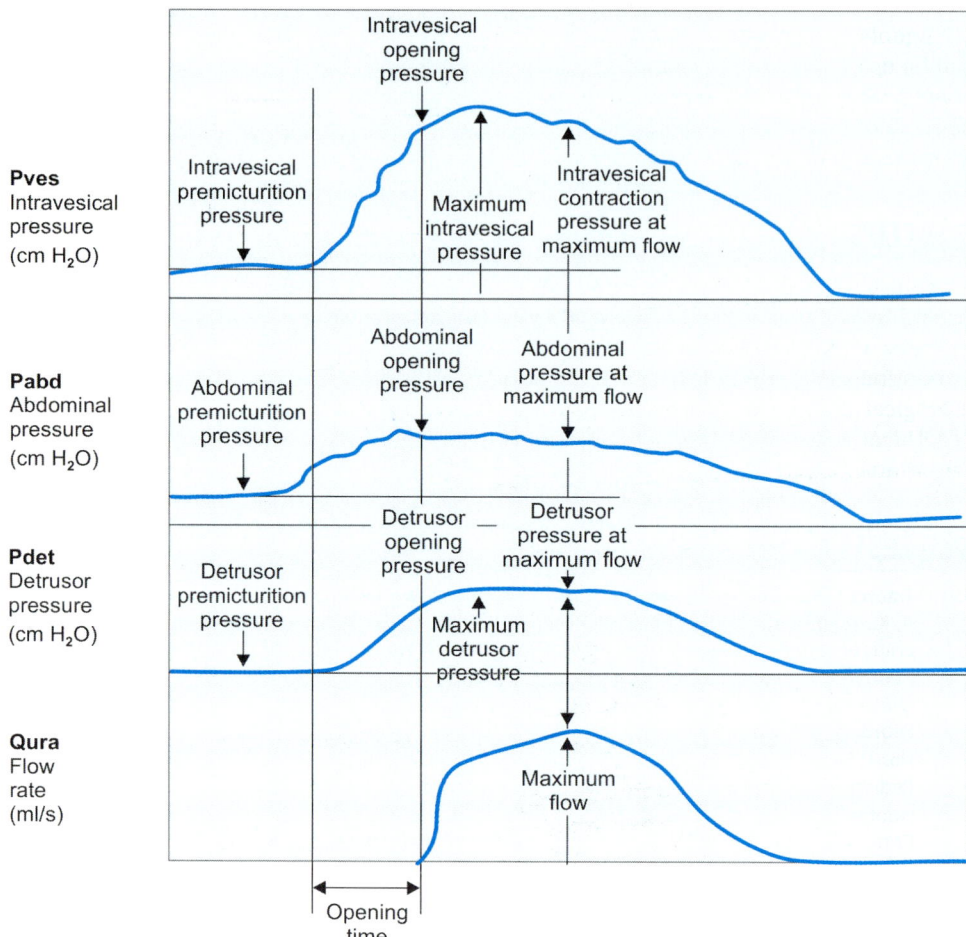

**FIG. 5:** Pressure flow study measurements.

evaluation and opinion should be sought in cases who do not respond. Cholinergic drugs (e.g., bethanechol) may be prescribed in cases with hypotonic bladder and may help to improve PVRU. The common side effects include excessive salivation, sweating, diarrhea, etc. Ideally, these agents should be used after documentation of the type of urological abnormality. Newer agents with effects restricted to the bladder are available with lesser incidence of systemic side effects and better patient tolerance.

Another important aspect is the choice of antibiotics. Most of the beta-lactams, aminoglycosides, fluoroquinolones (except moxifloxacin), and carbapenams achieve good concentration in urine. However, in patients with advanced CKD, the urinary concentration may be impaired and hence antibiotics such as nitrofurantoin may not be effective in the treatment of UTI in patients with estimated glomerular filtration rate (eGFR) <30 mL/min/1.73 m$^2$. Renal dose modification should be done as per creatinine clearance for antibiotics. For most of the practical purposes, the eGFR calculation may suffice as weight-based estimation that may be difficult in patients who may not be able to record weight and it may be confounded by presence of edema.

Agents such as cranberry and D-mannose have doubtful benefit. Urinary alkalizers can be used to control dysuria, but only after carefully ruling out some calculus diseases-related UTIs, e.g., Proteus infections in staghorn calculi, which exacerbates in alkaline pH. Adequate duration of therapy should be stressed. Suppressive prophylaxis with cotrimoxazole may help in some patients.

## CONCLUSION

To summarize, the management of UTI, particularly complicated and recurrent UTI should follow a systematic approach. Timely referral to an expert should be considered in cases with suspected structural or functional abnormalities of bladder. Thorough evaluation should include hematological, biochemical, microbiological, radiological, and urological assessment. Causes of pyuria other than UTI should be considered. Correlation of clinical profile with laboratory workup should be done. Patient education is very important.

## SUGGESTED READING

1. Trautner BW, Gupta K. Urinary tract infections, pyelonephritis and prostatitis. In: Longo D, Fauci A, Kasper D, Hauser S, Jameson J, Loscalzo J (Eds). Harrison's Principles of Internal Medicine, 18th edition. New York: McGraw-Hill Professional; 2011. p. 2800.
2. Centers for Disease Control and Prevention (CDC). (2019). Antibiotic Prescribing and Use in Doctor's Office. [online] Available from https://www.cdc.gov/antibiotic-use/community/. [Last accessed February, 2020].
3. Hari P, Srivastava RN. Urinary tract infections. In: Avner ED, Harmon WE, Niaudet P, Yoshikawa N (Eds). Pediatric Nephrology, 6th edition. Berlin Heidelberg: Springer-Verlag; 2009. p. 2063.
4. Hootan T. Urinary tract infections in adults. In: Johnson RJ, Feehally J, Floege J, Tonelli M (Eds). Comprehensive Clinical Nephrology, 6th edition. Canada: Elsevier; 2019. p. 1360.
5. Raja A, Hori S, Armitage JN. Hormonal manipulation of lower urinary tract symptoms secondary to benign prostatic obstruction. Indian J Urol. 2014;30(2):189-93.
6. Women's Health and Education Center (WHEC). (2009). Urodynamic Assessment: Voiding Studies. [online] Available from https://www.womenshealthsection.com/content/urog/urog013.php3. [Last accessed February, 2020].
7. Jacob CK, Alexender S. Principles of drug dosing and modifications in renal failure. In: Visveswaran RK (Ed). Prescribing Drugs in Renal Diseases. Philadelphia: Elsevier; 2005.

# CHAPTER 5

# Challenges of Renal Transplant in Females

*Suceena Alexander, Elenjickal Elias John, Santosh Varughese*

## ABSTRACT

The women when compared to males are deprived of a fair chance for the standard of care renal replacement therapy due to many reasons. The partiality faced by women in this patriarch world also reflects in the scenario of kidney transplantation worldwide, where women are most common donors but rarely recipients. Logistic issues such as higher risk of sensitization due to multiple pregnancies impair the scenario even further. The challenges faced by women continue post-transplant in the form of cautions before conception, poor pregnancy outcomes, and hurdles to breastfeeding. Transplant also narrows down the contraceptive choices for women. Even the donors can face difficult pregnancies postdonation.

## INTRODUCTION

Women face enormous challenges in kidney transplant compared to men, especially in developing countries such as India where economic, social, and cultural barriers are unfavorable toward them as compared to men. Majority of living kidney donors (LKDs) are women whereas they are overshadowed by men when it comes to receiving LKDs. This disparity is seen even in developed countries but is seemingly large in low-income countries.

## BARRIERS FOR KIDNEY TRANSPLANTATION

With more families becoming nuclear, spousal donations are one of the most common living donor kidney transplants in India. Pregnancy induces alloantibodies in women and greater the number of live births, higher is the frequency of sensitization with offspring-specific human leukocyte antigen (HLA) antibodies. There was a 3-fold reduction in offspring and spousal living kidney donation in women with a history of pregnancy. So, women face a great challenge due to pregnancy-induced incompatibility with spouse, widening the gender disparity among kidney transplant recipients. Some of the options available for overcoming this biological challenge is through desensitization prior to kidney transplant or thorough paired kidney exchanges depending on the availability of donors, cost of the desensitization procedures, and long-term graft outcome in various centers. Compounding this biological barrier, there are social, cultural, and economic disparities that are disadvantageous to women when they need LKDs.

## CONTRACEPTION FOLLOWING TRANSPLANTATION

Most popular methods recommended by transplant physicians are barrier contraceptives. Intrauterine devices are less effective due to immunosuppressive drugs and more prone for infections. Among oral contraceptive pills, progestin-only pills are safer, though combined pills have been used in women with well-controlled blood pressures. Post-transplant contraception should be discussed before transplantation in women of reproductive age.

## PREGNANCY OUTCOMES

Proportion of pregnant women having live births is around 70–75% and is higher than the general population in various studies. This may be because of selection bias resulting in healthier women opting for pregnancy after kidney transplant and better postdelivery care. Also, the live birth rate was calculated differently in various studies.

Maternal complications in the peripartum period are high and include abortions, miscarriages, stillbirths, ectopic pregnancies, preeclampsia, gestational diabetes, pregnancy-induced hypertension, cesarean section, and preterm deliveries.

The best time of conception in renal allograft recipients is usually 1–2 years post-transplant according to the American Society of Transplantation, but the European Best Practice Guidelines advise waiting for at least 2 years post-transplant. Pregnancy could be considered safe about 2 years after transplantation in women with good renal function, without proteinuria, without arterial hypertension, with no evidence of ongoing rejection, and with normal allograft ultrasound. If complications (usually hypertension, renal deterioration, and/or rejection) occur before 28 weeks, then successful obstetric outcome is reduced by 20%.

Pregnancy after transplantation should be considered a high-risk pregnancy and should be monitored by both an obstetrician and the transplant physician. Pregnancy should be diagnosed as early as possible. The principal risks are infection, proteinuria, anemia, arterial hypertension and acute rejection for the mother, and prematurity and low birth weight for the fetus. Pregnant women and transplanted patients are at increased risk of infections, especially bacterial urinary tract infections and acute pyelonephritis of the graft. Vaginal delivery is recommended, but cesarean section is required in at least 50% of cases. Delivery should occur in a specialized center.

## BREASTFEEDING

Low birth weight and preterm deliveries occur frequently in transplant recipients and breastfeeding can potentially reduce the risk of sepsis and necrotizing enterocolitis in the perinatal period and help in the overall growth of the infant.

Breastfeeding is the recommended norm in infants of healthy women, but is it any different in women postrenal allograft? It is well known that immunosuppressive drugs are present in varying amounts in breast milk. But what is more critical is whether the amount of drug present in the breast milk and absorbed by the infant has any adverse consequences on the infant? A three-pronged approach has been suggested to circumvent the complete stop to breastfeeding. Firstly, if the immunosuppressive drugs are known to be toxic without a safety threshold such as mycophenolic acid, then breastfeeding should not be advised. Secondly, if the immunosuppressive drugs are known to be safe at low or undetectable quantities in the infant's blood, such as cyclosporine, tacrolimus, steroids, azathioprine, etc., then monitoring of serum levels for these drugs in infants after 1–2 weeks of breastfeeding may help decide on continuation of breastfeeding. Thirdly, if immunosuppressive drugs have unknown safety profile such as sirolimus, everolimus, belatacept, etc., then caution is advised.

## KIDNEY DONOR AND PREGNANCY

Kidney donors are left with one functioning kidney which then compensates by glomerular hyperfiltration that may predispose them to hypertension long-term. Pregnancy further accentuates these changes and so, development of preeclampsia can have negative long-term consequences for both the mother and the baby. It has been shown that fetal and maternal outcomes in postkidney donation pregnancies are comparable to the rates in the general population. But, donating a kidney places a woman at a higher risk for complications compared to predonation pregnancies.

The Food and Drug Administration's categories for drugs in pregnancy are listed in **Table 1**.

## IMMUNOSUPPRESSIVE DRUGS AND GENDER DISPARITY

There are major differences in how immunosuppressive drugs are handled by men and women and reflect the need to consider gender, especially in the dosing guidelines of drugs with narrow therapeutic indices. Many immunosuppressive drugs used in the postkidney transplant setting such as cyclosporine, tacrolimus, mycophenolic acid, everolimus, etc., undergo therapeutic drug monitoring, and so, sex-related dosing adjustment will probably help in reaching therapeutic ranges quickly. But, for drugs such as prednisolone and azathioprine, sex-related dosing may help improve the pharmacokinetics and pharmacodynamics. The 6-mercaptopurine, which is a metabolite

**TABLE 1:** Food and Drug Administration's pregnancy categories for immunosuppressive drugs commonly used in transplant.

| Drugs | Pregnancy categories |
| --- | --- |
| Corticosteroids | B or C |
| Azathioprine | D |
| Cyclosporine | C |
| Tacrolimus | C |
| Mycophenolate mofetil | D |
| Enteric-coated mycophenolate sodium | D |
| Sirolimus | C |
| Belatacept | C |
| Antithymocyte globulin | C |
| Muromonab-CD3 | C |
| Basiliximab | B |

of azathioprine, is inactivated faster in men as compared to women, pointing to lower dose requirements in women. Prednisolone has lower clearance leading to increased exposure in women.

## GRAFT OUTCOME

Reports in pediatric transplants show inferior graft survival among girls compared to boys. In adult kidney transplants, the outcome in women is determined by the age of the recipients and the sex of the donors. With men donors, women recipients of all age group had inferior graft outcome compared to men recipients. With women donors, only women in the 14–15 age groups had inferior graft outcome compared to their men counterparts, whereas women aged ≥45 years had better graft outcomes than their men counterparts. It has been also reported that women have a higher risk of acute rejection, but reduced risk of chronic allograft injury compared to men. A meta-analysis done on gender mismatch and graft survival showed that women recipients had worse short-term graft survival, but the best long-term graft survival.

The gender differences in kidney allograft outcomes have several explanations. In general, the humoral and the cellular immune activation is much vigorous in women due to the immune enhancing effects of estrogen compared to the immune suppressing effects of androgen in men and this activity decreases when women reach menopause. Secondly, medication adherence varies between the genders. Thirdly, the small body size and lower metabolic needs may confer better graft outcomes in women compared to men. Fourthly, immune recognition of sexually determined minor histocompatibility antigens (H-Y antigens) may be a potential cause for inferior graft outcomes in women recipients of men donor kidneys. Lastly, at least in the developing world, there are significant dropouts among women than men for post-transplant follow-up care.

## CONCLUSION

Renal transplantation in the women is full of challenges from inception to post-transplant care. Unfortunately, both the society and nature's norms have been unfair to the fairer sex in this regard.

## SUGGESTED READING

1. Hart A, Smith JM, Skeans MA, Gustafson SK, Stewart DE, Cherikh WS, et al. OPTN/SRTR 2015 annual data report: Kidney. Am J Transplant. 2017;17 (Suppl 1):21-116.
2. HoÃànger G, Fornaro I, Granado C, Tiercy JM, HoÃàsli I, Schaub S. Frequency and determinants of pregnancy-induced child-specific sensitization. Am J Transplant. 2013;13(3):746-53.
3. Bromberger B, Spragan D, Hashmi S, Morrison A, Thomasson A, Nazarian S, et al. Pregnancy-induced sensitization promotes sex disparity in living donor kidney transplantation. J Am Soc Nephrol. 2017;28(10):3025-33.
4. August P, Suthanthiran M. Sex and Kidney Transplantation: Why Can't a Woman Be More Like a Man? J Am Soc Nephrol. 2017;28(10):2829-31.
5. McKay DB, Josephson MA, Armenti VT, August P, Coscia LA, Davis CL, et al. Reproduction and transplantation: report on the AST consensus conference on reproductive issues and transplantation. Am J Transplant. 2005;5(7):1592-9.
6. Coscia LA, Constantinescu S, Moritz MJ, Frank AM, Ramirez CB, Maley WR, et al. Report from the National Transplantation Pregnancy Registry (NTPR): outcomes of pregnancy after transplantation. Clin Transpl. 2010;2(3):65-85.

7. Shah S, Venkatesan RL, Gupta A, Sanghavi MK, Welge J, Johansen R, et al. Pregnancy outcomes in women with kidney transplant: Meta-analysis and systematic review. BMC Nephrol. 2019;20(1):24.
8. EBPG Expert Group on Renal Transplantation. European best practice guidelines for renal transplantation. Section IV: Long-term management of the transplant recipient. IV.10. Pregnancy in renal transplant recipients. Nephrol Dial Transplant. 2002;17 (Suppl 4):50-5.
9. Davison JM, Bailey DJ. Pregnancy following renal transplantation. J Obstet Gynaecol Res. 2003;29(4):227-33.
10. Constantinescu S, Pai A, Coscia LA, Davison JM, Moritz MJ, Armenti VT. Breast-feeding after transplantation. Best Pract Res Clin Obstet Gynaecol. 2014;28(8):1163-73.
11. Thiagarajan KM, Arakali SR, Mealey KJ, Cardonick EH, Gaughan WJ, Davison JM, et al. Safety considerations: breastfeeding after transplant. Prog Transplant. 2013;23(2):137-46.
12. Ibrahim HN, Akkina SK, Leister E, Gillingham K, Cordner G, Guo H, et al. Pregnancy outcomes after kidney donation. Am J Transplant. 2009;9(4):825-34.
13. Reisaeter AV, Røislien J, Henriksen T, Irgens LM, Hartmann A. Pregnancy and birth after kidney donation: the Norwegian experience. Am J Transplant. 2009;9(4):820-4.
14. Momper JD, Misel ML, McKay DB. Sex differences in transplantation. Transplant Rev (Orlando). 2017;31(3):145-50.
15. Foster BJ, Dahhou M, Zhang X, Platt RW, Samuel SM, Hanley JA. Association between age and graft failure rates in young kidney transplant recipients. Transplantation. 2011;92(11):1237-43.
16. Kaboré R, Couchoud C, Macher MA, Salomon R, Ranchin B, Lahoche A, et al. Age dependent risk of graft failure in young kidney transplant recipients. Transplantation. 2017;101(6):1327-35.
17. Lepeytre F, Dahhou M, Zhang X, Bouquemont J, Sapir-Pichhadze R, Cardinal H, et al. Sex differences in kidney graft failure risk differ by age. J Am Soc Nephrol. 2017;28(10):3014-23.
18. Meier-Kriesche HU, Ojo AO, Leavey SF, Hanson JA, Leichtman AB, Magee JC, et al. Gender differences in the risk for chronic renal allograft failure. Transplantation. 2001;71(3):429-32.
19. Zhou JY, Cheng J, Huang HF, Shen Y, Jiang Y, Chen JH. The effect of donor-recipient gender mismatch on short- and long-term graft survival in kidney transplantation: a systematic review and meta-analysis. Clin Transplant. 2013;27(5):764-71.
20. Bouman A, Heineman MJ, Faas MM. Sex hormones and the immune response in humans. Hum Reprod Update. 2005;11(4):411-23.
21. Frazier PA, Davis-Ali SH, Dahl KE. Correlates of noncompliance among renal transplant recipients. Clin Transplant. 1994;8(6):550-7.
22. Denhaerynck K, Steiger J, Bock A, Schäfer-Keller P, Köfer S, Thannberger N, et al. Prevalence and risk factors of non-adherence with immunosuppressive medication in kidney transplant patients. Am J Transplant. 2007;7(1):108-16.
23. Oh CK, Lee BM, Jeon KO, Kim HJ, Pelletier SJ, Kim SI, et al. Gender-related differences of renal mass supply and metabolic demand after living donor kidney transplantation. Clin Transplant. 2006;20(2):163-70.

# SECTION 8

# Pulmonology

SECTION EDITORS
Shibba Takkar Chhabra, Akashdeep Singh

# CHAPTER 1

# Pulmonology: Salient Issues in Women

*Battu Chaithanya, Jayasri Helen Gali*

## ABSTRACT

Female gender impacts the prevalence and presentation of various respiratory diseases such as asthma, chronic obstructive pulmonary disease (COPD), pulmonary arterial hypertension (PAH), pulmonary thromboembolism (PTE), lymphangioleiomyomatosis (LAM), and autoimmune diseases. Various factors such as anatomical, genetic, environmental, occupational, sociocultural differences in women attribute to the varied presentation of respiratory diseases. Women are at higher risk of exposure to household air pollutants, especially due to biomass fuels as they are more homebound due to their family and domestic commitments which leads to COPD on long-term. Increasing trends of smoking have been observed in women in developing countries causing decline in respiratory health in women. Certain respiratory diseases such as LAM, postpartum hypertension (HTN), thoracic endometriosis (TES), Meigs syndrome, amniotic fluid embolism, and tocolytic pulmonary edema occur exclusively in women and are often missed or diagnosis is delayed unless there is adequate clinical acumen to suspect and investigate these diseases. Respiratory diseases such as asthma, connective tissue disease (CTD)-associated interstitial lung diseases (ILDs), pulmonary embolism, pulmonary artery HTN, COPD in nonsmokers occur with increased frequency in women. Tuberculosis (TB) poses special diagnostic and therapeutic challenges in pregnant women and has to be carefully addressed. Management of drug resistant TB in pregnancy poses great risk to both the mother and fetus as most of the second-line drugs are contraindicated in pregnancy, safety of newer drugs such as bedaquiline and delamanid are not known.

## INTRODUCTION

Gender has shown marked impact on the prevalence of several lung diseases, such as lung cancer, bronchial asthma, chronic obstructive pulmonary disease (COPD), pulmonary arterial hypertension (PAH), lymphangioleiomyomatosis (LAM), and various autoimmune diseases. Pulmonary diseases pose a challenge in women as they affect women differently and with varying degrees of severity than in men. This disparity may be attributed to the unique biological cycle of women and also in part to anatomic, genetic, environmental, occupational, sociocultural aspects of women.

The purpose of this chapter is to give an overview on the unexplored territory of respiratory diseases, which manifest differently in women.

# FACTORS ATTRIBUTING TO INCREASING RESPIRATORY DISEASES IN WOMEN

## Developmental and Anatomical Factors

Presence of estradiol (E2) in female fetuses contributes to rapid lung maturation, resulting in smaller size of lungs in females. Alveolar volume and number of alveoli per unit area do not differ in both genders. Though few differences in airway caliber exist, with women having better FEF rates, high FEV1/ FVC ratios, it adds a little to the functional advantage.

Predominant changes in anatomy occur during pregnancy. Mucosal changes consist of hyperemia, edema, and hyper secretion of upper airway, predominantly during third trimester. Airway changes are usually confined to larger airways, mediated by estrogen, leading to tissue hydration, edema through an increase in hyaluronic acid, capillary congestion, mucous gland hypertrophy, and hyperplasia.

## Hormonal Factors (Progesterone and Estrogen)

Female sex hormones have a significant impact on the respiratory system.

### Progesterone

Progesterone is a respiratory stimulant, stimulates breathing at the level of peripheral chemoreceptors. Hyperventilation and reduced upper airway collapsibility during sleep occur during luteal phase of menstrual cycle when progesterone levels are high. Hypothesis suggests that progesterone and its metabolites can bind to GABA-A receptors and modulate their function.

### Estrogen

Lung is the target tissue for estrogen, as it expresses estrogen receptor (ER) subtypes, ERα and ERβ. Estrogen supports cell growth via interaction with both receptors by directly binding to estrogen response elements or through nongenomic pathways. Together they can contribute to obliterative lesions via cell proliferation.

Reactive oxygen species (ROS) generated from redox cycling of both stilbene and catechol estrogens can act as signaling messengers that are also involved in cell growth.

## Environmental Factors: Household Air Pollution

Household air pollution (HAP) is a leading cause of disability-adjusted life years in Southeast Asia and the third leading cause globally. It is a daunting problem in India, as many rural households still lack access to cleaner cooking options. Women are significantly at higher risk of exposure to various household air pollutants as they are more home bound due to their family and domestic commitments, especially cooking, leading to significant and chronic exposures.

More than 60 sources have been identified to be causing household pollution worldwide. As far as India is concerned, biomass fuel and tobacco remain the major sources of household pollutants.

## Household Air Pollution Secondary to Cooking

The fuel used for cooking and heating food remains major source of HAP in developing nations such as India. It is not unusual to see the use of biomass fuel such as crop residue, animal dung, wood, and charcoal being used for cooking purposes. Rather around half of the world's population is considered to be using this source. It will be surprising to note that this accounts for burning of around 2 million kilograms of biomass per day. Understandably, extremely high levels of pollutants and particulate matter such as carbon particles, iron, cadmium, silica, lead, phenols and free radicals, carbon monoxide (CO), nitrogen dioxide, sulfur dioxide, formaldehyde, hydrocarbon complexes, and other inorganic and organic substances [polycyclic aromatic hydrocarbons (PAHs), volatile organic compounds, and chlorinated dioxins] have been found in these households.

## Household Air Pollution Secondary to Tobacco Smoke

The exposure to smoking can be first hand (smokers themselves) or second hand (when other occupants smoke) or third hand (due to the presence of smoke particulate residue). It is prudent to note that the smoke particles remain suspended in the environment for a substantial time even after the primary smoker exits the premises. Homebound individuals, who are usually women, are hence much prone to be affected by this described type of smoke.

## Effect of Household Air Pollution on Women

*Young females*: While COPD and lung cancer are well-recognized complications, the oxidative stress caused by these pollutants also has effects on fertility. It may not just cause infertility or reduced fertility but also affects the zygote quality. Even PCOD and insulin resistance has been implicated to smoke particulates.

*Pregnant women*: The risks of eclampsia and preeclampsia increases (around 2-fold) in the pregnant women exposed to smoke produced from biomass and solid fuels.

# Sociocultural Effects

## Increasing Smoking Trends in Women

Gender also impacts consumption levels and prevalence rates of smoking, with women generally smoking fewer cigarettes. Few reasons accounting for gender lag include social processes such as proscriptive norms against smoking uptake by women, ascription of negative cultural stereotypes to women who smoke, and a strong socially circulated awareness on incompatibility with women's reproductive roles. Despite such powerful social barriers, consistent and powerful gender targeted advertising and marketing by tobacco industries over the past century has led to the pervasive uptake of smoking among girls and women in middle and higher income countries.

Women are at increased risk of developing more smoking-related adverse effects compared to men with same pack years because of smaller size of female lungs, which retain more amount of smoke per cigarette and delayed metabolism of nicotine.

## Effects of Smoking in Women

*Pregnancy*: Risk of stillbirth, small for gestational babies, neonatal death, and sudden infant death syndrome (SIDS) is high in off springs of mothers who smoke. Breastfeeding is less common or of shorter duration among women smokers.

*Reproduction and menstrual function*: Primary and secondary infertility, delay in conceiving, early menopause, and dysmenorrhea are commonly seen.

*Cardiovascular diseases*: Increased risk of cardiovascular diseases including coronary heart disease (CHD), ischemic stroke, and subarachnoid hemorrhage. Women smokers on oral contraceptives have a particularly elevated risk of CHD.

*Respiratory system*: Women smokers have markedly increased risks of developing and dying of COPD. Risk increases with the number of cigarettes smoked per day and higher in women compared to men with same pack years. Smoking is directly linked to 80% of COPD deaths in women each year. There is an increased risk of developing lung cancer than men.

## Occupational

Urbanization is creating more career opportunities for woman. Women are choosing both industrial and nonindustrial occupations with increased occupational exposure to various agents, resulting in rise in occupational lung diseases. Exposure to passive smoking at work places is also leading to increased tobacco-related complications in women.

## WOMEN AND RESPIRATORY DISEASES

Due to various reasons cited above, women are vulnerable to develop certain types of respiratory diseases uniquely and other with increased frequency and varying severity.

## Respiratory Diseases Which Occur Exclusively in Women

### Lymphangioleiomyomatosis

Lymphangioleiomyomatosis is a rare multisystem disorder that mostly affects young women. Sporadic LAM is LAM without tuberous sclerosis complex (TSC), while TSC-LAM refers to LAM that occurs in patients with TSC.

### *Pathogenesis*

Excessive proliferation of LAM cells occurs due to mutations in TSC genes, in particular, *TSC2*. Additional factors that may contribute to cellular proliferation in sporadic LAM include aberrant stimulation of LAM cell growth by estrogen and other growth factors.

The presenting symptoms and signs of LAM vary depending upon the organs affected by the disease. Patients may present with either pulmonary or extra pulmonary symptoms, especially pertaining to renal angiomyolipomas (AMLs) and the lymphatic vasculature.

### *Clinical Presentation (Table 1)*

*Evaluation*:
- *Clinical*: Should be suspected in women with a spontaneous pneumothorax or unexplained dyspnea, chylous effusion especially nonsmoking women of reproductive age.
- *High-resolution computed tomography (HRCT) chest*: Diffuse, round, bilateral well-defined thin-walled cysts, which are uniform in size, with no lobar predilection, typically devoid of internal structures (e.g., centrilobular vessels or septae) or consistent relationships with adjacent vessels, airways, or interlobular septae.

- *Pulmonary function test (PFT)*: Reveals either obstructive or restrictive or mixed.
- *Thoracentesis*: For chylous effusion
- Vascular endothelial growth factor D Levels > 800 pg/mL
- Video-assisted thoracoscopic surgery (VATS) lung biopsy if initial tests are inconclusive.

### Treatment and Prognosis

*Sirolimus*: The key treatment for parenchymal lung disease due to sporadic LAM is inhibition of the mechanistic target of rapamycin (mTOR) with sirolimus. It is indicated for symptomatic patients with abnormal lung function ($FEV_1$ <70%), evidence of rapidly progressive disease, or problematic chylous accumulations.

*Lung transplantation*: May be the only option for patients with advanced LAM or in those refractory to mTOR inhibitors.

*General*: Minimize exogenous estrogen.
Avoid pregnancy and use nonestrogen-based birth control measures

## Postpartum Pulmonary Hypertension

Although rare, it may be because of either high hemodynamic demands impairing a ventricle with little reserve, its subsequent appearance at the time of delivery or a previously asymptomatic pulmonary hypertension (PH) period that was triggered by physiological stress of labor or because of hyper coagulation, placental hypoxia or amniotic fluid embolism. Postpartum PAH carries a bad prognosis, especially in nonvasoreactive patients. They may end up in lung transplantation after failed medical management with pulmonary vasodilators.

## Thoracic Endometriosis

It is a rare disease characterized by the presence of functioning endometrial tissue in pleura, lung parenchyma, airways, and diaphragm. TES encompasses mainly four clinical entities.
1. Catamenial pneumothorax (CP)
2. Catamenial hemothorax (CHt)
3. Catamenial hemoptysis (CH)
4. Lung nodules

### Etiopathogenesis

Various hypotheses have been postulated:
- Open connection between the atmosphere and the peritoneal cavity during menstruation allows air to migrate into the thoracic cavity through diaphragmatic fenestrations and porosities.
- Endometrial tissue causes diaphragmatic defects.
- Metastatic spreading of endometriosis through the uterine veins into the venous system.
- Prostaglandin F2 which can be found in the plasma of some women during menstruation may destroy alveolar tissue due to vasospasm, leading to pneumothorax.

### Clinical Presentation

The most common presentation of TES is CP, which accounts for almost 80% of cases. Less frequent clinical entities include CHt (14%), CH (5%), and lung nodules. CP is defined

**TABLE 1:** Clinical presentation of lymphangioleiomyomatosis (LAM).

| General features | Pulmonary | Others |
|---|---|---|
| Premenopausal | • Fatigue (2/3rd) | • Renal angiomyolipomas |
|  | • Progressive dyspnea (2/3rd) | • Lymphatic |
| *Average age*: Mid 30s and 40s | • Spontaneous pneumothorax (1/3rd) | • Chylothorax, Chyloperitoneum, |
|  |  | • Chyluria |
|  | • Pleural effusion (1/4th) (chylous effusions) | • Chylopericardium |
|  |  | • Chylometrorrhea |
| May present in patients on ERT or pregnant women | • Chest pain (<15%) | • Chylocorporrhea |
|  | • Cough or phlegm (<15%) | • Lymphatic pulmonary congestion |
|  | • Pulmonary hypertension (<7%) | • Lymphangioleiomyomatosis |

as spontaneous, recurrent pneumothorax of women in reproductive age group occurring within 72 hours from the onset of menstruation. Though it is typically cyclic, noncyclic recurrences occurring in the immediate premenstrual period or ovulatory phase have also been reported. In most cases, CP is right sided with the left side being rarely involved.

### Diagnosis

The delays in the diagnosis are often due to low index of suspicion. While it is not unusual to see delays up till 8 months. Cyclic constellations of symptoms may be considered pathognomonic. It is important to rule out malignancy, infection, and other pathologies by carrying our relevant investigations such as chest radiology, bronchoscopy or thoracentesis. The diagnostic yield is however, variable with inconsistent findings.

Video-assisted thoracoscopic surgery is the gold standard modality for both, definitive diagnosis and surgical treatment of CP. Diaphragmatic abnormalities (fenestrations or endometriosis, alone or combined) are the most commonly described lesions (38.8%), followed by endometriosis of the visceral pleura (29.6%), discrete lesions, such as bullae, blebs, and scarring (23.1%), or no findings (8.5%) are noted.

Diaphragmatic fenestrations range from a few millimeters to 2 cm. Endometrial deposits in both the diaphragm and pleura have a similar appearance and range from a few millimeters to 1 cm. Their color ranges from violet to brown, depending on the day of menstrual cycle.

Performance of a combined VATS and laparoscopy procedure in a single session is another diagnostic approach to assess both the thoracic cavity as well as the pelvis and subdiaphragmatic region.

### Management

In patients developing recurrent pneumothorax despite effective hormone suppression with leuprolide 11.25 mg (administered intramuscularly 3 monthly), a detailed surgical exploration is advised in order to inspect and close the visible/identifiable defects. Ethinyl estradiol and norethisterone acetate low-dose formulations with selective serotonin reuptake inhibitor (SSRIs) can be used to avoid and treat mood changes due to hormonal suppression.

### Meigs Syndrome

It is defined as triad of benign ovarian tumor, ascites, and pleural effusion that resolves after resection of tumor. Approximately 70% of pleural effusions are right sided, 15% left sided, and 15% are bilateral, and occur due to filtration of interstitial fluid into peritoneum through the ovarian tumor capsule, which then enters pleural cavity through the transdiaphragmatic pores or lymphatic channels. It is uncommon before third decade and incidence increases thereafter and peaks at seventh decade.

It is a diagnosis of exclusion. Ascitic and pleural fluids are similar and can be either exudative or transudative. Tumor size (>10 cm) is an important factor for the formation of fluid than the histological type of tumor.

## Amniotic Fluid Embolism

It is one of the gravest complications of pregnancy, where the amniotic fluid, fetal cells, hair, and other debris enter the maternal pulmonary circulation resulting in cardiovascular failure. It is exceedingly rare and occurs in about 1 in 8,000 to 1 in 80,000 deliveries.

Though it can occur in healthy women, certain risk factors such as older maternal age, multiparity, eclampsia, placenta previa, induction of labor, C-section, and intense contractions during labor have been identified. It typically occurs during labor, soon after vaginal or cesarean delivery or during dilatation and evacuation procedures and is associated with very high mortality rates.

Symptoms are cough, dyspnea, hypotension, cyanosis, fetal bradycardia, acute PH, and coagulopathy.

Basic investigations are lung scan, serum tryptase, and zinc coproporphyrin levels.

Treatment is mainly supportive; however, exchange transfusion, extracorporeal membrane oxygenation (ECMO), and uterine artery embolization can be done.

## Tocolytic Pulmonary Edema

Tocolytics are drugs used to prevent preterm labor as they suppress premature uterine contractions and cause smooth muscle relaxation. The commonly used agents are ritodrine, terbutaline, salbutamol, isoxsuprine, etc., which have relatively specific b2 action but also can cause cardiovascular effects which can cause pulmonary edema. Tocolytic pulmonary edema typically occurs during oral or intravenous use or within 24 hours after discontinuation of β2 agonists. Women with high-risk pregnancies such as multipara, cardiac disease, steroid usage, etc., are at high-risk.

They present with dyspnea, cough with pink frothy sputum, bilateral crackles, and normal cardiac examination.

The close differentials are amniotic fluid or air embolism, sepsis, preeclampsia with pulmonary edema, and peripartum cardiomyopathy.

Treatment is oxygen supplementation under close monitoring and invasive ventilation, if required. The response to treatment is usually rapid, rarely requires mechanical ventilation.

# Respiratory Diseases Which Occur with Increased Frequency in Women

## Connective Tissue Disease-associated Interstitial Lung Diseases

Connective tissue diseases are a group of diseases characterized by circulating autoantibodies and systemic manifestations considered to be related to autoimmune-mediated organ damage. The spectrum of CTD encompasses rheumatoid arthritis (RA), systemic sclerosis (SSc), systemic lupus erythematosus, primary Sjögren's syndrome, inflammatory idiopathic myopathy (dermatomyositis, polymyositis, myositis associated with antisynthetase antibodies), and mixed CTD, each of them with international consensus diagnostic criteria. The autoimmune diseases are more common in women than in men. The actual prevalence ranges from as high as 10–15 females for each male for systemic lupus erythematosus to four females for every male with RA.

Interstitial lung disease can occur in any of the CTD with varying frequency and severity.

Interstitial lung diseases occur in 15% of all patients with CTDs, with higher rates in certain conditions such as SSc and RA, and they are associated with varying rates of mortality.

The risk of CTD-ILDs appears to be higher in women <50 years of age. Any patient with ILD who is younger than 50 years and who are females should be screened for CTDs.

Management includes treating primary connective tissue disorder along with addition of antifibrotics in certain scenarios.

## Pulmonary Artery Hypertension

The PAH predominantly affects women; they are 1.8 times more likely to be affected compared to men. Heritable PAH and idiopathic PAH occur twice as frequently in females compared to males. Similarly, PAH associated with CTD is reported to occur in a female-to-male ratio of 3.8:1. In addition, women with SSc are eight times more likely than men to suffer from PAH.

Estrogen has pro-proliferative properties that have been associated with reduced expression of BMPR2 in patients with PAH, regardless of their genotype, have also demonstrated that the presence of estrogen predisposes to PAH.

### Pregnancy Counseling

Pregnancy is ill advised and contraindicated in PAH due to high maternal and fetal mortality. Maternal survival and fetal outcomes are noted to be worse in patients with severe PAH compared to those with mild disease, with right heart failure (RHF) being the main cause of poor outcomes. Pregnancy is associated with physiologic changes that increase pulmonary flow, such as increased circulating volume and cardiac output. Unlike normal pulmonary vasculature, the remodeled vasculature of a patient with PAH cannot accommodate and compensate for the increased pulmonary blood flow. Labor and childbirth cause further volume shifts and resultant hemodynamic changes that add stress to the already compromised right ventricle in PAH patients, resulting in worsening PH and RHF. Patients and their families should be counseled regarding contraception and the need to avoid pregnancy as soon as PAH is diagnosed. Further assessment to determine individual risk during pregnancy should be conducted at a PH center experienced in managing pregnant women with PAH.

### Contraceptive Methods

Hormonal contraception is available in progestin-only or combined estrogen and progestin formulation. Use of contraceptives containing estrogen is relatively contraindicated in patients with PAH due to the increased risk of venous thromboembolism (VTE) associated with their use. Given that pulmonary embolism can be fatal in the setting of pre-existing RV dysfunction, estrogen-containing contraceptives are avoided in PAH. Progestin-only contraception, however, is a suitable alternative for patients who cannot use permanent methods of contraception. Progestin-only contraception is available in the form of pills, injections, implants, and intrauterine devices (IUDs), although injections are generally avoided in PAH due to the increased risk of VTE (**Fig. 1**).

Several barrier methods including diaphragms and cervical caps can be used in patients with PAH. However, given the high failure rate of these methods, they are not recommended as the only method of contraception in PAH patients.

Since no temporary form of contraception is 100% effective, some PH centers favor permanent contraception such as tubal ligation or device implantation into the fallopian tube for their patients. These procedures require careful assessment and evaluation regarding the modes of anesthesia and surgical approach and should be done in a centre with a multidisciplinary PH team.

Despite counseling, patients with PAH may choose to become pregnant, or those with no prior diagnosis may present with an initial diagnosis of PAH during pregnancy. In either condition, elective termination of pregnancy should be offered regardless of their functional class. With the overall high-risk in these patients, it is advised that therapeutic abortion be carried out at an experienced PH centre. The procedure is safest when carried out in the first trimester but can be performed during the second trimester until fetal viability is achieved.

If patients refuse termination, it is imperative that care be transitioned to a team of specialists that include a PH specialist, obstetrician, intensivist, and neonatologist at an experienced PH center. Close follow-up is advised to monitor the fetus for appropriate growth and the mother for worsening PH, with the mother also receiving regular echocardiograms. Concurrent evaluation for lung transplantation, especially in high-risk patients, should be conducted as it may be warranted emergently in the event of decompensation. If indicated and required, early delivery after the second trimester should be considered in high-risk patients.

It is essential to treat pregnant PAH patients with PAH-specific medications. As endothelin receptor antagonists (ERAs) have teratogenic side effects, their use during pregnancy is contraindicated in patients with PAH. Once an appropriate regimen is determined, it is vital to continue monitoring and making adjustments to the dose since certain physiologic changes and complications of pregnancy can affect the absorption and bioavailability of these medication.

## Bronchial Asthma

Bronchial asthma affects about 300 million people worldwide, asthma incidence and severity are higher in women than in men, and highest in women between the 4th and 6th decade. However, during childhood boys have nearly twice the risk of developing asthma over girls which shifts to female predominance in adulthood and these gender-based disparities fade in elderly.

The mechanisms for this gender differences are not fully understood, but are mostly hormonal and due to differences in lung capacity. Sex hormones have an impact on the asthma symptoms and progression. Estrogen promotes bronchial hyper reactivity. Women have more marked symptoms during various life stages such as menstruation, pregnancy, and menopause.

During pregnancy, it is known that about one-third of women show improvement in asthma symptoms, one-third show no change, and one-third show deterioration. Exacerbation and poor asthma control during pregnancy are due to mechanical or hormonal changes or due to reduction or stopping of asthma medications due to various concerns. Optimal control of asthma is vital during pregnancy as both symptom control of pregnant mother and the fetal oxygenation should be attained. Uncontrolled asthma has deleterious effects on mother (preeclampsia) and fetus (preterm delivery, low birth weight, increased perinatal mortality).

Treatment of asthma during pregnancy poses a great challenge due to various myths linked with usage of inhalers especially with steroids. The advantages of active treatment of asthma in pregnancy far outweigh the risks of controller or reliever medications. All inhaled medications and theophylline can be used safely in pregnancy.

## Chronic Obstructive Pulmonary Disease

Chronic obstructive pulmonary disease was previously a common disease among elderly smoking men, however, there is a paradigm shift recently in women due to rising smoking prevalence in women worldwide.

Women are more vulnerable to develop COPD than men and tend to have more severe and early-onset disease (<60 years). Early onset of smoking in women causes greater deterioration of lung function in women owing to their smaller lung size than men. COPD in nonsmokers is high in women due to exposure to biomass fuels which are commonly used for cooking purposes in developing nations. Global statistics also have shown a recent rise in smoking trend among women causing increased COPD burden in women. Women smokers with COPD also have a greater annual decline in FEV1 percent compared to males. Women also have more hospitalizations and exacerbations even with same FEV1, better oxygenation, better carbon dioxide tension, and less comorbid illnesses.

## Respiratory Diseases Which Require Change in Treatment

### Tuberculosis

Women of reproductive age group are more vulnerable to develop TB, which not only impacts their health but also affects the health of their family and children. Women

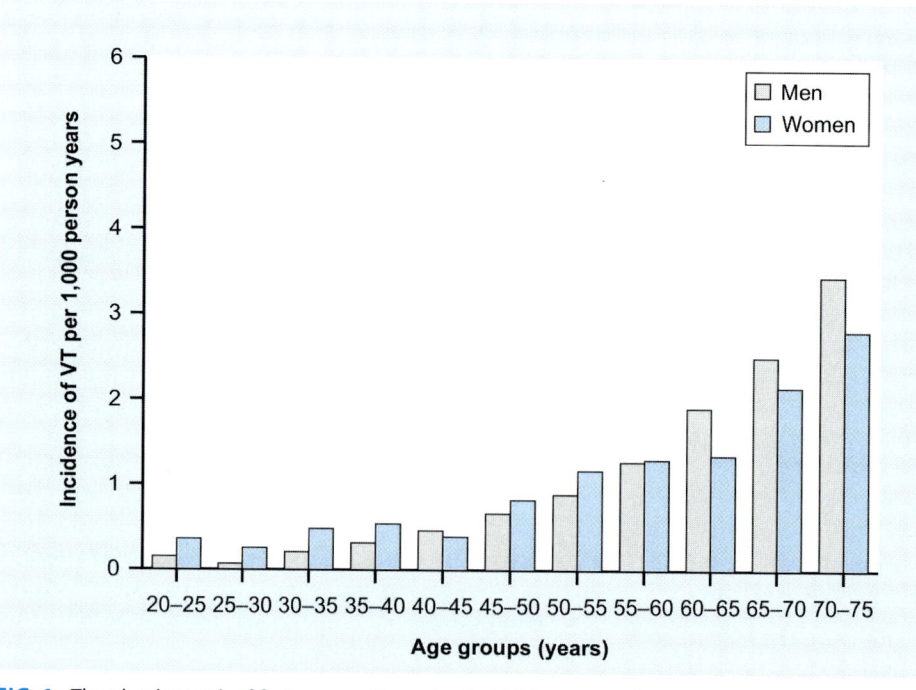

**FIG. 1:** The absolute risk of first venous thrombosis (VT) in men and women.

usually postpone their visit to healthcare facility due to the social stigma, lower literacy rates, household work, and dependence on spouse or children to accompany them.

Tuberculosis in pregnancy poses many diagnostic and therapeutic challenges even for an experienced person. Multitude of risks such as low birth weight, preterm births, abortions, increased fatal and maternal mortality, and preeclampsia can occur in pregnancy associated with TB. TB can be transmitted to the fetus either through hematogenous route or by aspiration or ingestion of infected amniotic fluid. Respiratory symptoms or relevant extrapulmonary symptoms with fever, reduced appetite, and inability to gain weight according to gestational age, history of contact are diagnostic pointers for TB. Upfront CBNAAT for all respiratory and nonrespiratory samples is recommended by RNTCP for diagnosis. Chest X-ray (CXR) is usually avoided, but if required, should be taken in second trimester after covering the abdomen with lead apron. Other supportive tests such as histopathological examination (HPE), cytology can be done in extra pulmonary TB. Appropriate tests for drug-resistant tuberculosis (DRTB) such as AFB culture sensitivity, LPA are done when DRTB is suspected.

Treatment for drug-sensitive TB is the same as nonpregnant persons with daily regimen of 2 months of intensive treatment with HREZ followed by 4 months of HRE with dosages according to the RNTCP weight bands.

Drug-resistant TB during pregnancy should be treated actively, but poses great risk to the mother and fetus. Women of childbearing age on DRTB treatment should be intensively advised on birth control measures to avoid pregnancy, preferred birth control measure is through barrier methods such as condoms, diaphragms or IUDs as oral contraceptive pills (OCPs) have drug interactions with DRTB drugs.

According to the PMDT 2019 Indian guidelines, management of DRTB in pregnant women depends on the gestational age. If the duration of pregnancy is <20 weeks, medical termination of pregnancy should be advised. For patients unwilling for MTP or have pregnancy >20 weeks, risk should be explained clearly and modified oral longer conventional MDR-TB regimen should be started (kanamycin and ethionamide are substituted with PAS). Safety of new drugs bedaquiline and delamanid is not yet established.

## CONCLUSION

Multiple factors play a vital role in the varied presentation of respiratory diseases in females. Awareness programs to curb smoking practices in women are most essential as it has both maternal and fetal adverse effects. It is also a pressing need to provide safer and cleaner cooking options for better respiratory health especially among women. In diseases which occur exclusively in women, diagnosis is often missed or delayed unless these diseases are particularly considered during evaluation. Pulmonary thromboembolism and PH are often fatal, early diagnosis and intervention are necessary. TB in pregnancy poses a diagnostic and therapeutic challenge which has to be addressed.

## SUGGESTED READING

1. Pinkerton KE, Harbaugh M, Han MK, Jourdan Le Saux C, Van Winkle LS, et al. Women and lung disease. Sex differences and global health disparities. Am J Respir Crit Care Med. 2015;192(1):11-6.
2. Buist S, Mapp CE, Rossi A. Respiratory Diseases in Women. Sheffield: European Respiratory Society Publications; 2008.
3. Behan M, Wenninger JM. Sex steroidal hormones and respiratory control. Respir Physiol Neurobiol. 2008;(1-2):213-21.

4. Apte K, Salvi S. (2016). Household air pollution and its effects on health. [online] Available from https://f1000research.com/articles/5-2593. [Last accessed February, 2020].
5. World Health Organization. (2003). Fact sheet on gender, health and tobacco. [online] Available from https://www.who.int/gender/documents/Gender_Tobacco_2.pdf. [Last accessed February, 2020].
6. Kalassian KG, Doyle R, Kao P, Ruoss S, Raffin TA. Lymphangioleiomyomatosis: new insights. Am J Respir Crit Carev Med. 1997;155:1183-6.
7. Matsui K, Tatsuguchi A, Valencia J, Yu Zx, Bechtle J, Beasley MB, et al. Extra pulmonary lymphangioleiomyomatosis Clinicopathologic features in 22 cases. Hum Pathol. 2000;31(10):1242-8.
8. Johnsosn SR, Cordier JF, Lazor R, Cottin V, Costabel U, Harari S, et al. European respiratory society guidelines for the diagnosis and management of lymphangioleiomyomatosis. Eur Respir J. 2010;35(1):14-26.
9. Escalante JP, Diez A, Figueroa Casas M, Lasave A, Cursack G, Poy C, et al. Medicina (B Aires). Postpartum pulmonary hypertension. 2015;75(1):44-7.
10. Nezhat C, Lindheim SR, Backhus L, Vu M, Vang N, Nezhat A, et al. Thoracic endometriosis syndrome: A review of diagnosis and management. JSLS. 2019;23(3):e2019.
11. Mason RJ, Broaddus VC, Murray JF, Nadel JA (Eds). Murray and Nadel's Textbook of Respiratory Medicine, 4th edition. Philadelphia: Elsevier Saunders; 2005. pp. 2277-8.
12. Saha S, Robertson M. Meigs' and Pseudo-Meigs' syndrome. Australas J Ultrasound Med. 2012;15(1):29-31.
13. Kaur K, Bhardwaj M, Kumar P, Singhal S, Singh T, Hooda S. Amniotic fluid embolism. J Anaesthesiol Clin Pharmacol. 2016;32(2):153-9.
14. Bhattacharya AK. A 24 year-old woman with pulmonary edema after labor and delivery. Lung India. 2006;23(3):133-4.
15. Cottin V, Hirani NA, Hotchkin DL, Nambiar AM, Ogura T, Otaola M, et al. Presentation, diagnosis and clinical course of the spectrum of progressive-fibrosing interstitial lung diseases. Eur Respir Rev. 2018;27:180076.
16. Memon HA, Park MH. Pulmonary arterial hypertension in women. Methodist Debakey Cardiovasc J. 2017;13(4):224-37.
17. Srivastava K, Narain A, Bajpai J, Kant S. Respiratory health hazards in women. J Assoc Chest Physicians. 2019;7:1-9.
18. Barnes PJ. Sex differences in chronic obstructive pulmonary disease mechanisms. Am J Respir Crit Care Med. 2016;193(8):813-24.
19. Guidelines on programmatic management of drug resistant tuberculosis in India–RNTCP 2019.

# SECTION 9

# Infectious Diseases

**SECTION EDITOR**
Mohanjeet Kaur

# CHAPTER 1

# HIV in Women

*Harbir Kaur Rao, Rajinder Singh Gupta, Rahul Purbey*

## ABSTRACT

Due to the stigma associated with human immunodeficiency virus (HIV), women affected with the disease often are hesitant to seek care which results in delay in treatment and increased incidence of opportunistic infections. More number of women are affected with HIV as compared to men. Hence, it becomes imperative that special significance be given to women with HIV so that there is greater awareness about the issue and steps can be taken to reduce barriers for women who seek care for themselves.

Human immunodeficiency virus has a number of obstetrical and gynecological complications which have a direct correlation with its severity and need to be managed properly in accordance with specific guidelines made to treat them.

Our chapter covers the special characteristics of HIV virus, discusses the magnitude of the infection in women and elaborates in detail the various problems HIV positive women face and the means and methods of managing them. We stress upon the need to confront HIV infection in women on priority basis to decrease the social and economic burden of this problem on society.

## INTRODUCTION

In 2013, nearly half of more than 40 million human immunodeficiency virus (HIV) infections worldwide were in women. Young people aged between 15 and 24 years account for 45% of the infections worldwide and approximately 2 million children are living with the virus. Women make up over 60% of 15–24 year-old living with HIV/AIDS. Sub-Saharan Africa is most affected with 67% of the people living with HIV/AIDS and 75% of the deaths due to AIDS worldwide; 97% of all new infections in 2009 occurred in middle or low-income countries.

This disease has had a significant impact on mankind in modern times. HIV is a retrovirus, which was unknown until the 1980s, when the first cases of this new disease were first identified in the US. The disease was named acquired immunodeficiency syndrome (AIDS) after its most characteristic features, death due to infectious diseases caused by immunodeficiency, and it has since then killed more than 25 million people worldwide. Antiretroviral therapy (ART) was introduced in resource-poor settings reluctantly for the fear of emerging resistance against antiretroviral drugs and lack of sustainability and human resources, but after public pressure and advocacy of international organizations such as Doctors Without Borders (MSF), introduction of adapted

ART and care and treatment schemes started to be rolled out with the support of UNAIDS from 2003 onward. In 2010, approximately 3 million people living with HIV/AIDS had access to ART from the 9 million needing it. The extent to which the epidemic spread in sub-Saharan Africa and Southeast Asia had significant impact on the economic and social development. The consequences can be seen at all levels of the economy, household and workforce, and at the macroeconomic level. As many societies' economies are based on subsistence farming and agricultural products, the impact of HIV/AIDS at the household level is most important. HIV/AIDS erodes social capital.

## CHARACTERISTICS OF HIV

Human immunodeficiency virus is a very simple organism, but its potential to survive, reproduce, and mutate is enormous. It is transmitted through hetero- and homosexual intercourse, from the pregnant mother to the fetus and during delivery and breastfeeding, through contaminated blood and by sharing contaminated needles or other sharp equipment. Globally, the most important way of transmission is heterosexual intercourse. People over 18 months of age can be tested for HIV with rapid field tests taking only a few minutes and more elaborate laboratory tests such as enzyme-linked immunosorbent assay (ELISA) or Western blot immunoassays. A test will become positive around 6–12 weeks after infection. The virus primarily infects CD4+ lymphocytes. In these lymphocytes, the two copies of the genome are turned into double-stranded deoxyribonucleic acid (DNA) genome by the virus reverse transcriptase, which is integrated in the host's own DNA genome. To produce new viruses, more RNA is transcribed to be integrated into new virions, which are released from the host cells which will gradually be destroyed. This will, in time (10–15 years) lead to a reduced immune response against diseases and eventually the person infected with HIV will die as his or her body will be overwhelmed by infectious diseases and certain forms of cancer. Today, most healthcare settings at district or regional level provide HIV counseling and testing. In most district hospitals, CD4 testing and ART are available and all countries have national guidelines on treatment and care for people living with HIV/AIDS.

## MAGNITUDE OF THE PROBLEM IN WOMEN

Women living with HIV/AIDS seek care for specific problems in obstetric and gynecological services all around the world. Recognizing and treating specific gynecological diseases can help to maintain the health of these women for a longer time. Women are diagnosed with HIV later than their male counterparts. Most women are diagnosed with HIV when pregnant, considering pregnancy, or admitted to hospital with acute illness. Once diagnosed, up to 25% of women postpone treatment. Most choose not to disclose their status. In addition, in low-resource settings, infants depend on their mothers' health and ability to take care of them to survive. Infant mortality and under-5 mortality in HIV exposed children is two to five times higher than in the non-exposed. These show the importance of women for the well-being of their families as caregivers and breadwinners.

## GYNECOLOGICAL PROBLEMS OF HIV/AIDS

Approximately 89% of female HIV patients experience at least one relevant gynecological problem in 5 years. Gynecological infections are the most common reason to seek care for

# CHAPTER 1: HIV in Women

the first time in HIV-infected women. HIV prevalence in gynecological services is often higher than average because women seek help for HIV-related gynecological problems. Frequent problems in HIV-positive women are:
- Sexually transmitted infections (STIs)
- Pelvic inflammatory disease (PID)
- Tuberculosis
- Cervical cancer
- Other HIV-related malignancies
- Menstrual disorders
- Miscarriages
- Family planning, infertility

These problems are discussed in detail below.

## Sexually Transmitted Infections/Reproductive Tract Infections

The most frequent way of transmission of HIV globally is heterosexual intercourse. This way of transmission is shared with other STIs such as chlamydia, trichomonas or syphilis. Those infections can facilitate the transmission of HIV during intercourse and at the same time HIV infection with low immunity can facilitate infection with other STIs. Thus, women with HIV should be routinely screened for other STIs or reproductive tract infections (RTIs) and all outpatient department (OPD) patients who come with symptoms of an STI should be counseled for HIV testing. Treatment of an STI is the same for HIV-positive and -negative patients but in HIV treatment sometimes needs to be prolonged:
- Vulvovaginal candidiasis was found in 30–70% of HIV-infected women. Severe vulvovaginal candidiasis tends to occur below a CD4 count of 350 cells/mm$^3$ and is often associated with oral or esophageal thrush which needs general treatment with oral antifungal tablets such as fluconazole.
- Genital herpes simplex may be the first manifestation of AIDS in an HIV-positive patient and is, if persisting for more than a month, an AIDS defining disease. Episodes tend to be more frequent, more severe, and persistent with falling CD4 counts.
- HIV-positive women have a higher prevalence of syphilis which does not respond to a single shot treatment with benzathine penicillin. Primary syphilis should thus be treated like secondary syphilis with benzathine penicillin 2.4 mega units once a week for 3 weeks.

## Pelvic Inflammatory Disease

Pelvic inflammatory disease is found more frequently in women living with HIV/AIDS and tends to be more severe with more frequent tubo-ovarian abscesses but often with less pain and lower blood leukocyte counts. Preoperative evaluation of the patient's health is very important since a patient with low CD4 counts tends to have more postoperative complications. There are two possibilities for treating such a patient without doing a laparotomy:
1. Medical treatment with ciprofloxacin tablets 250 mg OD for 14 days or chloramphenicol tablets 500 mg BD for 14 days. After this, another ultrasound should be done to assess response to treatment.
2. If the tubo-ovarian masses on ultrasound are in the pouch of Douglas, a culdotomy can be performed under local or general anesthesia.

## Tuberculosis

Tuberculosis is a big problem for people living with HIV and can easily lead to rapid progression to AIDS and death if untreated. Multidrug resistant tuberculosis bacilli are emerging more frequently especially in Southern Africa and South East Asia. Almost one-third of people living with HIV suffer from tuberculosis and one-third of people suffering from tuberculosis are HIV-positive. Tuberculosis can affect the cervix, uterus, tubes, and ovaries as well, causing endomyometritis with menstrual irregularities and amenorrhea, infertility or ectopic pregnancies, and early ovarian failure with early menopause. Peritoneal involvement can mimic ovarian cancer with ascites and miliary implantations leading to unnecessary surgery with serious complications for women living with HIV whose immune system is already low.

Tuberculosis should always be thought of in women living with HIV but unfortunately it is very difficult to diagnose, as sputum and Mantoux tests are often negative. If tuberculosis is suspected, a syndromic treatment can be worthwhile initiating for the above-mentioned negative impact of tuberculosis on disease progression.

## Cervical Cancer

This is the second most common cancer in women worldwide. More than 80% of the cases occur in low- resource settings with the highest rate in Asia, especially in India. Most cases of cervical cancer are caused by human papillomavirus (HPV).

The HIV and HPV have common ways of transmission and risk factors. As the immune system has a major role in clearing HPV infections, scientists expected a rise in the rate of cervical cancer with increasing HIV rates, and included cervical cancer in the WHO classification as an AIDS-defining disease, and a decrease with the onset of ART. However, this has not been the case, so the link between HIV and cervical cancer seems to be more complex.

Current evidence shows that women living with HIV have a higher risk for cervical HPV infection and higher rates of viral persistence which increases the risk of cervical intraepithelial neoplasia (CIN), the precursor of cervical cancer. This indeed seems to correlate to CD4 counts as the risk for persistence is two-fold in CD4 counts <200 cells/μL. As the rate of women with cervical cancer and HIV is high in many resource-poor settings, many patients will have both diseases and it is worthwhile considering screening for cervical cancer in HIV-positive women and proposing voluntary counseling and testing (VCT) to women with cervical cancer especially when they are young. Screening tools are the same for HIV-positive and -negative women—PAP smear. Due to higher risk for CIN, women living with HIV need more frequent examinations and should be screened at their first visit once they have tested positive for HIV. If the result is negative, repeat after 6 months and if the result is negative again, repeat at yearly intervals. The threshold for specialist colposcopic examination in women living with HIV should be low. CIN can be treated using cryotherapy, large loop excision of the transformation zone (LLETZ) or electric or knife conization. Invasive cancer should be treated with either surgery (radical hysterectomy) or radio (chemo) therapy which almost always needs referral to specialist care.

## Other HIV-Related Tumors

Experience from industrialized countries shows that people living with HIV/AIDS have an increased risk for developing cancer. Some are very specific for HIV, such as Kaposi

sarcoma and are thus classified as AIDS-defining diseases, others only show a higher frequency in people living with HIV/AIDS.
- Non-Hodgkin lymphoma (NHL) and adult Burkitt lymphoma are AIDS-defining diseases and are also associated with immunodepression (CD4 <100 cells/L). Hodgkin lymphoma (HL) shows the same association with immunodepression. Where ART is introduced, the prevalence of NHL, HL, and adult Burkitt lymphoma is declining. "Gynecological" presentations of lymphoma can be abdominal masses with or without acute abdominal pain or kidney problems due to enlarged intra-abdominal lymph nodes. The treatment for lymphoma is chemotherapy and the initiation of ART. NHL can be treated using the COP scheme (cyclophosphamide + vincristine+ prednisolone every 3 weeks for six courses, after this every 3 months).
- Cancers associated with HPV, such as vulval and anal cancer and their precursor lesions, intraepithelial neoplasia, are also associated with HIV/AIDS infection. Their prevalence is linked to immunosuppression as with the other previously described cancers. Gynecological presentations of vulval and anal cancer are commonly chronic ulcers or chronic genital itching and pain with skin changes, such as decoloration, hardening of the skin, and easy bleeding. The treatment is the same as for HIV-negative patients but with a higher rate of treatment failure and recurrence.
- Kaposi sarcoma is associated with herpes simplex virus type 8. It is associated with immunodepression and low CD4 counts. Its frequency is declining with ART. HIV patients with Kaposi sarcoma often have visceral organ involvement and gynecological symptoms can be acute abdominal pain mimicking pelvioperitonitis with ileus. The treatment for Kaposi sarcoma is the initiation of ART and radiotherapy.

## Menstrual Disorders

Menstrual disorders are a common problem in HIV infection and with women on ART. Especially in advanced stages and progression to AIDS, many women stop having their menstrual period (amenorrhea for more than 6 months). This can be due to wasting with extreme weight loss and stress but also due to underlying chronic diseases such as tuberculosis either generalized or affecting the female genital organs as described above. With ART or antituberculous treatment the amenorrhea is often reversible leading to ovulation and unplanned pregnancies as fertility and health are restored. If the period does not reoccur for more than a year although the patient is treated and puts on weight, she is likely to be postmenopausal. There seems to be an increased rate of early ovarian failure with early menopause in HIV although this is not proven by studies.

Another menstrual problem in HIV is a higher rate of heavy menstrual bleeding (hypermenorrhea) and irregular heavy bleeding (metrorrhagia) mostly due to low platelet counts as a result of ART and infection itself. Also these patients suffer from anemia more often than patients who are not HIV infected.

Heavy bleeding can be avoided by using injectables, progesterone implants or levonorgestrel intrauterine devices (IUDs). Many women stop having their periods while using these contraceptive methods. Another way of avoiding menstruation is to continuously use the pill; however, oral contraceptives decrease the bioavailability of ART in the body.

## Miscarriage

Women living with HIV/AIDS have a higher risk of miscarriage due to malfunctioning of the placenta and ascending infections when the mother's immune system is weak. Malaria seems to be more common in HIV-infected pregnant women and can cause miscarriage too. Women with recurrent spontaneous abortion should be offered HIV counseling and testing. Safe methods to deal with incomplete or missed abortion like misoprostol or manual vacuum aspiration (MVA) can be used in HIV-infected women.

## Reproductive Health

The majority of women living with HIV are of reproductive age and with the increased availability of ART, healthcare personnel face issues around conception and the desire for children in their HIV-positive patients. A gynecological service is a good place to detect as many HIV infections as possible in order to attach these clients to a care and treatment center (CTC) for HIV as early as possible to receive ART once they become eligible for it. Unfortunately, many healthcare workers lack knowledge about issues around procreation in people living with HIV and especially in women with HIV. For a long time women in low-resource settings were, and still are, advised not to become pregnant at all regardless of their age and parity at the time of diagnosis. This advice can lead to harmful consequences as most women feel the need to become pregnant in order to fulfill their role in their society. In some areas with a high prevalence of HIV, women who do not become pregnant are discriminated against by saying that this is because they have HIV. As a consequence many women with HIV will try to become pregnant regardless of the health providers' advice but will fail to go for antenatal care to the very provider for fear of trouble and discrimination. The prospect of a future planned and well-monitored pregnancy can be a powerful factor for adherence to ART; the advice not to become pregnant could be a cause for depression and ill-adherence. It is more and more recognized that people on ART in resource-poor settings are able to adhere to treatment and can lead a longer and healthier life. The risk of mother-to-child transmission (MTCT) without any preventive measures is 30–40%; using single nevirapine during labor and after delivery has an MTCT rate of 15–20%. The risk of MTCT under ART with high CD4 counts and low viral load, however, can be decreased to <2%. An HIV-positive woman who is well attached to her clinic and feels she can freely speak about her desire for pregnancy to the providers without being harassed has no reason to hide away with this desire and to attempt a pregnancy in secret with all the harmful effects on her family such as partner transmission, new HIV infection, MTCT, adverse pregnancy outcomes, and premature death.

## CONTRACEPTION

*Contraception is used as dual protection*: Against HIV transmission and STI, and unwanted pregnancy. It is important for HIV-positive individuals to protect themselves against an infection with other HIV viruses as this will hamper their immune system and increase the chance of resistance once they take ART. STIs can facilitate new infections through ulcers and local inflammation. The best contraceptive devices to protect against a new HIV infection are condoms which are unfortunately not very reliable in preventing conception unless they are used correctly. Thus, it is important to use condoms and another method for contraception and HIV prevention (dual protection or contraceptive method mix).

*Women with HIV can use the following contraceptives*:
- *IUD*: In 2004 WHO changed their guidelines about the use of IUD for women with HIV. There is no increased risk of PID or change in CD4 counts in HIV-positive women or women with AIDS who are well on ART. Levonorgestrel IUDs have the advantage that blood loss is absent or slight.

- The method with the lowest failure rate for multiparous women is *tubal ligation* feasible even on district level by mini-lap at any time or postpartum.
- *Progesterone-based contraceptives* such as Norplant® or injectables can be used by women with HIV but the evidence of risk of HIV acquisition is inconclusive at the moment. However, WHO and CDC still recommend progestin-only injectables and implants as contraceptives for women living with HIV. Many women on implants or injectables stop having their period (amenorrhea) which is beneficial to the anemia and thrombocytopenia often associated to HIV and even ART.
- The contraceptive pill should be used with caution in women on ART as the use of antiretrovirals lessens contraceptive action as does rifampicin, an antituberculous drug. Apart from this, it can be used safely and effectively in HIV-positive women.
- Microbicides when applied either in the vagina or rectum can reduce the transmission of STIs and HIV. They act as a physical barrier, maintain acidic pH, and prevent viral replication and entry. They come in the form of gels, creams, suppositories, films, lubricants, sponges or vaginal rings. They are cheap and nontoxic.

## SUGGESTED READING

1. Joint United Nations Programme on HIV and AIDS (UNAIDS). Status of the global HIV epidemic. [online] Available at http://www.unaids.org/globalreport/Epi_slides.htm. [Last accessed January, 2020].
2. Piot P, Bartos M, Ghys PD, Walker N, Schwartländer B. The global impact of HIV/AIDS. Nature. 2001;410:868-73.
3. Newell ML, Coovadia H, Cortina-Borja M, Rollins N, Gaillard P, Dabis F et al. Mortality of infected and uninfected infants born to HIV-infected mothers in Africa: a pooled analysis. Lancet. 2004;364(9441):1236-43.
4. Schäfer A. HIV in gynecology and obstetrics. Gynäkologe. 1999;32:540-51.
5. Massad LS, Seaberg EC, Watts DH, Minkoff H, Levine AM, Henry D, et al. Long-term incidence of cervical cancer in women with HIV. Cancer. 2009;115:524-30.
6. Palefsky J. HPV infection and HPV-associated neoplasia in immunocompromised women. Int J Gyn Obst. 2006;94(Suppl 1):S56-64.
7. Palefsky J. Human papillomavirus-related disease in people with HIV. Curr Opin HIV AIDS. 2009;4: 52-6.
8. Centers for Disease Control and Prevention (CDC). Update to CDC's U.S. Medical Eligibility Criteria for Contraceptive Use, 2010: Revised recommendations for the use of hormonal contraception among women at high risk for HIV infection or infected with HIV. MMWR Morb Mortal Wkly Rep. 2012;61(24):449-52.
9. Curtis C. Meeting health care needs of women experiencing complications of miscarriage and unsafe abortion: USAID's postabortion care program. J Midwifery Womens Health. 2007;52:368-75.
10. Cejtin HE. Gynecologic issues in the HIV-infected woman. Infect Dis Clin North Am. 2008;22:709-39.

# Approach to Fever in a Pregnant Women

*Savita Kapila, Ena Sharma, Jeji Pukhraj*

## ABSTRACT

Fever is a common complaint in pregnant women and needs special consideration. Malaria, viral hepatitis, urinary tract infections (UTI), typhoid, sexually transmitted diseases (STDs), and tuberculosis are the common causes. In this chapter we will review these causes along with their diagnosis and management.

## INTRODUCTION

Living in a tropical climate, fever is a common complaint for which patients seek medical opinion. An AM temperature of >37.2°C (>98.9°F) or a PM temperature of >37.7°C (>99.9°F) would define a fever with normal daily temperature variation being 0.5°C (0.9°F). A temperature above 38.8°C during pregnancy is a frequent reason to seek for obstetrician advice. Fever causes and consequences are variable depending on timing of occurrence (pregnancy term, labor or postnatal period) (**Table 1**). The threshold for intrapartum fever has generally been considered to be a maternal temperature ≥38°C (≥100.4°F) orally. This is based, in part, on a study of temperature in normal parturients, which ranged from 34.6 to 37.6°C (94.3–99.7°F) upon admission to the labor unit.

## CLINICAL EVALUATION

Detailed history and physical examination are a norm. It should be remembered that the syndromic associations of infections do not change in pregnancy, hence, initial evaluation is similar to nonpregnant patients. General investigations to be done at initial stages are given in **Box 1**. Imaging modalities should be chosen judiciously, and X-ray and CT should be avoided. Specific investigations have to be tailored (as discussed here) depending upon the suspected organism.

## Specific Considerations in Pregnancy

### Malaria in Pregnancy

Malaria is suspected when expecting mother complains of fever with chills. Fever can by typically tertian or quartan, with or without rash or body aches. Diagnosis can be confirmed

## CHAPTER 2: Approach to Fever in a Pregnant Women

**TABLE 1:** Causes of fever during pregnancy.

| Systemic diseases | Infections | Non-infectious diseases |
|---|---|---|
| • Tuberculosis<br>• Gall bladder<br>  ○ Cholecystitis<br>  ○ Cholangitis<br>  ○ Empyema<br>• Abscesses<br>  ○ Subphrenic<br>  ○ Hepatic<br>  ○ Pelvic<br>  ○ Cerebral<br>  ○ Dental<br>  ○ Breast<br>• Gastrointestinal<br>  ○ Appendicitis<br>  ○ Diverticulitis<br>• Urinary tract infections<br>• Retroperitoneal infection<br>• Septicemia<br>  ○ Meningococcal<br>  ○ Streptococcal<br>  ○ Staphylococcal<br>  ○ Gonococcal<br>  ○ Listeriosis<br>  ○ Vibriosis<br>  ○ Brucellosis<br>• Endocarditis<br>• Breast<br>  ○ Mastitis | • Gonococcal<br>  ○ Septicemia<br>  ○ Salpingitis<br>  ○ Arthritis<br>• Secondary syphilis<br>• Gas gangrene<br>• Tetanus<br>• Opportunistic-associated with immune deficiency syndrome<br>  ○ Candidiasis<br>  ○ Cryptococcosis<br>  ○ Coccidiomycosis<br>• Viral Infections<br>• Q-fever<br>• Amebiasis<br>• Leptospirosis | • Neoplasms<br>  ○ Lymphoma<br>  ○ Leukemia<br>  ○ Melanoma<br>  ○ Metastasis<br>  ○ Retroperitoneal sarcoma<br>  ○ Tumors of the lung, kidney, pancreas, and liver<br>• Connective tissue disease<br>  ○ Rheumatic fever<br>  ○ Systemic lupus erythematosus<br>  ○ Rheumatoid arthritis<br>• Other<br>  ○ Drug fever<br>  ○ Thromboembolism<br>  ○ Sarcoidosis |

---

**BOX 1** | **General investigations in a patient with fever.**

- Complete blood counts (CBC) with differential counts, platelets, erythrocyte sedimentation rate (ESR) and C-reactive protein (CRP)
- Peripheral blood film (including malarial parasite)
- Blood glucose
- Renal function tests
- Liver function tests
- Urinalysis and culture
- Blood Culture
- Widal test
- Swabs depending upon the suspected organism and site of infection

---

by Giemsa stained thick and/or thin peripheral blood smear and rapid diagnostic tests (RDT). Polymerase chain reaction (PCR) can be used to diagnose placental infection in asymptomatic women. Treatment is similar in nonpregnant as *Plasmodium vivax* is treated with Chloroquine 600 mg base orally followed by 300 mg base orally at 6, 24, and 48 hours. Resistant cases can be treated with Quinine. *P. falciparum* infections can be treated with tablet Quinine 10 mg/kg TDS for 7 days + Clindamycin 20 mg/kg/day TDS × 7 days. It should be remembered that ACT therapy should be avoided in first trimester but is used for *P. falciparum* infections in second and third trimesters.

## Viral Hepatitis

The most common cause of fever with jaundice in pregnancy in the tropic is acute viral hepatitis. Associated symptoms such as decreased appetite, lethargy, and generalized body aches are not clear-cut symptoms seen in pregnancy. Hepatitis is mostly restricted to the ill-nourished mothers, living in unhygienic environment. In the tropics, it often occurs as an epidemic form. There is also increased incidence of its affection in the pregnant state compared to the nonpregnant one. At present six distinct types of highly contagious hepatitis virus have been identified. Each type (mentioned here) has different clinical effect to the pregnant women and her fetus.

*Hepatitis A (HAV):* Diagnosis is confirmed by detection of immunoglobulin M (IgM) antibody to hepatitis A. Although the virus is not teratogenic, and perinatal transmission is rare; still the pregnant woman exposed to HAV infection should receive immunoglobulin 0.02 mL/kg within 2 weeks of exposure. Hepatitis A vaccine single dose of 0.06 mL given intramuscular (IM) is safe in pregnancy. The incidence of chronic career state in newborn is nil.

*Hepatitis B virus (HBV):* The virus is transmitted rarely through breast milk. The risk of transmission to fetus ranges from 10% in first trimester to as high as 90% in third trimester and it is especially high (90%) from those mothers who are seropositive to hepatitis B surface antigen (HBsAg) and "e"-antigen (HBeAg). These tests are also used to diagnose hepatitis B infection.

There are chances of neonatal transmission during delivery. About 25% of neonates affected will die from complications such as cirrhosis and carcinoma on a later stage.

*Hepatitis C (HCV):* Perinatal transmission (10–40%) is high when viral load is high and presence of coinfection with human immunodeficiency virus (HIV) and HBV. Detection is by antibody to HCV by enzyme immunoassay (EIA), which develops usually late in the infection. Confirmation is done by recombinant immunoblot assay (RIBA-3). Chronic carrier state is present. No effective vaccine against HCV is available. Women should be immunized against hepatitis A and B if not immune. Breastfeeding is not contraindicated.

*Hepatitis D (HDV):* This occurs either as a coinfection with HBV or super infection. It results in perinatal transmission. Neonatal immune prophylaxis for HBV is almost effective against HDV. Acute infection with fulminant course results in high maternal mortality (2–20%) due to hepatic failure.

*Hepatitis E (HEV):* This is similar to hepatitis A virus infection. A higher incidence is observed in Asia (Kashmir) and South America. It may lead to fulminant hepatitis. Enzyme-linked immunosorbent assay (ELISA) can detect HEV specific immunoglobulin G (IgG) and IgM antibodies or by PCR. Chronic carrier state is present. Perinatal transmission is uncommon. Maternal mortality following acute infection is high (15–20%).

## Human Immunodeficiency Virus Infection

*Perinatal transmission of HIV:* Vertical transmission to the neonates is about 14–25%. Transplacental transmission occurs: 20% before 36 weeks, over 80% of transmissions occur around the time of labor and delivery. Vertical transmission is more in cases with preterm birth and with prolonged membrane rupture. Risks of vertical transmission is directly related to maternal viral load (measured by HIV RNA) and inversely to maternal immune status (CD4+ count). Maternal antiretroviral therapy reduces the risk of vertical transmission by 70%. Breastfeeding doubles the risk of mother-to-child transmission (MTCT) transmission (14–28%).

*Diagnosis:* HIV diagnosis is made by detecting HIV viral RNA in blood by PCR testing (HIV RNA PCR) or by detecting antibodies to HIV. The EIA is used as a screening test for HIV antibodies which is then confirmed with western blot or HIV RNA PCR test.

## MANAGEMENT

### Prenatal Care

- Integrated counseling and testing (ICT) in the antenatal clinic (ANC) to all pregnant women with an "opt out" approach is offered.
- In seropositive cases the following additional tests should be done.
  - Test for other sexually transmitted diseases (STDs)—such as hepatitis B and C viruses, syphilis, chlamydia, herpes and rubella
  - Serological testing for cytomegalovirus and toxoplasmosis
  - Tuberculosis (TB)
  - Fungal opportunistic infection
  - Husband should be offered serological testing for HIV
- Counseling with education to the patient is done about the impact of HIV infection on pregnancy; perinatal transmissions, side effects of medications and mode of delivery.
- Highly active antiretroviral therapy (HAART) to HIV 1 positive women is effective in reducing the viral (HIV RNA) load. Triple chemotherapy is preferred as a first line defense and to be started any time between 14 and 28 weeks and then continued throughout pregnancy, labor, and postpartum period.
- *Principles of HAART are to*:
  - Suppress viral multiplication maximally
  - Reduce perinatal transmission
  - Reduce the risk of drug resistance. Efavirenz is avoided in the first trimester due to its teratogenic risk

## URINARY TRACT INFECTIONS IN PREGNANCY

Common symptoms of urinary tract infections (UTI) are dysuria, urinary frequency, urgency, painful urination, lower abdominal discomfort, and sometimes hematuria.

### Asymptomatic Bacteriuria

Presence of positive urine culture in given women without any clinical manifestation is labeled as asymptomatic bacteriuria (ASB). The ASB may progress to acute cystitis or urethritis 3-4 times more frequently in pregnant women. Recurrent ASB responds to empirical treatment with Amoxicillin, Cephalosporin or Nitrofurantoin.

## Pyelonephritis

Symptoms such as high-grade fever (>38°C) with chills, nausea, vomiting, and lumbar pain may give a clue to a diagnosis, e.g., acute pyelonephritis. Pyelonephritis patients are usually toxic looking with no urinary symptoms. Septicemia may complicate the disease. Usually manifesting in the second and third trimester, acute pyelonephritis is preferably managed with higher antibiotics in a multidisciplinary setting.

## TUBERCULOSIS IN PREGNANCY

Tuberculosis should be suspected in cases of fever (usually low grade) with presence of evening rise and night sweats, productive cough for >2 weeks, lymphadenopathy, altered bowel habits or unexplained weight loss with decreased appetite.

Pregnancy has got no deleterious effect on the course of the disease; nor has the disease any adverse effect on the course of pregnancy.

*Diagnosis:* Raised ESR or CRP can indicate a chronic infection such as TB.
- Tuberculin skin test with purified protein derivative (PPD) induration ≥5 mm is considered positive especially in presence of risk factors (HIV)
- X-ray chest (after 12 weeks)
- Early morning sputum (three samples) for acid-fast bacilli
- Gastric washings
- Diagnostic bronchoscopy
- Extrapulmonary site biopsies—lymph nodes, bones (rare in pregnancy)
- Direct amplification tests for 16S ribosomal DNA and gene probe can detect *M. tuberculosis* with greater sensitivity and specificity19

*Management:* Women with active TB should receive the ATT drugs orally daily for a minimum period of 9–18 months. It should be remembered that TB is not an indication for termination of pregnancy nor is a contraindication for breastfeeding.

## TORCH INFECTIONS

This group of infectious diseases present as fever with rash and ocular findings. These include:
- Toxoplasmosis
- Other (syphilis)
- Rubella
- Cytomegalovirus (CMV)
- Herpes simplex virus (HSV)

## Toxoplasmosis

Acute maternal infection by *Toxoplasma gondii* is usually asymptomatic (≥80% of cases). If symptoms occur, they are usually nonspecific and mild: Fever, chills, sweats, headaches, myalgias, pharyngitis, hepatosplenomegaly, and/or a diffuse nonpruritic maculopapular rash. The febrile episodes usually last 2–3 days. Bilateral, symmetrical, nontender lymphadenopathy (usually cervical) is the most common symptom.

*Diagnosis:* IgM antibodies appear as early as 2 weeks after the patient gets infection and many a times, it may persist for years together. IgG antibodies on the other hand peak after 6–8 weeks and then decline over next 2 years. The diagnosis of recent toxoplasmosis can be made with certainty when both IgM and IgG seroconversion are documented on serial testing. Probability of infection after conception is 1–3% for women who are initially screened at the end of the first trimester (and have positive IgM and IgG). Confirmatory tests must be obtained to be sure whether the positive IgM and IgG antibodies reflect recent or chronic infection or a false-positive result. High IgG avidity is a hallmark of chronic infection (>4 months old). If a highly suspected mother has positive tests, amniotic fluid should be sent for PCR for *T. gondii* to evaluate spread to baby.

*Management:* Disease is usually self-limiting. Pyrimethamine 25 mg orally daily and oral sulfadiazine 1 g four times a day is effective. Leucovorin is added to minimize toxicity. 4–6 weeks course is usually given. Pyrimethamine is not given in the first trimester and spiramycin (3 g orally daily) can be used as an alternative.

# Rubella

This disease is asymptomatic in 25–50% of cases. Prodromal symptoms include low grade fever, sore throat with cough.

Headache, conjunctivitis, generalized tender lymphadenopathy, and rose spots on the soft palate called Forchheimer spots are other clinical features. Erythematous maculopapular rash characteristically starts on the face and within hours spreads to trunk and extremities.

*Diagnosis:* Following tests are available:
- ELISA
- Immunofluorescent antibody assays
- Rapid and sensitive commercial IgG and IgM assays
- Passive hemagglutination antibody (PHA)
- Latex agglutination test
- Complement fixation test
- Hemagglutination inhibition (HI) assays

*The diagnosis of acute rubella syndrome is made by:*
- Fourfold rise in IgG titer between acute and convalescent serum specimens
- Presence of rubella specific IgM
- Positive rubella culture

*Management:* Management mostly includes conservative management, but patients should be offered pregnancy termination considering serious fetal effects.

# Cytomegalovirus

Primary CMV infection may cause a mild febrile illness and other nonspecific symptoms (rhinitis, pharyngitis, myalgia, arthralgia, headache, fatigue), but is not clinically apparent in most cases. CMV mononucleosis can be accompanied by dermatologic manifestations in approximately one-third of patients including macular, papular, maculopapular, rubelliform, morbilliform, and scarlatiniform eruptions.

*Diagnosis:* In clinically suspected maternal primary CMV infection, seroconversion of CMV-specific IgG in paired acute and convalescent sera collected 3–4 weeks apart is diagnostic of a new acute infection. The presence of CMV immunoglobulin M is not helpful for timing the onset of infection because: (1) It is present in only 75–90%, (2) it can remain positive for over 1 year, (3) it can revert from negative to positive in women with CMV reactivation or reinfection with a different strain, and (4) it can become positive in response to other viral infections, such as Epstein–Barr virus.

*Management:* Disease is usually managed symptomatically along with antiviral agents, e.g., ganciclovir.

## SEXUALLY TRANSMITTED DISEASES IN PREGNANCY

### Syphilis

Incidence rates for congenital syphilis generally mirror those of rates for women.

#### Implications for Pregnancy

Primary and secondary syphilis are the similar to nonpregnant patients as far as clinical manifestations are concerned. Focus is to prevent fetal infection. As per the recent literature *T. pallidum* can cross the placenta as early as 6 weeks, as against the earlier beliefs.

Clinical features include fever with enlarged lymph nodes (especially inguinal). A painless sore (chancre) on the skin may be seen, may also be inside rectum or vagina. The sore will heal on its own in about 3–6 weeks. This is followed by secondary syphilis which is associated with fever, ulcers in mouth, vagina or anus, skin rashes, and non-specific symptoms like weight loss, hair loss, and headache.

*Diagnosis:* Screening for syphilis must be done in all pregnant patients. The high-risk patients should be rescreened in the third trimester, e.g., patients with multiple sexual partners, patients having suspicious lesions on examination, history of multiple sexual partners, and sexual contact with patients diagnosed to be having syphilis.

*Treatment:* Drug of choice is benzathine penicillin or penicillin G.

### Gonorrhea

The affected women can be totally asymptomatic or may present with dysuria, vaginal discharge, and fever.

It is caused by *Neisseria gonorrhoeae* infects columnar and pseudostratified epithelium. Sexual contact is the mode of transmission.

*Implications for Pregnancy:* In neonates, it causes ophthalmia neonatorum.

*Diagnosis*:
- *Gram Stain*: The Centers for Disease Control and Prevention (CDC) considers the Gram stain to be insufficient to detect infection in endocervical, pharyngeal, and rectal specimens.
- The diagnostic test of choice is culture test with 100% specificity.
- *NAAT*: Nucleic acid amplification techniques (NAATs) use polymerase chain reaction technology to detect fewer organisms. These are highly sensitivity and specificity, can provide results in hours, and do not require special handling. NAATs cannot provide information on antibiotic resistance; therefore, in cases of treatment failures, testing needs to be augmented by use of culture.

*Treatment:* Ceftriaxone or azithromycin are treatment of choice, as recommended by CDC.

## Herpes

Herpes simplex virus infections can be caused by either the type I (HSV-1) or the type II (HSV-2) virus. Most infections of the oral cavity and upper torso are due to HSV-1. Historically, most genital infections have been caused by HSV-2. There is considerable overlap, however, and the virus can be transmitted by masturbation, urogenital contact, or poor hygiene.

*Clinical Manifestations*: This can be
- Primary
- Nonprimary first episode
- Recurrent
  Clinical manifestations can range from fever to characteristic skin lesions over various parts of the body.

*Diagnosis:* Most of the times, diagnosis is possible on clinical presentation only.
   The diagnostic is made by cell culture. Fresh vesicles yield better results. Pap smear yields positive results in three-fourths of the cases. PCR is more sensitive.

*Treatment:* There are various recommended regimens for each trimester, but drug of choice remains acyclovir.

## Chlamydial Infections

*Chlamydia trachomatis* is an obligate intracellular bacterium that has several serotypes, including those that cause lymphogranuloma venereum. It is the most common reported STD in the United States in pregnant women.
   Most pregnant women have asymptomatic infection, but one-third of women have fever with urethral syndrome, urethritis, or Bartholin gland infection. Mucopurulent cervicitis may be due to chlamydial or gonococcal infection or both. Other chlamydial infections not usually seen in pregnancy are endometritis, salpingitis, reactive arthritis, and Reiter syndrome.

*Diagnosis:* Diagnosis is made predominantly by culture or NAAT. Cultures are more expensive and less accurate than newer NAATs. Vaginal or cervical samples are preferred. As with gonorrhea, the first portion of the urine stream is collected.

*Management:* Treatment preferences can vary but preferred drug remains Azithromycin 1 g as a single dose.

## CONCLUSION

As evident from above discussion, fever in pregnant woman living in tropics requires special attention because of effect on both maternal and fetal health. Apart from good clinical history and examination, availability of good diagnostic tests makes these etiologies fully treatable with good clinical outcomes.

## SUGGESTED READING

1. Kasper D, Fauci A, Hauser S, Longo D, Jameson J, Loscalzo J. Harrison's principles of internal medicine, 19th edition. New York: McGraw-Hill Professional Publishing; 2018.
2. Le Gouez A, Benachi A, Mercier FJ. Fever and pregnancy. Anaesth Crit Care Pain Med. 2016;35:S5-12.

## SECTION 9: Infectious Diseases

3. Acker DB, Schulman EB, Ransil BJ, Sachs BP, Friedman EA. The normal parturient's admission temperature. Am J Obs Gynecol. 1987;157(2):308-11.
4. Dashe JS, Bloom SL, Spong CY, Hoffman BL. Williams Obstetrics. New York: McGraw Hill Professional; 2018.
5. World Health Organization. Practical manual for malaria programme review and malaria strategic plan midterm review. Geneva: WHO; 2016.
6. D'Alessandro U, Hill J, Tarning J, Pell C, Webster J, Gutman J, et al. Treatment of uncomplicated and severe malaria during pregnancy. Lancet Infect Dis. 2018;18(4):e133-46.
7. Desai M, Hill J, Fernandes S, Walker P, Pell C, Gutman J, et al. Prevention of malaria in pregnancy. Lancet Infect Dis. 2018;18(4):e119-32.
8. Rac MW, Sheield JS. Prevention and management of viral hepatitis in pregnancy. Obstet Gynecol Clin North Am. 2014;41(4):573-92.
9. American College of Obstetricians and Gynecologists. Viral hepatitis in pregnancy. Practice Bulletin No. 86. Obstet Gynecol. 2007;110(4):941-56.
10. Drake AL, Wagner A, Richardson B, John-Stewart G. Incident HIV during pregnancy and postpartum and risk of mother-to-child HIV transmission: a systematic review and meta-analysis. PLoS medicine. 2014;11(2):e1001608.
11. Fihn SD. Acute uncomplicated urinary tract infection in women. New Engl J Med. 2003;349(3):259-66.
12. Banhidy F, Ács N, Puho EH, Czeizel AE. Pregnancy complications and birth outcomes of pregnant women with urinary tract infections and related drug treatments. Scandinavian J Infect Dis. 2007;39(5):390-7.
13. Mignini L, Carroli G, Abalos E, Widmer M, Amigot S, Nardin JM, et al. Accuracy of diagnostic tests to detect asymptomatic bacteriuria during pregnancy. Obs Gynecol. 2009;113(2):346-52.
14. Cox SM, Cunningham FG. Acute focal pyelonephritis (lobar nephronia) complicating pregnancy. Obs Gynecol. 1988;71(3 Pt 2):510-1.
15. Snider D. Pregnancy and tuberculosis. Chest. 1984;86(3):10s-3s.
16. Ormerod P. Tuberculosis in pregnancy and the puerperium. Thorax. 2001;56(6):494-9.
17. Snider Jr DE, Layde PM, Johnson MW, Lyle MA. Treatment of tuberculosis during pregnancy. Am Rev Respir Dis. 1980;122(1):65-79.
18. Maldonado YA, Read JS, Committee on Infectious Diseases. Diagnosis, treatment, and prevention of congenital toxoplasmosis in the United States. Pediatrics. 2017;139(2):e20163860.
19. Best JM, O'Shea S, Tipples G, Davies N, Al-Khusaiby SM, Krause A, et al. Interpretation of rubella serology in pregnancy—pitfalls and problems. BMJ. 2002;325(7356):147-8.
20. Centers for Disease Control and Prevention. Knowledge and practices of obstetricians and gynecologists regarding cytomegalovirus infection during pregnancy--United States, 2007. MMWR. 2008;57(3):65.
21. Ash SJ, O'Keane J. Syphilis in Pregnancy. JSOGC. 1995;17(1):17-25.
22. Workowski KA, Berman SM. Centers for Disease Control and Prevention sexually transmitted disease treatment guidelines. Clin Infect Dis. 2011;53(Suppl 3):S59-63.
23. Centers for Disease Control and Prevention. Sexually transmitted disease surveillance, 2006. Atlanta: US Department of Health and Human Services; 2007. pp. 7-36
24. Kjaer HO, Dimcevski G, Hoff G, Olesen F, Østergaard L. Recurrence of urogenital Chlamydia trachomatis infection evaluated by mailed samples obtained at home: 24 weeks' prospective follow up study. Sex Transm Infect. 2000;76(3):169-72.

# CHAPTER 3

# Vaccination in Adolescent Girls and Women

*Mary John*

## ABSTRACT

Adolescent vaccination has been neglected due to various reasons namely financial, lack of an immunization schedule and this group being considered a relatively healthy one. However, the importance of understanding the need to vaccinate the adolescents cannot be undermined, as this will definitely have a positive health impact on these individuals. The Indian Academy of Pediatrics (IAP) has devised a separate immunization schedule for adolescents to use in the private sector, some of which can be applied to the adolescent group as a whole.

## INTRODUCTION

The importance of vaccinating adolescent girls and women has been a neglected domain in the practice of preventive medicine in India. Adolescents are in the age group of 10–19 years as defined by the WHO and UNICEF. India has a very robust Universal Immunization Programme (UIP). However, there is no follow-up immunization schedule or awareness amongst the medical profession on the concept and usefulness of vaccine preventable diseases (VPDs).

Although adolescents are considered to be a relatively healthy group, they are also vulnerable to various infections which may be prevented with immunization. High-risk behavior like IV drug abuse and sexual promiscuity are also prevalent in this group. There are around 243 million adolescents in India in whom booster or primary vaccination need to be administered. Adolescents also form a large proportion of the reproductive age group and there is need to immunize this group as they are not included in the UIP. There is a need to immunize adolescents against VPD's like hepatitis A, varicella, rubella, mumps, and meningococcal infection. Adolescent girls would benefit with HPV vaccination before going in for pregnancy. Since there are no Indian Immunization Programs for adolescents, the Indian Academy of Pediatrics (IAP) has devised an adolescent immunization schedule for the private sector, and categorized the schedule into three groups as follows:
1. *"Mandatory" vaccines* : Human papillomavirus (HPV) and tetanus, diphtheria and pertussis (Tdap)
2. *"Catch-up" vaccines*: Measles, mumps, and rubella (MMR), varicella, typhoid, hepatitis B and A

## SECTION 9: Infectious Diseases

3. *Vaccines given under "Special circumstances"*: Influenza, Japanese encephalitis, pneumococcal polysaccharide vaccine, and rabies.

The *IAP-ACVIP* recommendations for 2018–2019 has revised its recommendations and has suggested prioritization of vaccines for adolescents in India as follows (**Table 1**):
- Human papillomavirus
- Dengue
- Tetanus-diphtheria (Td)
- Mumps/MMR
- Hepatitis A
- Typhoid
- Varicella
- Hepatitis B

*Before vaccination,* a detailed history about the following should be undertaken:
- Past vaccination history
- Health status
- Coexisting diseases
- Immunosuppressive state
- Past history of the disease to be vaccinated for
- Past allergies or adverse effects of vaccination
- Pregnancy status

*Immunization in pregnant women*: The following general points are to be noted:
- Live attenuated virus and live bacterial vaccines are contraindicated during pregnancy; women should avoid conception for at least 4 weeks after vaccination.
- Immune globulin preparations are safe
    - In India, *tetanus toxoid* is the only vaccine routinely recommended in pregnancy.
      *Two doses*: About 0.5 mL, intramuscular (IM): 6–8 weeks apart
      *First dose*: About 22–24 weeks, one booster dose needed if previous pregnancy was within 3 years and if mother received complete prophylaxis in previous pregnancy.
    - *Influenza vaccination* is recommended by the CDC and Advisory Committee on Immunization Practices (ACIP) in all to be pregnant/pregnant women in any trimester during the influenza season.
      Trivalent influenza vaccine (TIV), single dose, annual; 0.5 mL IM.
    - *Measles, Mumps, Rubella*: Not to be administered in pregnancy, women to be counseled against conceiving for 28 days after vaccination with MMR vaccine.
    - *Hepatitis B vaccine*: Given to all women who are identified at risk for HBV infection during pregnancy and having more than one sex partner during previous 6 months, been evaluated or treated for an STD, recent or current injection drug use or having had an HBsAg-positive sex partner.
    - *Tetanus, diphtheria and pertussis/Td*: Tdap to be administered during each pregnancy irrespective of prior immunization with Tdap; administer vaccine between 27 to 36 weeks/anytime/immediately postpartum.
    - *Varicella vaccine*: Not given in pregnancy though pregnant women are at higher risk for severe varicella complications. Varicella zoster immunoglobulin (VZIG) strongly recommended in pregnant women without evidence of immunity, who have been exposed to varicella. This is to prevent complications in the mother but does not prevent viremia in fetus, congenital varicella syndrome or neonatal varicella. Following VZIG administration, varicella vaccine is given 5 months later (if not contraindicated).
        Vaccine—live attenuated varicella-zoster virus (VZV) (oka strain); 2 doses; 0.5 mL univalent varicella vaccine SC, 6 weeks apart.

**CHAPTER 3:** Vaccination in Adolescent Girls and Women

**TABLE 1:** Adolescent immunization.

| Vaccine | Rationale | Indication | Contraindication | Dose | Side effects |
|---|---|---|---|---|---|
| HPV (QHPV– HPV4 or BHPV–HPV2) | Decreases incidence of cervical cancer by 70% and genital warts | • Before commencement of sexual activity in females 11–12 years age; given even at 9 years and up to 26 years if unvaccinated<br>• HIV positive and immunocompromised | Pregnancy | • 3 doses 0, 1–2 and 6 months<br>• Catch-up vaccine up to 45 years | |
| Tdap (Boostrix or Adacel) Td | Protects in recurrent outbreaks | • Vaccinate in anticipation of local outbreak as it provides only short-term protection (1–2 years)<br>• In pregnancy, protects young infants (27–33 weeks)<br>• In unvaccinated or if status unknown | Encephalopathy within 7 days of previous dose<br>Anaphylaxis contains latex<br>Unstable neurological disease<br>LGBS (6 weeks after TT or diphtheria vaccine | • 3 doses<br>1st—Tdap;<br>4 weeks—Td;<br>6–12 months<br>• Booster at age 10–11 years and then every 10 years | Fever |
| Mumps/MMR | Highest incidence in adolescence | Single dose of mumps/MMR for every adolescent irrespective of past vaccination status | Pregnancy; anaphylaxis | 0.5 mL SC in upper arm | • Fever<br>• Malaise<br>• Arthralgia<br>• Arthritis<br>• LGBS<br>• Aseptic meningitis<br>• SSPE |

*Continued*

# SECTION 9: Infectious Diseases

*Continued*

| Vaccine | Rationale | Indication | Contraindication | Dose | Side effects |
|---|---|---|---|---|---|
| Hepatitis A (Vaqta–Merck Or Havrix-GSK) | • Higher attack rate in adolescents than children (4.6 vs. 3.1%)–eating out frequently<br>• Higher rates of hepatic failure | • "Catch-up" immunization for unvaccinated at 2–18 years<br>• Travel to or working in endemic countries – start 1 month before travelling<br>• MSM, Illicit drug users<br>• Food handlers<br>• Laboratory workers<br>• Persons who receive clotting factor concentrates<br>• Chronic liver disease; Persons infected with other hepatitis viruses | • Serious adverse reaction to previous dose of vaccine<br>• Moderately or severely ill persons | • 2 doses 0, 6–18 months<br>• Vaqta- 0.5 mL IM<br>• Havrix 0.5 mL IM | • Soreness at site of injection<br>• Headache<br>• Malaise<br>• Vaqta-Anaphylaxis<br>• LGBS<br>• Transverse myelitis<br>• Multiple sclerosis<br>• Erythema multiforme<br>• Havrix— no serious side effects |
| Typhoid (Vi-PS Polysaccharide and Ty21a oral vaccine | High incidence of typhoid fever | • Children 5–15 years and adolescents at greater risk with high mortality<br>• 2 weeks before travel<br>• Outbreak control | Ty21a not given below 6 years age | 0.5 mL IM, repeat once every 3 years<br><br>Oral—3 doses, alternate days | Local swelling<br><br>• Ty21a—fever, rash, abdominal pain, nausea, vomiting,<br>• Demyelinating disease |

*Continued*

*Continued*

| Vaccine | Rationale | Indication | Contraindication | Dose | Side effects |
|---|---|---|---|---|---|
| Varicella Varilrix Or Okavax | • VZV infection common in tropical countries<br>• Varicella disease more severe in adolescents and adults<br>• Seroprevalence increases with age | • Child-bearing age<br>• Household contacts of immune-immunocompromised people<br>• HCW<br>• Persons exposed to a case | • Pregnancy<br>• Primary and secondary immunodeficiency states<br>• HIV (avoid salicylates 6 weeks after immunization) | 2 doses; 0.5 mL, SC at 0 and 4 weeks | Skin rash |
| Hepatitis B Recombivax-HB | Indulgence in sexual activities and other high-risk behavior | • High risk groups<br>• Persons requiring multiple transfusions<br>• HIV<br>• ESRD<br>• Chronic liver disease<br>• HCW | HBsAg positive persons | 3 doses; 0.5 mL; 0,1 and 6 months | |

(ESRD: end-stage renal disease; HBsAg: hepatitis B virus surface antigen; HCW: healthcare worker; HIV: human immunodeficiency virus; IM: intramuscular; LGBS: Landry-Guillain-Barré syndrome; MSM: men who have sex with men; Td: tetanus-diphtheria; Tdap: tetanus, diphtheria and pertussis; VZV: varicella-zoster virus; SSPE: subacute sclerosing panencephalitis; TT: tetanus toxoid)

## CONCLUSION

Vaccination in adolescent girls and women remains an important health issues. Although, IAP has revised vaccination in this group as mandatory vaccines, catch up vaccines and vaccines under "special circumstances". HPV vaccine, dengue, tetanus diphtheria, mumps/MMR, hepatitis A, typhoid, varicella and hepatitis B are the vaccines on priority list. Tetanus toxoid is the only vaccine routinely recommended in pregnancy. Live attenuated virus and bacterial vaccines are contraindicated during pregnancy and women should be advised to avoid conception for at least one month after receiving the vaccine.

## SUGGESTED READING

1. Verma R, Khanna P, Chawla S. Adolescent vaccines: Need special focus in India. Hum Vaccin Immunother. 2015;11(12):2880-2.
2. Ministry of Health and Family Welfare. (2015-2016). National Family Health Survey, India. NFHS-4 Publications. [Online] Available from http://rchips.orginfhs/NFHS-4Reports/India.pdf. [Last accessed January, 2020].
3. Vashishtha VM. Adolescent immunization schedule: Need for a relook. Indian Pediatr. 2019;56(2):101-4.
4. Choudhury P. Immunization of adolescents. In: Vashishtha VM, Chodhury P, Bansal CP, et al. IAP Guidebook on Immunization 2013-2014. Gwalior: Gwalior National Publication House, Indian Academy of Pediatrics; 2014. pp. 357-63.
5. Balasubramanian S, Shah A, Pemde HK, Chatterjee P, Shivananda S, Guduru VK, et al. Indian Academy of Pediatrics (IAP) Advisory Committee on Vaccines and Immunization Practices (ACVIP) Recommended Immunization Schedule (2018-19) and Update on Immunization for Children Aged 0 Through 18 years. Indian Pediatr. 2018;55:1066-74.
6. Singla S, Agarwal AK, Singal RK. Adolescent immunization. In: Muruganathan A, Mathai D, Sharma SK, Nadkar MY, Munjal YP. Adult Immunization 2014; 2nd edition. New Delhi: Jaypee Brothers Medical Publishers (P) Ltd; 2014. pp. 8-12.
7. Sharma SK, Ruhela V. Immunization in pregnant women. In: Adult Immunization 2014, 2nd edition. Muruganathan A, Mathai D, Sharma SK, New Delhi: Jaypee Brothers Medical Publishers (P) Ltd; 2014. pp. 126-33.
8. Mast EE, Margolis HS, Fione AE, Brink EW, Goldstein ST, Wang SA, et al. A comprehensive immunization strategy to eliminate transmission of hepatitis virus infections in the United States: recommendations of the Advisory Committee on Immunization Practices (ACIP) part 1: Immunization of infants, children and adolescents. MMWR Recomm Rep. 2005;54(RR-16):1-31.
9. Centre for Disease Control and Prevention. Updated recommendations for use of tetanus toxoid and acellular pertussis vaccine (Tdap) in pregnant women–Advisory Committee on Immunization Practices(ACIP), 2012. MMWR Morb Mortal Wkly Rep. 2013;62(7):131-5.
10. Marin M, Güris d, Chaves SS, Schmid S, Seward JF; Advisory Committee on Immunization Practices, Centers for Disease Control and Prevention (CDC) . Prevention of varicella: Recommendations of the Advisory Committee on Immunization Practices (ACIP). MMWR Recomm Rep. 2007;56(RR-4);1-40.
11. Federation of Obstetric and Gynaecological Societies of India (2010). Recommendations for vaccination against human papilloma virus (HPV) infection for the prevention of cervical cancer. [Online] Available from www.fogsi.org/images/stories/pdf. [Last accessed January, 2020).
12. Broder KR, Cortese MM, Iskander JK, Kretsinger K, Slade BA, Brown KH, et al. Preventing tetanus, diphtheria, and pertussis among adolescents: use of tetanus toxoid, reduced diphtheria toxoid and acellular pertussis vaccines recommendations of the Advisory Committee on Immunization Practices (ACIP). MMWR Recomm Rep. 2006;55(RR-3):1-34.
13. Vashishtha VM, Yadav S, Dabas A, Bansal CP, Agarwal RC, Yewale VN, et al. IAP position paper on burden of mumps in India and vaccination strategies. Indian Pediatr. 2015;505(15):505-14.
14. Arankalle V, Mitra M, Bhave S, Ghosh A, Balasubramanian S, Chatterjee S, et al. Changing epidemiology of hepatitis A virus in Indian children. Vaccine: Development and therapy. 2014:4:7-13.
15. Ochiai RL, Acosta CJ, Danovaro-Holliday MC, Baiqing D, Bhattacharya SK, Agtini MD, et al. Study of typhoid fever in five Asian countries: Disease burden and implications for controls. Bull World Health Organ. 2008;86:260-8.

# CHAPTER 4

# Tuberculosis in Women: Unaddressed Issues

*Mohanjeet Kaur, Rupinder Kaur, Jyoti Jindal*

## ABSTRACT

Tuberculosis (TB) is the leading cause of mortality among young and middle-aged females. Many unaddressed issues like socioeconomic factors, lack of education, and gender barriers inhibit the women from seeking care, and that further leads to poor diagnostic rate and greater mortality rate. This further only affects women's health physically and mentally but it has also negative effects on family and society. Women empowerment, integration of various women health programs with TB programs, improvement in diagnostic tests, and research projects taking into consideration women concerns is the need of the day.

## INTRODUCTION

Tuberculosis (TB) is a contagious airborne disease. TB can have severe consequences for women especially during their reproductive years. So, we need to discuss these issues. This will further generate the positive health impacts, which is good for society and overall economy.

## TUBERCULOSIS BURDEN IN WOMEN

Women's health is a good indicator of economic development in the country. That means if women are healthy, economies tend to be healthier.

In 2008, one in five women with TB disease died. Among that, 700,000 women who died from TB in 2008, 200,000 had HIV.

It is one of the top five killers of women among adult women aged 20–59 years. 480,000 women died from TB in 2014 and among that, 140,000 women were HIV-positive (**Table 1**).

**TABLE 1:** Women mortality due to TB and HIV.

|  | Mortality due to TB cases | Mortality (TB + HIV) |
|---|---|---|
| 2008 | 700,000 | 200,000 |
| 2014 | 480,000 | 140,000 |

(HIV: human immunodeficiency virus; TB: tuberculosis)

In 2018, 3.2 million women had suffered TB and among that half million died, 95,000 deaths had both HIV and TB.

## UNADDRESSED ISSUES

### Socioeconomic Factors and Gender Barriers

As TB is considered as man dominant disease, this fear not only delays a woman from seeking medical care, but also cause many problems in the personal and professional life. Women, especially young women and girls, make up a larger proportion of the world's extreme poor and two-thirds of the world's illiterate are women.

*Contributing factors are*:
- Poverty
- Low socioeconomic status
- Lack of education, and
- Poor healthcare access
- Lack of independence

In some of the communities women are not free to travel on their own and must be accompanied, such things lead to delay in seeking care, diagnosis, and poorer prognosis. As per WHO report, since 70% of health workers are women, their health issues need to be catered well.

## CLINICAL MANIFESTATIONS OF TUBERCULOSIS

*Clinical manifestations of TB include:*
- Primary TB
- Reactivation TB
- Endobronchial TB, and
- Tuberculoma

*Pulmonary complications of TB are:*
- Hemoptysis
- Pneumothorax
- Bronchiectasis
- Extensive pulmonary destruction
- Chronic pulmonary aspergillosis
- Progressive primary disease with TB pneumonia, and
- Hilar lymphadenopathy
- Distant sites commonly with cervical lymphadenopathy, meningitis, pericarditis, or miliary dissemination.

## TUBERCULOSIS AND PREGNANCY

Tuberculosis is a cause of overall infertility as it can affect the genitals; it causes between 1 and 16% of overall infertility. Recent pregnancy is a risk factor in developing active TB in women living with HIV.

Pregnant women with TB have increased incidence of complications during and after pregnancy.

CHAPTER 4: Tuberculosis in Women: Unaddressed Issues

*Tuberculosis increases the risk of:*
- Miscarriage
- Insufficient weight gain
- Premature labor
- Transmission of TB to the fetus during the pregnancy or birth
- Newborns of mothers with TB are at an increased risk of death, low birth weight, and contracting TB after birth.

## TUBERCULOSIS AND BREASTFEEDING

Breast milk is very important for a newborn baby as it not only provides nutrition but also has immunological benefits. As per AAP recommendations, expressed milk should be given to babies, in mothers with pulmonary TB who are contagious, untreated or treated (<3 weeks) with isolation. According to WHO guidelines, breastfeeding should be continued under all circumstances.

## TUBERCULOSIS AND HIV

Both HIV and TB are leading cause of death among infectious diseases. Coinfection of HIV along with TB is very common globally due to the comprised immunity in HIV people. Therefore, antiretroviral therapy in HIV patients should be started as early as possible to prevent the progression of TB. All HIV people should be closely monitored for active signs and symptoms of TB so that necessary investigations and treatment can be done.

## MULTIDRUG-RESISTANT TUBERCULOSIS IN WOMEN

Multidrug-resistant tuberculosis (MDR-TB) mainly affects young adults, including women of reproductive age group. MDR-TB treatment is controversial in pregnant ladies. The management options include termination of pregnancy, use of second-line antitubercular drugs during pregnancy or reduction, and suspension of treatment during pregnancy. All pregnant women with MDR-TB should be given right to choose among these options.

## TREATMENT OF TUBERCULOSIS

Various treatment regimen for tubercular patients as per Revised National TB Control Programme (RNTCP) guidelines are depicted in **Tables 2** and **3**.

## IMPACT OF TUBERCULOSIS ON WOMEN

Tuberculosis is considered as "man's disease" and the stigma and fear attached to the disease is responsible for its greater impact on women as compared to men.

As tubercular patients, women have to face many concerns due to discredit status given by the society. There are reduced chances of marriage or chances of no marriage at all in girls whereas as married women faces the risk rejection by husband, harassment by in-laws family, and even divorce. This leads not only delay in seeking medical care but also significant effect on treatment adherence in women. In his study, Rajeswari R et al. found that both rural and urban female patients faced rejection by their families in (15%) of cases.

TABLE 2: Treatment regimen for drug-susceptible tuberculosis as per RNTCP.

| Treatment regimens | | |
|---|---|---|
| Category of treatment | Type of patient | Regimen |
| Category I | All new pulmonary (smear-positive and negative), extra pulmonary and 'others' TB patients | $2H_3R_3Z_3E_3 + 4H_3R_3$ |
| Category II | • TB patients who have had more than one month anti-tuberculosis treatment previously<br>• Relapse, failure, treatment after default, others | $2H_3R_3Z_3E_3S_3 + 1H_3R_3Z_3E_3 + 5H_3R_3E_3$ |

(E: ethambutol; H: isoniazid; R: rifampicin; RNTCP: Revised National TB Control Programme; S: streptomycin; TB: tuberculosis; Z: pyrazinamide)

TABLE 3: Treatment regimen for drug-resistant tuberculosis as per RNTCP: If INH resistance is not known or DST result shows sensitivity to INH, then addition of INH in the above-mentioned regimen of antitubercular drugs is to be done.

| Type of TB Case | Treatment regimen in IP | Treatment regimen CP |
|---|---|---|
| Rifampicin resistant + Isoniazid sensitive or unknown | (6–9) Km LfxEto Cs Z E H | (18) LfxEto Cs EH |
| MDR-TB | (6–9) Km LfxEto Cs Z E (Modify treatment based on the level of INH resistance as per the footnote) | (18) LfxEto Cs E |

(Cs: Cycloserine; CP: continuation phase; E: ethambutol; Eto: ethionamide; H: isoniazid; IP: intensive phase; Km: kanamycin; Lfx: levofloxacin; MDR-TB: multidrug-resistant tuberculosis; Z: pyrazinamide)

Negative impact of TB may lead to infertility, menstrual disorders, and chronic pain in females in reproductive age group. There is 6-fold increase in perinatal deaths and a 2-fold increased risk of premature birth and low birth-weight in mothers with TB.

There is strong association between HIV and TB. Presence of TB in HIV-positive mothers increases maternal and infant mortality rates by 300%.

The delay in seeking medical care and poor adherence to treatment in women affects not only women's health physically as well as mentally but it has also negative effects on family and society. There is increased risk of spread of disease from mother to child in their growing period and child may have to leave school to take care of mother, if father is earner. TB in women has adverse effect on child's survival also and thus leads to increase in number of orphans. It gives birth to deprived families and reduces the economic development of society.

In certain industries, female workers constitute the main workforce. These unaddressed issues can affect those workplaces adversely in various ways like low productivity, absenteeism, and high medical costs.

# WHAT CAN BE DONE?

## Women Empowerment

This is the key to change the current scenario of TB in women. Education and gender equity is its main element. Development programs should be focused on these aspects to ensure women empowerment.

## Commitment, Collaboration, and Integration

Mobilization of support at global and national level to ensure gender equitable access to all the facilities from diagnosis of TB to treatment, counseling, prevention, and supportive care. There should be collaboration and integration among the different global and national maternal and child healthcare programs and the TB programs to ensure adequate screening, early diagnosis of TB, and treatment adherence in female patients.

## Improvement in Data Collection and Monitoring System

Under notification of female patients with TB is a major issue. Social and cultural factors account for leading cause in under notification of female cases as compared to male but biological mechanism also may have important role in sexual inequity in TB. So improvement in TB data collection on the basis of sex and age is required to be maintained by promoting data recording and reporting programs. Integrated patient monitoring systems for TB, HIV should be strengthened to ensure successful follow-up of all the patients.

## Advance Diagnostic Techniques

Gender-equitable and easy accessibility of advanced diagnostic techniques like genexpert MTB/RIF is the need of the day. The use of xpert MTB as initial step for diagnosis of TB should be scaled up especially for the patients with HIV and patients suspected of multidrug resistant TB.

## Research

Research projects for the development of new diagnostic techniques and newer drugs, taking into consideration the specific needs of women should be advocated.

# CONCLUSION

As women's health is an indicator of the health of the family, the issues regarding the diagnosis, availability of treatment and notification of tuberculosis is very important. The issues of infertility, chronic pelvic inflammatory disease (PID), fetal outcome, breastfeeding need to be settled. The integration of woman and child healthcare programme should incorporate TB control programme for more effective culmination of this disease. TB with HIV and MDR TB also need special attention.

# SUGGESTED READING

1. Boudet AMM, Buitrago P, de la Briere BL, Newhouse D, Matulevich ER, Scott K, et al. Gender differences in poverty and household composition through the life-cycle: a global perspective. Washington, D.C: The World Bank; 2018.
2. United Nations. (2015). The World's Women 2015: Trends and Statistics. [online] Available from https://unstats.un.org/unsd/gender/worldswomen.html. [Last accessed January, 2020].
3. OECD. (2014). Gender, Institutions and Development Database. [online] Available from https://stats.oecd.org/Index.aspx?DataSetCode=GIDDB2014. [Last accessed January, 2020].
4. American Academy of Pediatrics. Tuberculosis. In: Pickering LK, (Ed). Red book: Report of the Committee on Infectious Diseases, 29th edition. Elk Grove Village, IL: American Academy of Pediatrics; 2012. pp. 736-56.

5. World Health Organization (WHO). Treatment of tuberculosis guidelines, 4th edition. Geneva: WHO; 2009.
6. Palacios E, Dullman R, Munoz M, Hurtado R, Chalco K, Guerra D, et al. Drug resistant tuberculosis and pregnancy. Clin Infect Dis. 2009;48(10):1413-9.
7. Chaudhuri AD. Recent changes in technical and operational guidelines for tuberculosis control programme in India–2016: A paradigm shift in tuberculosis control. J Assoc Chest Physicians. 2017;5(1):1-9.
8. Rajeswari R, Balasubramanian R, Muniyandi M, Geetharamani S, Thresa X, et al. Socio-economic impact of tuberculosis on patients and family in India. Int J Tuberc Lung Dis. 1999;3(10):869-77.
9. Connolly M, Nunn P. Women and tuberculosis. World Health Stat Q. 1996;49(2):115-9.
10. Neyrolles O, Quintana-Murci L. Sexual inequality in tuberculosis. PLoS Med. 2009;6(12):e1000199.

# SECTION 10

# Miscellaneous

## SECTION EDITOR
Anubha Rathi

**CHAPTER 1**

# Women and Eye Health

*Anubha Rathi, Madhushmita Mahapatra, Supriya Sharma, Namrata Sharma*

## ABSTRACT

Worldwide, two-thirds of the visually impaired individuals are women. The age-standardized adult prevalence of blindness in women is 1.26 times that in men. Several eye disorders such as thyroid eye disease, dry eye, uveitis, and angle closure glaucoma are seen more commonly in women. Most of these diseases cause avoidable blindness. In this chapter, we present an overview of various ocular diseases and discuss their gender predilection. We also highlight the gender gap in treatment-seeking behavior among the genders, especially when it comes to non-life-threatening ocular morbidities.

## INTRODUCTION

The most crucial social determinant of the health situation in a country is gender equity. Most of the times, due to non-life-threatening nature of the disease, eye health takes a further back seat in this regard. Worldwide, two-thirds of the visually impaired individuals are women. The age-standardized adult prevalence of blindness in women is 1.26 times that in men. Eye diseases are not only more commonly seen in women; they also tend to be more severe at presentation in the female gender. The burden of female blindness bears special importance as it affects the development and upbringing of the future generations as well. Various socioeconomic factors are associated with the higher incidence of blindness and visual impairment in women than men. Women are less likely to seek healthcare, especially eye care for themselves. In developing nations, the poor access to healthcare makes it even more difficult for women to seek appropriate eye care. Women tend to live longer than men, so the incidence of some diseases like age-related macular degeneration (ARMD) is higher in women. It is also possibly related to estrogen withdrawal after menopause. Autoimmune conditions and associated eye changes are also more commonly seen in women. This chapter highlights the pertinent gender gap seen in eye disorders and eye health-related conditions.

**Where does India stand?**
In the last few decades, two large population-based surveys have been conducted in India. One was a detailed eye examination survey (1999–2001) and the other was a rapid

assessment of blindness survey conducted in 2006–2007. Both surveys studied a total of over 1 lac participants ≥50 years of age and defined blindness as presenting visual acuity <3/60 in both eyes. The prevalence of blindness in 1999–2001 was 5.36% while it was 3.82% in 2006–2007. Male blindness was 4.19% in 1999–2001 which dropped to 3.05% in 2006–2007, while in females it was 6.4% in 1999–2001 and dropped to 4.44% in 2006–2007. Hence, though there was a significant reduction in overall blindness between 1999 and 2001 and 2006–2007 among both the genders, yet a significant difference in the prevalence of blindness between males and females was seen. The risk of blindness in women in urban areas was 1.41 times higher compared to males, while in rural areas it was 1.51 times higher. Overall, after adjusting for region and year of survey, it was observed that females had a 1.76 times higher risk of blindness compared to males. In both the surveys, it was seen that males had a 40% lower risk of being cataract blind compared to females. This gender inequity has both biological and social determinants. The aim of this chapter is to highlight them in order to understand the gravity of the situation and take appropriate measures to bridge the gender gap.

**A woman's eye: Is it biologically different?**
Most of the previous ophthalmic research considers women and men as a sex neutral form as patients and give results for a homogenous population. Richards et al. found that the results of same cataract surgery procedure with intraocular lens (IOL) implantation are seen to be worse in women than men. They attributed this to error in IOL power calculation as the same formulae cannot be considered for the two widely different genders. Women are noted to have shorter axial length and steeper keratometry. This could be due to their short stature and shallow orbit volumes. Because of these structural and anatomic differences, women are more prone to develop certain ocular conditions such as cataract and angle closure glaucoma (ACG).

Hormonal changes in the course of a woman's life span especially pregnancy and menopause further affect the ocular biometry and ask for special considerations while treating eye diseases in this subset of population. Similarly, lacrimal disorders such as nasolacrimal duct (NLD) obstruction are more commonly seen in women owing to the shorter and straighter placement of NLD in women.

## EYE DISORDERS AND GENDER PREDILECTION

Several eye ailments are seen to have a gender predisposition with most of them affecting women more both epidemiologically and in severity. For the ease of understanding, these disorders have been classified as under:
- Disorders of the orbit, lids, lacrimal apparatus, and adnexa
- Diseases of conjunctiva and sclera
- Diseases of cornea
- Diseases of the lens
- Glaucoma
- Diseases of retina and uvea
- Neuro-ophthalmologic disorders

## Disorders of the Orbit, Lids, Lacrimal Apparatus, and Adnexa

Among the various disorders of eyelids, lacrimal apparatus, and adnexa which have a female gender predisposition, thyroid eye disease is the most common. Other disorders affecting women more in number include vascular malformations, hemangiomas, orbital

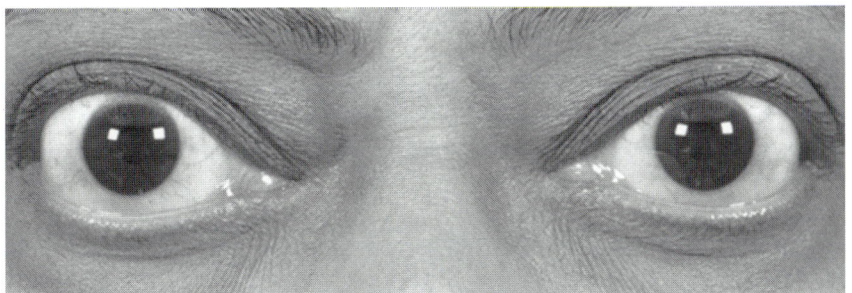

**FIG. 1:** Clinical photograph of bilateral axial proptosis in a woman with thyroid eye disease (TED). *(For color version, see Plate 6)*

meningioma, lacrimal gland adenoid cystic carcinoma, sebaceous cell carcinoma of the lids, and primary acquired NLD obstruction.

Thyroid eye disease (TED) (**Fig. 1**) is an autoimmune inflammatory disorder of the orbit. It may be associated with both Graves' disease and Hashimoto's thyroiditis. TED involves autoimmune activation of preadipocytic orbital fibroblasts by circulating thyroid-stimulating hormone (TSH) receptor-directed antibodies and infiltration of inflammatory cells. The increase in the bulk of orbital tissue leads to proptosis and other clinical signs of TED. Although TED is more commonly seen in women, the female-to-male ratio is reversed at 1:4 in severe TED.

Among eyelid tumors, benign lid tumors have no gender predilection while malignant tumors are more commonly seen in women. Basal cell carcinoma is the most common lid tumor with a higher rate of occurrence in women. Sebaceous cell carcinoma has the worst prognosis among various lid tumors and is also seen more commonly in females. Squamous cell carcinoma of the lid has a male preponderance on the other hand.

Proptosis is more commonly seen in women with TED being the most common etiology. Other than TED, meningioma, hemangioma, and lacrimal gland mass are other causes of proptosis in women.

Epiphora is also more commonly reported by females as compared to males. The characteristic shorter route of a thinner NLD in the female gender along with the higher incidence of associated deviated nasal septum, rhinitis, and sinusitis leads to more predisposition to development of primary acquired NLD obstruction (PANDO) in women.

## Disorders of Conjunctiva and Sclera

Disorders of conjunctiva such as pinguecula and pterygium (**Fig. 2**) have been attributed to several environmental risk factors particularly ultraviolet (UV) exposure. Gender predilection for the development of pterygium has been studied with mixed results. It is majorly confounded by other factors such as the nature of study population, lifestyle, and grade of outdoor exposure to environmental risk factors. Most studies have shown that men have higher prevalence of pterygium and are attributed to the nature of work with more hours spent outdoors. With the nature of a woman's work changing and several women doing prolonged outdoor work as well, this equation does not hold true for all spheres of society. In a study done in rural setting in China, the prevalence in females was much higher than that in males. It was done in the Bai minority community of China where they have a matriarchal society with women involved in outdoor work, particularly in farming or fishing and men are usually engaged in business, as drivers or in various indoor jobs.

SECTION 10: Miscellaneous

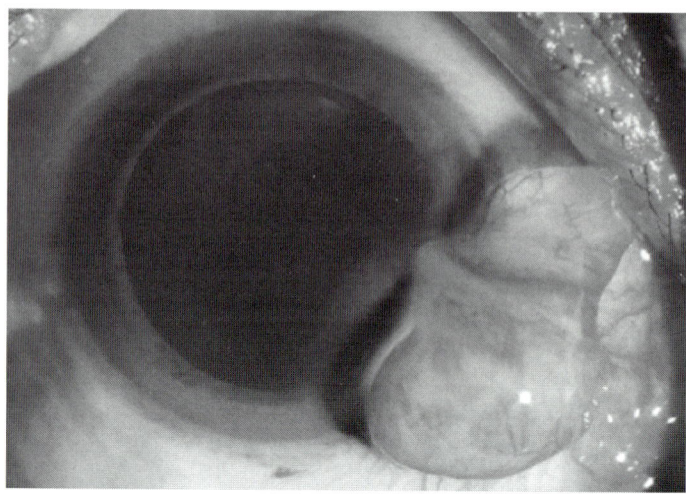

FIG. 2: Clinical photograph of pterygium with cystic degeneration. *(For color version, see Plate 6)*

Hence, there is no particular gender predisposition for pterygium and pinguecula and it is mainly governed by other factors such as inflammation, environmental factors, etc.

Vitamin A deficiency (VAD) is characterized by conjunctival xerosis and Bitot's spots. Bitot's spots are usually located temporally and appear as dry triangular patches with a foamy surface. There is a metaplasia of the conjunctival epithelium and presence of keratin mixed with *Corynebacterium xerosis* in the stratum corneum of the conjunctiva. The gas production from the bacteria gives the typical foamy appearance. Malnourishment is relatively more common in female gender as compared to males especially in the developing world. Hence, they are more likely to develop VAD and its sequelae. Moreover, pregnant and lactating women are at even greater risk of developing VAD and its ocular complications.

Ocular conjunctival melanocytic lesions range from benign conjunctival nevi to malignant melanoma. Benign conjunctival nevi are fairly common. They are more often seen in light-colored individuals and generally located at the nasal or temporal limbus. The melanocytic lesions have been seen to change in color, texture, and size with hormonal changes including puberty and pregnancy. No gender predilection has been noted for both benign and malignant conjunctival melanocytic lesions.

Ocular surface squamous neoplasia (OSSN) (**Fig. 3**) is a malignant lesion of conjunctiva and ocular surface. It has varying presentations. In the Western countries, it is seen more in fair-skinned males while in Africa and Asia, there is no definite gender predilection reported.

Episcleritis and scleritis (**Fig. 4**) are commonly seen in females, especially in association with various connective tissue disorders such as rheumatoid arthritis (RA) and systemic lupus erythematosus (SLE). They are common causes of acute red eyes in women and must be differentiated from other causes of red eye as their presence may require systemic workup to rule out associated autoimmune disorders. Both episcleritis and scleritis tend to recur. They can be differentiated on the basis of a simple phenylephrine test where 2.5% or 10% phenylephrine drops instilled in the inflamed eye blanches the episcleral vessels while it has no effect on the scleral vessels. Scleritis may be associated with deep boring pain and often requires corticosteroid therapy once the cause is established and is noted to be noninfective.

CHAPTER 1: Women and Eye Health

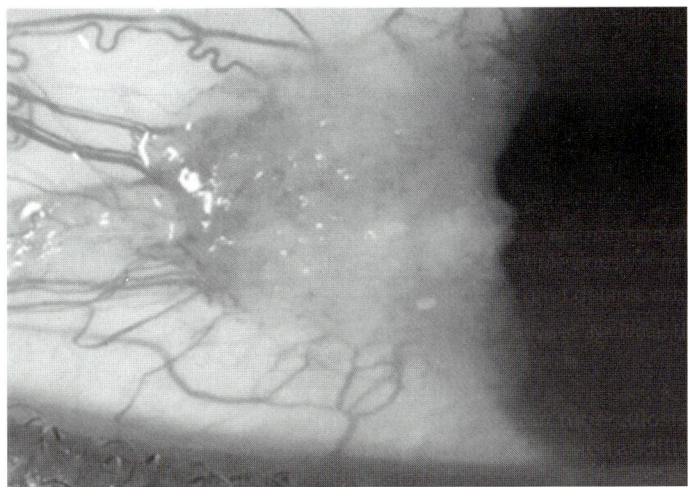

**FIG. 3:** Clinical photograph of an eye with ocular surface squamous neoplasia (OSSN). *(For color version, see Plate 6)*

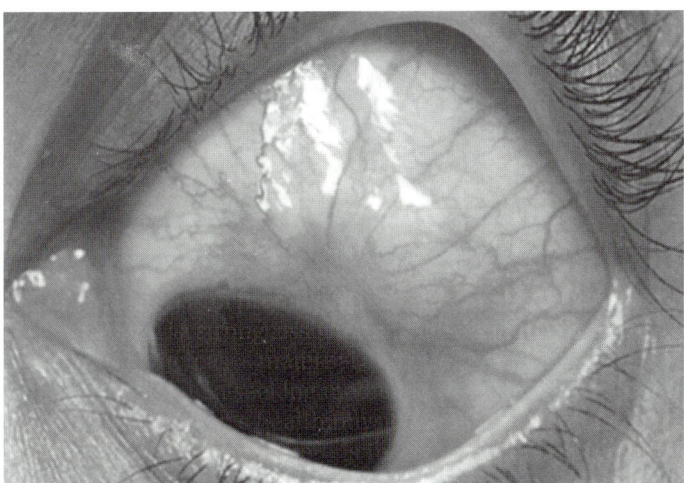

**FIG. 4:** Clinical photograph of an eye with nodular scleritis. *(For color version, see Plate 7)*

# Disorders of Cornea

Among the various disorders of cornea afflicting the females, corneal dystrophies and degenerations need a special mention. Corneal degenerations are typically age related and are usually present bilaterally. They are usually peripheral or may involve the entire cornea. Several degenerations are known to affect the cornea such as arcus senilis, Terrien's marginal degeneration (TMD), and Salzmann's nodular degeneration (SND). While arcus senilis and TMD show male preponderance, SND is more commonly seen in middle-aged females. Typically, these degenerations are not associated with significant vision loss. If extensive, they may lead to vision deprivation and need surgical treatment.

Corneal dystrophies (**Fig. 5**) are usually bilateral and typically more central as compared to degenerations. Most of the corneal dystrophies affect both genders equally, except Fuchs endothelial corneal dystrophy (FECD). FECD is seen in middle-aged females and

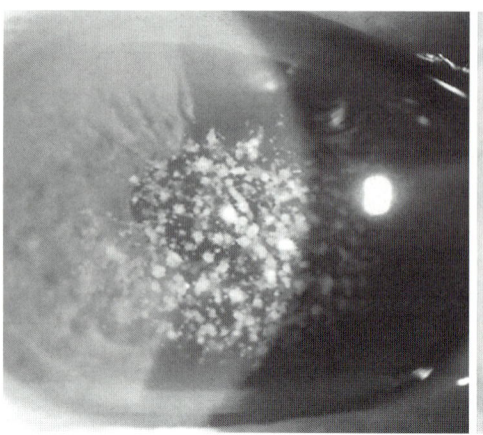 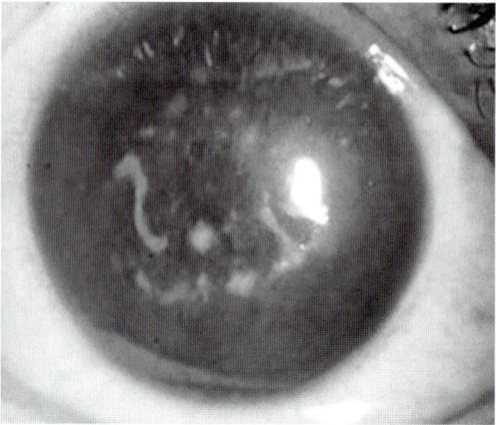

**FIG. 5:** Clinical photograph of eyes with corneal dystrophies. *(For color version, see Plate 7)*

is mostly sporadic. The inherited form of FECD shows autosomal dominant inheritance. FECD is gradually progressing and typically presents with early morning blurring of vision. It is initially managed medically but in advanced stages, surgical treatment in the form of posterior lamellar or full-thickness corneal transplantation may be needed.

Corneal ulcer or keratitis is seen more commonly in the male gender and is related to more outdoor work. These ulcers could be infective or noninfective. Infective or microbial keratitis could be caused by bacteria, fungus, virus, or parasite. Several atypical microorganisms are also known to cause corneal ulcers. A case of corneal ulcer typically needs an elaborate workup and diagnostic evaluation to determine the cause of the ulcer and provide treatment accordingly. A delay in treatment or incorrect or incomplete treatment can lead to permanent visual disability. In rural areas where females work at the farms, fungal corneal ulcers due to trauma to the eye by vegetative matter are fairly common in women as well. Lack of proper and timely eye care in such cases very often leads to permanent visual loss in these women making them visually dependent for life. Corneal blindness is avoidable and treatable. Several programs for the elimination of corneal blindness are targeted at timely referral of such cases to hospitals equipped with cornea services and functional eye bank, so that these precious eyes can be saved. It has been seen that in the developing countries, females with corneal ulcers usually present later as compared to their male counterparts. They are also less compliant with medications and follow-up possibly owing to social and economic constraints.

Peripheral ulcerative keratitis (PUK) is a form of noninfectious keratitis. It is seen in association with many autoimmune systemic diseases. Almost half of PUK is due to various collagen vascular diseases with RA being most common. Other associations include Wegener granulomatosis, microscopic polyangiitis, relapsing polychondritis, polyarteritis nodosa, and Churg–Strauss syndrome. PUK has no gender preponderance and affects both genders equally. Before initiating therapy, the presence of any focus of infection associated with PUK needs to be completely ruled out. Further management includes systemic workup and immunosuppressive therapy or corticosteroid therapy once the diagnosis is established.

Dry eye disease (DED) is more common in females, especially in postmenopausal age group. Several hormonal factors play a role in DED. It is the most common complaint which brings women to the ophthalmologist, especially in the developed world and in urban areas of developing nations as well. The diagnosis, presentation, and management of DED is discussed in detail in the next chapter.

Refractive errors in the form of myopia, hypermetropia, and astigmatism are known to affect both genders. What sets women apart in this regard is the social stigma of spectacles that is rampant in our society. The footfall of girls in marriageable age in the refractive surgery clinics around the world is proof enough. While myopia and astigmatism are seen more commonly in males, hyperopia is more commonly encountered in females. Amblyopia is also more commonly seen in females possibly due to lack of prescribed spectacle use in early childhood. With the advent of safe and affordable options in refractive surgery, the number of individuals opting for these is increasing day by day. While it is a welcome change, yet the fact that most of the girls who opt for these are doing so under parental or societal pressure only to get married, as the spectacled look is not acceptable to the community, is a matter of concern. A refractive surgery is an elective procedure and should be purely the decision of the person who goes for it and not governed by social norms.

## Disorders of the Lens

Cataract is the leading cause of avoidable blindness worldwide. It has been seen to be more common in women than men. Several studies show that women have more prevalence of lenticular opacification, mostly cortical cataract. One such study revealed 24–27% prevalence in women in the age group between 65 and 74 years as compared to 14–20% in age-matched males. The possible role of estrogen in cataract formation is being studied in this regard. As hormone replacement therapy (HRT) in postmenopausal females is associated with decreased risk of cataract, it has been hypothesized that the reduction in estrogen after menopause may be the culprit for increasing the possibility of cataract formation in women. It is not the presence or amount of estrogen, but the withdrawal effect which seems to be responsible. As cataractogenesis is related to oxidative stress, the protective effect of 17 beta-estradiol against the oxidative stress may also have a role.

Ectopia lentis refers to dislocation of crystalline lens from its natural position. It can be hereditary or acquired. Among the acquired causes, trauma and inflammation are common. Hereditary causes of ectopia lentis include Marfan syndrome, Weill–Marchesani syndrome, and homocystinuria. While traumatic ectopia lentis is more common in males, hereditary causes of ectopia do not show any particular gender predisposition.

Congenital cataract is seen to occur equally in both genders. Congenital cataract surgical rate is higher in boys as compared to girls. This is possibly due to the gender disparity in seeking care for children, especially in developing nations.

## Glaucoma

Due to anatomic differences, women in general are more prone to develop ACG while no specific gender predilection has been found for open angle glaucoma (OAG). Female gender is also considered an important risk factor for developing normal tension glaucoma (NTG). Similar to cataract, this risk is attributed to estrogen withdrawal around menopause. Hence, HRT is being studied for protective role for glaucoma as well. A review of United Healthcare database showed that females are 24% less likely to be seek treatment for glaucoma. As glaucoma is an irreversible cause of blindness, late presentation can lead to permanent visual disability.

## Diseases of Retina, Vitreous, and Uvea

Female sex hormones exert a neuroprotective action on the retina. Endogenous estrogens are seen to be protective against ARMD. The extent of estrogen exposure depends on menarche, age at menopause, number of pregnancies, use of HRT, and oral contraceptives. Central serous chorioretinopathy (CSCR) is linked to exogenous testosterone therapy. Macular hole is more common in women especially postmenopausal females and is possibly linked to withdrawal of estrogen. The neuroprotective action of progesterone has been thought to protect the female retina and its photoreceptors. Studies are underway exploring its role in treatment of retinitis pigmentosa (RP).

Uveitis or the inflammation of iris and ciliary body is fairly common in females. It may have several systemic associations. Uveitis is dealt with in detail in a subsequent chapter.

## Neuro-ophthalmologic Abnormalities

Optic neuritis or the inflammation of the optic nerve sheath is known to affect young and middle-aged women more as compared to men. It can be seen in association with infections such as Lyme disease or diseases such as multiple sclerosis or vitamin and nutritional deficiencies.

Benign intracranial hypertension (BIH) can present with bilateral disk edema or papilledema in the absence of any intracranial lesion or specific cause. It is seen more in young obese females. The therapy involves lowering intracranial pressure and reducing weight.

# PREGNANCY AND EYE

Pregnancy may induce several changes in a woman's eye. Most of these changes are reversible. They could be physiological or pathological. Discoloration or pigmentation of eyelid skin is fairly common along with pigmentation around the cheek which is referred to as chloasma. Transient corneal edema or thickening is noted with corneal steepening, especially in the late trimesters. Pregnancy-related dry eye is attributed to the hormonal changes. A slight myopic shift is noted due to change in curvature of the crystalline lens. Hence, refraction may change during pregnancy. This change is usually reversed after delivery and further more after breastfeeding is over. There is a risk of postrefractive surgery ectasia in some females due to corneal changes in pregnancy. This risk is higher in females who have associated hormonal disorders or thyroid disturbances. Refractive surgery is contraindicated in pregnancy. Intraocular pressure (IOP) has been seen to reduce in pregnancy.

# CONCLUSION

Gender equity is the most crucial social determinant of the health situation in a country. In the present day and era, most of the world's nations are still far from achieving this gender equity. It is attributed to lack of awareness, lack of healthcare-seeking behavior as also the anatomic difference and disease presentation in the female gender.

## SUGGESTED READING

1. Bourne RRA, Flaxman SR, Braithwaite T, Cicinelli MV, Das A, Jonas JB, et al. Magnitude, temporal trends, and projections of the global prevalence of blindness and distance and near vision impairment: a systematic review and meta-analysis. Lancet Glob Health. 2017;5:e888-97.
2. Murthy GV, Gupta SK, Bachani D, Jose R, John N. Current estimates of blindness in India. Br J Ophthalmol. 2005;89:257-60.
3. Neena J, Rachel J, Praveen V, Murthy GVS. Rapid Assessment of Avoidable Blindness in India. PLoS One. 2008;3:e2867.
4. Tan AG, Wang JJ, Rochtchina E, Mitchell P. Comparison of age-specific cataract prevalence in two population-based surveys 6 years apart. BMC Ophthalmol. 2006;6:17.
5. Friedman DS, Nordstrom B, Mozaffari E, Quigley HA. Variations in treatment among adult-onset open-angle glaucoma patients. Ophthalmology. 2005;112:1494-9.

# Dry Eye in Women

*Manpreet Kaur, Swapna Shanbhag, Anubha Rathi, Namrata Sharma*

## ABSTRACT

Dry eye disease (DED) results from disharmony in the tear film homeostasis. It is significantly more common in women, especially in the postmenopausal age group. The increased prevalence in women may be attributed to various factors such as hormonal changes, increased prevalence of autoimmune disorders in females, and a difference in treatment-seeking behavior. The clinical symptoms and signs, diagnosis, and treatment modalities are similar in men and women; however, the management approach may vary among the sexes. The management involves a more holistic approach. In this chapter, we discuss the various predisposing factors, clinical presentation, signs, and management approaches to DED in women.

## INTRODUCTION

The TFOS-DEWS II (Tear Film and Ocular Surface Society Dry Eye Workshop II) report defines dry eye disease (DED) as a multifactorial disorder of the ocular surface characterized by a loss of the tear film homeostasis accompanied by ocular symptoms, in which tear film instability, hyperosmolarity, ocular surface inflammation, damage, and neurosensory abnormalities play etiological roles.

Dry eye disease is significantly more common in women as compared with men, especially in the postmenopausal age group. The increased prevalence in women may be attributed to various factors such as hormonal changes, increased prevalence of autoimmune disorders in females, and a difference in treatment-seeking behavior. The chronicity of the disorder often adversely impacts the quality of life of women. The Women's Health Study and the Physicians' Health Studies have observed a disproportionately greater impact of DED on the activities of daily living among women as compared with men and an increased likelihood of dissatisfaction due to the treatment adverse effects. Timely detection and institution of appropriate therapy are essential to ensure the well-being of patients. The clinical symptoms and signs, diagnosis, and treatment modalities are similar in men and women; however, the management approach may vary among the sexes.

We herein discuss the various predisposing factors, clinical presentation, signs, and management approaches to DED in women.

## EPIDEMIOLOGY

Dry eye disease affects disproportionately more women than men with an earlier onset of the disease process in women. The overall prevalence of DED ranges from 6.7 to 28.7% with women affected two to three times more often than men. The TFOS-DEWS II epidemiology report highlighted an increase in prevalence of DED in women with age from 14% at 50 years to 22% in 80+ years. In contrast, the prevalence in men was reported to be 7% at 60–69 years of age which gradually progressed to 13% at 80+ years.

## PATHOPHYSIOLOGY OF DRY EYE DISEASE

The tear film is composed of a precorneal mucoaqueous subphase and a superficial lipid layer. The mucoaqueous subphase is formed by the secretions of lacrimal glands, goblet cells, and tarsal glands. The lipid layer is composed of secretions of the meibomian glands.

The main underlying pathophysiology of DED is tear film instability and hyperosmolarity caused due to evaporation of the tear film, which damages the ocular surface either directly or by inducing an inflammatory response. The two main subtypes of dry eyes include the evaporative dry eye (EDE) and aqueous deficient dry eye (ADDE). The ADDE and EDE exist as a continuum as per the new classification scheme of DED, rather than being mutually exclusive. Conditions affecting lacrimal gland function such as Sjögren's syndromes and other autoimmune conditions that result in lacrimal gland infiltration and reduced aqueous secretion predominantly lead to ADDE, whereas, ocular surface, lid, and meibomian gland-related causes predominantly lead to the development of EDE.

## PREDISPOSING FACTORS

Dry eye disease has a multifactorial etiology and various environmental, systemic, and ocular factors play a contributory role. Environmental pollutants and allergens are related to tear film dysfunction and DED. In addition, systemic autoimmune and collagen vascular diseases, chronic diseases such as diabetes, and prolonged administration of various systemic as well as topical medications also adversely affect the health of the tear film. Ocular adnexal and surface disorders result in DED due to decreased secretion of tears, improper and uneven distribution of the tear film on ocular surface, and instability of the tear film. In addition, various behavioral, systemic, and hormonal factors have been linked to an increased prevalence of dry eyes in women, which are discussed below:

- *Hormonal factors*: The hormonal fluctuations occurring in females during their life span, including menstruation, pregnancy, lactation, and menopause may adversely impact the ocular surface and tear film dynamics and lead to an increased propensity to develop DED in women.

    Perimenopausal DED has been linked to androgen insufficiency in recent studies. Androgens have been observed to be involved in the optimal functioning of meibomian and lacrimal glands and the decreased androgen levels in females explains the higher propensity of DED in women. Moreover, the androgen levels further decrease in perimenopausal females which may result in an increased incidence of DED. Postmenopausal females on hormone replacement therapy (HRT) are more likely to experience symptoms related to DED. Of note, estrogen-only therapy is four to seven times more likely to cause DED than no HRT or combination HRT with both estrogen and progesterone. Oral contraceptive pill usage is also linked to an increased incidence of DED.

- *Autoimmune diseases*: Various autoimmune and chronic inflammatory disorders such as thyroid disease, lupus, rheumatoid arthritis, and Sjögren's syndrome are more common in women and are associated with the development of DED.
- *Iatrogenic causes*: Various iatrogenic factors may predispose to the development of DED or aggravate pre-existing dry eyes. Chronic systemic medications such as oral contraceptives and HRT, topical medications with preservatives, contact lens usage, facial cosmetics, permanent cosmetic tattoos on lash line, cosmetic lid surgeries, and refractive surgeries may disturb the ocular homeostasis, lead to destruction of meibomian glands and tear film instability. Contact lens use is associated with DED. Females use contact lenses more commonly and are less likely to discontinue contact lens use on developing early signs of dryness and ocular irritation.

  Heavy cosmetic usage such as eyeliners and kohl on the waterline leads to blockage of meibomian gland ducts and aggravates the symptoms of DED. Eyelash extensions applied with toxic formaldehyde glue and eyeliner tattoos also cause DED. Incomplete removal of eye cosmetics at night contributes to the development of DED.

  Women are more likely to undergo refractive surgeries, lid surgeries such as blepharoplasty, injection of botulinum toxin for the cosmetic correction of wrinkles, face lifts, and brow lifts, all of which have been linked to an increased risk of developing DED. Corneal ablative procedures such as laser-assisted in situ keratomileusis and small incision lenticule extraction lead to DED due to transection of the subepithelial nerve fiber layer and a subsequent decrease in corneal sensations.
- *Behavioral factors*: Women are more likely to seek treatment than men, which may account for a higher incidence of DED.

## CLINICAL PRESENTATION AND DIAGNOSIS

The patients with DED may present with complaints of ocular grittiness or discomfort, burning or stinging sensation in the eye, pain, photophobia, redness, and blurring of vision.

There is no universally acceptable "gold standard" to establish a definitive diagnosis of DED. Different diagnostic criteria exist for DED based on the presence of a combination of symptoms and signs.

The objective assessment of symptoms may be performed using patient reported outcome questionnaires, such as the OSDI (Ocular Surface Disease Index) questionnaire (**Fig. 1**), the Dry Eye Questionnaire 5 (DEQ-5), McMonnies Questionnaire (MQ), Impact of Dry Eye on Everyday Life (IDEEL) questionnaire, DEQS (Dry Eye-Related Quality-of-Life Score), Symptom Assessment in Dry Eye (SANDE), and Standard Patient Evaluation of Eye Dryness (SPEED), etc.

Signs of DED include tear film instability, increased tear osmolarity, decreased secretion of tears, ocular surface staining, increased tear inflammatory mediators, and abnormal impression cytology, which may be evaluated using a number of diagnostic tests as detailed below.
- *Tear film stability*: Tear breakup time (TBUT) and noninvasive breakup time (NIBUT) are commonly performed to assess the stability of the tear film. TBUT is the duration of time from a complete blink to the appearance of the first dry spot on the cornea. It is generally performed after instillation of 1% sodium fluorescein in the conjunctival fornix to enhance the visibility of the tear film. NIBUT is a noninvasive diagnostic modality wherein the specular reflection of an illuminated grid pattern or placido rings from the ocular surface is observed. A value of <10 seconds on TBUT or NIBUT is indicative of tear film instability.

## Ocular Surface Disease Index© (OSDI©)

Ask your patient the following 12 questions, and circle the number in the box that best represents each answer. Then, fill in the boxes A, B, C, D, and E according to the instructions beside each.

| Have you experienced any of the following *during the last week?* | All of the time | Most of the time | Half of the time | Some of the time | None of the time | |
|---|---|---|---|---|---|---|
| 1. Eyes that are sensitive to light? | 4 | 3 | 2 | 1 | 0 | |
| 2. Eyes that feel gritty? | 4 | 3 | 2 | 1 | 0 | |
| 3. Painful or sore eyes? | 4 | 3 | 2 | 1 | 0 | |
| 4. Blurred vision? | 4 | 3 | 2 | 1 | 0 | |
| 5. Poor vision? | 4 | 3 | 2 | 1 | 0 | |

Subtotal score for answers 1 to 5 (A)

| Have problems with your eyes limited you in performing any of the following *during the last week?* | All of the time | Most of the time | Half of the time | Some of the time | None of the time | N/A |
|---|---|---|---|---|---|---|
| 6. Reading? | 4 | 3 | 2 | 1 | 0 | N/A |
| 7. Driving at night? | 4 | 3 | 2 | 1 | 0 | N/A |
| 8. Working with a computer or bank machine (ATM)? | 4 | 3 | 2 | 1 | 0 | N/A |
| 9. Poor vision? | 4 | 3 | 2 | 1 | 0 | N/A |

Subtotal score for answers 6 to 9 (B)

| Have your eyes felt uncomfortable in any of the following situations *during the last weeks?* | All of the time | Most of the time | Half of the time | Some of the time | None of the time | N/A |
|---|---|---|---|---|---|---|
| 10. Windy conditions? | 4 | 3 | 2 | 1 | 0 | N/A |
| 11. Places or areas with low humidity (very dry)? | 4 | 3 | 2 | 1 | 0 | N/A |
| 12. Area that are air conditioned? | 4 | 3 | 2 | 1 | 0 | N/A |

Subtotal score for answers 10 to 12 (C)

Add subtotals A, B, and C to obtain D
(D = sum of scores for all questions answered) (D)

Total number of questions answered
(do not include questions answered N/A) (E)

**FIG. 1:** The Ocular Surface Disease index (OSDI) questionnaire used for objective assessment of dry eye symptoms.

**SECTION 10:** Miscellaneous

- *Tear volume*: Tear meniscometry (tear meniscus height and volume) may be performed to assess tear volume. Slit lamps, digital meniscometers, and optical coherence tomography (OCT) devices may be used to perform tear meniscometry and provide a noninvasive assessment of tear volume. Conventionally, the characteristics of the tear meniscus in the center of the lower eyelid are assessed after a complete blink without manipulation of the eyelid.

   Schirmer test employs a 5 × 35 mm Schirmer strip which is placed in the temporal one-third of the lower fornix to assess tear secretion. The wetting of the strip in 5 minutes is assessed. It may be performed without anesthesia, with topical anesthesia, or with nasal stimulation. Schirmer test without anesthesia provides an estimate of stimulated reflex tearing and a value <5 mm is indicative of severe aqueous deficiency, as in Sjögren's-associated DED. Schirmer test is invasive in nature with variable test readings, thereby limiting its use as a routine diagnostic test in evaporative DED.

- *Tear osmolarity*: Tear hyperosmolarity is the underlying pathophysiology of DED and raised tear osmolarity values have been observed to be most specific to the diagnosis of DED. A cutoff value of 316 mOsm/L is diagnostic of moderate-to-severe DED whereas a cutoff value of 308 mOsm/L is more sensitive for the diagnosis of mild-to-moderate DED, especially when used in conjunction with other tests. The TFOS-DEWS II diagnosis report suggests a value over 308 mOsm/L in either eye or at least 8 mOsm/L difference in osmolarity between the two eyes as indicative of disturbance in tear film homeostasis and ocular surface instability.

- *Ocular surface assessment*: Ocular surface staining is routinely performed for the diagnosis and management of DED (**Fig. 2**). Punctate staining of the cornea or conjunctiva is indicative of DED. The dyes used to stain the cornea and conjunctiva include sodium fluorescein, rose bengal, and lissamine green. Various grading systems are available to ensure consistent evaluation of the ocular surface staining including the van Bijsterveld system, the Oxford grading, the National Eye Institute/Industry Workshop guidelines, and the Collaborative Longitudinal Evaluation of Keratoconus (CLEK) grading. A combination of sodium fluorescein (for cornea) and lissamine green (for conjunctiva) is preferred to evaluate ocular surface staining.

   Conjunctival impression cytology may be performed to assess squamous metaplasia and goblet cell density of the conjunctiva. It is useful in establishing the severity of disease and monitoring response to treatment.

   Corneal sensations may be assessed using a cotton wisp or Cochet-Bonnet esthesiometers. The test has low sensitivity for DED, but the specificity increases with disease severity.

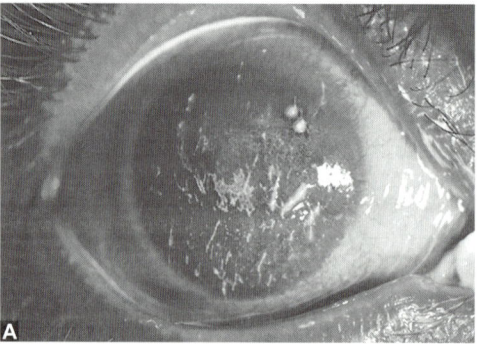 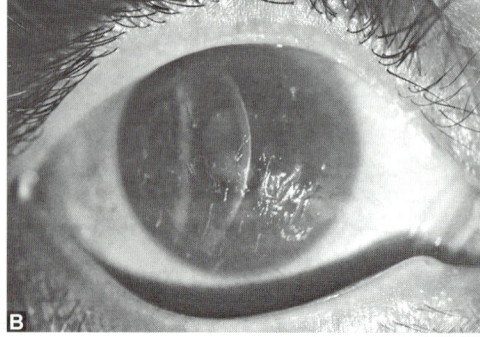

**FIG. 2:** (A) Clinical photograph of an eye with severe dryness after fluorescein staining under cobalt blue filter. (B) Clinical photograph of an eye with severe dryness showing a lustreless cornea. *(For color version, see Plate 7)*

- *Ocular surface inflammation*: Various inflammatory markers present in the tear film may be used as indicators of chronic ocular surface inflammation, including matrix metalloproteinases (MMPs), tear cytokines and chemokines, and HLA-DR expressions. A rapid screening assay has been developed for the quantification of MMP-9 levels in the tear film within 10 minutes, with values above 40 ng/mL indicative of ocular surface inflammation. However, these tests are not specific for the diagnosis of DED, require specialized equipment, and are costly, limiting their widespread usage.
- *Interferometry and meibography*: Thickness of the lipid layer of the tear film may be assessed using interferometry. The LipiView interferometer allows automated assessment of lipid layer thickness and establishes a cutoff of 75 nm for diagnosis of meibomian gland dysfunction.

Meibomian gland morphology may be assessed using meibography which gives information regarding gland dropout, truncation of glands, etc.

## MANAGEMENT

A stepwise algorithm is recommended for the management of DED. Firstly, the patients must be educated regarding their ocular condition and explained regarding the chronicity of the disease. It is essential to determine the underlying causative factor for the DED and correct it if possible. Estrogen-only HRT is strongly associated with DED in postmenopausal women and the patients may be advised to shift to a combination therapy containing both estrogen and progesterone. DED associated with chronic systemic medications may benefit from shifting to an alternative systemic drug if feasible. Similarly, preservative-associated DED in patients using topical eye drops for prolonged periods may improve after shifting to preservative-free eye drops. Lifestyle changes such as decreasing cosmetic usage, avoiding contact lenses, and limiting screen time also alleviate the symptoms of DED. Topical lubricants form the mainstay of therapy and a variety of topical formulations are available constituting of carboxymethyl cellulose (CMC), dextran, hyaluronic acid (HA), HP-Guar, hydroxypropyl methylcellulose (HPMC), polyvinyl alcohol (PVA), and polyethylene glycol. The patients should be encouraged to maintain proper lid hygiene and warm compresses may be advised in cases with coexisting meibomian gland dysfunction.

Temporary or permanent occlusion of the puncta may be required in more severe cases for conservation of tears. Moisture chambers and dark goggles also help to maintain a localized humidified environment around the eyes. Various pressure, heat, and light-based therapies are available for meibomian gland dysfunction including LipiFlow and intense pulsed light therapy. In addition, a brief course of oral macrolide or tetracycline antibiotics may be prescribed.

Topical corticosteroids and topical immunosuppressants help to control the underlying inflammation in persistent cases. Oral secretagogues may be prescribed to facilitate aqueous secretion. A combination of various therapeutic modalities with a more aggressive approach may be required in severe cases including bandage contact lenses, amniotic membrane grafts, surgical punctal occlusion, minor salivary gland transplants, and tarsorrhaphy.

Women are likely to be more compliant in following the treatment regimen.

## CONCLUSION

To conclude, DED is a chronic ocular problem that is widely prevalent among post-menopausal women and adversely impacts their quality of life. Androgen insufficiency, hormonal fluctuations, autoimmune diseases, and increased use of cosmetics or cosmesis-

## SECTION 10: Miscellaneous

related surgeries have been linked to an increased propensity to develop DED in women. The investigations and management of DED in women are as per standard protocol. It is also essential to determine the underlying cause to enable a holistic treatment of DED in women.

## SUGGESTED READING

1. Craig JP, Nichols KK, Akpek EK, Caffery B, Dua HS, Joo CK, et al. TFOS DEWS II definition and classification report. Ocul Surf. 2017;15:276-83.
2. Caffery BE, Richter D, Simpson T, Fonn D, Doughty M, Gordon K. The Canadian Dry Eye Epidemiology Study. Adv Exp Med Biol. 1998;438:805-6.
3. Schaumberg DA, Sullivan DA, Buring JE, Dana MR. Prevalence of dry eye syndrome among US women. Am J Ophthalmol. 2003;136:318-26.
4. Chia EM, Mitchell P, Rochtchina E, Lee AJ, Maroun R, Wang JJ. Prevalence and associations of dry eye syndrome in an older population: the Blue Mountains Eye Study. Clin Exp Ophthalmol. 2003;31:229-32.
5. Moss SE, Klein R, Klein B. Prevalence of and risk factors for dry eye syndrome. Arch Ophthalmol. 2000;118:1264-8.
6. Matossian C, McDonald M, Donaldson KE, Nichols KK, MacIver S, Gupta PK. Dry Eye Disease: Consideration for Women's Health. J Womens Health (Larchmt). 2019;28:502-14.
7. Gagliano C, Caruso S, Napolitano G, Malaguarnera G, Cicinelli MV, Amato R, et al. Low levels of 17-beta-oestradiol, oestrone and testosterone correlate with severe evaporative dysfunctional tear syndrome in postmenopausal women: A case–control study. Br J Ophthalmol. 2014;98:371-6.
8. Sriprasert I, Warren DW, Mircheff AK, Stanczyk FZ. Dry eye in postmenopausal women: A hormonal disorder. Menopause. 2016;23:343-51.
9. Ablamowicz AF, Nichols JJ, Nichols KK. Association between serum levels of testosterone and estradiol with meibomian gland assessments in postmenopausal women. Invest Ophthalmol Vis Sci. 2016;57:295-300.
10. Schaumberg DA, Uchino M, Christen WG, Semba RD, Buring JE, Li JZ. Patient reported differences in dry eye disease between men and women: impact, management, and patient satisfaction. PLoS One. 2013;8:e76121.
11. Stapleton F, Alves M, Bunya VY, Jalbert I, Lekhanont K, Malet F, et al. TFOS DEWS II Epidemiology Report. Ocul Surf. 2017;15:334-65.
12. Bron AJ, de Paiva CS, Chauhan SK, Bonini S, Gabison EE, Jain S, et al. TFOS DEWS II pathophysiology report. Ocul Surf. 2017;15:438-510.
13. Fortune MD, Guo H, Burren O, Schofield E, Walker NM, Ban M, et al. Statistical colocalization of genetic risk variants for related autoimmune diseases in the context of common controls. Nat Genet. 2015;47:839-46.
14. Silpa-Archa S, Lee JJ, Foster CS. Ocular manifestations in systemic lupus erythematosus. Br J Ophthalmol. 2016;100:135-41.
15. Patel S, Lundy D. Ocular manifestations of autoimmune disease. Am Fam Physician. 2002;66:991-8.
16. Gomes JAP, Azar DT, Baudouin C, Efron N, Hirayama M, Horwath-Winter J, et al. TFOS DEWS II iatrogenic report. Ocul Surf. 2017;15:511-38.
17. Wolffsohn JS, Arita R, Chalmers R, Djalilian A, Dogru M, Dumbleton K, et al. TFOS DEWS II Diagnostic Methodology report. Ocul Surf. 2017;15:539-74.
18. Bron AJ, Tomlinson A, Foulks GN, Pepose JS, Baudouin C, Geerling G, et al. Rethinking dry eye disease: a perspective on clinical implications. Ocul Surf. 2014;12:s1-31.
19. Kaufman HE. The practical detection of MMP-9 diagnoses ocular surface disease and may help prevent its complications. Cornea. 2013;32:211-6.
20. Finis D, Pischel N, Schrader S, Geerling G. Evaluation of lipid layer thickness measurement of the tear film as a diagnostic tool for Meibomian gland dysfunction. Cornea. 2013;32:1549-53.
21. Jones L, Downie LE, Korb D, Benitez-Del-Castillo JM, Dana R, Deng SX, et al. TFOS DEWS II Management and Therapy Report. Ocul Surf. 2017;15:575-628.

# CHAPTER 3

# Uveitis in Women

Supriya Arora, Anubha Rathi, Somashiela Murthy

## ABSTRACT

Inflammatory autoimmune disorders of the eye can potentially lead to blindness or severe visual impairment. Uveitis refers to inflammation of uvea which includes iris and ciliary body. Uveitis may be infective or noninfective. Noninfective uveitis is generally due to autoimmune etiology and occurs more frequently in women compared to men, though it tends to be more severe in men. Noninfectious uveitis may be associated with systemic autoimmune conditions such as systemic lupus erythematosus (SLE), rheumatoid arthritis (RA), multiple sclerosis (MS), sarcoidosis, etc. The management in such cases needs to be holistic and not just eye centric.

## INTRODUCTION

Women account for 64.5% of blindness worldwide. This gender imbalance could be partially explained by delay in seeking treatment, poor access to care as well as lack of family support. Other than that, it is important to highlight certain ocular disorders which are predominantly seen in women and affect women in more severe forms too.

Inflammatory disorders of the eye or its various parts are basically autoimmune conditions wherein the organ is attacked by the immune system of the body, potentially leading to blindness or severe visual impairment. Uveitis is the third leading cause of blindness worldwide. Women are more predisposed to developing uveitis and this gap widens in older age groups.

Based on etiology, uveitis can be classified into noninfectious (mostly autoimmune) or infectious. Since prevalence of autoimmune diseases is higher in women, similarly uveitides due to autoimmune etiology occurs more frequently in women as compared to men.

## ROLE OF SEX HORMONES AFFECTING AUTOIMMUNE RESPONSE

The B and T cells have estrogen receptors. While the cell-mediated immune response involves Th1 subtype of cells, humoral-mediated immunity involves the Th2 cells. Th2-mediated response predominates in women while men have a stronger Th1 response. This disparity among the genders can partly explain the higher prevalence of Th2-mediated autoimmune disorders in females.

Estrogen may have a dose-dependent effect on the autoimmunity. Higher estrogen levels are related to several autoimmune disorders in women. Estrogen stimulates the Th2 immune response and decreases the cell-mediated immune response. It also increases the production of interferon-gamma and interleukin-10.

Not only does the prevalence of autoimmune uveitides vary between men and women, but they also present with differing severity of the same cause of uveitis.

## NONINFECTIOUS UVEITIS WITH SYSTEMIC INVOLVEMENT

### Juvenile Idiopathic Arthritis

The International League of Associations for Rheumatology (ILAR) has set diagnostic criteria for juvenile idiopathic arthritis (JIA) which includes age <16 years with presence of an unexplained arthralgia for 6 or more weeks. Anterior uveitis is the most common extra-articular feature of JIA. Oligoarthritis variant of JIA is the most common subtype and is more frequently seen in girls than boys.

Almost 50–80% of JIA patients are female and uveitis occurs in 10–45% of JIA patients. Evidence suggests that girls under the age of 7 years at diagnosis of JIA have a greater risk of developing uveitis, as do antinuclear antibody (ANA)-positive children. Although females have higher likelihood of developing uveitis, but uveitis in males with JIA is more severe and is associated with more severe ocular complications as well. This trend of more severity but reduced prevalence in the male gender holds true for most autoimmune disorders.

### Systemic Lupus Erythematosus

Systemic lupus erythematosus (SLE) is a chronic autoimmune disease which affects women disproportionately more. During the childbearing years, female: male prevalence ratio is 9:1. Prior to puberty, this ratio is 2–6:1 and after menopause, this ratio is 3–8:1. It has been suggested that the threshold for disease initiation is lower in women. However, once disease develops in males, it is more severe in them as compared to females. The most common ocular manifestation of SLE is keratoconjunctivitis sicca (KCS). The involvement of retina, choroid, or optic nerve can result in vision-threatening complications.

Systemic lupus erythematosus patients have higher levels of estrogen and active estrogen metabolites in serum and majority of symptoms occurred during luteal phase of menstrual cycle. Also, symptomatic episodes were more common during or immediately after pregnancy. Studies have shown that hormone replacement therapy (HRT) or oral contraceptive estrogen dose doubles the risk of developing SLE.

This may suggest that for same women, higher level of estrogens have a triggering effect for development of SLE. A study has also described previously healthy women developing SLE after repeated cycles of ovulation induction.

In known SLE patients with anticardiolipin antibodies, repeated ovulation induction may result in severe or even fatal flares. Some clinical trials have shown modest clinical improvement in moderate disease with supplementation of exogenous dehydroepiandrosterone sulfate (DHEAS). This therapeutic success could be attributed to modulation of T-cell activity and cytokines secretion in vivo.

## Rheumatoid Arthritis

Rheumatoid arthritis (RA) is a chronic autoimmune disease in which the female to male prevalence has been noted to be 2–3:1. The peak incidence of RA is around 45–55 years which coincides with the perimenopausal age group suggesting that there may be an association between estrogen deficiency and disease development.

After the age of 45 years, the incidence of RA increases in men and approaches age-matched women. This is probably because below the age of 45 years, higher level of androgens may have a protective effect against RA.

Ocular manifestations of RA include KCS, episcleritis, scleritis, corneal changes, and retinal vasculitis.

## Multiple Sclerosis

Multiple sclerosis (MS) is an autoimmune disease affecting young women more frequently and causes demyelination of the central nervous system. It affects a variety of body functions. As the nerve tissue and eye tissue have similar embryonic origin, MS, and uveitis are often seen in association with each other.

## Sarcoidosis

Sarcoidosis is a chronic granulomatous disorder with prominent epithelioid and giant cell granulomas in the absence of any caseous necrosis. It is more common in women and shows a bimodal age distribution with peaks at 25–29 years age and 65–69 years age.

Uveitis is seen in 20–50% cases of sarcoidosis and is usually an early feature. It is characterized by mutton-fat keratic precipitates and typical iris nodules along with anterior and posterior synechiae. Posterior segment of the eye may also be involved with the presence of vitritis, retinal vasculitis, or choroidal lesions. Sight-threatening sequelae of chronic inflammation such as cystoid macular edema may be seen.

Ocular involvement in sarcoidosis is more common in females. Women are also known to have a worse visual outcome.

## Vogt–Koyanagi–Harada Disease

Vogt–Koyanagi–Harada (VKH) is characterized by granulomatous posterior uveitis or panuveitis which is usually bilateral and is associated with a sunset glow fundus. Serous retinal detachments and disk edema may also be seen. VKH is associated with vertigo, tinnitus, hearing loss, vitiligo, poliosis, and meningismus.

Vogt–Koyanagi–Harada is more prevalent in females. In India, 84.4% of VKH patients were females, in Brazil 70% were females, and in USA 78.7% were females.

Gender also affects the prognosis of the patient, similar to other uveitis conditions with systemic involvement. Pregnancy and menstruation appear to be protective in females.

## NONINFECTIOUS UVEITIS WITHOUT SYSTEMIC INVOLVEMENT

## Birdshot Chorioretinopathy

Birdshot chorioretinopathy (BCR), a form of posterior uveitis, is strongly associated with the human leukocyte antigen (HLA)-A29 and is characterized by multiple discrete hypopigmented choroidal lesions. A female preponderance of the disease has been reported and the mean age of presentation was 53 years.

## White Dot Syndromes

Multiple evanescent white dot syndrome (MEWDS) is a self-limiting condition characterized by multiple small, ill-defined white dots at the level of the retinal pigment epithelium or outer retina with a distinct granular appearance in the fovea.

It predominantly affects young myopic women between the age of 20–45 years.

Multifocal choroiditis (MFC) predominantly affects young myopic white women and unlike MEWDS, it is more likely to have irreversible visual damage and impairment. MFC is frequently associated with sight-threatening choroidal neovascular (CNV) membranes.

Punctate inner choroidopathy (PIC) also affects young myopic women more frequently. It is characterized by the presence of small, multiple yellowish white fundus lesions which are mostly limited to the posterior pole of retina. Inflammatory cells are absent in anterior chamber or vitreous. In most of the cases, the disease does not threaten vision, so treatment is not required. However, when subfoveal CNV ensues, rapid loss of sight occurs warranting immediate treatment.

Acute zonal occult outer retinopathy (AZOOR) is also seen in young women predominantly. Almost 28% of AZOOR patients have other associated autoimmune conditions such as Hashimoto's thyroiditis.

Among the white dot syndromes, female predominance, in order of most to least, is PIC > AZOOR > MFC > MEWDS.

However, despite gender differences, no clinical differences or differences in treatment/prognosis have been described between the sexes.

## IMPORTANCE OF STUDYING ROLE OF GENDER IN UVEITIS

It is important for general physicians and other practitioners to know the role of gender in uveitis, so that appropriate patients can be referred to ophthalmologists.

Hormone therapy can be used efficaciously and judiciously in specific patients. For example, use of supplemental estrogen in the form of oral contraceptive pills has been shown to increase flare of SLE. Sarcoidosis has a second peak in postmenopausal women. Hormonal replacement therapy could possibly be utilized as an adjuvant therapy for late-onset sarcoidosis.

## CONCLUSION

Uveitis has a very strong female predilection among various eye disorders. It has a significant association with several autoimmune conditions. Hence it is very important for holistic management of a patient to be aware of possible signs and symptoms of uveitis and look out for it.

## SUGGESTED READING

1. Abou-Gareeb I, Lewallen S, Bassett K, Courtright P. Gender and blindness: A meta-analysis of population-based prevalence surveys. Ophthalmic Epidemiol. 2001;8:39-56.
2. Gritz DC, Wong IG. Incidence and prevalence of uveitis in Northern California; the Northern California Epidemiology of Uveitis Study. Ophthalmology. 2004;111:491-500.

3. Fairweather D, Frisancho-Kiss S, Rose NR. Sex differences in autoimmune disease from a pathological perspective. Am J Pathol. 2008;173:600-9.
4. Pennell LM, Galligan CL, Fish EN. Sex affects immunity. J Autoimmun. 2012;38:J282-91.
5. Yeung IY, Popp NA, Chan CC. The Role of Gender in Uveitis and Ocular Inflammation. Int Ophthalmol Clin. 2015;55:111-31.
6. Verthelyi D. Sex hormones as immunomodulators in health and disease. Int Immunopharmacol. 2001;1:983-93.
7. Choudhary MM, Hajj-Ali RA, Lowder CY. Gender and ocular manifestations of connective tissue diseases and systemic vasculitides. J Ophthalmol. 2014;2014:403042.
8. Ucar-Comlekoglu D, Fox A, Sen HN. Gender Differences in Behçet's Disease Associated Uveitis. J Ophthalmol. 2014;2014:820710.
9. Petty RE, Southwood TR, Manners P, Baum J, Glass DN, Goldenberg J, et al. International League of Associations for Rheumatology Classification of Juvenile Idiopathic Arthritis: Second Revision, Edmonton, 2001. J Rheumatol. 2004;31:390-2.
10. Heiligenhaus A, Heinz C, Edelsten C, Kotaniemi K, Minden K. Review for disease of the year: Epidemiology of juvenile idiopathic arthritis and its associated uveitis: The probable risk factors. Ocul Immunol Inflamm. 2013;21:180-91.
11. Ravelli A, Felici E, Magni-Manzoni S, Pistorio A, Novarini C, Bozzola E, et al. Patients with antinuclear antibody-positive juvenile idiopathic arthritis constitute a homogeneous subgroup irrespective of the course of joint disease. Arthritis Rheum. 2005;52:826-32.
12. Saurenmann RK, Levin AV, Feldman BM, Laxer RM, Schneider R, Silverman ED. Risk Factors for Development of Uveitis Differ Between Girls and Boys With Juvenile Idiopathic Arthritis. Arthritis Rheum. 2010;62:1824-8.
13. Ballou SP, Khan MA, Kushner I. Clinical features of systemic lupus erythematosus: differences related to race and age of onset. Arthritis Rheum. 1982;25:55-60.
14. Lu LJ, Wallace DJ, Ishimori ML, Scofield RH, Weisman MH. Review: male systemic lupus erythematosus: a review of sex disparities in this disease. Lupus. 2010;19:119-29.
15. Mohan C. Environment versus genetics in autoimmunity: a geneticist's perspective. Lupus. 2006;15:791-3.
16. Lahita RG, Bradlow L, Fishman J, Kunkel HG. Estrogen metabolism in systemic lupus erythematosus: patients and family members. Arthritis Rheum. 1982;257:843-6.
17. Folomeev M, Dougados M, Beaune J, Kouyoumdjian JC, Nahoul K, Amor B, et al. Plasma sex hormones and aromatase activity in tissues of patients with systemic lupus erythematosus. Lupus. 1992;13:191-5.
18. Bruce IN, Laskin CA. Sex hormones in systemic lupus erythematosus: a controversy for modern times. J Rheumatol. 1997;24:1461-3.
19. Sánchez-Guerrero J, Liang MH, Karlson EW, Hunter DJ, Colditz GA. Postmenopausal estrogen therapy and the risk for developing systemic lupus erythematosus. Ann Intern Med. 1995;122:430-3.
20. Ben-Chetrit A, Ben-Chetrit E. Systemic lupus erythematosus induced by ovulation induction treatment. Arthritis Rheum. 1994;371:1614-7.
21. Van Vollenhoven RF. Dehydroepiandrosterone in systemic lupus erythematosus. Rheum Dis Clin North Am. 2000;26:349-62.
22. Wilder RL. Adrenal and gonadal steroid hormone deficiency in the pathogenesis of rheumatoid arthritis. J Rheumatol. 1996;44:10-2.
23. Cimmino MA, Salvarani C, Macchioni P, Montecucco C, Fossaluzza V, Mascia MT, et al. Extra-articular manifestations in YZ Italian patients with rheumatoid arthritis. Rheumatol Int. 2000;19:213-7.
24. Jamilloux Y, Kodjikian L, Broussolle C, Séve P. Sarcoidosis and uveitis. Autoimmun Rev. 2014;13: 840-9.
25. Judson MA, Boan AD, Lackland DT. The clinical course of sarcoidosis: Presentation, diagnosis, and treatment in a large white and black cohort in the United States. Sarcoidosis Vasc Diffuse Lung Dis. 2012;29:119-27.
26. Lobo A, Barton K, Minassian D, du Bois RM, Lightman S. Visual loss in sarcoid-related uveitis. Clin Exp Ophthalmol. 2003;31:310-6.
27. Murthy SI, Moreker MR, Sangwan VS, Khanna RC, Tejwani S. The spectrum of Vogt-Koyanagi-Harada disease in South India. Int Ophthalmol. 2007;27:131-6.

## SECTION 10: Miscellaneous

28. Junior BR, Nishi M, Hayashi S, Abreu MT, Petrilli AM, Plut RC. Vogt–Koyanagi–Harada's disease in Brazil. Jpn J Ophthalmol. 1988;32:344-7.
29. Lertsumitkul S, Whitcup SM, Nussenblatt RB, Chan CC. Subretinal fibrosis and choroidal neovascularization in Vogt–Koyanagi–Harada syndrome. Graefes Arch Clin Exp Ophthalmol. 1999;237:1039-45.
30. Gass JD, Agarwal A, Scott IU. Acute zonal occult outer retinopathy: a long-term follow-up study. Am J Ophthalmol. 2002;134:329-39.
31. Faia LJ. Gender differences in birdshot chorioretinopathy and the white dot syndromes: Do they exist? J Ophthalmol. 2014;2014:146768.
32. Birnbaum AD, Rifkin LM. Sarcoidosis: sex-dependent variations in presentation and management. J Ophthalmol. 2014;2014:236905.

# CHAPTER 4

# Otolaryngorhinology in Women

*Bhumika Sharma, Neha Chauhan*

## ABSTRACT

Ear, nose, and throat (ENT) disorders are very commonly encountered among women. Due to lack of accessibility or ignorance, most of the times women present late to the doctor with ENT issues and try home-based remedies to no avail for a long time. Otalgia, blocked ears, ear discharge, decreased hearing, and tinnitus are few common ear-related complaints among women. Nasal obstruction, nasal discharge, postnasal drip, epistaxis, facial pain, and headache secondary to sinusitis are also fairly common among women. This chapter describes the various ENT disorders which are encountered frequently among women.

## INTRODUCTION

Health of an individual contributes to economic and social growth of a country; more so if an individual is a woman. Women's health focuses on the treatment and diagnosis of various diseases and conditions that affect a woman's physical and emotional well-being. Despite several initiatives and efforts worldwide, women from the poorer classes and backward areas experience differential access to healthcare services. In developing nations such as India, women's health takes a further back seat.

Although ear, nose, and throat (ENT) related complaints are one of the common causes for visiting a doctor, most individuals especially females try to manage their problems by home remedies. This can be attributed to lesser number of otolaryngologists, especially in remote areas and less awareness of society regarding the symptoms of sometimes sinister ENT problems.

## COMMON EAR PROBLEMS

Otalgia, blocked ears, ear discharge, decreased hearing, and tinnitus are few common ear-related complaints with which patients present in a clinic. For most of these complaints, patients would have sought multiple consultations (if chronic), that too with physicians and in few, would have tried some or the other home remedies. Prescribing any type of ear drops without knowing the pathology is quite common. Any ear-related complaint actually requires a thorough examination by a trained and experienced ENT surgeon and

SECTION 10: Miscellaneous

many times very simple treatment is required for correcting the underlying pathology. Quite a few numbers of patients require surgical intervention. Surgical treatment is still not a preferred choice by many patients, more so in female population as the household duties and responsibilities come into their way and they rather prefer to live with the disease for many years, sometimes lifelong before actually putting themselves under the knife.

Most of ear diseases do not have a sex predilection, except a few like otosclerosis, glomus tympanicum, and glomus jugulare. They present as decreased hearing, tinnitus, vertigo, and nerve palsies (in glomus). Detailed examination by a specialist is required for diagnosis. Timely intervention can prevent morbidities. Only few cases are managed nonsurgically and rest of them requires surgical intervention.

Presbycusis (age-related hearing loss) requires a special mention. Using hearing aids is still a social taboo. Patients will prefer to be deaf rather than using hearing aids and society calling them deaf. In India, where most of the females are still housewives, do not consider hearing as essential part of their lives and prefer to live with their morbidity. We need to educate and convince them to use hearing aids to make them self-sufficient.

Another chronic ear-related problem is tinnitus, i.e., ringing sensation in ears which may cause a spectrum of symptoms starting from just ringing in ear to severe depression sometimes leading to suicidal tendencies. Quite a few numbers of females present to us with tinnitus. Tinnitus may have "n" number of causes. Any organic cause should be ruled out before commencing treatment. Many drugs have been tried for treating tinnitus, but the most important part of treatment is counseling and psychotherapy, missed out most of the times. Tinnitus matching and masking by a trained professional may help the patients to deal with it.

## COMMON NOSE PROBLEMS

As explained in ear diseases, most of the nose pathology also does not have sex predilection except a few. Patients mostly present with nasal obstruction, nasal discharge, postnasal drip, epistaxis, facial pain, and headache. Ophthalmological involvement secondary to nasal pathology is not uncommon. A detailed ENT examination by a professional is required to reach a diagnosis. Treatment may be medical or surgical depending on the pathology. Irrational and prolonged use of topical decongestants to treat nasal obstruction can be harmful as it leads to rhinitis medicamentosa, a disease more difficult to treat.

Benign intracranial hypertension and spontaneous cerebrospinal fluid (CSF) rhinorrhea have a female preponderance. Combined approach by a team of ENT surgeon, neurologist, and ophthalmologist is required for their treatment.

Atrophic rhinitis (AR) is another chronic disease more commonly seen in females and is characterized by nasal crusting, purulent discharge, nasal obstruction, halitosis, and roomy nasal cavities. Treatment for AR is extensive and not always successful. The main goals of treatment are to rehydrate the inside of nose and to alleviate the crusting that builds up in the nose. In few cases, surgical intervention may be required.

## COMMON THROAT PROBLEMS

Common throat-related symptoms include pain, foreign body sensation, dysphagia, odynophagia, recurrent sore throat, and sometimes symptoms related to voice. Most of these patients do not have serious ailments. Quite a few number of female patients present with the abovesaid symptoms in outpatient department (OPD) and most of them have gastroesophageal reflux disease, globus hystericus, or neuralgia. But the importance of detailed ENT examination including videolaryngoscopy cannot be denied. In addition to medical treatment, counseling and psychotherapy play an important role in these patients. Oral, oropharyngeal, and hypopharyngeal except postcricoid and laryngeal malignancies are more common in males as compared to females but in recent times, increase use of tobacco and alcohol in females will soon be changing the trends. Health education and awareness of women regarding harmful effects of tobacco and alcohol can prevent them from these debilitating diseases.

## VERTIGO AND WOMEN

Dizziness is another common complaint with which patients present in OPD and can be a symptom in any systemic illness. Females presenting with vertigo contribute to a significant number. Diagnosis of a vertigo patient can sometimes be tricky and it needs a thorough neuro-otological examination and a battery of tests including pure tone audiometry, videonystagmography, and sometimes magnetic resonance imaging of brain to reach to a diagnosis. Vertigo can be a symptom in various diseases including migraine-related vertigo at one end to a morbid intracranial pathology at other end. Labyrinthine vertigo is rotatory most of the times and is associated with nausea or vomiting. Aural symptoms are often associated. Treatment of labyrinthine vertigo is disease specific and may not even require antivertigo medicines as is the case with benign positional paroxysmal vertigo where repositioning maneuvers are the basis of treatment. Vestibular rehabilitation forms important part of therapy, especially in case of vestibular neuritis and Meniere's disease. Nonlabyrinthine vertigo requires evaluation by a team of otolaryngologist, neurophysician, orthopedician, and ophthalmologist. Apart from disease-specific treatment, physiotherapy and psychotherapy form essential part of treatment.

## EAR, NOSE, AND THROAT TRAUMA AND WOMEN

In spite of implementation of domestic violence act, it still has its roots deep down in our society. The victims of domestic violence are overwhelmingly women and women tend to experience more severe forms of violence. In our clinical practice, we tend to see victims with tympanic membrane perforation, nasal bone and facial fractures, black eye, and sometimes laryngotracheal trauma (LTT). Later is also seen in road traffic accidents in females wearing dupatta. The long floating end of the dupatta may get entangled in a rotating wheel or machinery and cause serious injuries, sometimes debilitating to larynx and other vital structures in neck. These can be avoided by simply educating cycle rickshaw and two wheeler riders against any loose clothing. Making females aware about the domestic violence act, seeking early legal help, and training females for self-defense can decrease the incidence of grievous injuries sustained as a result of domestic abuse.

## CONCLUSION

In recent times, increased level of education, awareness, and improvement in health infrastructure have helped in early diagnosis and treatment of various ENT diseases. This actually holds true for urban population. In rural and backward population deficiency of experts, lack of awareness, old beliefs, and taboos still prevent the patients especially females in reporting to the health personals which cause increase in the morbidity and hence the economic burden of country. Targeting and educating this group of population will help India to progress in a healthy and progressive way.

## SUGGESTED READING

1. Morrison AW. Otosclerosis: a synopsis of natural history and management. Br Med J. 1970;2:345-8.
2. O'Leary MJ, Shelton C, Giddings NA, Kwartler J, Brackmann DE. Glomus tympanicum tumors: A clinical perspective. Laryngoscope. 1991;101:1038-43.
3. Sanna M, Fois P, Pasanisi E, Russo A, Bacciu A. Middle ear and mastoid glomus tumors (glomus tympanicum): An algorithm for the surgical management. Auris Nasus Larynx. 2010;37:661-8.
4. Carlson ML, Sweeney AD, Pelosi S, Wanna GB, Glasscock ME, Haynes DS, et al. Glomus tympanicum: A review of 115 cases over 4 decades. Otolaryngol Head Neck Surg. 2015;152:136-42.
5. Bunnag C, Jareoncharsri P, Tansuriyawong P, Bhothisuwan W, Chantarakul N. Characteristics of atrophic rhinitis in Thai patients at the Siriraj Hospital. Rhinology. 1999;37:125-30.
6. Bist SS, Bisht M, Purohit JP. Primary atrophic rhinitis: A clinical profile, microbiological and radiological study. ISRN Otolaryngol. 2012;2:404075.

# Ear, Nose, and Throat Disorders in Pregnancy

*Neha Chauhan, Bhumika Sharma*

## ABSTRACT

Pregnancy is associated with a variety of metabolic and hormonal changes in a woman's body. Ear, nose, and throat (ENT) changes seen with pregnancy are fairly common. They can be troublesome as most of the drugs instituted for these conditions otherwise are not safe for use in pregnancy. Most of these changes are self-limiting and hence need only symptomatic treatment.

## INTRODUCTION

Pregnancy induces various metabolic, endocrinological, and physiological changes affecting every system of the body. This chapter briefly describes the multifarious ear, nose, and throat (ENT) manifestations of pregnancy.

Knowledge of these conditions is essential for diagnosis, management, and reassurance of the expecting female. Special considerations should be given while prescribing any medications to safeguard the mother and fetus against any possible adverse effects. The specialist should not hesitate to consult the attending obstetrician for the same. Many of these conditions are self-limiting.

Pregnancy-related physiological ENT changes are described in the following section.

## EAR CHANGES

Hearing impairment during pregnancy may be due to Eustachian tube dysfunction, sudden sensorineural hearing loss, and otosclerosis.

Eustachian tube dysfunction may be due to mucosal edema or patulous Eustachian tube leading to obstruction, otitis media with effusion, autophony, and tinnitus. Tympanic membrane examination reveals fluttering during respiration or retraction, however the pure tone audiogram is usually normal. Management includes reassurance and steam inhalation as the condition usually resolves following delivery.

A pregnant female near term or postpartum may present with complaints of decreased hearing and tinnitus either in one ear or both suggesting otosclerosis. Estrogen in pregnancy stimulates the otosclerotic focus leading to the abovementioned symptoms. Pure tone audiogram reveals mixed hearing loss with Carhart's notch and impedance shows type A curve. Sodium fluoride is contraindicated due to detrimental effects on fetal growth. Patient can be reassured and counseled for surgical treatment in the form of stapedotomy in postpartum period.

Gestation and associated estrogen changes cause hypercoagulability that may affect the inner ear circulation rarely leading to sudden sensorineural hearing loss. It may be related to viral causes as well. Presentation may be in the form of complaints of sudden decreased hearing and there may be associated tinnitus and vertigo. Diagnosis is confirmed by pure tone audiogram. Corticosteroids may be given in the third trimester.

Vertigo due to Ménière's disease may be seen due to fluid retention. Worsening of symptoms may probably be attributed to estrogen and progesterone. Dimenhydrinate and meclizine can be safely given in pregnancy to manage an acute attack. Diuretics and histamines should be avoided as they may lead to hypovolemia, hypotension, and low cardiac output. Metoclopramide which belongs to Category B may be used for intractable vomiting.

Third trimester or postpartum period may witness sudden onset of deviation of face and inability to close the eye completely with other associated symptoms indicating Bell's palsy. The possible causes include perineural edema and mechanical compression, viral [herpes simplex virus (HSV)] inflammatory reactivation, and subsequent demyelination. Treatment is with corticosteroids if it presents in third trimester. Acyclovir which is a Category B drug may be used if viral etiology is suspected.

## NASAL CHANGES

Pregnancy rhinitis may be seen in as many as 30% of pregnant women. Nasal blockage and nasal discharge if persistent may lead to sinusitis and exacerbate asthma. It may affect normal sleep and appetite. It is attributable to raised estrogen levels causing vascular engorgement and increased mucous gland activity. Symptoms increase in third trimester. Oral decongestants like pseudoephedrine may be used. Intranasal steroids are best avoided as they are Category C drugs. Topical decongestants lead to rebound rhinitis and rhinitis medicamentosa, so treatment for long durations should be avoided. In case of sinusitis, penicillin, cephalosporins, clindamycin, and erythromycin being Category B drugs may be used. Allergic rhinitis may be managed with antihistamines like chlorpheniramine, cetirizine, and loratadine (Category B).

Epistaxis in pregnancy may be due to nasal congestion, hypertension, lesions like hemangioma, or pyogenic granuloma of nasal mucosa. Recurrent epistaxis needs endoscopic evaluation of nasal cavity. Treatment with saline nasal drops, control of hypertension, and topical application of neosporin ointment is seen due to vascular congestion. In severe epistaxis, nasal packing with antibiotic cover may be performed.

## THROAT/ORAL CAVITY CHANGES

Pregnancy tumor or granuloma gravidarum is a hyperplastic lesion of oral mucosa mostly gingiva comprising of loose granulation tissue with capillary vessels, endothelial cells, and inflammatory cells with a thin epithelial layer that may be ulcerated. These are painless sessile or pedunculated lesions with rapid progression in size. Symptoms include bleeding that occurs spontaneously or following brushing. Management may be conservative consisting of reassurance, clinical observation, and follow-up if the lesion is small and has no bleeding. However, in case of recurrent and severe bleeding or pain, surgical removal is recommended.

About 50–75% of expecting females may complain of heartburn, throat discomfort, and voice change indicating gastroesophageal reflux disease. Third trimester of pregnancy may show worsening of symptoms as abdominal pressure rises, lower esophageal sphincter pressure falls, and gastric emptying time increases. Patient should be counseled for small frequent meals, head end elevation while sleeping, and dietary modification in addition H2 blockers like famotidine (Category B) or proton pump inhibitors like lansoprazole, pantoprazole, and rabeprazole may be advised.

## LARYNGOPATHIA GRAVIDARUM

The endocrinological changes during pregnancy also affect the larynx causing changes in fluid content in the lamina propria layer of true vocal cords. Abdominal distension during later part of pregnancy affects the abdominal muscle function affecting phonation. Symptoms as change in voice or hoarseness may be presenting complaints. Professional singers may particularly observe restriction in range of pitch and change in voice. It mostly resolves in postpartum period.

## CONCLUSION

Most of the ENT conditions during pregnancy described above are reversed after the postpartum period. The ENT surgeon can help the expectant mothers by correct and timely diagnosis, reassurance, and various medical therapies may be used for the management.

## SUGGESTED READING

1. Gonca S, Eml B. Audiological findings in pregnancy. J Laryngol Otol. 2001;115:617-21.
2. Bhagat DR, Chowdhary A, Verma S, Jyotsana V. Physiological changes in ENT during pregnancy. Indian J Otolaryngol Head Neck Surg. 2006;58:268-70.
3. Sherlie VS, Varghese A. ENT Changes of Pregnancy and Its Management. Indian J Otolaryngol Head Neck Surg. 2014;66:6-9.
4. Weissman A, Nir D, Shenhav R, Zimmer EZ, Joachims ZH, Danino J. Eustachian tube function during pregnancy. Clin Otolaryngol Allied Sci. 1993;18:212-4.
5. Gristwood RE, Venables WN. Pregnancy and otosclerosis. Clin Otolaryngol Allied Sci. 1983;8:205-10.
6. Markou K, Goudakos J. An overview of the etiology of otosclerosis. Eur Arch Otorhinolaryngol. 2009;266:25-35.
7. Koichi T, Shizue T, Minako T, Yoshitaka S. The influence of pregnancy on sensation of ear problems—ear problems associated with healthy pregnancy. J Laryngol Otol. 1999;113:318-20.
8. Uchide K, Suzuki N, Takiguchi T, Terada S, Inoue M. The possible effect of pregnancy on Ménière's disease. ORL J Otorhinolaryngol Relat Spec. 1997;59:292-5.
9. Vrabec JT, Isaacson B, Van Hook JW. Bell's palsy and pregnancy. Otolaryngol Head Neck Surg. 2007;137:858-61.
10. Ellegård E, Karlsson G. Nasal congestion during pregnancy. Clin Otolaryngol. 1999;24:307-11.
11. Ellegård EK. Clinical and pathogenetic characteristics of pregnancy rhinitis. Clin Rev Allergy Immunol. 2004;26:149-59.
12. Incaudo GA. Diagnosis treatment of allergic rhinitis, sinusitis during pregnancy, lactation. Clin Rev Allergy Immunol. 2004;27:159-77.
13. Schatz M, Petitti D. Antihistamines and pregnancy. Ann Allergy Asthma Immunol. 1997;78:157-9.
14. Hardy JJ, Connolly CM, Weir CJ. Epistaxis in pregnancy—not to be sniffed at! Int J Obstet Anesth. 2008;17:94-5.

## SECTION 10: Miscellaneous

15. Sills ES, Zegarelli DJ, Hoschander MM, Strider WE. Clinical diagnosis and management of hormonally responsive oral pregnancy tumor (pyogenic granuloma). J Reprod Med. 1996;41:467-70.
16. Gill SK, Maltepe C, Koren G. The effect of heartburn and acid reflux on the severity of nausea and vomiting of pregnancy. Can J Gastroenterol. 2009;23:270-2.
17. Aselton P, Jick H, Milunsky A, Hunter JR, Stergachis A. First-trimester drug use and congenital disorders. Obstet Gynecol. 1985;65:451-5.
18. Abrams RS. Will It Hurt the Baby? The Safe Use of Medications during Pregnancy and Breastfeeding. United States: Addison-Wesley; 1990. pp. 1-5.
19. Brodnitz FS. Hormones and the human voice. Bull NY Acad Med. 1971;47:183-91.
20. Sataloff RT, Hoover CA. Endocrine dysfunction. In: Sataloff RT (Ed). Professional Voice: the Science and Art of Clinical Care, 2nd edition. San Diego: Singular; 1997. pp. 293-5.

# CHAPTER 6

# Women and Mental Health

*Navkiran Mahajan*

## ABSTRACT

Women and men differ in physical and physiological attributes as well as in the psychological makeup. Gender is a critical determinant of mental health and mental illnesses. This chapter discusses various mental illnesses that affect women during life, starting from pubertal to peripartum and menopausal phase.

## INTRODUCTION

One in four persons suffers from mental illnesses in the world, whereas, in India, it is one in seven people. A 2017 study estimates that 14.3% of Indian population is living with some mental disorder which contributes to 4.7% of the total disability adjusted life years (DALYs). The leading contribution to DALYs is from depressive disorders followed by anxiety disorders, intellectual disability, schizophrenia, bipolar disorder, and conduct disorder.

Women and men differ in physical and physiological attributes as well as in the psychological makeup. Gender is a critical determinant of mental health and mental illnesses. Sex and gender differences impact the prevalence, cause, presentation, intervention, and response to treatment in women seeking help for mental illness. Women are more likely to be treated for mental health problem than men, which reflects their greater emotional literacy and willingness to acknowledge the problem and get support.

*The social factors affecting women's health include*:
- Women are mostly the main caregivers in the family that affects their physical and emotional health as well as their social activities and finances.
- Women play multiple roles in a family; balancing work and household.
- Poverty and concerns about personal safety can make a woman stay indoors and isolated.
- Physical and sexual abuse impacts mental health especially if no support was received in past.

The behavioral difference amongst the women lies in the fact that some women internalize their feelings and then express emotional pain through self-harm while others externalize and act out through violence and aggression.

There are various underlying factors which contribute to the causation of mental illnesses.

# NEUROENDOCRINE BASIS OF MENTAL HEALTH AND ILLNESSES

Changes in the levels of estrogen (E) and progesterone during menstrual cycle and pregnancy as well as thyroid imbalance increase the risk for mental illness in women.

## Prenatal Factors

The elevated levels of cortisol and maternal depression during pregnancy as well as the elevated milk cortisol during lactation are associated with more fearful and reactive behavior in female infants than male offspring.

## Childhood Factors

The risk factors including stress, substance use, maternal deprivation, abuse or neglect pose greater risk for mental illnesses in a child especially in developing countries like India, where the female child is mostly unwanted. Prepubertal girls have 2-fold higher rates of separation anxiety, specific and social phobias.

## Pubertal Factors

Puberty is related to emerging sexuality, identity issues, parental conflicts, and peer pressure. The Tanner stage III, ovarian cycling, rising estrogen levels, and increased rate of interpersonal stress are associated with increased rates of onset of major depression in girls.

## Factors Related to Menstrual Cycle

Premenstrually (in luteal phase), women are more likely to experience emotional symptoms of irritability, tension, and mood lability; physical symptoms of fluid retention, increased appetite, and fatigue; and psychological symptoms of anxiety and depression due to increasing progesterone during the period.

### Premenstrual Dysphoric Disorder (PMDD)

- Happens mostly in the 7–14 days of luteal phase as this phase is more reactive to progesterone.
- There is a note of selective response to selective serotonin reuptake inhibitor (SSRI) and serotonin-norepinephrine reuptake inhibitor (SNRI) because of dysregulation of serotonergic systems. SSRI induces 3-alpha reductase, the enzyme producing anxiolytic metabolite allopregnanolone.

Other affective disorders are also seen to exacerbate premenstrually. Schizophrenia symptom severity is highest perimenstrually and in early follicular phase when estrogen and progesterone levels are the lowest. Increased reactivity to hypothalamic-pituitary-adrenal (HPA) axis and decreased sensitivity to glucocorticoid feedback relate to luteal phase of menstrual cycle for pharmacological or stress challenges.

## Pregnancy-related Factors

There is much increase in estrogen, androgen, progesterone, allopregnanolone, prolactin, cortisol, corticotropin-releasing hormone (CRH), oxytocin, sex hormone binding globulin, and cortisol binding globulin during pregnancy.

Third trimester up to 4 weeks after childbirth is the peripartum onset specifier for occurrence of major depression.

Free thyroxine (T4) is decreased during pregnancy. The decreased T4 is responsible for increase in depressive symptoms in third trimester.

Postpartum illnesses include postpartum blues, postpartum depression, postpartum psychosis, and others.

- *Postpartum blues* (*also known as baby blues or maternity blues*): It is a phase of emotional lability following childbirth, characterized by frequent crying episodes, irritability, confusion, and anxiety. It is seen in around 50–75% of postpartum women. It is a self-limiting phase which requires no active intervention except for the social support and reassurance from the family members.
- *Postpartum major depression*: It is observed in 10–13% of new mothers.
  - One-third have chronic depression.
  - One-third have onset during pregnancy.
  - One-third have actual postpartum onset of depression.
- *Postpartum psychosis*: Postpartum psychosis has an incidence of 2.5–5 per 10,000 deliveries. It is both an obstetric and psychiatric emergency. Most common symptoms include elation, lability of mood, disorganized behavior, hallucinations, and/or delusions. Infanticide and suicide are observed in 4% and 5% of the women suffering from postpartum psychosis.
- Women with postpartum manic episodes have more disorganization, disturbed sensorium, bizarre behavior, and sense of persecution than seen in typical manic episodes. Childbirth is the trigger for hypomanic episode in 10–20% of women and in early postpartum period.
- *Other postpartum psychiatric disorders*: About 32% of adult women with obsessive-compulsive disorder (OCD) report that their OCD symptoms began either during pregnancy or early postnatal period and worsening of symptoms is seen in perinatal period and premenstrually (exacerbation usually seen in hormonally sensitive women).

Postpartum period is also a high risk of onset/relapse of panic attacks in cases of panic disorder.

## Factors Related to Lactation and Breastfeeding

Increase in oxytocin and prolactin causes central activity that has anxiolytic effects. It includes suppression of HPA axis and autonomic responses to stress which decrease the rate of depression and anxiety in lactating women. SSRI, SNRI, and valproic acid are considered safe whereas, antipsychotics are considered relatively safe during the breastfeeding period.

## Menopausal Factors

Variability of estrogen and progesterone levels during perimenopausal period poses risk for major depressive episode. The risk is 4- to 6-fold with no history of major depression during childbearing years. The age-dependent decline in cognition during menopausal transition is also noticed.
- Estradiol (E2) (50–100 mg/day) is effective than placebo in treating major depression with perimenopasual onset but not major depression that onsets after menopause.

- Raloxifene (SERM) benefits in schizophrenia both in perimenopausal and post-menopausal women as there is a protective effect of reproductive hormones in schizophrenia. The second peak of schizophrenia is seen in approximately 45–49-year-old women.

## DEPRESSIVE AND ANXIETY DISORDERS

The contribution of depressive disorder to the percentage of total DALYs is 38.6% whereas, the prevalence of these disorders is 3.9%.

In the windows of vulnerability, i.e., reproductive age-related depressive episodes are associated with increased sensitivity experienced by women to changes in hormonal milieu that occur during luteal phase of cycle, during postpartum and menopause.

## RISK FACTORS FOR MIDLIFE DEPRESSION

- Demographic/socioeconomic (unemployment, low education, being black etc.).
- Health related (greater body mass index (BMI), substance abuse).
- Psychological (poor social support, history of anxiety or stressful life event).
- Past history of depressive episode is the strongest predictor.
- Hormonal variations in follicle-stimulating hormone (FSH) and E2.
- Menopausal related symptom [vasomotor symptoms(VMS), sleep issues].
- Overall health (chronic medical condition).
- Psychosocial stressors.
- Others—gender discrimination, violence, sexual abuse, and antenatal and postnatal stress.

Anxiety and sleep problems are major contributing factors to psychiatric morbidity among midlife women.

Women with depression and VMS have been found to have poorer perceived sleep quality. Increase in depressive symptoms is associated with changes in sleep patterns, i.e., nocturnal hot flashes are more closely associated with depression in women who are estrogen deprived (naturally or surgically).

Treatment modalities include antidepressants (SSRI are the first line drugs) with/without psychotherapy [cognitive behavioral therapy (CBT), interpersonal therapy (IPT), and psychodynamic therapy].

### Role of Estrogen

Interaction of estrogen on serotonin and norepinephrine (NE) systems causes depressive symptom in women. Prefrontal cortex, hippocampus are involved in mood and cognitive regulation with estrogen receptors and estrogen activity there.

Estradiol limits monoamine oxidase (MAO)-A and B activity, thereby increasing serotonin availability. Estrogen also increases serotonin receptor density in hypothalamus and amygdala, downregulates 5HT1A, and upregulates 5HT2A receptors.

Estrogen promotes NE availability by decreasing MAO expression; also promotes brain-derived neurotrophic factor (BDNF; neuroprotective factors) in depression.

Menopausal women with significant VMS and depressive symptoms could benefit from initial, brief (2–4 week) trial of transdermal E2 with/without an antidepressant, but for RDD, antidepressants are first choice even during midlife years.

## Dementia

The 2013 meta-analysis estimated doubling of prevalence of dementia every 5–7 years due to increasing population of older adults.

In women, rate of dementia doubles every 5 years after 65 years in both developed and developing countries. Women outnumber men in adults older than 60 years and in prevalence of dementia with increasing age especially older than 80 years.

## Gender Differences

- Alzheimer is more common in women (both in prevalence and severity).
- Women have more pronounced cognitive defects.
- Survival rate is greater for women.
- Women have more concern and fears about developing dementia, loss of independence, inability to help family members with their care needs.
- Depressive symptoms are common in mild cognitive impairment (MCI)/mild stage of dementia and in advanced stages, it is missed and mistaken for the dementia process itself.
- Urinary tract infections (UTIs) are one of most common causes of behavior disturbance in females with dementia.

About 60–70% of caregivers for patients with dementia are women, mostly adult daughters/spouses and mostly >65 years of age.

Maintenance of identity for patients with dementia and their families helps them connect to their prior roles, past identity, and life.

## Eating Disorders

Lifetime prevalence of eating disorders is 0.3% with anorexia nervosa (AN), bulimia nervosa (BN), and binge eating disorder (BED) in 0.9%, 1.5%, and 3.5%, in women, respectively. Mood (54.2%), anxiety (37.1%), and substance use (24.8%) are most common psychiatric comorbidities with BED. Obesity and metabolic syndrome are medical comorbidities along with menstrual dysfunction, long duration of labor, and polycystic ovarian disease (PCOD).

Female:male in AN and BN is 9:1 and in BED, it is 6:4 due to effect of biological and sociocultural factors on sexes. E during puberty in females facilitates development of BED.

High levels of estrogen and progesterone are associated with increased episodes of binge eating and emotional eating. BN and BED are under-recognized among women.

Binge eating disorder screener-7 should be applied to screen and diagnose women with it. Psychotherapy is first line of treatment if BED symptoms are mild without any comorbidity. CBT and IPT are the specific ones. In moderate and severe BED, pharmacotherapy including antidepressants and antiobesity drugs, is found to be effective with psychological interventions. Lisdexamfetamine is the only medication approved for treating BED. The aim is to treat psychiatric and medical comorbidities along with BED.

## FEMALE SEXUAL DYSFUNCTION

The changes in DSM-5 include:
- Female sexual arousal disorder (FSAD) and female hypoactive sexual desire disorder (HSDD) have been included together as female sexual interest/arousal disorder (FSIAD).

- Dyspareunia and vaginismus are merged into genitopelvic pain/penetration disorder (GPPD).
- Sexual aversion disorder eliminated.
- Frequency and severity criteria included in diagnostic criteria.
- Sexual dysfunction due to general medical condition and combined factors has been eliminated.

Incidence of female sexual dysfunction ranges from 25.8 to 91% with about desire difficulties in 64%, arousal difficulties in 31%, orgasm difficulty in 35%, and sexual pain in 26%. HSDD is most prevalent sexual complaint (8.9% in aged 18–44 years, 12.3% in aged 45–64 years, and 7.4% in aged 65 years and above).

## Female Orgasmic Disorder

- Second most common sexual disorder in women.
- Orgasm is most commonly achieved by clitoral/vaginal stimulation.

Psychological aspects include body image, self-esteem, relationship conflict, preoccupation with genital appearance, any past history of sexual abuse, low EQ, and emotional instability which lead to perception of lack of orgasm as a failure followed by depression and anxiety.

## Female Sexual Pain Disorders

Prevalence of dyspareunia ranges from 6.5 to 45% in older women and 14–35% in younger women whereas, vulvar pain is prevalent in 7.8% and vaginismus in 1–6% of women.

A comprehensive pain and psychosocial assessment is required along with physical examination. A cotton swab test is standard for diagnosis of provoked vulvodynia. The causes for the same can be irritative, anatomic, and infections.

Treatment options include hormonal topical products, systemic estrogen, and oral ospemifene (in postmenopausal women) and psychological interventions, pelvic floor physical therapy, and surgical vulvar vestibulectomy in case of failure of conservative management.

Male partner's responses to sexual pain are prognostic factors to sexual functioning.

Therapeutic modalities for vaginismus are sex therapy and systematic desensitization.

## SEXUAL MINORITY AND TRANSGENDER WOMEN

Sexual minority women are nonheterosexual in one of the three dimensions of sexual orientation, namely sexual identity, sexual attraction, and sexual behavior. Mental health disparities are seen among them in the area of body image, eating disorders, mood and anxiety, suicidality, self-harm, and substance abuse. Lifetime suicidal risk is 3-fold in bisexual women and 2-fold in lesbians. These women experience several barriers in accessing quality care because of their concerns that medical personnel would treat them differently. A study in 2011 reveals that medical schools, on average, teach only 5 hours of sexual minority and transgender-related content over 4 years.

## CONCLUSION

All through their life, women are prone to developing affective mental disorders. It is important to encourage a healthy lifestyle along with good mental health for the caregiver of the family.

## SUGGESTED READING

1. Krienger N. Discrimination and Health. In Berkman LF, Kawachi I, editors. Social epidemiology. Oxford (United Kingdom) Oxford U Press, 2000.
2. Gater R, Tansella M, Korten A, Tiemens BG, Mavreas VG, Olatawura MO. Sex differences in the prevalence and detection of depressive and anxiety disorders in general health care settings: report from the World Health Organization Collaborative Study on Psychological Problems in General Health Care. Arch Gen Psychiatry. 1998;55:405-13.
3. Buss C, Davis E, Shahbaba B, Pruessner JC, Head K, Sandman CA. Maternal cortisol over the course of pregnancy and subsequent child amygdala and hippocampus volumes and affective problems. Proc Natl Acad Sci U S A. 2012;109:1312-9.
4. Grey K, Davis E, Sandman C, Glynn LM. Human milk cortisol is associated with infant temperament. Psychoneuroendocrinology. 2012;38:1178-85.
5. Angold A, Costello E, Worthman C. Puberty and depression: the roles of age, pubertal status and pubertal timing. Psychol Med. 1998;28:51-61.
6. Schmidt PJ, Nieman LK, Danaceau MA, Adams LF, Rubinow DR. Different behavioral effects of gonadal steroids in women and with an in those without premenstrual syndrome. N Engl J Med. 1998;338:209-16.
7. Teatro M, Mazmanian D, Sharma V. Effects of the menstrual cycle on bipolar disorder. Bipolar Disord. 2014;16:22-36.
8. Roca C, Schmidt P, Altermus M, Deuster P, Danaceau MA, Putnam K, et al. Differential menstrual cycle regulation of hypothalamic-pituitary-adrenal axis in women with premenstrual syndrome and controls. J Clin Endorinol Metab. 2003;88:3057-63.
9. Wisner K, Sit D, McShea M, Rizzo DM, Zoretich RA, Hughes CL, et al. Onset timing, thoughts of self-harm, and diagnoses in postpartum women with screen-positive depression findings. JAMA Psychiatry. 2013;70:490-8.
10. Munk-Olsen T, Laursen T, Pedersen C, Mors O, Mortensen PB. New parents and mental disorders. JAMA. 2006;296:2582-9.
11. Heron J, Haque S, Oyebode F, Craddock N, Jones I. A longitudinal study of hypomania and depression symptoms in pregnancy and the postpartum period. Bipolar Disord. 2009;11:410-7.
12. Altemus M, Neeb C, Davis A, Occhiogrosso M, Nguyen T, Bleiberg KL. Phenotypic differences between pregnancy-onset and postpartum-onset major depressive disorder. J Clin Psychiatry. 2013;73:e1485-91.
13. Wisner K, Peindl K, Gigliotti T, Hanusa BH. Obsessions and compulsions in women with postpartum depression. J Clin Psychiatry. 1999;60:176-80.
14. Glinoer D. The regulation of thyroid function in pregnancy: pathways of endocrine adaptation from physiology to pathology. Endocr Rev. 1997;18:404-43.
15. Watson J, Mednic S, Huttunen M, et al. Prevalence of autoimmune thyroid dysfunction in postpartum psychosis. Br J Psychiatry. 2011;198:264-8.
16. Neumann ID, Torner L, Wigger A. Brain oxytocin: differential inhibition of neuro-endocrine stress responses and anxiety-related behaviour in virgin, pregnant and lactating rats. Neuroscience. 2000;95:567-75.
17. Cohen L, Soares C, Vitonis A, et al. Risk for new onset of depression during the menopausal transition: the Harvard Study of Moods and Cycles. Arch Gen Psychiatry. 2006;63:375-82.
18. Morrison M, Kallan M, Have T, Katz I, Tweedy K, Battistini M. Lack of efficacy of estradiol for depression in postmenopausal women: a randomized, controlled trial. Biol Psychiatry. 2004;55:406-12.
19. Usall J, Huerta-Ramos E, Labad J, Cobo J, Núñez C, Creus M, et al. Raloxifene as an Adjunctive Treatment for Postmenopausal Women with Schizophrenia: A 24-Week Double-Blind, Randomized, Parallel, Placebo-Controlled Trial. Schizophr Bull. 2016;42:309-17.
20. McEwen BS, Alves SE. Estrogen actions in the central nervous system. Endocr Rev. 1999;20(3):279-307.
21. Prince M, Bryce R, Albanese E, Wimo A, Ribeiro W, Ferri CP. The global prevalence of dementia: a systematic review and metaanalysis. Alzheimers Dementia. 2013;9(1):63-75.
22. Erol R, Brooker D, Peel E. Alzheimer's Disease International. Women and dementia: a global research review. 2015. Available at: https://www.alz.co.uk/sites/default/files/pdfs/Women-and-Dementia.pdf. Accessed May 5, 2016.
23. The burden of mental disorders across the states of India: the Global burden of disease study 1990-2017. The Lancet Psychiatry (2019).
24. Kessler RC, Berglund PA, Chiu WT, et al. The prevalence and correlates of binge eating disorder in the World Health Organization World Mental Health Surveys. Biol Psychiatry. 2013;73(9):904-14.
25. Wright JJ, O'Conor KM. Female sexual dysfunction. Med Clin North Am. 2015;99:607-28.

# Women and Skin Ailments

*Aditi Jha, Parul Verma, Divya Seshadri*

## ABSTRACT

Skin disorders are more commonly seen in women majorly owing to the hormonal milieu. Several sexually transmitted diseases, autoimmune and allergic skin diseases are more common in women. Dermatological ailments also bring with them psychosomatic issues as the women since time immemorial are expected to be fair and lovely! This chapter highlights the various skin ailments encountered in women and briefly describes their presentation and management.

## INTRODUCTION

The skin is the largest multifunctional organ in the body. It functions as a protective physical barrier by absorbing ultraviolet radiation and preventing microorganism invasion and chemical penetration. The skin also controls the passage of water and electrolytes and has a major role in the thermoregulation of the body, in addition to its immunological, sensory, and autonomic function.

There is sex-related difference in anatomy, physiology, epidemiology, and the manifestations of several diseases. With regard to skin disorders, infectious diseases are presented more in men but psychosomatic problems, pigmentary disorders, certain hair diseases, and autoimmune and allergic diseases are more common in women. Indeed, there are more sex-associated dermatoses in women and the occurrence and prognosis of certain skin malignancies are related to sex-related differences. The mechanisms that underlie sex-related differences in skin diseases are mostly unknown. Sex hormones, behavioral factors, ethnicity, and differences in environment may all contribute to these differences. Studies have shown that sebum content is higher in men because sebum is highly influenced by sex hormones. Also, skin pigmentation and thickness are significantly higher, facial wrinkles are deeper, and facial sagging is more prominent in the lower eyelids of men, but there is no significant difference in skin elasticity between the sexes.

Disorders which are specific to women may be very few and not very common. Hence, this chapter would focus primarily on dermatosis which is commonly seen in women and dermatological conditions specific to pregnancy.

## CHAPTER 7: Women and Skin Ailments

# COMMON DERMATOLOGICAL CONDITIONS

## Melasma

Melasma is a common acquired pigmentary skin disorder of the sun-exposed areas like the face. Melasma affects females much more commonly than males and majority of patients are in the third and fourth decades of their life. Several factors such as genetics, sunlight, cosmetics, pregnancy, hormonal treatments, thyroid dysfunction, and drugs have been implicated in the pathogenesis of melasma.

### Presentation

Melasma is usually asymptomatic and patients often seek medical attention owing to cosmetic concerns.

Melasma typically presents as symmetric, hyperpigmented macules on the face and usually has well-demarcated borders (**Figs. 1A and B**). The most common pattern of pigmentation in melasma is centrofacial (cheeks, forehead, upper lip, and nose). Other presentations are malar (cheeks and nose) and mandibular (mandibular area of cheeks). The areas of pigmentation may appear over several weeks to months and is aggravated by sun exposure.

### Diagnosis

Diagnosis of melasma is usually based on clinical examination and history. Wood's lamp examination and dermoscopy are a helpful tool for diagnosing and determining the depth of pigmentation and hence are helpful in guiding the treatment accordingly. A skin biopsy is occasionally required when there are very close differentials, treated cases, and more than one dermatosis occurring concurrently over the same area. Other laboratory tests are generally not required.

Differential diagnosis of melasma are postinflammatory hyperpigmentation where patient has a history of preceding dermatosis over the affected areas and solar lentigines which are generally seen in fifth or sixth decade and involve the face and other sun-exposed areas. Some drugs like anticonvulsants, amiodarone, antipsychotics, and minocycline

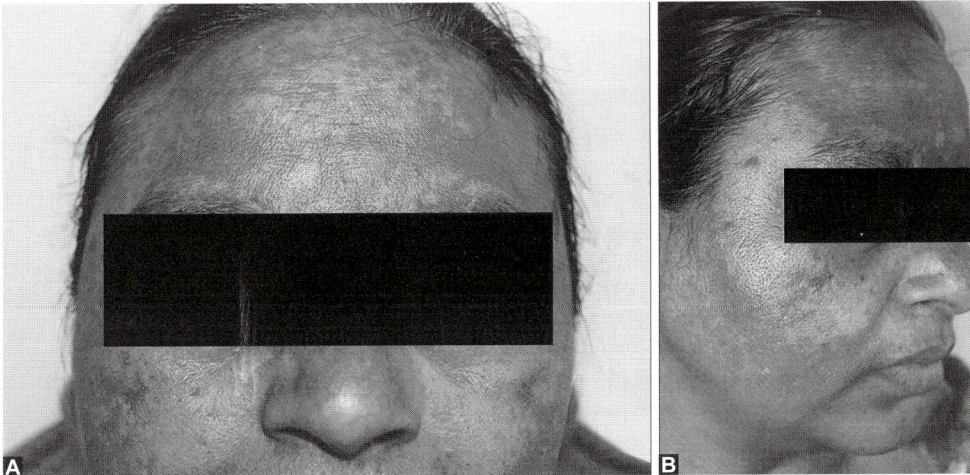

**FIGS. 1A AND B:** Well-demarcated brownish macules present over the forehead and malar areas of a middle age female with melasma. *(For color version, see Plate 8)*

can also induce pigmentation over the unexposed areas. Freckles are smaller light brown discrete macules over the cheeks and generally fade over a period of time.

## Treatment

Treatment should focus on eliminating underlying etiological factors if any (drugs, hormonal imbalance, etc.). Patients of melasma should be advised to liberally apply a broad-spectrum sunscreen with a minimum sun protection factor (SPF) of 30 and which also covers UVA, UVB, and visible light. The sunscreen application should be repeated every 2–3 hourly.

Topical treatment with skin-lightening agents remains the first line of therapy. Topical retinoids, hydroquinone, kojic acid, azelaic acid, deoxyarbutin, ascorbic acid, and triple combination therapy (hydroquinone, a retinoid, and a fluorinated corticosteroid) can be used either alone or in combination depending on the extent and type of melasma. Caution should be exercised and appropriate counseling should be done when using these formulations especially the corticosteroid and hydroquinone-containing regimens as they have a potential of being abused by the patient and can lead to lasting complications when used unsupervised.

Chemical peels like lactic acid, salicylic acid, glycol acid, and trichloroacetic acid are used as second line of therapy. However, the medium-depth peels should be used with caution and deep peels should be avoided in patients with Fitzpatrick skin types IV–VI due to the risk of scarring and hyperpigmentation.

Lasers and light-based therapies are considered as third-line agents and further research is still required in this area.

## Prognosis

There may be a variable clinical course in patients with melasma. It may fade spontaneously over months to years or may be persistent. Melasma which develops during pregnancy usually fades postpartum. The most important aspect of prevention is rigorous photoprotection.

## Acne

Acne is a chronic inflammatory condition affecting the pilosebaceous unit. It is most frequently associated with adolescents and hence is known as acne vulgaris. However, acne vulgaris may persist from adolescence beyond the age of 25 years when it is known as "persistent acne" or it may manifest for the first time after the age of 25 years when it is labeled as "late-onset adult acne". The prevalence of female acne is estimated to be between approximately 40% in women between the ages of 25 and 40 years. The etiopathogenesis of acne vulgaris involves a complex interaction between the main factors such as: Genetic predisposition; androgenic hormone stimulation leading to an increase in sebaceous secretion; alteration of the lipid composition; follicular hyperkeratinization; and bacterial colonization mainly by *Propionibacterium acnes* (*P. acnes*) and periglandular dermal inflammation. Several other factors have been postulated as triggers or aggravating factors such as: Exposure to ultraviolet radiation, stress, obesity, diet, smoking, sleep disorders, cosmetics, medications, and endocrine disorders.

## Presentation

Acne manifests as a polymorphic eruption consisting of noninflammatory lesions which includes both open and closed comedones ("blackheads" or "whiteheads", respectively) and inflammatory (papules, pustules, and nodules) over the forehead, cheeks, and chin (**Fig. 2**). Lesions of acne may result in postinflammatory hyperpigmentation and various types of scarring over the affected areas. Adult female acne lesions are located mainly on the lower part of the face, including the mandibular region, the perioral region, and the chin, conferring a U-shape, in addition to the anterior cervical region. If a hyperandrogenic state is the cause of acne, signs of irregular menses, excess facial hair, hyperhidrosis, and acanthosis nigricans may be present.

## Diagnosis

The diagnosis of acne is mostly clinical. Close differential diagnosis are folliculitis and rosacea which can be easily differentiated by the absence of comedones. A history of other concomitant drug intake is essential to rule out drug-induced acne (e.g., phenytoin, lithium, and isoniazid) or steroid-induced acne. In the presence of other clinical signs of hyperandrogenism, it is advisable to order plasma concentrations of free and total testosterone, dehydroepiandrosterone sulfate (DHEA-S), luteinizing hormone (LH), follicle-stimulating hormone (FSH) and, in some cases, when suspecting polycystic ovary syndrome (PCOS) and transvaginal ultrasound for visualization of the ovaries. These investigations should always be performed in the follicular phase, preferably between the 1st and 5th day of the menstrual cycle and the serum samples collection should be done in the morning between 8 and 10 AM.

## Treatment

Selection of therapy differs depending on the type/severity of acne and the patient's skin type. For mild or moderate, noninflammatory or comedonal acne, therapy begins with topical retinoids (tretinoin, adapalene, and tazarotene). Topical antimicrobials like benzoyl peroxide, clindamycin, and erythromycin should be added in cases of inflammatory acne. Due to the potential for development of resistant strains of *P. acnes* to clindamycin and erythromycin, it should be used in combination with other topical agents such as benzoyl peroxide or retinoids. Systemic tetracyclines may be added if clinical improvement is

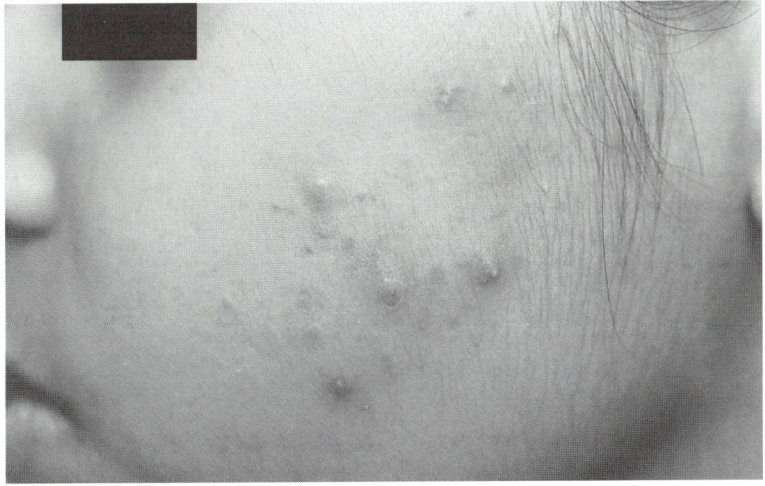

**FIG. 2:** Comedones, erythematous papules, and pustules on the cheeks of an adolescent female with acne vulgaris. *(For color version, see Plate 8)*

not noted after 2–3 months of topical therapy. For severe acne, a combination of topical therapy and systemic antibiotic is preferred. Isotretinoin, an oral retinoid, is the treatment of choice for severe nodulocystic acne. It should be used with extreme caution in women of childbearing age given its potential for teratogenicity (pregnancy Category X) and can also cause dyslipidemia, pancreatitis, hepatotoxicity, and pseudotumor cerebri. Other therapies which have been used are combined oral contraceptives and antiandrogens depending upon the underlying condition.

## Prognosis

The prognosis is generally good with treatment. Adult-onset acne may be more persistent than typical adolescent acne and patients may require maintenance topical treatments for a variable period of time. The goal of treatment is to prevent the formation of new lesions as scars can develop from even small comedones.

# Alopecia

Alopecia/hair loss is a common condition that may cause significant emotional and psychosocial distress. Alopecia can be described as either nonscarring when there is no evidence of tissue destruction or scarring alopecia. Scarring alopecia generally appears secondary to a dermatosis affecting the scalp and rarely de novo.

Hair loss may be diffuse or localized. In women, the two most common causes of diffuse hair loss are female pattern hair loss (FPHL) and telogen effluvium (TE). Some variants of alopecia which occur as a result of hair care practices are traction alopecia, hair shaft disorders, and central centrifugal alopecia. Some common localized causes of hair loss include alopecia areata, tinea capitis, and trichotillomania.

## Presentation

Female pattern hair loss presents as loss of hair on the central and bitemporal regions of the scalp and affects roughly one-half of women in their 50s. It usually starts presenting as visible midline parting and gradually may progress to involve the central and temporal regions of the scalp. Frontal hairline is however, spared unlike male androgenetic alopecia. When a diagnosis of FPHL is suspected, other signs of androgen excess like acne, hirsutism, irregular menses, and virilization should also be looked upon. The degree of hair loss in FPHL is most severe between ages 30 and 50 years with subsequent slowing of hair loss.

Telogen effluvium is an acute, generalized hair loss that presents several months after physical or psychological stressors which may include childbirth, major surgery, medications, crash dieting, thyroid abnormalities, and nutritional deficiencies. In a large portion of cases, no clear cause can be determined. The patient's health and well-being and diet over the preceding 6–12 months should be elucidated in a patient presenting with generalized hair loss. It is a self-limiting condition that usually resolves within 2–6 months, although it may be prolonged if the trigger is not resolved. In some patients, chronic TE (i.e., TE lasting >6 months) can develop.

Alopecia areata presents as localized areas of complete hair loss from the scalp, but may involve other body areas. Generalized involvement can lead to alopecia totalis (entire scalp) or alopecia universalis (all body areas).

With a history suggestive of hair breakage along the shaft, prompt investigation should be made into the patient's hair care practices; most common culprits being chemical relaxers, permanent waves, or hair straighteners.

## Diagnosis

A detailed history and careful examination of the scalp will usually result in a preliminary diagnosis.

*Other tests which can help to supplement the diagnosis are*:
- A hair-pull test.
- *Hormonal tests*: Serum testosterone, DHEA-S, and prolactin.
- *Others*: Thyroid function tests, iron studies, a complete blood count, and antinuclear antibodies.
- *Trichoscopy*: It has emerged as a valuable handheld noninvasive method and can be very helpful in supplementing the diagnosis.
- *Scalp biopsy*: It is generally not necessary for nonscarring alopecia but may be helpful to demonstrate the presence, character, and location of inflammation.

## Treatment

Common treatments for alopecia are presented in **Table 1**.

## Prognosis

The prognosis of hair loss depends on the cause and responsiveness to available treatments.

# Pregnancy Dermatosis

Pregnancy is witnessed by many physiological skin changes such as melasma, striae gravidarum, along with many hair, nail, and vascular changes. Some pre-existing skin conditions may either improve or exacerbate in pregnancy due to immunological changes. There may be increased severity and frequency of skin infections as candidiasis because of depressed cell-mediated immunity (CMI). Apart from all these, there are a few inflammatory skin dermatoses which are specific to pregnancy and are seen only in pregnancy.
- *Atopic eruption of pregnancy*: It consists of eczema in pregnancy (women presenting with atopic eczema), prurigo of pregnancy (excoriated papules and nodules over extensors of arms, legs, and abdomen), and pruritic folliculitis (pruritic, 2–4 mm,

**TABLE 1:** Commonly used treatments for alopecia.

| Etiology | Treatment |
|---|---|
| Female pattern hair loss | • Topical minoxidil<br>• Antiandrogens (cyproterone acetate, spironolactone, finasteride, and flutamide) |
| Telogen effluvium | • Identification and withdrawal of triggering factors<br>• Reassurance |
| Alopecia areata | • Topical potent corticosteroids<br>• Intralesional corticosteroids<br>• Oral immunosuppressives (extensive and rapidly progressive AA)<br>• Contact immunotherapy |

*Source*: Torres F, Tosti A. Female pattern alopecia and telogen effluvium: figuring out diffuse alopecia. Semin Cutan Med Surg. 2015;34:67-71; Alkhalifah A, Alsantali A, Wang E, McElwee KJ, Shapiro J. Alopecia areata update: part II. Treatment. J Am Acad Dermatol. 2010;62:191-202.

follicular papules or pustules typically on the shoulders, upper back, arms, chest, and abdomen).
- *Polymorphic eruption of pregnancy*: Also known as pruritic urticarial papules and plaques of pregnancy (PUPPP), it presents with pruritic, polymorphous, erythematous, nonfollicular papules, plaques, and sometimes vesicles over the abdomen, commonly involving striae gravidarum with sparing of the periumbilical region. The lesions resolve near term or in the early postpartum period. The maternal and fetal prognosis is excellent.
- *Pruritus gravidarum and intrahepatic cholestasis of pregnancy (ICP)*: Pruritus gravidarum is classically associated with itching, without any skin lesions and occurs in the first trimester; ICP (also called obstetric cholestasis) is seen in third trimester and is characterized by pruritus with or without jaundice, absence of primary skin lesions, and with laboratory markers of cholestasis (elevated serum bile acids and alkaline phosphatase). The skin lesions are usually secondary linear excoriations and excoriated papules which are caused by scratching. The condition is associated with a higher risk of fetomaternal complications and hence an early identification and management along with close obstetric surveillance are required in cases of ICP.
- *Pemphigoid gestationis (PG)*: It is a rare autoimmune disorder characterized by pruritic, urticarial, and vesiculobullous eruption starting in the periumbilical region. It begins in the second or third trimester, may resolve late in pregnancy, but classically flares up again at delivery.

## Treatment

Polymorphic eruption of pregnancy and atopic eruption of pregnancy are not associated with any adverse fatal outcomes and are benign in nature. They usually resolve in early postpartum period. Topical emollients and midpotent steroids along with antihistamines can be used for treatment. Pruritic folliculitis responds well to topical benzoyl peroxide. Patients with PG and ICP carry fetal risk and require specific treatment. Oral antihistamines are used to control pruritus but more severe cases of PG require systemic corticosteroids. For ICH, ursodeoxycholic acid is the drug of choice and has been shown to decrease both maternal pruritus and fetal mortality.

## CONCLUSION

Several pigmentary, hair-related, and autoimmune disorders are seen more in women as compared to men. Due to the general perception of looks being attributed to the fairer sex, it is imperative that women get emotionally and physically more affected because of skin aliments. Complete holistic management of the patient is usually the right way ahead.

## SUGGESTED READING

1. Chen W, Mempel M, Traidl-Hofmann C, Al Khusaei S, Ring J. Gender aspects in skin diseases. J Eur Acad Dermatol Venereol. 2010;24:1378-85.
2. Rahrovan S, Fanian F, Mehryan P, Humbert P, Firooz A. Male versus female skin: What dermatologists and cosmeticians should know. Int J Womens Dermatol. 2018;4:122-30.
3. Miot LD, Miot HA, Silva MG, Marques ME. Physiopathology of melasma. Ann Bras Dermatol. 2009;84:623-35.
4. Sheth VM, Pandya AG. Melasma: a comprehensive update: Part I. J Am Acad Dermatol. 2011;65: 689-97.

5. Handel AC, Lima PB, Tonolli VM, Miot LD, Miot HA. Risk factors for facial melasma in women: a case-control study. Br J Dermatol. 2014;171:588-94.
6. Boukari F, Jourdan E, Fontas E, Montaudié H, Castela E, Lacour JP, et al. Prevention of melasma relapses with sunscreen combining protection against UV and short wavelengths of visible light: A prospective randomized comparative trial. J Am Acad Dermatol. 2015;72:189-900.
7. Sarma N, Chakraborty S, Poojary SA, Rathi S, Kumaran S, Nirmal B, et al. Evidence-based review, grade of recommendation, and suggested treatment recommendations for melasma. Indian Dermatol Online J. 2017;8:406-42.
8. Sarkar R, Gokhale N, Godse K, Ailawadi P, Arya L, Sarma N, et al. Medical management of melasma: A review with consensus recommendations by Indian pigmentary expert group. Indian J Dermatol. 2017;62:558-77.
9. Bhate K, Williams HC. Epidemiology of acne vulgaris. Br J Dermatol. 2013;168:474-85.
10. Collier CN, Harper JC, Cafardi JA, Cantrell WC, Wang W, Foster KW, et al. The prevalence of acne in adults 20 years and older. J Am Acad Dermatol. 2008;58:56-9.
11. Yentzer BA, Hick J, Reese EL, Uhas A, Feldman SR, Balkrishnan R. Acne vulgaris in the United States: a descriptive epidemiology. Cutis. 2010;86:94-9.
12. Preneau S, Dreno B. Female acne—a different subtype of teenager acne? J Eur Acad Dermatol Venereol. 2012;26:277-82.
13. Dréno B, Thiboutot D, Layton AM, Berson D, Perez M, Kang S. Global Alliance to Improve Outcomes in Acne. Large-scale international study enhances understanding of an emerging acne population: adult females. J Eur Acad Dermatol Venereol. 2015;29:1096-106.
14. Bhat YJ, Latief I, Hassan I. Update on etiopathogenesis and treatment of Acne. Indian J Dermatol Venereol Leprol. 2017;83:298-306.
15. Yarak S, Bagatin E, Hassun KM, Parada MO, Filho TS. Hyperandrogenism and skin: polycystic ovary syndrome and peripheral insulin resistance. Ann Bras Dermatol. 2005;80:395-410.
16. Tan AU, Schlosser BJ, Paller AS. A review of diagnosis and treatment of acne in adult female patients. Int J Womens Dermatol. 2018;4:56-71.
17. Harfmann KL, Bechtel MA. Hair loss in women. Clin Obstet Gynecol. 2015;58:185-99.
18. Torres F, Tosti A. Female pattern alopecia and telogen effluvium: figuring out diffuse alopecia. Semin Cutan Med Surg. 2015;34:67-71.
19. Mirmirani P, Huang KP, Price VH. A practical, algorithmic approach to diagnosing hair shaft disorders. Int J Dermatol. 2011;50:1-12.
20. Dhurat R, Saraogi P. Hair evaluation methods: merits and demerits. Int J Trichology. 2009;1:108-19.
21. Alkhalifah A, Alsantali A, Wang E, McElwee KJ, Shapiro J. Alopecia areata update: part II. Treatment. J Am Acad Dermatol. 2010;62:191-202.
22. Sachdeva S. The dermatoses of pregnancy. Indian J Dermatol. 2008;53:103-5.
23. Ambros-Rudolph CM, Mullegger RR, Vaughan-Jones SA, Kerl H, Black MM. The specific dermatoses of pregnancy revisited and reclassified: Results of a retrospective two-center study on 505 pregnant patients. Am Acad Dermatol. 2006;54:395-404.
24. Matz H, Orion E, Wolf R. Pruritic urticarial papules and plaques of pregnancy: Polymorphic eruption of pregnancy (PUPPP). Clin Dermatol. 2006;24:105-8.
25. Palma J, Reyes H, Ribalta J, Hernandez I, Sandoval L, Almuna R. Ursodeoxycholic acid in the treatment of cholestasis of pregnancy: A randomized, double-blind study controlled with placebo. J Hepatol. 1997;27:1022-8.
26. Kondrackiene J, Beuers U, Kupcinskas L. Efficacy and safety of ursodeoxycholic acid versus cholestyramine in intrahepatic cholestasis of pregnancy. Gastroenterology. 2005;129:894-901.

# Medical Ailments in Adolescent Girls

*Puneet A Pooni, Sujata Bhatti*

## ABSTRACT

Adolescence (10–19 years' age) is a period of rapid physical and psychological development and the child moves from dependency to autonomy in many domains. With various physical changes that an adolescent girl encounters at this age, several physical and mental concerns arise. There is a risk of several diseases with lack of proper information about these physiological changes. Hence this chapter highlights the various adolescent-related changes and the possible pathologies that could occur.

## INTRODUCTION

Human life completes its journey through various stages and one of the most important stages is adolescence, in which transition from puberty to legal adulthood happens. This is the age group between 10 and 19 years ([World Health Organization (WHO) definition]. This phase is a period of rapid physical and psychological development and the child moves from dependency to autonomy in many domains. In India, most of the adolescents do their work independently but final decisions are usually taken by their parents or caregivers. About 21% of population in India is contributed by adolescents. They have specific needs and face challenges such as poverty, poor health and lack of healthcare facilities, unsafe environments, nutritional deprivation, psychosocial stress etc. This chapter focuses on problems faced by adolescent females related to physical and mental health.

Physical development represents only the gross picture of changes that occur in adolescence. More significant are the development of skills and mental strength. Physical changes occurring in girls are:
- Development of breasts
- Changes in body shape and increase in height
- Growth of body and pubic hair
- Menstruation

*Health problems in adolescent females are categorized into following headings*:
- *Infections*: Sexually transmitted infections (STIs), urinary tract infections (UTIs)
- Teenage pregnancy
- Menstrual problems and menstrual hygiene

- *Endocrine problems*: Thyroid disorders, diabetes
- Nutritional deficiencies
- *Mental health issues*: Depression and behavioral problems, and eating disorders.

## INFECTIONS

Examples of STIs are syphilis, hepatitis B, herpes, HIV, trichomonas, chlamydia, and genital warts. Special relevance to HIV and AIDS in adolescents can be attributed to adventurous and risk-taking behavior which makes them susceptible to unsafe sexual practices. Young females are at risk for unsafe sex and acquisition of sexually transmitted diseases (STDs); above that, they are deprived of healthcare facilities or medical aid on time due to social taboo or inability to communicate regarding their problems. As per National Family Health Survey (NFHS-3) data, 2.7% boys and 8% girls reported sexual debut before the age of 15 and most of the sexual activity happens in context of marriage which leads to teenage pregnancy. UTIs are particularly common in adolescent females and they often have concurrent sexual activity or a complication of that activity. It is as important to counsel adolescents about sexual activity and its consequences as it is to treat UTIs. In all adolescents with UTI, evidence of STDs should be sought and counseling for STDs and responsible sexual activity is recommended.

Pelvic inflammatory diseases (PIDs), infertility, fetal loss, cervical cancer, newborn health issues, and HIV can all result because of untreated infections. Gynecological morbidity in these females also leads to severe emotional distress. Early detection and management is crucial as most of these problems can become chronic later. Very few studies are available which analyzed the prevalence of reproductive tract infections (RTIs) in the adolescent age group. Only when we know the extent of the problem can we come up with possible solutions. One such study conducted in Tamil Nadu, India included young married women aged 16–22 years in a rural community and showed that more than half of the women were suffering from at least one or more RTIs. This is attributed to the poor health seeking behavior for reproductive morbidity of adolescent women mainly because of the social taboo.

## TEENAGE PREGNANCY

Pregnancy in a female under the age of 19 is very frequent. Approximately 16 million girls aged 15–19 years and 2.5 million girls under 16 years give birth each year in developing regions. Complications during pregnancy and childbirth are the leading cause of death for 15–19-year-old girls globally. Every year, some 3.9 million girls undergo unsafe abortions. Adolescent mothers face higher risks of eclampsia, puerperal endometritis, and systemic infections. Some 3.9 million unsafe abortions among girls aged 15–19 years occur each year, contributing to maternal mortality and lasting health problems. Furthermore, the emotional, psychological, and social needs of pregnant adolescent girls can be greater than those of other women.

Babies born to adolescent mothers have more risk to have low birthweight, preterm delivery, and severe neonatal conditions with long-term potential effects. Even decreased time gap between two pregnancies can put both the mother and child at risk.

Adolescent pregnancy also bears negative social and economic effects on girls, their families and communities with the social stigma associated with these. These girls not only face rejection by parents and peers but also receive threats of violence. There are several such cases of honor killings reported in news every day. For most of these girls leave school, their overall growth and future possibilities of being socially and financially dependent suffers. Child marriage reduces future earnings by 9% in these girls.

## MENSTRUAL PROBLEMS AND MENSTRUAL HYGIENE

Most commonly faced menstrual problems are dysmenorrhea and premenstrual syndrome which lead to school absenteeism, decreased social activities, disturbed sleep, and decreased appetite. Poor menstrual hygiene is one of the leading causes of RTIs and contributes to adolescent morbidity significantly. Most of the adolescent girls in villages use old clothes or rags during menstruation increasing chances of infections. In June 2010, the Government of India proposed a new scheme toward menstrual hygiene by provision of subsidized sanitary napkins to rural adolescent girls. But there are various other issues such as awareness, availability and quality of napkins, regular supply, privacy and water supply, disposal of napkins, reproductive health education, and family support which need simultaneous attention for promotion of menstrual hygiene.

Due to the relative immaturity of the hypothalamic–pituitary–ovary axis in the first 2 years following menarche, more than half of the menstrual cycles are anovulatory. This results in irregular cycles where cycle frequency can vary from <20 days to >90 days. After the first 1–2 years, the capacity for estrogen-positive feedback on the anterior pituitary develops with the subsequent mid-cycle luteinizing hormone (LH) surge and ovulation, resulting in regulation of the menstrual cycle.

Anovulatory cycles are often heavy and prolonged with some girls bleeding for several weeks at a time. This can lead to iron deficiency anemia and, in rare cases, cardiovascular collapse requiring admission and blood transfusion. Initial anovulatory cycles tend to be pain-free, although heavy menstrual loss can result in an element of dysmenorrhea. When regular ovulatory cycles commence, the periods often become more painful due to the increased levels of circulating prostaglandins.

## ENDOCRINOLOGICAL PROBLEMS

Type 1 diabetes mellitus and type 2 diabetes mellitus is increasingly being seen in adolescents due to genetic susceptibility, lifestyle, behavioral problems, etc. Education of the patient by participation of multidisciplinary team including physicians, nurse, nutritionist, and psychologist should include family, teachers, friends, and partners. Accepting a chronic disease is a long process of maturation and several psychological reactions have been reported such as denial, revolt, bargaining, sadness, and finally acceptance.

Another group of endocrinal disorders which are common in adolescent females are thyroid disorders. Most common is goiter which could be idiopathic, due to dyshormonogenesis, hormone resistance, Hashimoto thyroiditis, Graves' disease, and, on the other hand, hypothyroidism due to iodine deficiency. Thyroid disorders are often missed due to lack of healthcare access or partly due to lack of awareness. Girls with untreated thyroid disorders face many complications like weight gain or loss, menstrual irregularities, temperature disturbances, etc.

## NUTRITIONAL DEFICIENCIES

Adolescence is a period of rapid physical growth, with a corresponding increase in nutritional requirements to support the increase in body mass and to build up stores of nutrients. The daily intake of nutritional requirements increases according to the following factors:

*Age*: At the beginning of puberty, with the increase of height and at the last stage of adolescence

*Gender*: Adolescent girls require 10% more nutrients, iron, and iodine, in particular, than boys

*Pregnancy*: During the second half, in particular, as well as during the first 6 months of breastfeeding, it is advised that the first pregnancy after marriage be postponed at least until the girl is over 18 years old because it might not be possible to meet additional requirements, especially among middle income and poor families.

Adolescent nutrition can be improved through several measures including:
- Recognition of the increased nutritional requirements of adolescents.
- Nutritional education for the promotion of healthy dietary habits stated below; an adequate diet at specific times.
- Control excessive indulgence in food, especially those foods high in sugar and fat; minimizing the intake of sweets and snacks between main meals, especially junk food snacks.
- Regular physical exercise to burn excess calories and to strengthen muscles.
- Always eating breakfast.
- Use of sugar replacement if prone to obesity.
- Ensuring that poultry and poultry products, as well as other meats, are well-cooked, ensuring the cleanliness.
- Food should be hygienically kept; vegetables and fruits should be washed with soap and water before use and milk should be brought to boiling point.

## MENTAL HEALTH ISSUES

With increase parental and peer pressure, mental disorders and mental health problems have risen significantly among adolescents in the last two decades.

Common disorders faced by them are depression, anxiety, eating disorders, conduct disorders, substance abuse, attention deficit, etc.

Early diagnosis with proper treatment along with family and peer support helps bring these kids out of the mental illnesses very effectively.

## CONCLUSION

Today's youth, especially adolescent girls, are exposed to many pressures and also have access to lot of information; misconceptions still prevail. Health issues need to be discussed and their concerns addressed in nonjudgmental manner. Good relationship with parents, other family members, teachers and easy access to adolescent friendly health facilities will help adolescents enjoy a positive health leading to healthy adulthood.

## SUGGESTED READING

1. Rashtriya Kishor Swasthya Karyakram. Adolescent Health Division. Ministry Of Health and Family Welfare. Government of India. (2014). Strategy Handbook. [online] Available from http://4dj7dt2ychlw3310xlowzop2.wpengine.netdna-cdn.com/wp-content/uploads/2016/09/RKSK_Strategy_Handbook.pdf [Last accessed January, 2020].

## SECTION 10: Miscellaneous

2. International Institute for Population Sciences (IIPS) and Macro International. (2007). National Family Health Survey (NFHS-3), 2005–06: India: Volume I. [online] Available from http://rchiips.org/nfhs/NFHS-3%20Data/VOL-1/India_volume_I_corrected_17oct08.pdf [Last accessed January, 2020].
3. Weir M, Brien J. Adolescent urinary tract infections. Adolesc Med. 2000;11(2):293-313.
4. Prasad JH, Abraham S, Kurz KM, George V, Lalitha MK, John R, et al. Reproductive tract infections among young married women in Tamil Nadu, India. Int Fam Plan Perspect. 2005;31(2):73-82.
5. Neal S, Matthews Z, Frost M, Fogstad H, Camacho AV, Laski L. Childbearing in adolescents aged 12-15 years in low resource countries: a neglected issue. New estimates from demographic and household surveys in 42 countries. Acta Obstet Gynecol Scand. 2012;91(9):1114-8.
6. WHO. Global Health Estimates 2015: Deaths by cause, age, sex, by country, and by region. 2000–2015. Geneva: WHO; 2016.
7. Darroch J, Woog V, Bankole A, Ashford LS. Adding it up: Costs and benefits of meeting the contraceptive needs of adolescents. New York: Guttmacher Institute; 2016.
8. Wodon Q, Male C, Nayihouba A, Onagoruwa A, Savadogo A, Yedan A, et al. Economic impacts of child marriage: Global synthesis report. Washington DC: The World Bank and International Center for Research on Women; 2017.
9. Garg R, Goyal R, Gupta S. India moves towards menstrual hygiene: subsidized sanitary napkins for rural adolescent girls-issues and challenges. Matern Child Health J. 2012;16(4):761-74.
10. Williams CE, Creighton SM. Menstrual disorders on adolescents: Review of current practice. Horm Res Pediatr. 2012;78(3):135-43.
11. Type 2 diabetes in children and adolescents. American Diabetes Association. Pediatrics. 2000;105(3 Pt 1):671-80.
12. Lazar L, Kalter-Leibovici O, Pertzelan A, Weintrob N, Josefsberg Z, Phillip M. Thyrotoxicosis in prepubertal children compared with pubertal and postpubertal patients. J Clin Endocrinol Metab. 2000;85(10):3678-82.
13. Branca F, Piwoz E, Schultink W, Sullivan LM. Nutrition and health in women, children, and adolescent girls. BMJ. 2015;351:H4173.
14. Costello EJ, Mustillo S, Erkanli A, Keeler G, Angold A. Prevalence and development of psychiatric disorders in childhood and adolescence. Arch Gen Psy. 2003;60(8):837-44.

# CHAPTER 9

# Sex Education of Adolescent Girls

*Ruchita Shah, Sana Yumnam Devi*

## ABSTRACT

Adolescence is a stage of life cycle where significant changes occur in physical, cognitive, social, sexual, and emotional domains. This developmental period opens up exciting vistas for the adolescent but also makes her vulnerable to risky or exploitative behaviors and relations. In this context, developmentally appropriate and accurate information regarding the various aspects and influencers of sexuality has been thought to help children and adolescents during this crucial stage of development. Sexuality education is defined as teaching about human sexuality including intimate relationships, human sexual anatomy, menstruation and sexual reproduction, sexually transmitted infections (STIs), sexual activity, sexual orientation, gender identity, abstinence, contraception, and reproductive rights and responsibilities. Moreover, comprehensive and effective sexuality education programs consider gender equality and human rights as core and over-arching components. There is adequate evidence that such programs reduce risky sexual behaviors and adverse sexual outcomes such as teenage pregnancy and infections; and do not increase sexual activity amongst adolescents. In India, there are school/curriculum-based initiatives such as the Adolescent Education Programme (AEP) and community-based programs such as the Rashtriya Kishore Swasthya Karyakram that provides for peer educators and adolescent friendly health clinics. Various aspects of sexuality education in adolescent girls with a special emphasis on the Indian scenario have been covered in this chapter. Finally, there is a need to consolidate the efforts to provide high quality and comprehensive sexuality education (CSE) to adolescent girls, both in and out-of-school, through co-ordination between departments of education and health, private and nongovernmental organizations, community, parents, and youth.

## INTRODUCTION

Adolescence is a developmental stage of life extending from 11 to 19 years of age. India is home to >243 million out of world's 1.2 billion adolescents, and these adolescents account for a quarter of the country's population. Adolescent girls constitute around 47% of this group in India, and needless to say, their development and well-being is of paramount importance. Development during adolescence can be grouped into five domains, namely, physical, cognitive, social, emotional, and sexual. Navigation through these domains in a developmentally appropriate manner facilitates entry into healthy adulthood. Sexuality is defined as a central aspect of human existence that evolves over the lifespan. Sexuality encompasses sex, gender identities and roles, sexual orientation, eroticism, pleasure, intimacy, and reproduction. It is experienced and expressed in thoughts, fantasies, desires, beliefs, attitudes, values, behaviors, practices, roles, and relationships. Importantly, it can be influenced by the interaction of biological, psychological, social, economic, political, cultural, legal, religious, and spiritual factors. During adolescence, experiences related to sexuality and sexual behavior typically precede knowledge and understanding about sexuality. Moreover, an adolescent's need for autonomy, experimentation, and need to fit in the peer group influences her/his sexuality-related values, thoughts, and behaviors. This raises the possibility of early, exploitative, or risky sexual activity among adolescent girls leading to various adverse consequences such as teenage pregnancy, unsafe abortion, sexual abuse, sexually transmitted infections (STIs), and human immunodeficiency virus infection and acquired immune deficiency syndrome (HIV/AIDS) as well as dropping out of school. According to a World Health Organization (WHO) report while postulating disease burden, the pattern for younger and older adolescents is different. Injury and communicable diseases are the common causes for the mortality in younger adolescents from 10 to 14 years; sexual behavior, and mental health for older adolescents from 15 to 19 years are the common causes of mortality. In this context, developmentally appropriate and accurate information regarding the various aspects and influencers of sexuality has been thought to help children and adolescents during this crucial stage of development.

## EVOLUTION OF SEXUALITY EDUCATION

Around 1970s and 1980s, sex education (as it was called then) was considered as a crucial element to fight the epidemic of HIV/AIDS at the international level. With a narrow focus, the earlier sex education programs emphasized on abstinence-only approach, i.e., sexual activity should be avoided by the youth. The emphasis was equally moral in nature and premarital sex was discouraged strongly through sex education. However, abstinence-only programs did not significantly reduce rates of STI including HIV/AIDS among this population. Moreover, teenage pregnancy was recognized as another potential outcome of these programs. So, sex education programs started including concepts of safe sex with information regarding use of condoms and oral contraceptives, i.e., the abstinence-plus approach.However, despite implementing above strategies, rates of teenage pregnancy and sexual abuse among this population remained alarmingly high. Moreover, it was realized that gender-based power differential in relations discourage informed and healthy decision-making among adolescent girls. Therefore, sexuality education programs based on principles of gender equality and rights evolved over time and have been shown to be more effective than abstinence and abstinence-plus. Moreover, it was recognized that it was important to impart education regarding life skills so as to empower adolescents to inculcate critical thinking, problem-solving, develop healthy social and emotion regulation skills, and finally, to maintain healthy sexual relationships without violating others' sexual rights. The current concept of sexuality education which is also termed comprehensive sexuality education (CSE) draws from all the above principles.

## Indian Realities

Indian adolescents, especially females of low to middle socioeconomic strata face numerous challenges to their healthy development from childhood into adulthood. These mainly include gender discrimination, lack of information, poor education, early marriage, and childbearing. As per National Family Health Survey information level on sexual health is poor among adolescents, with girls and boys ratio of 47/16. Use of contraception among married teenagers is only 13% while the unmet need for contraception in the age group of 15–19 years is 27%. About 8% of the girls and 2.7% of the boys in this age group had sexual intercourse before 15 years of age. Only 3% of the girls and 19% of the boys had used condoms. These figures are actually disturbing and show how important this sexuality education is in Indian scenario.

## DEFINITION, CONTENT, AND DELIVERY OF SEXUALITY EDUCATION

Sexuality education is more than providing mere information and instruction regarding anatomy and physiology of human reproductive system. It encompasses healthy sexual development, gender identity, interpersonal relationships, affection, sexual development, intimacy, and body image for all adolescents, including adolescents with disabilities, chronic health conditions, and other special needs. As per United Nations Educational, Scientific and Cultural Organization (UNESCO), CSE is defined as teaching about human sexuality including intimate relationships, human sexual anatomy, sexual reproduction, STIs, sexual activity, sexual orientation, gender identity, abstinence, contraception, and reproductive rights and responsibilities. There is a growing emphasis on human rights and gender equality as core components of sexuality education.

As per UNESCO (2018), the major objectives of sexuality education are to equip adolescents with knowledge, skills, attitudes, and values that will empower them to: (1) Realize their health, well-being and dignity; (2) Develop respectful social and sexual relationships; (3) Consider how their choices affect their own well-being and that of others; and (4) Understand and ensure the protection of their rights throughout their lives.

## CONTENT OF COMPREHENSIVE SEXUALITY EDUCATION (UNESCO, 2018)

There are eight major areas that need to be covered in a developmentally appropriate manner as identified by UNESCO (2018). These areas are described briefly below:

1. *Relationships*: CSE should involve discussions regarding relationships involving different kinds of love and that love can be expressed in many different ways. Families can promote gender equality through parental roles and responsibilities; help children to acquire values and guide in decision making.
2. *Values, rights, culture, and sexuality*: For successful adoption of the program, focus should be on the values, rights, and attitudes of the population as well.
3. *Understanding gender*: Gender inequality and power differences have an influence on sexual behavior and may increase the risk of sexual abuse and gender-based violence. Understanding of these issues is important to empower the adolescent girls.
4. *Violence and staying safe*: Right to privacy and bodily integrity are fundamental rights, and respecting and protecting these rights is essential.
5. *Skills for health and well-being*: Negative influences on sexual decisions should be challenged and methods to promote health and well-being should be encouraged.

## SECTION 10: Miscellaneous

6. *The human body and development*: Menstruation is a normal biological process in a woman's physical development and should not be considered as stigma.
7. *Sexuality and sexual behavior*: Sexual behavior should be associated with responsibilities of health and well-being of self and partner as well.
8. *Sexual and reproductive health*: Access to contraceptives, regardless of ability, marital status, gender, gender identity or sexual orientation to young population who are sexually active should be there.

## Delivery Forms of Comprehensive Sexuality Education

The mode of delivery of CSE should be in an interactive manner that engages the learner, promote critical thinking, decision making, and improves communication skills. This can be delivered by teachers, counselors, health professionals, parents and even community members and trained peers in a safe and healthy learning environment.

## Role of Media in Sexuality and Sexuality Education

Media has a crucial role as it can influence values, attitudes, and norms about sexuality and gender in both positive and negative ways. As per UNESCO (2018), CSE should "define different types of media (e.g., social media, traditional media); share examples of how men and women and relationships are portrayed in the media; describe the impact of media upon personal values, attitudes and behavior relating to sexuality and gender; and recognize the power of media to influence values, attitudes, and behavior relating to sexuality and gender." Media should promote gender equality and safe sexual practices and avoid inaccurate portrayals of sexuality and sexual practices.

## Effectiveness of Comprehensive Sexuality Education

There are two types of outcomes of CSE, namely primary outcomes and secondary outcomes.

The primary outcomes include sexual behavior and health, and the secondary outcomes include sexual knowledge, attitudes, and other behavioral outcomes. These outcomes have been studied by various systematic reviews and meta-analytic studies that demonstrate effectiveness of CSE on both the outcomes.

Sexuality education has shown to have positive effects, including increasing young people's knowledge and improving their attitudes related to sexual reproductive health (SRH) and behaviors thus lowering the STI/HIV infection rates. School-based programs should be complemented with community elements including access to contraceptives (condom); providing training for health providers to deliver youth-friendly services; and involving parents/guardians and teachers, to make sexuality education effective.

## SEXUALITY EDUCATION FOR ADOLESCENT GIRLS—INDIAN SCENARIO

The need for sexuality education to adolescent girls has been recognized by health and education ministries of India and so efforts have been taken to provide the same through school/curriculum based education and community based programs.

## Curriculum-based/School-based
### Adolescent Education Programme
Developed by the Ministry of Human Resource Development (MHRD), this program is meant to provide young population, accurate, age appropriate, and culturally relevant information to develop healthy attitudes and learn skills to respond to real life situations in positive and responsible ways. Following themes are covered: Changes during adolescence, body image, positive relationships, gender and sexuality based stereotypes and discrimination, violence and abuse, reproductive tract infection (RTI)/STI, HIV/AIDS, substance use. Six national agencies that have implemented it are:
1. National Council of Educational Research and Training (NCERT),
2. Council of Boards of School Education (COBSE),
3. National Institute of Open Schooling (NIOS),
4. Central Board of Secondary Education (CBSE),
5. Kendriya Vidyalaya Sangathan (KVS), and
6. Navodaya Vidyalaya Samiti (NVS).

Trained teachers deliver the education through a 16–23 hour model to students in classes 8, 9, and 11, i.e., between ages 13–18 years.

National Education Programme (NEP), in his draft of 2019, has emphasised that "sex education will also be included in secondary school for future judgment surrounding consent, harassment, respect for women, safety, family planning, and sexually transmitted disease (STD) prevention."

The CBSE has decided to introduce sexuality education in a more comprehensive and developmentally appropriate manner through the regular curriculum, after it faced resistance in 2005 when it was included in curriculum.

Lack of knowledge and competence, preconceived notions, and reluctance amongst school teachers to deliver sexuality education are some of the reasons why adolescent education programme (AEP) has not delivered to its full potential.

## Community-based
National level health programs for adolescents in some manner facilitate sexuality education as well as connect it to sexual and reproductive healthcare services. The Reproductive, Maternal, Newborn, Child and Adolescent Health (RMNC+A) program has as its major component the Rashtriya Kishor Swasthya Karyakram (RKSK). Amongst others, the major objectives of the RKSK are to improve knowledge, attitudes, and behavior in relation to SRH to promote healthy menstrual hygiene practices among adolescent girls, to improve birth preparedness and complication readiness among adolescents, and to reduce teenage pregnancies. There are a host of counseling and clinical services as well as provision of commodities, i.e., weekly iron and folic acids, sanitary napkins, contraceptives, and medicines. Three components of the RKSK need special mention in context of sexuality education.
1. *Peer education program*: It was started as a part of the "Saathiya resource toolkit" which was launched in 2017. This is a peer educator program and the adolescents in the population are covered by it. The peer educators under this program are called "Saathiya". They are being trained across the country in a phased manner, ensuring optimum use of the resource kit specially designed to help them to be recognized and respected as "saathiya," a good friend for the adolescents. In addition, a mobile app "Saathiya Salah" has been developed which acts as a ready information source for

the adolescents. Saathiya help in the organization of the quarterly adolescent health days (AHD) and participate in the Adolescent Friendly Club (AFC) meetings also. The sexual and reproductive education and health related aspects are covered under this peer education program.
2. *Adolescent Friendly Health Clinics (AFHC)*: This is the component of RKSK with facility-based approach. AFHC entails a whole gamut of clinical and counseling services on diverse adolescent health issues ranging from SRH to nutrition, substance abuse, injuries, and violence (including gender-based violence, noncommunicable diseases and mental health). Services are delivered through trained service providers—medical officers (MO), auxiliary nurse midwife (ANM), and counselors at AFHCs located at primary health centers (PHCs), community health centers (CHCs) and district hospitals (DHs), and medical colleges. These clinics provide the clinical support needed for practical effectiveness of peer-based or curriculum-based sexuality education.
3. *Menstrual hygiene scheme*: It focuses on adolescent girls in rural areas, creating awareness on menstrual hygiene, use of high quality sanitary napkins, and their safe disposal.

### Adolescent Life Skill Training Program Developed by NIMHANS, Bengaluru

The life skills training program targets vulnerable population which includes street and working children, orphan and abandoned children, children infected/affected with HIV, and children affected by gender and sexuality vulnerabilities.

Series II–focus is on gender, sexuality, and relationship for sexually-abused children, children in conflict with the law or those who have ran away from house to marry or be in mutually consenting relationships.

Its purpose is to develop an understanding of emotions, awareness, and recognition of sexual abuse and coercion and the learning of skills such as problem solving, refusal (not giving consent), and negotiation (practicing safe sex).

## BARRIERS TO ACCESS SEXUALITY EDUCATION

There are certain beliefs and norms that may hinder the successful implementation of sexuality education which is life skills based and rights based. Some of them are:
- A false belief that increased awareness will lead to promiscuity in young people.
- Gender discrimination of young women that prevent them to take ownership of their bodies and sexual behaviors.
- Few social norms which believe that access to such programs will make women lose their purity. Women are forced to limit their choices, restrict their movement, dress conservatively, and silence any question regarding their bodies and sexuality. CSE program that is contextualized and actively involves the community and the youth may be able to overcome some of these barriers.

## CONCLUSION

Sexuality education, which is comprehensive, rights-based, and fosters gender equality can facilitate healthy sexual development and decrease risky and exploitative sexual behaviors. Toward this end, concerted efforts are needed so that sexuality education is introduced in a developmentally appropriate manner and in synchrony with family and cultural values. Sexuality education programs should target universal adolescent populations as well as high-risk or vulnerable groups, albeit with varying emphasis as well as both in and out-of-school youth. Sexuality education must go hand-in-hand with adolescent friendly healthcare services. Coordination between governmental departments of education and health, private and nongovernmental agencies, community, parents and last but extremely important, the youth themselves is essential.

## SUGGESTED READING

1. Government of India. Census of India 2011. Post enumeration survey. Registrar General and Census Commissioner of India, Ministry of Home Affairs, New Delhi, India. [Online] Available from http://censusindia.gov.in/2011census/population_enumeration.html. [Last accessed February, 2020].
2. Sadock BJ, Sadock VA, Ruiz P. Kaplan & Sadock's Comprehensive Textbook of Psychiatry, 10th edition. Philadelphia: Wolters Kluwer; 2015.
3. World Health Organization. Sexual and reproductive health. Geneva: World Health Organization; 2006.
4. American Academy of Pediatrics. Sexuality education for children and adolescents. Committee on psychosocial aspects of child and family health and committee on adolescence. Pediatrics. 2001;108(2):498-502.
5. World Health Organization. Factsheet on adolescent health, India. Geneva: World Health Organization; 2011.
6. Cora CB, Gerri M. Sexuality education for children and adolescents. Committee on adolescence and committee on psychosocial aspects of child and family health. American Academy of Pediatrics Clinical report. 2016;138(2).
7. Santelli J, Ott MA, Lyon M, Rogers J, Summers D, Schleifer R. Abstinence and abstinence-only education: a review of U.S. policies and programs. J Adolesc Health. 2006;38(1):72-81.
8. Boonstra HD. Advancing sexuality education in developing countries: Evidence and implications. Guttmacher Policy Review. 2011;14(3):17-23.
9. Haberland NA. The case for addressing gender and power in sexuality and HIV education: a comprehensive review of evaluation studies. Int Perspect Sex Reprod Health. 2015;41(1):31-42.
10. International Institute for Population Sciences (IIPS) and Macro International. (2007) National family health survey (NFHS-3), 2005–06. [online] Available from http://rchiips.org/nfhs/nfhs3.shtml. [Last accessed February, 2020].
11. UNESCO. (2018). International technical guidance on sexuality education, an evidence-informed approach. Revised edition. [online] Available from https://unesdoc.unesco.org/ark:/48223/pf0000260770. [Last accessed February, 2020].
12. UNFPA. (2014). Operational guidance for comprehensive sexuality education, a focus on human rights and gender. [online] Available from https://www.unfpa.org/sites/default/files/pub-pdf/UNFPA_OperationalGuidance_WEB3.pdf. [Last accessed February, 2020].
13. UNESCO. Review of the evidence on sexuality education. Report to inform the update of the UNESCO international technical guidance on sexuality education. [online] Available from https://unesdoc.unesco.org/ark:/48223/pf0000264649. [Last accessed February, 2020].
14. Fonner VA, Armstrong KS, Kennedy CE, O'Reilly KR, Sweat MD. School based sex education and HIV prevention in low- and middle-income countries: A systematic review and meta-analysis. PLoS One. 2014;9(3):e89692.
15. Chhabra R, Springer C, Rapkin B, Merchant Y. Differences among male/female adolescents participating in a School-based Teenage Education Program (STEP) focusing on HIV prevention in India. Ethn Dis. 2008;18((2 Suppl 2):123-7.
16. Chandra-Mouli V, Lane C, Wong S. What does work in adolescent sexual and reproductive health: A review of evidence on interventions commonly accepted as best practices. Glob Health Sci Pract. 2015;3:333-40.
17. Ministry of health and family welfare, Government of India. Adolescence education programme. Government of India; 2005.
18. Ministry of health and family welfare, Government of India. Implementation guidelines Rashtriya Kishore Swasthiya Karyakram (RKSK). National Health Mission;GOI:2018.
19. Chaitra GK, Shekhar S. Life Skills for Children aged 8 to 12 years. Bengaluru: NIMHANS; 2017.
20. Khubchandani J, Clark J, Kumar R. Beyond controversies: sexuality education for adolescents in India. J Fam Med Primary Care. 2014;3(3):175.

# Medical Problems in Women Undergoing Infertility Treatment

*Suman Puri, Rupinder Kaur*

## ABSTRACT

For eons, a woman is meant to be a mother at some point of life. That is how things have been and that is how we are told things should be. But with late marriage age and couples leading a stressful work life, infertility is on the rise. More than 50 million couples worldwide suffer from infertility. Several drugs and treatment regimens are available for inducing conception in such couples. Most of these target the would be mother. Some of these therapies are double edged swords and may produce intolerable side effects and complications. This chapter highlights the various medical issues a woman faces in her journey to win over infertility and have a successful pregnancy.

## INTRODUCTION

For thousands of years, a lot of studies have been done on infertility. Based on our information regarding hypothalamic-pituitary axis, a variety of therapies that use gonadotropins have been developed for stimulating the ovulation. This has helped us to be capable of treating anovulatory infertility; for in vitro fertilization (IVF), it can also help in induction of superovulation. But this has also resulted in consequences like increased rate of multiple pregnancies and various other health problems. Progression of the treatment modalities for infertility had opened majority of the locks in the way of problems related to infertility; however, it also lead to some complications.

As defined by Shaw, "Infertility stands for evident failure of a couple to conceive following 1 year of regular and unprotected intercourse."

Primary infertility is designated to those individuals who never conceived. Secondary infertility includes those individuals who have conceived in the past at some time.

## INCIDENCE

According to the existing data, infertility is experienced by at least 50 million couples globally. Most common cause of anovulatory infertility is considered to be polycystic ovary syndrome (PCOS). Among the anovulatory women who present to infertility clinics, nearly 90–95% have PCOS.

## CAUSES OF INFERTILITY

Conception relies on the capacity of the male and female partners for fertility. In nearly 40–55% of cases, female is responsible, male in approximately 30–40% of cases, and in 10% cases both are responsible. Rest of the 10% are not explained despite detailed investigations.

## MANAGEMENT OF INFERTILITY

Investigations of the male and female partners should be initiated by the general practitioner. Couple should be referred to specialist clinic at appropriate time by the general practitioner.

## INVESTIGATIONS FOR FEMALE INFERTILITY (NICE GUIDANCE)

- Full examination including body mass index (BMI).
- Basal hormonal profile [follicle-stimulating hormone (FSH), luteinizing hormone (LH), thyroid-stimulating hormone (TSH), prolactin, anti-Müllerian hormone (AMH) levels] and others depending upon symptoms.
- Cervical cytology and screening
- Tubal patency
- Imaging of pelvis.

## PRINCIPLES OF FERTILITY TREATMENT

Advice regarding infertility treatment advice should be provided in relation to the preparation of pregnancy, which includes both physical approach as well as psychological approach.

## INFERTILITY TREATMENT OPTIONS

- Ovulation induction
- Artificial reproductive techniques [intrauterine insemination (IUI), IVF + embryo transfer (ET), and intracytoplasmic sperm injection (ICSI)]
- Other drugs
- Surgical techniques (laparoscopy/hysteroscopy)

### Ovulation Induction

Ovulation induction stands for the stimulation of ovulation; this include therapeutically restoring the release of one egg per cycle in the woman who is not ovulating frequently or is not ovulating at all. The ovulation of >2 eggs should be avoided for minimizing the risk of ovarian hyperstimulation syndrome (OHSS) as well as multiple gestations. In infertility patients, for determining the success of ovulation induction, correct selection of patient can be a significant determinant.

### Ovulation Induction Drugs

In infertile women, the main treatment is fertility drugs and the cause of infertility is ovulation disorder. These drugs are associated with benefits as well as risks. Most commonly employed drugs are:

SECTION 10: Miscellaneous

- *Selective estrogen receptor modulators (SERMs)*: Clomiphene citrate
- *Aromatase inhibitors*: Letrozole

### Clomiphene Citrate

The first-line ovulation-inducing agent is clomiphene citrate for the women suffering from PCOS and infertility. Clomiphene citrate is a nonsteroidal triphenylethylene derivative; it has estrogen agonist as well as antagonist properties.

Dose of clomiphene citrate is 50–150 mg/day.
The various side effects associated with the use of clomiphene citrate include:
- Nonspecific side effects like nausea and vomiting and antiestrogenic side effects such as hot flushes, sweating, osteopenia, and osteoporosis.
- Abdominal pain due to abnormal ovarian enlargement has been seen in up to 10% of cases, multiple pregnancies in 6% of cases, and OHSS in 5% of cases.
- Visual disturbances and scotomas.
- Breast tenderness, hair loss, and rashes
- Increased risk of epithelial ovarian cancer if clomiphene citrate or other ovulating drugs are given for >1 year.
- Mood swings, depression, and headaches

### Aromatase Inhibitors (Letrozole)

In women with PCOS (anovulatory infertility), the most effective aromatase inhibitor for ovulation induction is letrozole; it is used as an adjunct to gonadotropin therapy for controlled ovarian hyperstimulation (COH) in women with ovulatory infertility. Presently, in women with PCOS, it is considered as the drug of choice for ovulation induction. Its dose is 2.5–7.5 mg/day.

Letrozole is associated with mild-to-moderate adverse events, which are rarely severe to be discontinued. The most commonly reported adverse effects with letrozole include:
- Arthralgia, hot flushes, nausea, fatigue, lethargy, malaise, asthma, headache, and back pain.
- Coronary artery disease, vaginal dryness, and osteoporosis are seen due to the antiestrogenic effect of letrozole.
- Visual disturbances and OHSS are relatively less as compared to clomiphene citrate.

## Gonadotropins

Gonadotropins are fertility drugs, which are administered by injection; these include:
- Follicle-stimulating hormone alone
- Combined with LH. Such drugs are provided at the beginning of the menstrual cycle for facilitating recruitment of multiple eggs to a mature size prior to IUI/IVF.
- Another important drug/injectable is human chorionic gonadotropin (hCG), which is used to trigger the release of eggs once mature.

Close monitoring of these drugs is required in order to minimize side effects. Most common side effects of these drugs include medical and pregnancy-associated side effects as follows.

### Ovarian Hyperstimulation Syndrome

This syndrome is characterized by enlargement of ovaries and accumulation of fluid in the abdomen following ovulation, which results due to stimulation by gonadotropins.
- Mild form is accountable for 10–20% of cycles. It leads to some discomfort that generally resolves fast with no complications.

- In nearly 1% of patients, severe form is found. The risk of OHSS is noticeably increased in women having PCOS and who get pregnant in the same cycle in which gonadotropins are provided. In severe form, OHSS can lead to nausea, vomiting, dehydration, coagulopathy, rapid weight gain, kidney dysfunction, torsion (twisting of an ovary), pleural effusion, ascites, and in rare cases, even death also. But, this condition is not permanent, which generally lasts for 1 or 2 weeks. However, hospitalization is usually required in severe cases for monitoring.

### *Prevention of Ovarian Hyperstimulation Syndrome*

A number of strategies exist to prevent or minimize clinical symptoms of OHSS. This includes:
- Human chorionic gonadotropin administration should be delayed till levels of hormone plateau or decline.
- Further gonadotropin stimulation should be withhold or even hCG should be withhold for preventing ovulation.
- In IVF cycles, where OHSS is susceptible to develop.
  - Cabergoline per orally may be given to lessen the severity of the clinical signs and symptoms.
  - Also, in IVF couples, it can be considered to delay the ET by freezing (cryopreserving) the embryos and transferring it at a later date when the OHSS symptoms are completely resolved.

However, as OHSS is diagnosed on basis of clinical criteria, clinicians must be aware of the signs and symptoms in all the women undergoing infertility treatment.

### *Management of Ovarian Hyperstimulation Syndrome*

All the women diagnosed with severe OHSS should be admitted for close monitoring. After taking the above preventive measures, investigations [complete blood count (CBC), packed cell volume (PCV), C-reactive protein (CRP), renal function test (RFT) and electrolytes, liver function test (LFT) including albumin, coagulation profile, beta-hCG, ultrasonography (USG), electrocardiogram (ECG), and chest X-ray] should be monitored. Daily weight monitoring, intake/output monitoring, abdominal girth, and vitals are to be monitored.

### *Treatment*

Treatment modalities include a multidisciplinary approach. A fluid intake of at least 1 L should be maintained. Nonsteroidal anti-inflammatory drugs (NSAIDs) are to be avoided as it compromise renal function. Patients with severe OHSS should receive thromboprophylaxis with low-molecular-weight heparin (LMWH). Paracentesis of ascitic fluid should be carried out in specific cases under USG guidance. Diuretics are to be avoided. Surgery is indicated only in cases when there is:
- Ovarian rupture
- Ectopic (tubal) pregnancies
- Adnexal torsion (ovarian twisting)

# Other Drugs

## Metformin

Metformin, an oral hypoglycemic agent, results in decrease in levels of circulating glucose by inhibition of the production of hepatic glucose, by reduction of lipid synthesis, by

## SECTION 10: Miscellaneous

enhancing fatty acid oxidation, and by inhibition of gluconeogenesis. It causes reduction in insulin resistance by increasing insulin sensitivity at the cellular levels; it also seems to be having direct effects within the ovary. Therefore, in patients with infertility, it would be reasonable to predict that lowering of insulin and insulin-sensitizing treatment would be beneficial.

### Side Effects and Medical Problems

Using metformin is always related with adverse effects specifically nausea, vomiting, as well as other gastrointestinal disturbances. The symptoms of lactic acidosis are as follows:
- Reduced appetite
- Abdominal or stomach discomfort
- Diarrhea
- General feeling of discomfort
- Fast or shallow breathing
- Unusual sleepiness, tiredness, or weakness
- Cramping or severe muscle pain

## Aspirin

Aspirin, an antiplatelet agent, in low doses (75 mg) results in vasodilation and improves blood perfusion via enhancing prostacyclin synthesis. Also, there are a number of studies which has determined the role of low-dose aspirin in improvement of the outcome of treatment with IVF/ICSI.

### Side Effects and Medical Problems

Various side effects noted are bleeding disorders, hearing problems, renal dysfunction, severe or persistent nausea/vomiting, dizziness, unexplained tiredness, dark-colored urine, and yellow eyes/yellow skin. Rarely, it can result in serious side effects such as gastrointestinal bleeding as well as intracranial hemorrhage. It is very rare that it results in serious allergic reaction that presents as severe dizziness; rash; itching or swelling particularly of the face, tongue, and throat; and difficulty in breathing.

## Progesterone

It helps in the fertilized egg implantation in the uterus and therefore, promotes establishment and maintenance of healthy pregnancy. Usually, it is given in IVF, the reason being that the medications provided in the process result in reduction of natural production of progesterone in a woman. It includes both synthetic as well as natural progesterone such as micronized progesterone, dydrogesterone, and medroxyprogesterone.

### Side Effects and Medical Problems

This includes weight gain, changes in appetite, fluid retention and swelling (edema), fatigue, acne, drowsiness or insomnia, allergic skin rashes, hives, fever, headache, and depression. It can also lead to premenstrual syndrome (PMS) such as symptoms, breast discomfort or enlargement, and altered menstrual cycles.

## Sildenafil

It is a phosphodiesterase inhibitor and is used to treat sexual dysfunction.
Sildenafil citrate enhances uterine blood flow and increases endometrial thickening for better implantation and improved pregnancy rates.

## Side Effects and Medical Problems
Various side effects include visual disturbance, headache, dyspepsia, and flushing. Other related side effects are nasal congestion, rhinitis, epistaxis, and insomnia. Sildenafil is hemodynamically safe; it may result in induction of significant vasodilation and, then, leading to harmful hypotension among patients who are susceptible. This product should be used with caution in patients with hypertension and cardiovascular disease.

## Estrogens
Estradiol is the most commonly used estrogen in IVF; it supports natural estrogen requirements such as uterine lining thickening, so that uterus gets able for implantation. It also boosts functioning of placenta, promotes blood flow to the uterus, and helps in preparation of the body for breastfeeding following birth.

## Side Effect and Medical Problems
Common side effects include headache, nausea/vomiting, stomach upset, bloating, breast tenderness, change in weight, etc.

This drug can also cause breast lumps, mental or mood changes (e.g., memory loss, depression), and unusual vaginal bleeding such as breakthrough bleeding, spotting, prolonged, or recurrent bleeding. It is very rarely found that it can cause thrombotic disorders such as strokes, heart attacks, pulmonary embolism, deep vein thrombosis, etc.

# Assisted Reproductive Techniques
The following are assisted reproductive techniques used for infertility treatment. Potential medical and related complications with these techniques are discussed below.

## Intrauterine Insemination
### Procedure
In the process of IUI, at the time of ovulation, healthy sperms are directly put in the uterus.

### Risks
Intrauterine insemination is reported to be a relatively simple as well as safe procedure, with low-risk of serious complications. Following are risks and medical problems seen in patients undergoing IUI:
- Ovulation drugs-induced side effects (OHSS)
- Infection (rare)
- Spotting
- Multiple pregnancies
- Pain
- Mild cramping
- Psychological side effects

## In Vitro Fertilization
### Procedure
The most common assisted reproductive technology (ART) technique is IVF. It requires ovarian stimulation for retrieving several mature eggs, fertilizing eggs with the sperm in a dish in laboratory, and implantation of the embryos in the uterus many days following fertilization.

## Risks

*Complications of IVF include the following*:
- Ovulation stimulation drugs side effects (OHSS)
- Bleeding
- Breast tenderness due to increased estrogen levels
- Infection
- Multiple pregnancies
- Psychological side effects
- Pregnancy-related complications

## Laparoscopy Procedure and Other Surgical Techniques

Infertility treatment may include various surgical interventions that are associated with some benefits and risks related to the procedure. Uterine problems such as intrauterine scar tissue, endometrial polyps, pelvic adhesions, a uterine septum, and some fibroids can be treated with the use of hysteroscopy technique. Laparoscopic surgery is required in endometriosis, pelvic adhesions, and larger fibroids.

### Risks, Complications, and Medical Problems

These techniques are associated with various medical and surgical complications which include: Infection, bleeding, perforation of a hollow viscus, metabolic acidosis, and cardiac irregularities (with uncontrolled pressures used in hysteroscopy).

Excessive absorption of the fluid, i.e., sorbitol and glycine that are used in hysteroscopy results in hyponatremia as well as hypervolemia. It manifests clinically as vomiting, nausea, headache, and agitation. If it is not treated, it may develop as bradycardia and hypertension and then hypotension, cerebral edema, pulmonary edema as well as cardiovascular collapse.

## INFERTILITY AND MENTAL HEALTH

In the life of infertile couples, infertility is a stressful event, which is associated with depressive symptoms. In both the infertile females and males, grief reactions are a common finding; in these individuals, mourning process is significant so that to resolve the crisis associated with infertility. In infertile couples along with the treatment of infertility, proper psychological consultations are required as they are at risk of psychosocial problems.

As per the World Health Organization (WHO), in fertility, health infertility is considered to be the main problem with diverse physical, social, and psychological dimensions. Treatment of infertility not only involves long-time strict medications but it has also resulted in psychosocial reaction because of the high cost of treatment involved. Also, diagnosis and long-term follow-up of infertility treatment lead to stress and can result in anxiety, depression as well as other physical and psychological illnesses. It also results in social abnormalities.

## MANAGEMENT

Infertile couples use more emotional-coping strategies because of the lack of control on the events of life, less social support, less self-esteem as well as high stress level.

## Psychotherapy

As reported by many studies conducted in couple of years in past, it has been reported that cognitive behavioral group psychotherapy leads to reduction in mood and stress symptoms. It also enhances rate of fertility.

## Pharmacotherapy

In women and men who develop depression because of infertility as well as its treatment, pharmacotherapy is still an important alternative. But it is avoided by several many patients as they fear that medication may have an impact on fertility or it may affect their pregnancy outcome. Also, there is little data available regarding role of pharmacologic treatment of patient with infertility, so more studies are required to be done for a conclusive result.

*The role of mental health professional (MHP) includes:*
- Tailoring evidence-based interventions for the management of emotional challenges and treatment burden (before, during, and after specific treatment).
- Helping patients to make informed decisions.
- Coping during waiting periods before pregnancy tests.
- Helping couples prepare for semen samples, multifetal reductions, and support in the gestational period after conception following fertility treatments.
- Offering specific services in complex programs (e.g., in surrogacy: Interventions for intended parents and gestational carriers in surrogacy).
- Providing consultancy for staff training in communication skills, empathy, and breaking the bad news.
- Ensuring extended periods of support and collaborative team programs for staff experiencing burnouts.
- Adaptive coping in patients, during critical times such as repeated treatment failures, ending treatments, and long-term psychological adjustment.
- Development of emotional support programs for patients who are vulnerable.

## CONCLUSION

With the social stigma centered around infertility, more and more young couples are desperate to get any treatment option available for them to successfully conceive. Several of these options come with their share of adverse effects. In a society like ours, the woman usually faces the brunt more. Psychosomatic issues surrounding infertility also affect a woman's health and well being. A judicious decision for possible management strategies after thorough investigation along with mental counseling of couple and family is of utmost importance in this regard.

## SUGGESTED READING

1. te Velde ER, Pearson PL. The variability of female reproductive ageing. Hum Reprod Update. 2002;8(2):141-54.
2. Shakhar K. The psychological implications of infertility. In: Shakhar K (Ed). The Infertility Manual, 3rd edition. New Delhi: Jaypee Brothers Medical (P) Pvt. Ltd.; 2016. p. 85.
3. Maternal Health Task Force. (2017). The Burden of Infertility: Global Prevalence and Women's Voices from Around the World. [online] Available from https://www.mhtf.org/2017/01/18/the-burden-of-infertility-global-prevalence-and-womens-voices-from-around-the-world/. [Last accessed February, 2020].

4. Barthelmess EK, Naz RK. Polycystic ovary syndrome: current status and future perspective. Front Biosci (Elite Ed). 2014;6(1):104-19.
5. Speroff L, Fritz MA. Clinical Gynecologic Endocrinology and Infertility. Lippincott: Williams and Wilkins; 2005. pp. 1013-69.
6. Balen AH, Rutherford AJ. Management of infertility. BMJ. 2007;335(7620):608-11.
7. Casper RF, Mitwally MF. Aromatase Inhibitors for Ovulation Induction. J Clin Endocrinol Metab. 2006;91(3):760-71.
8. Practice Committee of the American Society for Reproductive Medicine. Use of clomiphene citrate in women. Fertil Steril. 2006;86(5):S187-93.
9. Practice Committee of the American Society for Reproductive Medicine. Use of clomiphene citrate in infertile women: a committee opinion. Fertil Steril. 2013;100(2):341-8.
10. Sallam HN, Abdel-Bak M, Sallam NH. Does ovulation induction increase the risk of gynecological cancer? Facts Views Vis Obgyn. 2013;5(4):265-73.
11. American College of Obstetricians and Gynecologists (ACOG). (2018). Aromatase Inhibitors in Gynecologic Practice. [online] Available from https://www.acog.org/Clinical-Guidance-and-Publications/Committee-Opinions/Committee-on-Gynecologic-Practice/Aromatase-Inhibitors-in-Gynecologic-Practice?IsMobileSet=false. [Last accessed February, 2020].
12. Webmd. (2019). Drugs and Medications: Letrozole. [online] Available from https://www.webmd.com/drugs/2/drug-4297/letrozole-oral/details. [Last accessed February, 2020].
13. Reproductive Facts. (2012). Side effects of injectable fertility drugs (gonadotropins). [online] Available from https://www.reproductivefacts.org/news-and-publications/patient-fact-sheets-and-booklets/documents/fact-sheets-and-info-booklets/side-effects-of-injectable-fertility-drugs-gonadotropins. [Last accessed February, 2020].
14. Royal College of Obstetricians and Gynaecologists (RCOG). (2016). The Management of Ovarian Hyperstimulation Syndrome Green-top Guideline No. 5. [online] Available from https://www.rcog.org.uk/globalassets/documents/guidelines/green-top-guidelines/gtg_5_ohss.pdf. [Last accessed February, 2020].
15. Metformin Therapy for the Management of Infertility in Women with Polycystic Ovary Syndrome. BJOG. 2017;124(12):e306-13.
16. Mayo Clinic. (2019). Metformin (Oral Route) Side Effects. [online] Available from https://www.mayoclinic.org/drugs-supplements/metformin-oral-route/side-effects/drg-20067074?p=1. [Last accessed February, 2020].
17. Madani T, Ahmadi F, Jahangiri N, Bahmanabadi A, Lankarani NB. Does low-dose aspirin improve pregnancy rate in women undergoing frozen-thawed embryo transfer cycle? A pilot double-blind, randomized placebo-controlled trial. J Obstet Gynecol Res. 2018;45(1):156-63.
18. Webmd. (2019). Drugs and Medications: Aspirin. [online] Available from https://www.webmd.com/drugs/2/drug-1082-3/aspirin-oral/aspirin-oral/details. [Last accessed February, 2020].
19. Webmd. (2019). Progesterone: Uses, Side Effects, Interactions, Dosage, and Warning. [online] Available from https://www.webmd.com/vitamins/ai/ingredientmono-760/progesterone. [Last accessed February, 2020].
20. Medscape. (2006). Hypotensive Potential of Sildenafil and Tamsulosin During Orthostasis. [online] Available from https://www.medscape.com/viewarticle/546917. [Last accessed February, 2020].
21. Webmd. (2019). Drugs and Medications: Estradiol. [online] Available from https://www.webmd.com/drugs/2/drug-5186/estradiol-oral/details. [Last accessed February, 2020].
22. Mayo Clinic. (2019). In vitro fertilization (IVF). [online] Available from https://www.mayoclinic.org/tests-procedures/in-vitro-fertilization/about/pac-20384716. [Last accessed February, 2020].
23. Tarneja P, Tarneja V, Duggal B. Complications of Hysteroscopic Surgery. Med J Armed Forces India. 2002;58(4):331-4.
24. Baghianimoghadam MH, Aminian AH, Baghianimoghadam B, Ghasemi N, Abdoli AM, Ardakani SN, et al. Mental health status of infertile couples based on treatment outcome. Iran J Reprod Med. 2013;11(6):503-10.
25. MGH Center for Women's Mental Health. (2018). Fertility and Mental Health—MGH—CWMH. [online] Available from https://womensmentalhealth.org/specialty-clinics/infertility-and-mental-health/. [Last accessed February, 2020].
26. Patel A, Sharma PVN, Kumar P. Role of mental health practitioner in infertility clinics: A review on past, present and future directions. J Hum Reprod Sci. 2018;11(3):219-28.

# CHAPTER 11

# Dental Health in Women

*Ena Sharma, Amit Lakhani, Savita Kapila, Divya Arora*

## ABSTRACT

Oral health concerns of women are unique and fluctuations in endocrinal profile further lead on to special oral requirements in women. Changes in gums and the oral cavity are noticeable during puberty, menstruation, pregnancy, and menopause. The need of oral hygiene instructions should be emphasized to every women undergoing above changes. Further presence of diabetes and other eating disorders increase the probability of oral infections and tooth decay. Regular brushing, flossing, and timely dentist visits are an important part to avoid complications. Special care should be ensued in rural areas with limited facilities.

## INTRODUCTION

Women have unique oral health concerns at different levels of life leading to a point of special oral health requirements during every unique phase of life. Hormones are the basic unit indicating the health changes and there is fluctuation in the hormone level changes seen in the body. Hormones such as estrogen, progesterone, and testosterone steroid hormones have profound effect on the oral cavity and its apparatus and have been linked with pathogenesis of various gum diseases.

Fluctuation in steroid sex hormones is seen throughout the women's menstrual cycle. Various changes include:
- Increase in gingival inflammation and discomfort, most commonly around the menses time.
- Ovulation can induce swelling of gums with redness and increased chance of bleeding.

## ORAL CONTRACEPTIVE PILLS AND THEIR EFFECT ON ORAL HEALTH

Women taking oral contraceptives have a higher risk of inhabiting organisms such as *Bacteroides* species in the oral cavity. These pills lead to changes in amount and nature of saliva which may cause gingivitis, periodontitis, and dental caries.

**SECTION 10:** Miscellaneous

## CHANGES SEEN IN PREGNANCY

Pregnancy does not cause gingivitis, but may aggravate pre-existing disease. The most marked changes are seen in gingival vasculature. Gingiva is dark red, swollen, smooth, and bleeds easily. Women with pregnancy gingivitis may sometimes develop localized gingival enlargements.

## CHANGES RELATED TO MENOPAUSE

With menopause, the withdrawal of estrogen can lead to several oral pathologies which include increased dental pain and dry mouth with gingivitis and mouth ulcers.

## PUBERTY-RELATED DENTAL ISSUES

- Increased level of progesterone leads to puberty-associated gingivitis characterized by swollen and bleeding gums.
- These soft tissue changes are transient and revert back to normal.
- Higher population of bacteria in subgingival pocket is present during puberty which may selectively accumulate estradiol and progesterone.

## SYSTEMIC DENTISTRY

Oral cavity health can be a pointer of many systemic issues such as:
- *Eating disorders*: With eating disorders leading to purging, vomiting, and regurgitation of acid into the oral cavity, tooth decay is very common.
- *Diabetes mellitus (DM)*: Women with DM are at a higher risk of dry mouth and gingival diseases. Tooth decay and infections are also more common with delayed healing in these patients.
- *Oral cancer*: Gingival cancer in women has a high correlation with high blood glucose levels. Both estrogen deficiency and elevated fasting glucose are being studied as possible risk factors for oral cancer in postmenopausal women.

## CONCLUSION

Since there are many hormonal fluctuations in every phase of a women's life, special care should be taken of the oral hygiene at every phase. Oral hygiene instructions should be emphasized to every women going through the changes. Extra emphasis should be made for women in the rural areas as provision and access to amenities are restricted and the people are not aware about the conditions and their consequences in the oral cavity. Thus, they should be made aware and made to practice good oral hygiene habits so that they can lead a healthy life.

## SUGGESTED READING

1. Mariotti A. Sex steroid hormones and cell dynamics in the periodontium. Crit Rev Oral Biol Med. 1994;5:27-53.
2. Machtei EE, Mahler D, Sanduri H, Peled M. The effect of menstrual cycle on periodontal health. J Periodontol. 2004;75:408-12.

3. Jensen J, Liljemark W, Bloomquist C. The Effect of Female Sex Hormones on Subgingival Plaque. J Periodontol. 1981;52:599-602.
4. Thomas Ek, Chitra N. Periodontal changes pertaining to women from puberty to post-menopausal stage. Int J Pharma Bio Sci. 2013;4:766-71.
5. Suri V, Suri V. Menopause and oral health. J Midlife Health. 2014;5:115-20.
6. Friedlander AH. The physiology, medical management and oral implications of menopause. J Am Dent Assoc. 2002;133:73-81.
7. Cao M, Shu L, Li J, Su J, Zhang W, Wang Q, et al. The expression of estrogen receptors and the effects of estrogen on human periodontal ligament cells. Methods Find Exp Clin Pharmacol. 2007;29:329-35.
8. Kisely S, Baghale H, Lalloo R, Johnson NW. Association between poor oral health and eating disorders: systematic review and meta-analysis. Br J Psychiatry. 2015;207:299-305.
9. Suba Z. Gender-related hormonal risk factors for oral cancer. Pathol Oncol Res. 2007;13:195-20.

# CHAPTER 12

# Women and Transfusion Medicine

*Kusum Thakur*

## ABSTRACT

There is a paucity of gender studies in the transfusion medicine. This is true regarding effect of gender on motivating potential donors, the selection of donors, and promotion of repeat donations, whether blood components collected from a man or a woman may have different effects on recipients and women as recipients' of blood/components. Blood can be taken from healthy donors in the age range of 18–65 years, weight >45 kg, and hemoglobin ≥12.5 g% for providing safe blood/component to the needy patients. So, ideally from men and women should contribute equally. Recently, the World Health Organization (WHO) data about the gender profile of blood donors shows that globally 32% of women are blood donors but with wide range and in 14 of the 119 reporting countries, <10% of women are blood donors. Another study in India shows that only 3.1% women are blood donors. Women are more eager to donate blood than men despite their limitations as they have 21% deferral rate as compared to men (6%) because of anemia. According to another study, men had more mortality and morbidity when given blood donated by women in reproductive age group. Women are most common recipients of blood/components due to anemia, abortions, pregnancy, labor, and their complications. To conclude, women in transfusion medicine are less energetic than men, so efforts should be made to make them eligible for blood donation by minimizing anemia prevalent in women which will further reduce need for blood transfusion during pregnancy, labor, and postpartum period and women in reproductive age group should not be encouraged to donate blood.

## INTRODUCTION

Gender medicine which comprises diversity in biological sex impacts on health and disease, many branches have tried to apply this concept to strictly biomedical fields (biology, genetics, internal medicine, cardiology, pharmacology, endocrinology, nephrology, orthopedics, epidemiology, gynecology, psychiatry, and psychotherapy). There are very few gender studies in the field of transfusion medicine which involves effect of gender on motivating a potential donor, the selection of donor, and promotion of repeat donations, whether blood components collected from a man or a woman may have different effects on recipients and women as recipients' of blood/components.

# CHAPTER 12: Women and Transfusion Medicine

Recent, the World Health Organization (WHO) data shows that globally 32% women are blood donors, although this ranges widely and 14 of the 119 reporting countries report lower than 10% of female donors. Another study in India shows that only 3.1% women are blood donors. Women are more eager to donate blood than men despite their limitations as they have 21% deferral rate as compared to men (6%) because of anemia. According to another study, men had more mortality and morbidity when given blood donated by women in reproductive age group. Women are most common recipients of blood/components due to anemia, abortions, pregnancy, labor, and their complications. Various pregnancy complications and disorders of labor present as risk factors for extra blood loss during pregnancy and due to abortion (spontaneous or induced) and ruptured ectopic pregnancy show up as conditions needing transfusion in the day-to-day practice of obstetrics. Another study shows that patients receiving red cell transfusions donated by women who are ever-pregnant as compared with a male donor were having increased mortality among male recipients but not among female recipients. Transfusions from never-pregnant female donors were not associated with increased mortality among male or female recipients.

## WOMEN AS BLOOD/COMPONENTS DONORS

### World Scenario (Table 1)

In an Italian study, various regions represent about 38% as women donors whereas at National level, it was about 32%. European countries had another picture of women as blood donors. In Spain, 46% of the donors are women, in Portugal 43%, in Belgium 45.4%, in the Netherlands 50%, in Denmark 50%, in France 50%, in the United Kingdom 53%, and in Finland 55%. Greece is the only European country in which the percentage of female donors, 33%, almost similar to that in Italy.

A Nigerian study shows that cultural and religious issues such as women's dependence on men, the erroneous belief that men are healthier than women, that women make monthly blood donations to nature through their menstrual cycle, and other factors such as pregnancy and breastfeeding further restrict many women from

**TABLE 1:** World scenario female blood donors (studies only).

|  | Male donors | Female donors |
|---|---|---|
| World Health Organization (WHO) | 90% | 10% |
| Nigeria | 99.4% | 0.64% |
| Italy | 68% | 32% |
| Spain | 54% | 46% |
| Portugal | 57% | 43% |
| Belgium | 55% | 45% |
| UK | 47% | 53% |
| Finland | 45% | 55% |
| Denmark | 50% | 50% |
| France | 50% | 50% |
| Netherlands | 50% | 50% |
| Greece | 67% | 33% |

**TABLE 2:** Indian scenario female blood donors.

|  | Male donors | Female donors |
|---|---|---|
| Gwalior* | 96.16% | 3.84% |
| Kashmir* | 95.56% | 4.44% |
| Ahmedabad* | 95.48% | 4.52% |
| Hyderabad* | 97.73% | 2.27% |
| Punjab# | 95.50% | 4.50% |
| Haryana# | 96.50% | 3.50% |
| Himachal# | 81.00% | 9.00% |
| Jammu# | 97.66% | 2.34% |
| Delhi# | 90.00% | 10.00% |
| Gujarat# | 96.42% | 3.58% |
| Maharashtra# | 94.42% | 5.58% |
| West Bengal# | 90.00% | 10.00% |

*studies; #State AIDS Prevention and Control Societies (SACS) data

donating blood. The total number of blood donors from January 2010 to July 2013 was 14,965. Donors included 14,871 males (99.4%) and 94 females (0.64%). The number of male donors was significantly higher (p = 0.0001) than that of female donors. A previous report that investigated donor rates in Germany and Switzerland between 1994 and 2010 suggested the need to motivate women to donate blood.

## Indian Scenario (Table 2)

In Gwalior from 2004 to 2014, data collected for all blood were male donors, 97.73% as compared to female donors, 2.27% only. Donation, compiled and analyzed on gender basis which showed male versus female ratio, was found to be 132,470 (96.16%) and 5,297 (3.84%), respectively and it was statistically significant (p < 0.00001) which shows that women contribution in Gwalior, India is lower as compared to women from developed countries so need to educate the females in this regard. In Kashmir, blood donors were majority males (95.56%) as compared to females (4.44%). Ahmadabad study conducted in Western part showed that 95.48% were male donors and 4.52% were females donors.

## WOMEN AS BLOOD/COMPONENTS RECIPIENTS

### Nigeria Study

Blood transfusion is an important part of obstetric care and even lifesaving. Improper blood transfusions for pregnancy and its complications lead to the risk of hemolytic disease of the newborn. If there is obstetric hemorrhage crystalloids and/or colloids with oxygenation given and taking all necessary steps to control bleeding and reduce the need for blood transfusion. The clinical and hematological condition of patient guides about need for transfusion. The recommended to be maintained at 21–24% while in active bleeding, target hematocrit should be 30%. To avoid delusional coagulopathy, concurrent replacement with coagulation factors and platelets may be necessary. Whole blood should be used in acute massive bleeding in case blood components are not available. When the blood group is unknown, O-negative red cells can be given.

## Pune Study

Transfusion of blood/components during pregnancy and labor is required, especially in placental problems like previa, abruption, accreta, retained placenta, in uterine overdistension due to multiple gestations, and polyhydramnios. Other conditions like preeclampsia, disseminated intravascular coagulation, preterm labor, and augmentation of labor and operative delivery vaginal or abdominal also require transfusion of blood/components. The cosmetic transfusion should be avoided. Component usage should be preferred. Clinical judgment should be correlated with hemoglobin (Hb) triggers for transfusion and massive transfusion protocols should be standardized.

The American Association of Blood Banks (AABBs), the Australian National Blood Authority, and the National Blood Transfusion Committee recommend Patient Blood Management (PBM) program which covers England and North Wales. PBM involves all steps to avoid unnecessary transfusion by optimizing preoperative/delivery Hb, using cell salvage where appropriate, accepting lower transfusion triggers, avoiding overtransfusion, and using intravenous (IV) which can have oral iron supplements in women who are not actively bleeding and are cardiovascular stable.

## WOMEN AS ADMINISTRATORS IN TRANSFUSION MEDICINE

Exact data is not available but in India, Director National Blood Transfusion Council (NBTC) and National Blood Cell incharge are women. Almost half of blood centers are headed by women in government as well as in private sectors. As per my knowledge, Government sector departments of transfusion medicine in North India such as PGIMER and GMCH Sector-32 Chandigarh, GMC Patiala, GMC Amritsar, GMC Jammu, GMC Bhopal, KGMC Lucknow, in Government sector and DMC, Ludhiana, SGRD Amritsar, PIMS Jalandhar, MAX Delhi, and MMIMSR Mullana, Haryana are headed by women of National and International repute

## CONCLUSION

Women are less energetic than men as far as transfusion medicine is concerned. Efforts should be made to make them eligible for blood donation by minimizing anemia prevalent in women, which will further reduce need for blood transfusion during pregnancy, labor, and postpartum period. They should not be encouraged to donate blood during reproductive period. Gender bias in society has to be improved to make women equal to men as far as diet is concerned. Women should be made independent by education facilities, jobs reserved so that they are equally participating in blood donation drives as well as donate blood/components and receive least blood components.

## SUGGESTED READING

1. Bani M, Giussani B. Gender differences in giving blood: a review of the literature. Blood Transfus. 2010;8:278-87.
2. World Health Organization (WHO). (2019). Global database on blood safety. [online] Available from https://www.who.int/bloodsafety/global_database/en/. [Last accessed January, 2020].

## SECTION 10: Miscellaneous

3. Chawla S, Bal HK, Vardhan BS, Jose CT, Sahoo I. Blood Transfusion Practices in Obstetrics: Our Experience. J Obstet Gynaecol India. 2018;68:204-7.
4. Sharma R. Psychosocial profiling of blood donors and assessing source of awareness of blood donation through a blood donation camp at a medical college, Ahmadabad, Gujarat. Asian J Transfus Sci. 2011;5:183-4.
5. Edgren G, Murphy EL, Brambilla DJ, Westlake M, Rostgaard K, Lee C, et al. Association of Blood Donor Sex and Prior Pregnancy with Mortality among Red Blood Cell Transfusion Recipients. JAMA. 2019;321:2183-92.
6. Wikipedia. (2019). Federación Española de Donantes de Sangre. [online] Available from https://es.wikipedia.org/wiki/Federaci%C3%B3n_Espa%C3%B1ola_de_Donantes_de_Sangre. [Last accessed January, 2020].
7. Instituto Português do Sangue e da Transplantação. (2008). Annual Report 2008. [online] Available from www.ipsangue.org. [Last accessed January, 2020].
8. Rode Kruis Vlaanderen. (2008). Annual Report Belgian Red Cross. [online] Available from www.rodekruis.be. [Last accessed January, 2020].
9. Sanquin Blood Supply Foundation. (2018). Personal communication: Annual Report 2018. [online] Available from https://www.sanquin.nl/binaries/content/assets/sanquinen/about-sanquin/annual-reports/sanquin_annual_report_2018.pdf. [Last accessed January, 2020].
10. Danish Blood Donor Association. (2019). Introduction. [online] Available from www.bloddonor.dk. [Last accessed January, 2020].
11. Rapport d'activité. (2007). Établissement Français du Sang. [online] Available from www.donnedusang.net. [Last accessed January, 2020].
12. NHS Blood and Transplant. (2007). Introduction. [online] Available from http://www.blood.co.uk. [Last accessed January, 2020].
13. Finland Red Cross. (2008). Annual Report 2008. [online] Available from www.bloodservice.finland. [Last accessed January, 2020].
14. Erhabor O, Isaac Z, Abdulrahaman Y, Ndakotsu M, Ikhuenbor DB, Aghedo F, et al. Female Gender Participation in the Blood Donation Process in Resource Poor Settings: Case Study of Sokoto in North Western Nigeria. J Blood Disorders Transf. 2013;5:176.
15. Tscheulin DK, Lindenmeier J. The willingness to donate blood: an empirical analysis of socio-demographic and motivation-related determinants. Health Serv Manage Res. 2005;18:165-74.
16. Koram SK, Sadula M, Veldurthy VS. Distribution of ABO and Rh-blood Groups in Blood Donors at Tertiary Care Centre. Int J Res Health Sci. 2014;2:326-30.
17. Bala SS, Handoo S, Jallu AS. Gender Differences in Blood Donation among Donors of Kashmir Valley. IOSR J Dent Med Sci. 2015;14:116-9.
18. Patel PA, Patel SP, Shah JV, Oza HV. Frequency and distribution of blood groups in blood donors in Western Ahmedabad—a hospital based study. Nat J Med Res. 2012;2:202-6.
19. Jadon A, Baga R. Blood transfusion practices in obstetric anesthesia. Indian J Anaesth. 2014;58:629-63.
20. Nyfløt LT, Sandven I, Stray-Pedersen B, Pettersen S, Al-Zirqi I, Rosenberg M, et al. Risk factors for severe postpartum hemorrhage: a case-control study. BMC Pregnancy Childbirth. 2017;17:17.
21. Prata N, Hamza S, Bell S, Karasek D, Vahidnia F, Holston M. Inability to predict postpartum hemorrhage: insights from Egyptian intervention data. BMC Pregnancy Childbirth. 2011;11:97.
22. Al-Zirqi I, Vangen S, Forsén L, Stray-Pedersen B. Effects of onset of labor and mode of delivery on severe postpartum hemorrhage. Am J Obstet Gynecol. 2009;201:273.e1-9.
23. Vachhani JH, Joshi JR, Bhanvadia VM. Rational use of blood: a study report on single unit transfusion. Indian J Hematol Blood Transfus. 2008;24:69-71.
24. Carson JL, Carless PA, Hebert PC. Transfusion thresholds and other strategies for guiding allogeneic red blood cell transfusion. Cochrane Database Syst Rev. 2010;10:CD002042.
25. Carson JL, Hill S, Carless P, Hébert P, Henry D. Transfusion triggers: a systematic review of the literature. Transfus Med Rev. 2002;16:187-99.
26. Goodnough LT, Shander A. Patient blood management. Anesthesiology. 2012;116:1367-76.

# CHAPTER 13

# Challenges for Lady Physicians in India

*Roopali Khanna, Vinita Mani Daniel*

## ABSTRACT

Gender disparity in medical education is well-known with very low numbers of females in field of medicine. Those who make a bold choice of entering the field of medicine the road ahead them is full of challenges. Even when one gets an opportunity to enter the field of male dominated branch, the female physician is subtly but surely excluded from the male bastions!! Considered as a weaker sex, the females are not given important responsibilities in their field of work. The exposure and opportunities for skill development for a female physician are less. Lady physicians have to face biases at work from their superiors as well. This is more pronounced in surgical or interventional fields, where the more complicated and challenging procedures. The key obstacles facing female physicians are lack of equal career opportunities and balancing family responsibilities. Women are also underrepresented in areas like conferences, leadership positions, journal editorial board, and speaker invitations compared with their male peers. To overcome these challenges, one has to change the mindset at the basic grassroot level which should also include change in the perspective of the society as a whole. Senior female physicians who have been role models should come forward and discuss the challenges faced by them and how they overcame these difficulties, rather than shying away or living in the denial of gender discrepancies. To attract and retain more women into the field of medicine, the medical community, including professional society leaders must all work to overcome these barriers.

## INTRODUCTION

Gender disparity in medical education in India is well-known. Women account for a third of all admissions to MBBS (undergraduate level) declining to 15–20% of admissions to MD (postgraduate course) internal medicine. This proportion further decreases to ~8% in the subspecialty branches. The scenario is not much different in developed world. In the USA, there have been underrepresentation of women in all medical fields, with the discrepancy being most evident in the surgical and procedural subspecialties. There has been decrease in the gap between male and female ratio over the years. According to the data in 1975, only 20% of medical students in the USA were women, whereas this number reached 50% in 2005 and has held steady since then. A survey by the UN Educational, Scientific and Cultural Organization's Women in Science data shows that <30% of the world's researchers are women. In medicine, imbalances in specialist training participation persist, with very few women opting for surgical specialties.

## CHALLENGES

Reasons for the underrepresentation of women in field of medicine are many and multilayered and reflect sociocultural influences and perceived gender roles. India being a patriarchal society, a woman's primary responsibility is toward tending the family and bearing and rearing children. Average age at marriage of female in India is 22 years. Consequently, most women tend to get married just after graduation. The predominant responsibility for childcare is still borne by women and the issue of balancing career and family seems to be of paramount importance for women. In many families, higher education is discouraged as many believe it causes delay in parenthood. Even those opting for postgraduation, prefer disciplines that are less demanding on time and require less interaction with males. Female physician opting for clinical disciplines prefer subjects such as Obstetrics and Gynecology and Pediatrics where the interaction is mostly with women clients. Surgical specialties continue to be chosen three times more frequently by men than by women doctors.

Even when one gets an opportunity to enter the field of male dominated branch, the female physician is subtly but surely excluded from the male bastions!! Considered as a weaker sex, the females are not given important responsibilities in their field of work. The exposure and opportunities for skill development for a female physician are less. The perception that women abstain from work during childbearing age leads to restrict the job opportunities. Lady physicians have to face biases at work from their superiors as well. This is more pronounced in surgical or interventional fields, where the more complicated and challenging procedures are preferably given to males rather than to females who are considered the weaker sex. Men who are junior often find it difficult to take orders from women, making work unpleasant and difficult. A survey of 30 Indian female cardiologists undertaken by me revealed that 88% believed they faced discrimination at work owing to their gender, but interestingly only 16% of them faced barriers at the patient level, highlighting the fact that patients seek only a competent and efficient doctor irrespective of the gender. In super specialty training, there are only a handful of women in institutes and often women find themselves one among many men in a department. This often leaves them feeling lonely and wanting for friends, leading frequently to sadness and depression.

The hard work of female physician is also not duly regarded. Data has shown that females are usually underpaid and this is seen across all the specialties. This gender pay gaps are not wholly explained by seniority, career breaks, and part-time work.

Another interesting observation is that the representation of females in different national organizations and societies of medicine is either very low or absent. Although the proportion of women in medicine is low, they are not represented in different societies in country in the same proportion. The national organizations have had very few or no female representatives on their executive boards. The number of female speakers is also less, even when adjusted for their low number in medicine itself.

Differences in work and opportunities, hierarchical and institutional support, lack of female mentor models, and institutional gender bias may contribute to the slow career progression and limited visibility of medical women with respect to their male colleagues. Due to underrepresentation of women in senior positions, it leads to less likely participation in decision-making processes. Their individual and collective opinions are usually ignored. In absence of women role models in medicine, young women will not be motivated to achieve top careers.

**Gender inequality: Why it is important?**
Female gender equality in medicine is not only about feminism, but it also has impact on the outcome of the patients. A gender diverse medical workforce translates into improved patient outcomes. A recent study by Greenwood et al. showed both male and female patients, treated by female physicians, experienced similar outcomes whereas, among those treated by male physicians, female patients had poorer outcome as compared to male patients. This study investigating mortality of female patients with acute myocardial infarction found higher mortality in women treated by male doctors than in those treated by female doctors. The effect was attenuated if male doctors had higher exposure to female patients and physician colleagues. Dahrouge S et al. conducted a study to investigate the relationship between family physician gender and quality of primary care. It showed that there were better patient outcomes under the care of female physicians. The reason given by authors for this observation was pointing to evidence that female doctors tend to follow guidelines more closely, spend more time with patients, and might have more effective communication skills than male doctors.

**How to overcome these challenges?**
It is important to change the mindset at the basic grassroot level which should also include change in the perspective of the society as a whole. Barriers erected by the society and inner barriers created by our mind should be broken. Senior female physicians who have been role models should come forward and discuss the challenges faced by them and how they overcame these difficulties, rather than shying away or living in the denial of gender discrepancies. There should be more female faces at different national level organization not only as speakers but also as members of the executive bodies. Conferences should have stand-alone women-oriented sessions which would encourage the younger female generation to come forward in the field of cardiology. Opinion leaders of leading national medical societies should actively come forward in response to these issues and help tackle them to maintain a gender equipoise in this field. Along with political and government initiatives to advance the position of women in medicine, the strategies to address gender inequality must be discussed by the institution. Seniors and colleagues should facilitate the working environment for the female physician. There should be provision of support during and on return from maternity leave, and finally, encouraging women to apply for appointments and promotions.

## CONCLUSION

There are many challenges a lady physician faces, but societal change can be achieved through a series of small steps made by individuals and institutions in pursuit of a better world. To utilize the full potential of the women physicians, there should be continuing efforts to improve the ways in which they are trained and mentored. Achieving gender equality is not simply instrumental for health and development, its impact has wide-ranging benefits and is a matter of fairness and social justice for everyone.

**SECTION 10:** Miscellaneous

# SUGGESTED READING

1. Current trends in medical education—AAMC diversity facts and figures 2016. Washington: Association of American Medical Colleges; 2016.
2. UN Educational, Scientific and Cultural Organization. (2018). Women in science. [online] Available from http://uis.unesco.org/en/topic/women-science. [Last accessed January, 2020].
3. Australian Institute of Health and Welfare. Medical Practitioners Workforce 2015. Canberra: Australian Institute of Health and Welfare; 2015.
4. Ministry of Statistics and Programme Implementation. (2016). Women and Men in India-2016. [online] Available from http://mospi.nic.in/publication/women-and-men-india-2016. [Last accessed January, 2020].
5. Kesavarapu K, Schwartz J, Ikonomi E, Ahmad A. What's holding women back? A review of gender inequality in gastroenterology in the USA. Lancet Gastroenterol Hepatol. 2019;4:898-900.
6. Khanna R. (2019). Taking the Road Less Traveled: A Female Cardiologist in India. [online] Available from https://www.acc.org/membership/sections-and-councils/women-in-cardiology-section/section-updates/2019/04/17/14/22/taking-the-road-less-traveled. [Last accessed January, 2020].
7. Connolly S, Holdcroft A. The pay gap for women in medicine and academic medicine: an analysis of the WAM* database. London: British Medical Association; 2009.
8. Greenwood N, Carnahan S, Huang L. Patient-physician gender concordance and increased mortality among female heart attack patients. Proc Natl Acad Sci USA. 2018;115:8569-74.
9. Dahrouge S, Seale E, Hogg W, Russell G, Younger J, Muggah E, et al. A comprehensive assessment of family physician gender and quality of care: a cross-sectional analysis in Ontario, Canada. Med Care. 2016;54:277-86.
10. Elta GH. The challenges of being a female gastroenterologist. Gastroenterol Clin North Am. 2011;40:441-7.
11. Arrizabalaga P, Abellana R, Vinas O, Merino A, Ascaso C. Gender inequalities in the medical profession: are there still barriers to women physicians in the 21st century? Gac Sanit. 2014;28:363-8.

# INDEX

Page numbers followed by *b* refer to box, *f* refer to figure, *fc* refer to flow chart, and *t* refer to table.

## A

Abortion
  incomplete 332
  missed 332
  unsafe 408
Abortive treatment plan 84
Abscesses 335
Abstinence 407
Acanthosis nigricans 119
Acetaminophen 190, 191*t*
*Acinetobacter* 221
Acne 119, 396
  diagnosis 397
  presentation 396
  prognosis 398
  treatment 397
  vulgaris 397*f*
Acquired immunodeficiency syndrome 327, 408
Acquired nasolacrimal duct obstruction, primary 359
Activated partial thromboplastin time 234
Active estrogen metabolites 374
Acute coronary syndrome 26, 32, 42, 43, 50
  non-ST segment elevation of 50
Acute fatty liver 230, 231, 233, 234, 238, 295
  diagnosis of 234*t*
Acute hepatic necrosis, drug-induced 245
Acute kidney injury 285, 291, 295
  diagnosis of 292
  network 292
Adalimumab 287
Adapalene 397
Adenocarcinoma 241
  esophageal 214
Adenoid cystic carcinoma 359
Adenomas, adrenal
  benign 142
Adenomyosis 131
Adenosine
  A1-agonists, partial 44

monophosphate, propionate activates 222
Adipogenicity 221
Adiposity, abdominal 26
Adnexa 358
  disorders of 358
Adnexal torsion 417
Adolescent education programme 407, 411
Adolescent Friendly Health Clinics 412
Adolescent girls
  medical ailments in 402
  sex education of 407
Adolescent Life Skill Training Program 412
Adrenal hyperplasia, nonclassic congenital 122, 142
Adrenocortical axis 142
Advanced disease, locally 255
Age-related macular degeneration 357
Airway 169
*Akkermansia muciniphila* 222
Alanine aminotransferase 234, 275, 277, 294
Alcohol 40
  consumption, moderate 26
  dehydrogenase 239
Aldosterone antagonist 124
Alemtuzumab 200
Alkaline phosphatase 231
Allopregnanolone 388
Alopecia 119, 398
  areata 398, 399
  diagnosis 399
  presentation 398
  prognosis 399
  treatments for 399, 399*t*
Alzheimer's disease 142
Amaurosis fugax 207
Amblyopia 363
Amebiasis 335
Amenorrhea
  functional hypothalamic 22
  hypothalamic 122

American Association of Blood Banks 429
American College of Cardiology 139
American College of Obstetricians and Gynecologists 127
American College of Rheumatology 148, 282
  Criteria 283
American Congress of Obstetrics and Gynecology 257
American Heart Association 19, 39, 139
American Society of Reproductive Medicine 118, 121
American Thyroid Association 108, 141
Amino-3-hydroxy-5-methyl-4-isoxazolepropionic acid 202
Aminoglycosides 304
Amiodarone 43, 103, 395
Amitriptyline 191
Amlodipine 27
Ammonia, high 234
Amniotic fluid embolism 319
Anakinra 287
Androgen 388
  excess society 118
  receptor 132
  secreting tumor 122
Anemia 21, 40, 42, 53
Anencephaly 93
Angina
  microvascular 33
  stable 50
  symptoms of 32
Angiogram 20
Angiotensin receptor
  blockers 42, 74, 296
  neprilysin inhibitor 42
Angiotensin-converting enzyme 23, 42, 50
  inhibitors 74, 153, 296
Angle closure glaucoma 358
Ankle swelling 38
Anorectal atresia 93

Anorexia nervosa 391
Anovulatory infertility, treating 414
Anthracyclines 256
Antiandrogens 399
Anti-AQP4 antibody, presence of 198
Antiarrhythmic drugs 70
Antibiotics 226, 303
  use of 222
Antibody testing 198
Anticardiolipin 152
Anti-CD20 monoclonal antibody 286
Anti-CD22 antibodies 287
Anticentromere 208
Anti-citrullinated peptide antibodies 157
Anticonvulsants 395
Anticyclic citrullinated peptide 148
Anticytokine therapy 148
Antiepileptic drugs 163, 166, 167, 169
  fetal risk of 167
  hormonal interactions of 166
  management 168
Antigen, prostate-specific 205
Antihypertensive medications 278
Antihypertensive treatment 20
Anti-müllerian hormone 165, 217, 415
Antineuronal nuclear antibody
  type 1 201
  type 2 201
Antineutrophil cytoplasmic antibody-associated vasculitis 205
Antinuclear antibody 283, 374
Antiphospholipid antibody
  role of 157
  syndrome 152, 156, 157, 207, 278, 295
Antiplatelet 50
  therapy 53
Antipsychotics 395
Antiretroviral therapy 327
Antirheumatic drugs, disease-modifying 148, 159
Antisynthetase antibodies 320
Antithrombotic therapy 51
Antithymocyte globulin 308
Antithyroid
  autoantibodies, presence of 104
  peroxidase antibodies 109

Antithyroidal drugs 100, 103
Antitumor necrosis factor-α inhibitors 287
Anxiety 143, 215
  disorders 387, 390
Aorta, coarctation of 71-74, 79, 93
Aortic dilatation 73
Aortic diseases, prevalence of 76
Aortic dissection 81
Aortic root dilatation 79
Aortic stenosis 59, 70-72, 74
  congenital 79
  severe symptomatic 69, 73
Aorto-left ventricular tunnel 8
Aorto-right ventricular tunnel 9
Apgar scores 167
Appendicitis 302
Aquaporin-4, extracellular domain of 196
Aromatase inhibitors 416
Arrhythmia 40, 43, 63, 80
  cardiac 83
  ventricular 72
Arterial thrombosis 207
Arteritis, coronary 156
Artery
  brachial 159
  disease, peripheral 25
Arthralgias 208
Arthritis, inflammatory 151
Artificial reproductive techniques 415
Ascites 233, 234
Aspartate aminotransferase 231, 234, 235, 275, 277
Aspergillosis, chronic pulmonary 350
Aspiration, manual vacuum 332
Aspirin 23, 25, 50, 53, 418
  high dose 191
  low dose 191
Assisted reproductive techniques 419
Asthma 313
  bronchial 313, 321
  treatment of 322
Astigmatism 363
Atenolol 191
Atherogenesis 157
Atherosclerosis 19, 20, 32
  accelerated 156
  multi-ethnic study of 20
Atherosclerotic diseases 17
Atopic eruption 399, 400
Atorvastatin 27
Atresia 71

Atrial appendage, left 58
Atrial fibrillation 20, 40, 42, 57, 80
Atrial flutter 80
Atrial septal defect 56, 71, 72, 93, 74
Atrioventricular valve regurgitation 74
Attack
  acute 190
  prevention 198, 200
Atypical hemolytic uremic syndrome 293
Australian National Blood Authority 429
Autoantibody 156
Autoimmune
  disease 31, 103, 155, 158, 160, 313, 360, 368, 375
  disorders 196, 206
  inflammatory 373
  encephalitis 169, 201, 201*t*, 202, 202*t*, 203*b*, 205*b*
  diagnosis of 203
  treatment of 204
  encephalopathies 195
  etiology 373
  inflammatory disorder 359
  systemic diseases 362
  uveitides, revalence of 374
Autonomic tone 216
Auxiliary nurse midwife 412
Azathioprine 209, 217, 247, 308

# B

Bacterial translocation 222
Bacteriuria, asymptomatic 337
*Bacteroides* 224, 423
Bad adipose tissue 221
Balanitis 302
Balloon mitral valvuloplasty 66
  management with 66
Balloon valvotomy 80
Bariatric surgery 227
Barrett's esophagus 214
Basal cell carcinoma 359
Basal hormonal profile 415
Basiliximab 308
B-cell 373
  targeted therapies 286
Belatacept 308
Bell's palsy 384
Benzathine penicillin 329
Beta-blockers 43, 50, 191
Beta-lactams 304
Bethanechol 304
Bevacizumab 260

# Index

*Bifidobacterium* 224, 225
Bile acid binder 233
Biliary cirrhosis, primary 239, 240, 245
Biliary diseases 231
Bilirubin, high 234
Binge eating disorder 391
Biochemistry 301
Biopsy, endomyocardial 42
Bipolar disorder 387
Birdshot chorioretinopathy 375
Birth
 anomaly 93
 control 126
 defects
  congenital 94
  risk of 93
 injury 94
Bitot's spots 360
Bivalirudin 51
Bladder 296
 relaxant agents 303
 ultrasonography of 302
Blindness 277, 358, 373
 causes of 363
 incidence of 357
Blood
 culture 335
 donors 426, 427, 427t
 film, peripheral 335
 glucose 41, 335
 pressure 13, 65, 128, 130, 273
  diastolic 26
  systolic 18, 19, 26, 293
 recipients 428
 smear, peripheral 235
 transfusion 428
 volume 65
B-lymphocyte
 stimulator blockers 287
 tolerogens 287
Body
 growth of 402
 mass index 20, 82, 120, 130, 225, 415
Bone
 health 129, 218
 mineral density 129, 139
Botulinum toxin 183
Bouchard's nodes 149
Bowel
 disease, inflammatory 213, 216
 syndrome, irritable 213, 215
Brachytherapy 257
Brain
 infarction, hypoperfusion-induced 206
 magnetic resonance imaging of 203f, 204f
 natriuretic peptide, measurement of 42
Brainstem 83
Breast 31
 calcification 21
 cancer 22, 31, 133, 253-255, 262
  diagnosis of 254
  risk of 131
  screening for 254
  surgery in 254
  syndrome, hereditary 258
 conservative surgery 255
 development of 402
Breastfeeding 307, 353, 389
Breath, shortness of 57, 69
Breathing 169
Breathlessness 38, 41
Bronchiectasis 350
B-type natriuretic peptide 79
Budd–Chiari syndrome 231, 245
Bulimia nervosa 391

## C

Cabergoline 417
Cadmium 315
Caffeine 191
Calcinosis cutis 208
Calcitonin gene-related peptide 188
Canadian Angiographic Study 31
Cancer 253
 adrenocortical 142
 early stage 258
 endometrial 117, 122, 132, 261, 262
 gingival 424
 gynecological 253, 262
 therapy 264
Candesartan 191
Candidiasis 300
Carbamazepine 166, 167
Carbapenams 304
Carbidopa 181
Carbon
 monoxide 315
 particles 315
Carboxymethyl cellulose 371
Carcinoma
 endometrial 114
 hepatocellular 238, 239, 241, 244
Cardiac disease 64
Cardiac lesions, congenital 70
Cardiac pathology, pre-existing 64
Cardiac resynchronization therapy 42
Cardiac shunts 69, 76
Cardiac surgery 66, 79
Cardiac tamponade 42
Cardiology 1
 beginning of 3
 development of 3
 pioneers in 4
Cardiometabolic risk factors 114
Cardiomyopathy 39, 80
 end-stage 42
 hypertrophic 33, 40
 idiopathic 40
 peripartum 22, 38, 40, 80, 81
 restrictive 40
Cardiovascular disease 13, 16, 17, 31, 36, 49, 56, 69, 76, 78, 82, 94, 114, 120, 128, 130, 136, 138, 155, 158, 316
 atherosclerotic 20, 158
 prevention 22
  primary 25
 primary prevention of 22, 23
Cardiovascular health 128, 138
Cardiovascular illnesses
 prevention of 70
 treatment of 70
Cardiovascular risk 117, 122
 assessment 13, 158
 factors 44
 management of 159
Carotid intima medial thickness 156, 159
Cataract 363
 blind 358
 congenital 363
 formation 363
Catch-up vaccines 343
Catechol-O-methyltransferase 181
Catheter-based interventions, journey of 10
Caudal regression syndrome 93
Centers for Disease Control and Prevention 73
Central nervous system 93, 169, 199, 286
 dysfunction of 276
 symptoms of 276
Cephalosporins 384
Cerebellar ataxia 207
Cerebral
 artery, middle 83
 venous thrombosis 169, 177

Cerebrospinal fluid 197, 199, 204
 analysis 197
 spontaneous 380
Cerebrovascular disorders 173
Certolizumab pegol 287
Cervical
 cancer 133, 256, 257, 329, 330
 cytology and screening 415
 intraepithelial neoplasia, risk of 330
Cesarean section 94
 hemodynamic effects of 65
Cetuximab 260
Chemical peels like lactic acid 396
Chemokines 371
Chemotherapy 257, 258, 260, 262, 264-266
 lesser effect of 265
Chest
 pain 32
 X-ray 42, 79, 323
*Chlamydia trachomatis* 341
Chlamydial infections 341
Chlorinated dioxins 315
Chlormadinone acetate 131
Cholelithiasis 231
Cholestasis 239
 infantile 234
 intrahepatic 230-233, 400
Cholesterol 15, 22
 lower total 156
Cholestyramine 233
Cholinergic drugs 304
Chorea 207
Chorioretinopathy, central serous 364
Choroid 374
Choroidal lesions 375
Choroidal neovascular membranes 376
Chronic inflammatory
 diseases 148
 disorders 368
Chronic obstructive pulmonary disease 313, 322
Churg–Strauss syndrome 362
Chylocorporrhea 318
Chylopericardium 318
Chyloperitoneum 318
Chylothorax 318
Chyluria 318
Ciliary body 373
Circulation 169
Cirrhosis 231, 239
 autoimmune linked 245
 cryptogenic 245

Cisplatin 257
Cladribine 200
Cleft
 lip 93
 palate 93
Clindamycin 384
Clinically isolated syndrome 197, 199
Clobazam 166
Clomiphene citrate 416
Clonazepam 166, 167
Clonus 277
*Clostridium difficile* 227
Clubfoot 93
Coagulation, tests of 277
Coarctation of aorta, severe 69
Cocaine 40
Codeine 191
Collagen vascular disease 40
Collapsin response mediator protein 5 201
Colony-forming units 226
Combined oral contraceptives 127, 267
 mechanism of action of 132*fc*
Compared menopausal hormone therapy 138
Complete blood count 41, 301
Comprehensive sexuality education 407
 content of 409, 411
 delivery forms of 410
 effectiveness of 410
Computed tomography
 cardiac 42
 contrast-enhanced 122
 guided image-based planning 255
Congenital heart block, complete 152
Congenital heart disease 9, 69, 71, 74, 81
 acyanotic 79
 birth prevalence of 70
 cyanotic 79
 prevalence of common 71*t*
Congestion, capillary 314
Conjunctiva 360, 370
 diseases of 358
 disorders of 359
 malignant lesion of 360
Conjunctival impression 370
Conjunctival nevi, benign 360
Connective tissue disease 313, 319, 335
 treatment of 151
Connective tissue disorders 209

Contact immunotherapy 399
Contactin-associated protein 2 202
Contraception 126, 166, 264, 266, 307, 332, 407
 devices, intrauterine 267
 estrogen-containing 267
 hormonal 133, 320
 method of 126
Contraceptive 332, 410
 estrogen-containing 320
 hormonal 126, 130*t*
 methods 320
 progesterone based 333
 types of 126*fc*
Copper chelation 184
Cornea
 diseases of 358
 disorders of 361
Corneal ablative procedures 368
Corneal dystrophies 362*f*
Corneal sensations 370
Coronary angiogram 35, 62*f*
Coronary angiography 42, 51
Coronary artery 51, 83
 bypass graft surgery 36
 calcification 20
 calcium 20
 disease 14, 32, 33, 34*fc*, 35*t*, 69, 70, 80, 120, 221
 management of 49, 50
 microvascular 36
 prevention of 19
 dissection, spontaneous 33, 50, 52, 52*f*, 81
 left main 51
 revascularization 26
 right 51
 risk development 20
 wall thickness 21
Coronary calcium
 evaluation of 20
 score 21
Coronary computed tomography angiography 35
Coronary flow reserve 159
Coronary syndromes 80
Coronary vasomotor disorders 31
Corticosteroids 308, 371
 intralesional 399
Corticotropin-releasing hormone 91, 388
Cortisol 388
*Corynebacterium xerosis* 360
Council of Boards of School Education 411

# Index

C-reactive protein 156, 417
  highly sensitive 19, 159
Crohn's diseas 216
Cryoglobulinemia 148, 205
Cryopreservation 266
Crystalline lens 363
Cushing's syndrome 122, 142
Cyclophosphamide 151
Cycloserine 352
Cyclosporine 308
Cyproterone acetate 131, 399
Cystadenoma, biliary 241
Cystic degeneration 360$f$
Cystitis, interstitial 302
Cytochrome 232
Cytokine inhibition 287
Cytomegalovirus 337, 339
Cytotoxic T-lymphocyte
  antigen-4 287

## D

Darifenacin 303
Data Collection and Monitoring
  System 353
de Quervain's thyroiditis 103
Death rate 31
Decarboxylase inhibitor,
  peripheral 181
Deep brain stimulation 182
Deep vein thrombosis, high-risk
  of 140
Dehydroepiandrosterone sulfate
  116, 122, 141, 397
Delirium 207
Dementia 391
Dengue 344
Dental
  health 423
  issues, puberty-related 424
Depression 117, 142, 215, 403, 421
  cortical spreading 188
  measures of 143
Depressive disorder 390
  contribution of 390
Depressive symptoms 391
Deprivation 20
Dermatomyositis 208, 319
*Desulfovibrio* 224
Device therapy 43
Dexamethasone 233
Dextran 371
  sulfate apheresis 294
Dextrocardia 93
Diabetes 13, 22, 89, 90, 90$t$
  mellitus 20, 22, 40, 50, 78, 80, 138, 157, 240, 301, 424

management of type 2 25
pre-existing 89
pregestational 278
risk of 114
type 1 15, 91
type 2 98, 122, 137, 221
  pregestational 93$t$
  study cardiac risk score 20
Diclofenac 191
Dienogest 131
Diet 225
  high-carbohydrate 222
  high-fat 222
  high-fiber 222
Dietary
  changes 96, 225
  fibers 222
  strategies 224
Dimethyl fumarate 200
Dipeptidyl peptidase-like
  protein 6 202
Diphtheria 343
Dipstick test 274
Director National Blood
  Transfusion Council 429
Disability adjusted life years 387
Disease-specific risk factors 156
Disseminated intravascular
  coagulation 236, 277, 294
Diverticulitis 302
Dizziness 381
Donors
  motivating potential 426
  selection of 426
Dopamine dysregulation
  syndrome 182
Dopa-responsive dystonia 183
Double outlet right ventricle 71
Double vessel disease 51
Double-stranded
  deoxyribonucleic acid 283
  genome 328
Doxylamine 232
Drospirenone 131
Drug 43, 227
  abuse 142
  fever 335
  use 142
Dry eye 366, 368
  deficient 367
  disease 362, 366, 367
    development of 368
    diagnosis of 370
    evaporative 367, 370
    higher propensity of 367
    holistic treatment of 372
    incidence of 367

management of 370, 371
mild-to-moderate 370
moderate-to-severe 370
pathophysiology of 367, 370
perimenopausal 367
preservative with 371
prevalence of 367
risk of developing 368
symptoms of 367, 368, 371
pregnancy related 364
related quality-of-life score 368
subtypes of 367
symptoms 369$f$
Dual antiplatelet therapy 52
Dual-energy X-ray 218
  absorptiometry 135, 139
Duodenal atresia 93
Dysbiosis 222
Dyslipidemia 15, 22, 24, 53, 240
Dyspareunia 268, 392
Dysphoric disorder,
  premenstrual 131, 388
Dystonia 181, 183
  common focal 183
  parkinsonism, X-linked 183

## E

Ear
  changes 383
  discharge 379
  diseases 380
  nose, and throat
    disorder 383
  trauma 381
  problems, common 379
Eating disorders 391, 403, 424
  lifetime prevalence of 391
Ebstein's anomaly 71, 80
Echocardiography 42
Eclampsia 31, 44, 53, 78, 81, 231, 234, 277
Ectopia
  lentis 363
  traumatic 363
Eculizumab 287, 293, 294
Edema 41
  peripheral 38
Eisenmenger syndrome 72
Ejection fraction 38
  preserved 43
Electrocardiogram 283
Electrocardiography 42
Electroencephalogram 204
Electrolytes 275
Eletriptan 191

Elevated jugular venous pressure 38
Embryo cryopreservation 265
Emotional support programs, development of 421
Enalapril 26, 74
Encephalocele 93
Encephalopathy 233, 234
Endocarditis 63, 335
  infective 72
Endocrinal profile 423
Endocrine
  changes 136
  disorders 40
Endogenous hormone levels 71
Endometrial cancer
  early stage 261
  risk of 131
Endometriosis 131, 318
Endothelial dysfunction 83, 158
Endothelin receptor antagonists 321
Endovascular dysfunction 82
Endovascular system 82
Entacapone 181
Enzyme-linked immunosorbent assay 283, 328
Epilepsy 163-166, 168, 170, 207
  catamenial 164, 165f
  localization-related 164
Epiphora 359
Episcleritis 360
Epistaxis 379, 384
Epithelial ovarian cancer 258
Eplerenone 42
Ergot derivatives 191
Erythematous papules 397f
Erythrocyte sedimentation rate, high 157
Erythromycin 384
*Escherichia coli* 299
Eslicarbazepine 166
Esophageal acid exposure 214
Esophageal dysmotility 213
Esophageal epithelial barrier function 214
Esophageal motility 214
  disorder, reflux-related 214
Esophageal nociception 214
Esophageal sphincter pressure, lower 214
Estimated glomerular filtration rate 304
Estradiol 138, 389
  limits monoamine oxidase 390
  presence of 314

Estrogen 101, 164, 214, 216, 314, 374, 388, 419
  contains pills 152
  high-dose 126
  in strokes, role of 174
  levels of 374, 388
  low-dose 126
  metabolism 241
  receptor 314
  role of 390
Ethambutol 352
Ethionamide 352
Ethosuximide 166
Eubiosis 222
European League Against Rheumatism 148, 155
European Society of Cardiology 15
European Society of Human Reproduction and Embryology 118
Eustachian tube dysfunction 383
Exercise 225
  electrocardiogram 42
Extensive pulmonary destruction 350
Extracellular antigens 202t
  antibody directed against 201
Extracorporeal membrane oxygenation 319
Extractable nuclear antigen 284
Eye 361f, 362, 370f
  blanches, inflamed 360
  diseases, treating 358
  disorders 358
  dryness, evaluation of 368
  examination survey 357
  health 357
    related conditions 357
  inflammatory disorders of 373
  movement, rapid 181
Eyelids, disorders of 358
Ezogabine 166

**F**

Facet joints 149
Facial
  defects, midline 93
  migraine 188
  pain 379
*Faecalibacterium prausnitzii* 228
Fair sex 45, 69
Family planning 329
Farnesoid X receptor 222, 223, 232
Fasting plasma glucose 90

Fastrointestinal disorders, functional 215
Fatigue 38, 57, 69, 240
Fatty acid
  infiltration of 240
  oxidation inhibitor 44
  short-chain 222
Fatty liver 234
Fecal microbiota transplant 227
Felbamate 166
Female orgasmic disorder 392
Female sexual
  arousal disorder 391
  dysfunction 391, 392
  pain disorders 392
Feminism 433
Fenestrations 318
Ferriman–Gallwey
  scoring system, modified 119f
  syndrome 120
Fertility 151, 217, 264
  management 124
  treatment, principles of 415
Fetal
  circulation, normal 57
  complications 94
  death, intrauterine 233, 294
  growth restriction 277
  thyroid gland 106
  toxicity, potential for 124
Fetus, recurrence in 74t
Fever 334, 335b
  causes of 335t
Fibrinogen 16
Fibromyalgia syndrome 150
Fibrosis, interstitial 285
Finasteride 124, 399
Fingolimod 200
Firmicutes 221
First venous thrombosis, absolute risk of 322f
Fish oil 25
  supplementation 25
Fluid-attenuated inversion recovery 203, 203f, 204, 204f
Fluorodeoxyglucose 204, 205
Fluoroquinolones 304
Flutamide 124, 399
Follicle-stimulating hormone 122, 135, 397, 415, 416
Food and Agriculture Organization 139
Formaldehyde 315
Fracture-risk assessment 140
Framingham Risk Score 13, 18
  interpretation of 14
  limitations of 14

# Index

Fuchs endothelial corneal dystrophy 361
Fundus examination 206
Fungal infections 301, 337

## G

Gabapentin 166, 167
Gallbladder 335
  malignancy 242
Gallstones 238, 239, 242
Gamma-aminobutyric acid 165, 202
Gamma-glutamyltransferase 231
Gas gangrene 335
Gastric acid 213
Gastroesophageal reflux disease 208, 213, 214
Gastrointestinal
  disorders 213, 230, 259
  physiology 213
  system 93
  tract 221
Generalized chronic musculoskeletal pain, causes of 150$t$
Genetic
  hemochromatosis 238, 241
  polymorphism 42
Genital
  graft versus host disease 264, 267
  herpes simplex 329
  host disease, management of 267
Genitourinary system 93
Gestational age
  large for 95
  small for 95
Gestational diabetes mellitus 31, 78, 81, 89, 90$t$
  pathogenesis of 92$f$
  risk of 117
Gestational hypertension 81, 274, 275, 277$b$, 279
  clinical diagnosis of 275
  diagnosis of 275
  transient 274, 275
Giant cell
  arteritis 205, 206
  granulomas 375
Glatiramer acetate 200
Glaucoma 358, 363
  tension 363
  treatment for 363
Glomerular filtration rate, lower 71

Glomerulonephritis 301
Glomerulosclerosis, focal segmental 286
Glucagon-like peptide-1 223
Glucose
  metabolism 127
  regulation 16
Glutamate, interstitial 83
Glycol acid 396
Glycosylated hemoglobin 90, 138, 225
Golimumab 287
Gonadotropic hormones, secretion of 165
Gonadotropin 416
  releasing hormone 115, 265
Gonorrhea 340
Gout 158
Graft
  outcome 309
  size of 246
Granuloma gravidarum 384
Granulomatosis 205
  eosinophilic 205
Granulomatous disorder, chronic 375
Graves' disease 103, 111, 359, 404
  management of 100
Graves' ophthalmopathy 105
Great arteries, transposition of 70, 71
Great vessels, transposition of 93
Growth factor 91
Gut microbiome 220
Gut microbiota 221, 222
  characteristics of 223$fc$
Gynecological malignancy 114
  risk 131

## H

Hair loss, female pattern 398, 399
Hashimoto's thyroiditis 101, 103, 359, 376, 404
Headache 187, 188, 188$t$
  causes of 192
  cluster 187
  disorders 187
  first 188
  new onset 188
  severe 277
  tension type 187
  type of 187
  worsening 188
  worst 188

Health
  assessment questionnaire 152
  problems 402
  status 344
Healthcare
  utilization of 75
  worker 347
Healthy diet 23, 26
Hearing impairment during pregnancy 383
Hearing loss
  age-related 380
  sensorineural 383, 384
Heart
  block, complete 80
  defect, congenital 56, 93
  disease 9, 25, 49, 64, 78
    acquired 63
    coronary 13, 14$t$, 17, 316
    cyanotic 79, 80
    etiology of 64
    ischemic 31, 32, 34, 35, 51, 82
    management of congenital 7
    prevalence of congenital 75
    risk of congenital 74$t$
    type of congenital 71
  failure 24, 38-40, 40$t$, 43-45, 50
    causes of 39, 40
    congestive 40, 57
    diagnosis of 41
    etiology of 40
    management of 43, 44
    medications 38
    pathophysiology of 41
    right 320
    signs of 39$t$, 41
    stages of 39
    symptoms of 39$t$, 41
    types of 38, 39$t$
  physiology of 76
  rate 65
    accelerated 65
  univentricular 72
Heat shock protein–60 159
Hemangioma, cavernous 239
Hematological malignancies 264
Hematology 301
Hematopoietic stem cell 264
  transplant 264
Hemochromatosis 239
Hemodynamic changes 65, 78
Hemoglobin 21, 275, 277

Hemolysis and elevated liver enzymes and low platelets syndrome 94, 230, 231, 235, 235t, 291, 293, 294
  complications of 236
Hemoptysis 350
  catamenial 317
Hemorrhage
  intracerebral 177
  subarachnoid 316
Henoch–Schönlein purpura 205
Heparin, unfractionated 51
Hepatic adenomas, reports of 129
Hepatic disorders 231t, 236
Hepatic failure, fulminant 232
Hepatic glucose production 138
Hepatitis
  A 231, 336, 344
    virus 240
    acute viral 231
    autoimmune 239, 240
  B 231, 344
    chronic 241
    infection 239
    vaccine 344
    virus 240, 336
  C 336
    infection 239
    virus 240
  D 336
    virus 241
  E 231, 336
    virus 240
Hepatobiliary disorders 238
Hepatotoxicity, drug-induced 231
Herpes simplex virus 268, 338, 341, 384
High-density lipoprotein 226
  cholesterol 13
Higher pulmonary artery pressures 72
Highly active antiretroviral therapy 337
High-resolution computed tomography chest 316
Hirsutism 119f
  management of 124
  score 119
Hoarseness 385
Hodgkin's lymphoma 264, 265
*Holdemania* 224
Holoprosencephaly 93
Homeostatic model assessment-insulin resistance 127
Homocystinuria 363

Honeymoon cystitis 299
Hormonal changes 358, 364
Hormonal disorders 364
Hormonal functions 35
Hormonal therapy 137, 265
  impact of 137
Hormone 100
  adrenocorticotropic 122
  replacement 174
    therapy 127, 138, 191, 215, 363, 367, 374
Household air pollution 314, 315
  effect of 315
Human body and development 410
Human chorionic
  gonadotropin 122, 231, 292
  somatotropin 91
Human immunodeficiency virus 267, 327, 347, 349, 349t, 351
  characteristics of 328
  diagnosis 337
  gynecological problems of 328
  infection 336, 408
  perinatal transmission of 336
  related malignancies 329
  related tumors 330
  treatment center for 332
Human leukocyte antigen 232, 306
Human papillomavirus 256, 268, 343, 344
Human placental lactogen 91
Human sexual anatomy 407
Huntington's disease 183
Hyaluronic acid 314, 371
Hydranencephaly 93
Hydrocarbon complexes 315
Hydrochlorothiazide 27
Hydronephrosis 93
Hydroxychloroquine 153
Hydroxyprogesterone 122
Hydroxypropyl methylcellulose 371
Hydroxytryptamine 188
Hyperandrogenism 116, 120, 132fc, 165
  clinical signs of 397
  symptoms of 131
Hyperbilirubinemia, neonatal 94
Hypercholesterolemia 82, 157
Hyperemesis gravidarum 230, 231, 292
Hyperglycemia 94t, 246
  classification of 90, 90fc

management of 95
  pathophysiology of 91
Hyperlipidemia 82, 83
Hypermetabolism, bilateral striatal 204
Hyperplasia 314
  congenital adrenal 131
  endometrial 131
  focal nodular 241
Hyperprolactinemia 122, 165
Hypertension 22, 24, 53, 81-83, 233-235, 240, 273-275, 301, 307
  benign intracranial 364, 380
  chronic 274, 275, 277, 278
  classification of 274, 274b
  control of 24, 278
  development of diastolic 273
  diagnosis of 274
  masked 274
  portal 231
  pregnancy induced 31, 78, 81, 94
  risk factor for 158
Hypertensive disorders 78, 273, 280
  diagnosis of 274
  management for 278
  pregnancy related 276b
Hyperthyroidism 105
  during pregnancy 111t, 112
  management of 100
  mild 292
  per se 100
  severity of 100
  subclinical 141
Hypertriglyceridemia 246
Hypertrophic obstructive cardiomyopathy 59
Hyperuricemia 158
Hypoactive sexual desire disorder 391
Hypocalcemia 94, 234
Hypoglycemia 94, 233, 234
  neonatal 94
  risk of 25
Hypopituitarism 103
Hypoplasia, femoral 93
Hypoplastic left heart syndrome 71
Hypoplastic pelvis, sacral agenesis with 93
Hypothalamic failure 103
Hypothalamic pituitary-ovarian axis 136
Hypothyroidism 101-103, 108, 108t, 109t, 122

causes of 104
management of 110
primary 103
secondary 103
subclinical 109, 135, 141
tertiary 103

**I**

Iatrogenic injuries 296
Ibuprofen 191
Ileal pouch-anal anastomosis 217
Immune
　aberrations 195
　complexes 284
　deficiency syndrome 335
　response 214
　　cell-mediated 374
　system 101
Immunoglobulin
　G 200
　intravenous 169
Immunosuppressive
　agents 207
　drugs 308, 308t
　state 344
Impulse control disorders 182
In vitro fertilization 265, 414, 419
In vitro maturation 265
Inclusion body myositis 208
India Ukieri Study 40
Indian Academy of Pediatrics 343
Indomethacin 191
Infarction 83
Infection 43, 94, 402, 403
Infertility 165, 329, 420
　causes of 415
　female 415
　management of 415
　treatment 414, 415
Inflammatory cells 376, 384
　infiltration of 359
Inflammatory demyelinating
　diseases 195
　disorders 196
Inflammatory disorders 206
Infliximab 287
Influenza vaccination 344
Inner ear circulation 384
Inositol 124
Insulin
　requirements 94
　resistance 24, 31, 119
　　and diabetes, management of 124

model assessment of 138
pregnancy with 92
therapy 97
Intellectual disability 387
Intercellular adhesion molecules 159
Interferons, types of 200
Interleukins 1 and 6 156
International Association of
　Diabetes and Pregnancy
　Study Groups 90
International Classification of
　Headache Disorders-3 187
International Diabetes
　Federation 89
International League
　of Associations for
　Rheumatology 374
International normalized ratio 275
International Society for Study of
　Hypertension 274
International Society of
　Hypertension 18, 19
International Society of
　Nephrology 285
　Classification 282
Interphalangeal joints and
　wrists, swelling of proximal 148f
Intestinal endocannabinoid
　system 223
Intracellular antigens 201t
　antibody directed
　　against 201
Intracranial pressure 364
Intracytoplasmic sperm
　injection 415
Intranatal screening 168
Intraocular lens 358
Intraocular pressure 364
Intrauterine devices 123, 320
Intrauterine insemination 415, 419
Iodine
　deficiency 101, 103
　therapy 103
Iris 373
　inflammation of 364
Iron 315
Irradiation, external 103
Ischemia 32, 83
　subendocardial 33, 51
Ischemic attacks, transient 207
Ischemic heart disease 31, 32, 34, 35, 51, 82
　risk of 82

stable 34
treatment of 35
Isoniazid 352, 397
Itching 268

**J**

Joints
　apophyseal 149
　interphalangeal 149
Juvenile idiopathic arthritis 374
Juxtacortical demyelinating
　plaque 203f

**K**

Kanamycin 352
Kaposi sarcoma 331
Kawasaki disease 205
Keratitis 362
Keratoconjunctivitis sicca 374
Ketoacidosis, diabetic 94
Ketorolac 191
Kidney
　biopsy 285
　disease, chronic 20, 221, 285, 292, 301
　donors 308
　injury
　　management of acute 296
　　postrenal acute 296
　　pregnancy related acute 291, 292
　transplantation 306
　ultrasonography of 302
Kupffer cells 239

**L**

Labor
　premature 351
　preterm 94
　stage of 75
Labyrinthine vertigo, treatment of 381
Lacosamide 166
Lacrimal apparatus 358
　disorders of 358
Lacrimal disorders 358
Lacrimal gland 359
　function 367
Lactate dehydrogenase 235, 275, 293
*Lactobacillus* 221, 225
　*acidophilus* 226
　*gasseri* 226
Lamina propria 385
Lamotrigine 166, 167
Landry–Guillain–Barré
　syndrome 347

Language deficits 167
Laparoscopy procedure 420
Laryngopathia gravidarum 385
Laryngotracheal trauma 381
Lead 315
Left ventricular
 aneurysm 58
 ejection fraction 39
 systolic dysfunction, severe 79
Lens
 diseases of 358
 disorders of 363
Leptospirosis 335
Lesions, milder 73
Letrozole 416
Leucine-rich glioma-inactivated protein 1 202
Leukemia, acute 264
 lymphoblastic 265
 myeloid 265
Leukocytosis 234
Levetiracetam 166, 167, 169
Levofloxacin 352
Levonorgestrel intrauterine devices 331
Levothyroxine treatment 109$t$
Lids, disorders of 358
Limbic encephalitis 202
Lipid metabolism 127
Lipopolysaccharides 223
Lipoprotein 156
 cholesterol, low-density 15
 levels of low-density 156
 low-density 156, 226
Lithium 397
Liver 129, 234
 biopsy 232, 234
 disease 230, 231
  alcoholic 238, 239
  autoimmune 231
  common 239$t$
  drug-induced 238, 241
  end-stage 239, 347
  hypertension-related 231
  immune-mediated 238, 240
 disorders 230, 231
 donors 247
 enzymes 277
  elevated 235
  values 275
 function test 41, 230, 275, 335, 417
 infarction 231
 injury, drug-induced 239, 241, 245

involvement 277
lesions, benign 239
mass lesions in 241
physiological changes in 230
rupture 231
transaminases 293
transplantation 244, 245, 247
tumors 231
Living donor liver transplantation 246
Living kidney donors 306
Losartan 27
Low birth weight 279
Low-fat mediterranean diet 222
Low-molecular-weight heparin 295, 417
Lung
 biopsy 317
 cancer 313
 crepitations 41
 disease, interstitial 209, 319, 320
 nodules 317
 transplantation 317
Lupus nephritis 282, 284, 285, 295
 diagnosis of 282, 284
 etiopathogenesis of 284
 treatment of 285
Luteinizing hormone 122, 132, 136, 397, 415
 mid-cycle 404
 resulting in 115
 secretion of 131
Lymphadenopathy, hilar 350
Lymphangioleiomyomatosis 313, 316, 318, 318$t$
Lymphatic pulmonary congestion 318

## M

Magnesium sulphate, infusions of 294
Magnetic resonance imaging 257
Malaria 334
Malarial parasite 335
Marfan's syndrome 73, 74, 79, 363
Mass lesions 238
Maternal and fetal demises 234
Maternal body mass index 278
Maternal complications 94
Maternal heart disease 64
Maternal hyperglycemia, uncontrolled 93$t$
Maternal insulin resistance 92

Maternal obesity 222
Maternal organ dysfunction 277
Maternal saturation 73
Maternoplacental syndrome 78, 81
Matrix metalloproteinases 371
Maturity onset diabetes of young 91
McDonald's diagnostic criteria, revised 199$t$
Measles 343
 mumps, rubella 344
Mechanical circulatory support 43
Mechanical thrombectomy 176
Medial temporal lobe hyperintensities, bilateral 204$f$
Medical community 431
Medical officers 412
Medical therapy, guideline-directed 43
Medicamentosa 384
Medication safety 217
Mediterranean diet 225
Medroxyprogesterone 262
Megestrol acetate 262
Meibography 371
Meibomian gland 367
Meibomian gland ducts 368
Meigs syndrome 318
Melanocytic lesions, malignant conjunctival 360
Melanoma, malignant 360
Melasma 395, 395$f$
 diagnosis 395
 differential diagnosis of 395
 presentation 395
 prognosis 396
 treatment 396
Memantine 191
Memory recall 143
Ménière's disease 384
Meningioma 359
Meningitis, aseptic 207
Meningomyelocele 93
Menometrorrhagia 267
Menopausal factors 389
Menopausal hormone therapy 139
Menopausal transition 135, 141
Menopausal women 140, 390
Menopause 31, 102, 135, 136, 138, 142, 218, 424
 and diabetes 136, 138$b$
 and osteoporosis 139
 correlated significantly 136

# Index

decision-support
    algorithm 139
  premature 165, 268
  timing of 137
  type of 137
Menorrhagia 267
Menstrual cycle 165*f*, 388, 397, 404
  phases, track of 165
Menstrual disorders 329, 331
Menstrual dysfunction 391
Menstrual function 316
Menstrual hygiene 402, 404
  scheme 412
Menstrual irregularity 22, 131
  management of 123
Menstrual migraine 189
  diagnostic criteria for 190*t*
Menstrual problems 402, 404
Menstruation 216, 402, 407
Mental health 387, 420
  and illnesses 388
  disparities 392
  issues 403, 405
  professional, role of 421
Mental illnesses 387
Mental status, altered 277
Mental stress 31
Mercaptopurine 217
Mesial temporal lobe epilepsy 164
Metabolic diseases 231, 241
Metabolic disorders 40
Metabolic dysfunction 117
Metabolic syndrome 158, 240
Metabolite
  estradiol exerts proconvulsant 164
  microbiota-derived 222
Metastatic disease 255, 256
Metatarsophalangeal joint 149, 151
Metformin 124, 227, 417
Metoclopramide 191, 384
Metoprolol 191
Metrorrhagia 267
Microangiopathic hemolytic anemia 293, 294
Microgenderome 216
Microsomal enzyme induction, degree of 166
Microvesicular steatosis 233, 234
Midlife depression, risk factors for 390
Migraine 82, 84, 84*f*, 187, 190, 191
  attack 83*f*

burden of 83
during breastfeeding 191*t*
headache 53, 85, 188
in perimenopausal
  period 191
  state 189
in pregnant women 189
management of 83
pain, reduction in 84
pathophysiology of 82, 188, 191
prevalence of 189
prevention of 83
prognosis of 190
prophylaxis, future of 85
risk factors for 83
role of hormones in 189
treatment 84
types of 188
  with aura 83, 84*t*, 188
  without aura 188
    menstrually-related 190
    pure menstrual 190
Miliary dissemination 350
Mineralocorticoid receptor antagonist 42
Minimal change disease 286
Minocycline 395
Minoxidil, topical 399
Miscarriage 329, 331, 351
  increased risk of 152
Misoprostol 332
Mississippi protocol 235
Mitochondrial enhancer 44
Mitochondrial trifunctional protein 233
Mitoxantrone 200
Mitral annular calcification 21
Mitral regurgitation 59, 63, 66
Mitral stenosis 58, 64, 66
Molecular studies 232
Monoamine oxidase 181
Monoclonal antibodies 84
Mood disorders 117
Mortality 73
Mother-to-child transmission, risk of 332
Motility 215
Mouth, dryness of 303
Movement disorder 180, 183, 207
Moxifloxacin 304
Mucosal edema 383
Mucous gland hypertrophy 314
Multidisciplinary care 151
Multidrug-resistant tuberculosis 351-353

Multifactorial disorder 366
Multifocal choroiditis 376
Multifunctional organ, largest 394
Multiple gestation 44, 277
Multiple pregnancies 419
Multiple sclerosis 132, 196, 198-200, 375
  clinical features of 197, 198*t*
  diagnostic criteria of 199*t*
  investigations 197
  pathogenesis of 196
  prevalence 196
  primary progressive 197
  progressive-relapsing 197
  relapsing-remitting 197
  secondary progressive 197
  treatment protocol for 198
  types of 196
Mumps 343
Murmur 41
Muromonab-CD3 308
Muscle function, abdominal 385
Musculoskeletal complications 208
Musculoskeletal pain, chronic 150
Musculoskeletal system 93
Myalgias 208
Mycophenolate 247
  mofetil 209, 308
  sodium, enteric-coated 308
Myelin oligodendrocyte glycoprotein 198
Myelopathy 207
  transverse 207
Myocardial dysfunction 157
Myocardial infarction 22, 32*t*, 33*fc*, 51, 81, 157
  acute 53
  history of 40
Myocardial ischemia, risk of 157
Myocarditis 40, 63, 156, 209
Myoclonus-dystonia 183
Myoma 131
Myopathy
  idiopathic inflammatory 208
  inflammatory idiopathic 319
Myopia 363
Myositis 319

# N

Nadolol 191
Nailfold capillary changes 208
Naproxen 191
Nasal changes 384
Nasal discharge 379

Nasal obstruction 379
Nasolacrimal duct 358
Natalizumab 200
National blood cell incharge 429
National Blood Transfusion
    Committee 429
National Council of Educational
    Research and Training 411
National Education Programme
    411
National Eye Institute 370
National Family Health
    Survey 403
National Health and Nutrition
    Examination Survey 83, 137
National Institute of Health 118
National Institute of Open
    Schooling 411
National Level Health Programs
    411
National Tuberculosis Control
    Programme, revised 352
Natriuretic peptides 41
Necrosis, acute cortical 296
Necrotizing autoimmune
    myositis 208
Neoadjuvant chemotherapy
    255, 260
Neonatal complications 94
Neonatal unit care 279
Neoplasms 335
Nephritis, interstitial 301
Nephropathy 25
    diabetic 94
Nervous system 195
    peripheral 206
    sympathetic 41
Neural tube defects 93, 167
Neurocognitive health 128,
    142
Neurodegenerative
    diseases 143
Neuroendocrine 388
Neuroimmunological disorders
    195, 196
Neuroimmunology 195
Neurological complications 277
Neurological disorders 180
Neurology outpatient
    department 187
Neuromyelitis optica 195, 196,
    198
    clinical features of 198*t*
    diagnostic criteria of 199*t*,
        200*t*
    spectrum disorders 196, 200
Neuronal injury, prevent 83

Neuro-ophthalmologic
    abnormalities 364
    disorders 358
Neuropathy 25
Nitrates 50
Nitric oxide 188
Nitrogen dioxide 315
Nitroglycerine mediated
    dilation 159
N-methyl-D-aspartate 165
    receptors 164, 202
Nodular scleritis 361*f*
Nodules
    autonomously functioning 105
    benign 105
Nonalcoholic fatty liver disease
    114, 220, 231, 238-240
    prevalence of 117
Nonalcoholic steatohepatitis
    240, 245
Noncardiac structural
    anomalies 73
Noncommunicable diseases, rise
    of 173
Noncontraceptive health 131
Nonerosive reflux disease 214
Nonhereditary ovarian
    cancer 260
Non-Hodgkin's lymphoma 264,
    331
Noninfectious keratitis 362
Noninfectious uveitis 373
    with systemic involvement
        374
    without systemic involvement
        375
Noninvasive breakup time 368
Nonmotor symptoms 182
Nonobstructive coronary artery
    disease 31, 32
Nonpharmacologic measures 24
Non-ST segment elevation
    myocardial infarction 35
Nonsteroidal anti-inflammatory
    drug 84, 157, 158, 417
    minimizing 159
Nortriptyline 191
Nose problems, common 380
Nutcracker esophagus 214
Nutritional deficiencies 403, 404

## O

Obesity 22, 116, 142, 220, 222*t*,
    223, 224, 227, 240
    abdominal 22
    increased risk of 222

Obsessive-compulsive disorder
    389
Obstetrics and gynecology 432
Obstructive lesions,
    symptomatic 79
Obstructive sleep apnea 114,
    117, 122
Obstructive uropathy 296
Ocrelizumab 200
Ocular conjunctival melanocytic
    lesions 360
Ocular exocrine dysfunction,
    evidence of 208
Ocular morbidities, non-life-
    threatening 357
Ocular surface
    assessment 370
    disease index 368, 369*f*
    inflammation 366, 371
    squamous neoplasia 360, 361*f*
Offspring complications 74
Oligoclonal immunoglobulin,
    synthesis of 198
Oligometastatic disease 255
Omphalocele 93
Onabotulinum toxin A 191
Onconeural antibody-mediated
    autoimmune encephalitis
    203
Oocyte cryopreservation 266
Open angle glaucoma 363
Operational taxonomic unit 225
Optic nerve 374
    inflammation of 364
Optic neuritis 364
Optic neuropathy, ischemic 207
Oral anticoagulants 74
Oral antihypertensive 279
Oral cancer 424
Oral cavity changes 384
Oral conjugated estrogen, effect
    of 138
Oral contraceptive 22, 364
    and risk of
        malignancies 132
        strokes 174
    effect of 127
    estrogen 374
    pills 50, 123, 131, 152, 323,
        423
    treatment remains 124
Oral health concerns 423
Oral hypoglycemic agents 97
Oral immunosuppressives 399
Oral infections and tooth
    decay 423
Orbit, disorders of 358

Organic heart valve 63
Orthopnea 41
Osteoarthritis 149
Osteoporosis 246, 264, 268
   treatment of 140
Otalgia 379
Otolaryngorhinology 379
Otosclerosis 383
Outpatient department 329
Ovarian cancer 132, 258, 259
   recurrent 260
   risk of 131, 260
   syndrome, hereditary 258
Ovarian cysts 131
Ovarian failure, primary 122
Ovarian hyperstimulation
     syndrome 265, 416
   management of 417
   prevention of 417
   risk of 415
Ovarian hyperthecosis 142
Ovarian rupture 417
Ovarian sex-cord stromal
     tumors 142
Ovarian tissue cryopreservation
     and reimplantation 266
Ovarian transposition 266
Ovarian twisting 417
Ovary, metastases to 142
Overlap syndromes 157
Overt hypothyroidism 109
Overweight
   and obesity 22
   subjects, treatment for 24
Ovulation disorder 415
Ovulation drugs-induced side
     effects 419
Ovulation induction 415
   drugs 415
Ovulatory dysfunction 116
Oxcarbazepine 166, 167
Oxford-Family Planning
     Association 133
Oxidative stress 363
Oxygen and ventilatory
     support 43
Oxytocin 388

## P

P2Y12 inhibitors 53
Packed cell volume 417
Pain 268
   abdominal 234
   chronic 150
   epigastric abdominal 277
   genitopelvic 392
Painless thyroiditis 103

Palpitations 57
Parieto-occipital cortices 204
Parkinson's disease 181
   clinical features 181
   epidemiology 181
   management issues 181
Parkinsonism 180
Paroxysmal nocturnal
     dyspnea 41
Paroxysmal vertigo 381
Patchy transverse myelitis 197
Patent ductus arteriosus 58, 71,
   74, 79, 93
Patent foramen ovale 57, 84
Patulous eustachian tube 383
Peer Education Program 411
Pelvic inflammatory disease
   131, 329, 403
   chronic 353
Pelvis, imaging of 415
Pemphigoid gestationis 400
Penetration disorder 392
Penicillin 384
Peptic ulcer disease 213
Perampanel 166
Percutaneous coronary
     intervention 36
   primary 50
   related complications 52
Percutaneous mitral balloon
     valvuloplasty 58
Percutaneous therapy 60
Pericarditis 40, 42, 63
Peridiskal neovascularization
   206
Perimenopausal women 170
Perineal injuries 94
Pertinent hemato-oncological
     issues 264
Pharmacological therapy 24, 97
Pharmacotherapy 421
Phenobarbitone 166
Phenols 315
Phenytoin 166, 167, 397
Physical activity 24, 96
Physical development 402
Physical inactivity 22
Physically active 26
Pinguecula 359
Pituitary tumor 103
Placental abruption 294
Placental defects 294
Placental growth
     factor 277
   hormone, secretion of 91
Plasma
   exchange 293

   regain, rapid 283
   volume 230
Plasmapheresis 234
Plasminogen activator
     inhibitor-1 128
*Plasmodium vivax* 335
Platelet 293
   aggregation 82
   count 235, 275, 277, 293, 294
     low 94, 235
   dysfunction 156
   transfusions 295
Pneumonia 42
Pneumothorax 350
   catamenial 317
Polyangiitis 205
   microscopic 362
Polyarteritis nodosa 205, 362
Polychondritis, relapsing 362
Polycyclic aromatic
     hydrocarbons 315
Polycystic ovarian disease 22,
   31, 391
Polycystic ovarian syndrome
   114, 117, 118, 118$t$, 120, 122,
   125, 142, 165, 397, 414
   clinical presentation 116
   complications in 122$t$
   core components of 115$f$
   diagnostic approach to 118
   differential diagnosis of 117
   management 123
   pathophysiology 115
   phenotypes of 118$t$
   women with 120$t$
Polycythemia 94
Polydipsia 234
Polyhydramnios 94
Polymorphic eruption 400
Polymyositis 208, 319
Polypill 26
   advantages of 26
Polyuria 234
Polyvinyl alcohol 371
Post-fibrinolysis 36
Postinflammatory
     hyperpigmentation 395
Post-liver transplantation state
   231
Postmenopausal
     hyperandrogenism 141
   causes of 142$t$
Postmenopausal women 35, 137
Post-myocardial infarction 31
Postnasal drip 379
Postnatal care and
     breastfeeding 169

Postpartum 279
　bleeding 294
　cardiomyopathy 40
　care 98
　hypertension 313
　major depression 389
　psychiatric disorders 389
　psychosis 389
　pulmonary hypertension 317
　thyroiditis 103
Postprandial glucose values 138
Potential reproductive
　consequences 163
Pramipexole 181
Prebiotics 225
Prednisolone 308
Preeclampsia 31, 44, 53, 78, 81,
　82, 94, 231, 234, 276, 277,
　278b, 293, 321
　antenatal 279
　conditions 277b
　diagnostic criteria of 293
　prediction of 277
　pregnant patients 83
　prevention of 277
　prior 277
Pregabalin 166
Pregnancy 136, 217, 230, 315
　and cardiac disease 66
　and congenital heart
　　disease 73
　and coronary intervention 53
　and eye 364
　and heart 78
　　failure 44
　and postpartum 102
　and rheumatological illness
　　151
　and stroke 175
　complications 152
　counseling 320
　dermatosis 399
　　treatment 400
　disorders, hypertensive 81
　ectopic 417
　implications for 340
　normal 73
　outcome, predictors of 295
　related factors 388
　rhinitis 384
　risks 152
　teenage 402, 403, 408
　tubal 417
　tumor 384
Premenopausal females 52
Premenopausal women,
　symptomatic 34

Premenstrual syndrome 131
Prenatal care 337
Prenatal counseling 168
Prenatal factors 388
Prepregnancy planning 95
Presbycusis 380
Preterm births 152
Primary disease, progressive 350
Primidone 166
Primigravida 44
Proangiogenic mediators,
　concentration of 294
Probiotics 226
Prochlorperazine 191
Professional Society Leaders 431
Progesterone 314, 388, 418
　only contraceptives 129
　receptor 255
Progestin only pills 123
Proinflammatory cytokines 156
Prolactin 101, 388, 415
　inhibitors, role of 44
Proliferative obliteration 156
Propranolol 191
Proptosis, bilateral axial 359f
Prostatitis 302
Prosthetic valves 79
Protein excretion, estimation
　of 275
Proteinuria 234, 274, 277, 293
Prothrombin time 234
Proton pump inhibitor 215, 227
Pruritus gravidarum 400
Psychological disturbances 114
Psychotherapy 421
Pterygium 359, 360f
　development of 359
　prevalence of 359
Pubertal factors 388
Puberty and menstruation 101
Pubic hair, growth of 402
Pulmonary arterial hypertension
　157, 313, 320
Pulmonary crackles 38
Pulmonary edema 42, 78, 293
Pulmonary embolism 42
Pulmonary function test 317
Pulmonary hypertension 42, 69,
　71, 79, 317
　severe 79
Pulmonary hypoplasia 93
Pulmonary stenosis 71, 74, 80
Pulmonary thromboembolism
　323, 313
Pulmonary vascular
　disease 72
　　obstructive 72

Pulmonology 313
Pulse, irregular 41
Pulseless disease 205
Punctate inner choroidopathy
　376
Purkinje cell cytoplasmic
　antibody type 1 201
Pyelonephritis 338
　acute 307
　chronic 301
Pyrazinamide 352

## Q

Q-fever 335

## R

Radiation
　chemotherapeutic
　　agents 40
　therapy 257
Radioiodine therapy 101, 103
Radiotherapy 255, 264
Ramipril 74
Rapamycin, mechanistic target
　of 317
Rasagiline 181
Rashtriya Kishor Swasthya
　Karyakram 411
Raynaud's phenomenon 151,
　208
Refraction 364
Refractive errors 363
Refractive surgery 364
Regurgitant lesions 80
Regurgitation, aortic 63
Renal abnormality 276
Renal agenesis 93
Renal angiomyolipomas 316,
　318
Renal calculi 296, 302
Renal deterioration 307
Renal disease 278
Renal dysfunction 246
Renal failure 234
　acute 291
Renal function 36
　test 41, 335, 417
Renal insufficiency 42
Renal Pathology Society 285
　classification 282
Renal transplant, challenges
　of 306
Renal transplantation 309
Renin–angiotensin–aldosterone
　system 41
Reproductive and sexual
　dysfunction 165

# Index

Reproductive health 332
Reproductive tract infections 329
Respiratory diseases 313, 314, 316, 319
  treatment 322
Respiratory system 316
Retina 374
  diseases of 264, 358
  posterior pole of 376
Retinal artery occlusion 207
Retinal vasculitis 375
Retinitis pigmentosa, treatment of 364
Retinoids, topical 397
Retinopathy 25
  acute zonal occult outer 376
Retroperitoneal infection 335
Reynolds risk score 18
Rheumatic diseases 147, 151, 153
  and safety 153*t*
  inflammatory 147
Rheumatic disorders 147
Rheumatic fever 67, 335
  acute 63
Rheumatic heart disease 39, 63, 64, 75, 81
  A to Z of 63
Rheumatic valvular lesion 64
Rheumatoid arthritis 20, 132, 148, 149*t*, 155, 156, 158, 319, 335, 360, 368, 375
  disease activity 152
Rheumatoid factor 148
Rheumatological diseases 150
Rhinitis, atrophic 380
Riboflavin 191
Rifampicin 352
Ringing sensation 380
Rituximab 286
Rontalizumab 287
Ropinirole 181
*Roseburia* 224
Roux-en-Y gastric bypass 228
Rubella 338, 339, 343
  syndrome, congenital 70
Rufinamide 166

## S

Salicylic acid 396
Salpingo-oophorectomy, bilateral 260, 261
Salzmann's nodular degeneration 361
Sarcoidosis 335, 375, 376
Schirmer test 370
Schistocytes 294
Schizophrenia 387
Sclera
  diseases of 358
  disorders of 359
Scleritis 360
Sclerodactyly 208
Scleroderma 208
Sclerosing cholangitis, primary 231, 239, 240
Sclerosis, benign multiple 197
Score risk charts 15
Sebaceous cell carcinoma 359
Seborrhea 119
Sedentary lifestyle 222
Seizure
  control 168
  cyclic exacerbation of 164
  exacerbation, risk for 169
  management of 169*fc*
Selective estrogen receptor modulators 140, 416
Selegiline 181, 182
Sepsis 42, 294
Septicemia 335
Serological testing 337
Seropositive cases 337
Serotonin reuptake inhibitor, selective 216, 318, 388
Serum 122
  albumin 275
  anti-müllerian hormone 121
  bilirubin 275
  creatinine 234, 275, 277
  electrolytes 41
  iron profile 41
  triglyceride levels 127
  uric acid 277
Sex hormone 163
  affecting autoimmune response, role of 373
  binding globulin 115, 131, 132, 388
  levels of 136
  female 176
Sex specific differences 70
Sexual abuse 408
Sexual activity 407
Sexual and reproductive health 410
Sexual attraction 392
Sexual behavior 392, 410
Sexual function assessment 268
Sexual health 264
  assessment 268
Sexual identity 392
Sexual minority 392
Sexual orientation 407
Sexual reproduction 407
Sexual reproductive health 410
Sexuality education 407, 409, 410, 412
  content of 409
  delivery of 409
  evolution of 408
  role of media in 410
Sexually transmitted disease 299, 334, 340, 403
  prevention 411
Sexually transmitted infections 329, 402, 407, 408
Sheehan's syndrome 103
Shock 82
  cardiogenic 43
Sifalimumab 287
Sildenafil 418
Silica 315
Sinusitis 384
Siponimod 200
Sirolimus 308, 317
Sjögren's syndrome 150, 208, 367, 368
  primary 151, 319
Skeletal muscle 234
Skin
  ailments 394
  disorders 394
  tags 119
Sleep
  behavior disorder 181
  sisturbed 181
Small vessel 158
  vasculitis 205
Smoking 22
  avoidance and cessation 23
Social issues 170
Social media 410
Sociocultural effects 315
Socioeconomic factors and gender barriers 350
Sodium fluoride 384
Solifenacin 303
Somatic nociception 215
Spina bifida 93
Spironolactone 42, 124, 399
Spondyloarthropathy 150, 156, 157
Spotting 419
Squamous cell carcinoma 359
*Staphylococcus saprophyticus* 299
Statin 23, 50, 83
  use of 176

Status epilepticus, management of 169fc
Stenotic lesions 80
Steroid
  low-dose 153
  sex hormones 423
  sparing agent 209
Streptomycin 352
Stress
  challenges 388
  tests 35t
Stroke 17, 25, 173, 174, 207, 277
  cryptogenic 57
  ischemic 83, 176, 316
  issues of 173
  occupy 173
  primary prevention of 26
  risk 174
  volume 65
Structural birth defects 93t
Structural heart
  disease 3, 56, 60
    spectrum of 56
    treatment of 59
  interventions 59
ST-segment elevation myocardial infarction 35
Sudden cardiac
  arrest 82
  death 82, 83
Sudden death 24
Sudden infant death syndrome 315
Sulfasalazine 153
Sulfur dioxide 315
Sumatriptan 191
Surgery 254
  and radiation 261
    therapy 257, 259
Swansea criteria 233
Sydenham's chorea 183
Symbiotics, use of 222
Syphilis 340
  congenital 340
  primary 329
  secondary 335
Systematic coronary risk evaluation 15-17, 158
Systemic dentistry 424
Systemic lupus erythematosus 148, 150, 155, 157, 205, 206, 207, 267, 278, 282, 283t, 284, 295, 319, 335, 360, 374
  diagnosis of 282
Systemic lupus international collaborating clinics 282, 283

Systemic sclerosis 151, 152, 155, 157, 208, 319
Systemic therapy 255
Systemic treatment 259
Systemic vascular resistance 65

## T

Tachyarrhythmias 80
Tachycardia 41
  ventricular 83
Tachypnea 41
Tacrolimus 308
Takayasu arteritis 205
Taxonomy 32
Tazarotene 397
T-cell 373
  target 287
Tear
  breakup time 368
  cytokines 371
  film 367
    homeostasis 366
    stability 368
  meniscometry 370
  meniscus 370
  volume 370
Telangiectasias, cutaneous 208
Telogen effluvium 398, 399
Teratogenicity 167
Teriflunomide 200
Terrien's marginal degeneration 361
Tetanus 335, 343
  diphtheria 344
  and pertussis 344
Tetralogy of Fallot 72, 74
Therapeutic lifestyle changes 23
Thermoregulation, role in 394
Thoracentesis 317
Thoracic endometriosis 317
Thoracoscopic surgery, video-assisted 317, 318
Thorough history taking 299
Throat problems, common 380
Thrombocytopenia 276, 277, 293
  therapy-induced 267
Thromboembolism 206, 335
Thrombolysis 175
  safety of 176
Thrombophilia 53
Thrombotic microangiopathy 223, 286
Thrombotic thrombocytopenic purpura 285, 295
Thyroid
  and menopause 140

antithyroglobulin antibody 110
  autoantibodies 104, 109
  binding globulin 107
  cancer 105, 106, 112
  disease 40, 100, 368
    autoimmune 104
    etiology of 140
    management of 110, 140
  disorders 100-102, 403, 404
    anatomical 105
    autoimmune 101
    functional 102
  disturbances 364
  dysfunction 100
    causes of 103t
    risk factors for 104b
  eye disease 358, 359, 359f
  function 101
    abnormal 102
    interpretation of 107
  function test 41, 110
    interpretation of 103t
  gland 101, 107
  hormone, regulation of 101f
  nodules 105
  peroxidase 103
  physiology during pregnancy 106, 107t
  stimulating activity 292
  stimulating hormone 101f, 103, 107-110, 359, 415
    level 140
    receptor antibodies 100
    trimester-specific 108t
Thyroidectomy 103
Thyroiditis 70
  atrophic 103
  autoimmune 101
  subacute 103
Thyrotoxicosis 103, 110
Thyrotropin-releasing hormone 101f
Thyroxine 103, 107, 110
Tiagabine 166
Tinnitus 379, 380
Tocilizumab 157, 287
Tocolytic pulmonary edema 319
Tooth decay and infections 424
Topiramate 166, 167, 191
TORCH infections 338
Total cholesterol 13
Tourette syndrome 183
Toxic
  adenoma 103
  cardiomyopathy 40
  nodular goiter 103

# Index

Toxoplasmosis 337, 338
Transformation zone, large loop excision of 330
Transforming growth factor-β 165
Transfusion medicine 426, 429
Transgender women 392
Transvaginal ultrasonography 258
Transvaginal ultrasound 397
Transverse myelitis, longitudinally extensive 200
Treatment regimen 352*t*
Tremor, essential 182
Tretinoin 397
Trichloroacetic acid 396
Triglycerides 16
Triiodothyronine 100, 102, 107, 110
  N-oxide 222, 223*f*
Trivalent influenza vaccine 344
Trivandrum Heart Failure Registry 40
Truncus arteriosus 93
Tubal patency 415
Tuberculoma 350
Tuberculosis 313, 322, 323, 329, 330, 334, 335, 337, 338, 349, 351, 352
  advance diagnostic techniques 353
  and breastfeeding 351
  and pregnancy 350
  burden 349
  clinical manifestations of 350
  diagnosis of 353
  drug-resistant 323, 352*t*
  drug-susceptible 352*t*
  impact of 351
  increases risk of 351
  negative impact of 352
  newborns of mothers with 351
  notification of 353
  pulmonary complications of 350
  treatment of 351, 353
  women mortality to 349*t*
Tuberous sclerosis complex 316
Tubo-ovarian masses 329
Tubular atrophy 285
Tumor necrosis factor 246
  alpha 156
Typhoid 334, 344

## U

Ulcer, corneal 362
Ulcerative colitis 216
Ulcerative keratitis, peripheral 362
Ultrasonography 122
Umbilical artery, abnormal 277
Unhealthy diet 22
Universal Immunization Programme 343
Ureter 296
  duplication 93
  ultrasonography of 302
Uric acid 275
  high 234
Urinalysis
  and culture 335
  and microscopy 275
Urinary tract
  anatomy 299*f*
  lower 300
    symptoms, causes of 300*f*
Urinary tract infection 94, 298, 299, 301, 334, 335, 337, 391, 402
  bacterial 307
  challenges of 298
  management of 305
Urine
  dipstick 302*f*
  human chorionic gonadotropin 122
  postvoid residual 302
  routine examination 301
Uroflow patterns 303
Urticarial vasculitis, hypocomplementemic 205
Uterine artery doppler 277
Uterine bleeding
  abnormal 264
  management of abnormal 267
Uterine pathology, local 52
Uteroplacental dysfunction 277
Uvea
  diseases of 358, 364
  inflammation of 373
Uveitis 364, 373, 375
  causes of 374
  role of gender in 376

## V

Vaccination, adolescent 343
Vaccine 344
  mandatory 343
  preventable diseases 343
Vaginal bleeding, abnormal 267
Vaginal delivery 75, 234, 307
Vaginal scarring, management of 268
Vaginitis 302
Valproate 166, 167
Valproic acid 191
Valvar obstruction 80
Valve surgery 66
Valvular heart disease 40, 58, 63, 80
Valvular lesions during pregnancy 66
Varicella 344
  vaccine 344
  zoster immunoglobulin 344
Vascular complications 82
Vascular disease 158
Vascular endothelial growth factor 294, 317
Vascular function, assessment of 159
Vascular thromboembolism, risk of 128
Vasculitic disorders 195, 205
Vasculitis 158, 205
  primary 205
  secondary 206
Vasomotor disorders 32
Vasomotor symptoms, treatment of 137
Vasospasm myocarditis, coronary 33
Venous thromboembolism 138, 320
Ventricular dysfunction 74, 80
  right 42
Ventricular function postpartum 80
Ventricular septal defect 57, 74, 79, 93
Verbal intelligence 167
Vertigo 82
  and women 381
Vessel disease, triple 51
Vessels pulse wave velocity, peripheral 159
Vestibular rehabilitation 381
Vigabatrin 166
Vigorous-intensity exercise 24
Vijaya's echo criteria 9
Violence and staying safe 409
Viral hepatitis 238, 240, 334, 336
Viral infections 335
Virgo classification system 32*t*
Visceral nociception 215
Visceral stimuli, central processing of 216
Vision-threatening complications 374
Visual disability, permanent 363

Visual impairment 357
  severe 373
Visual scotomata, persistent 277
Vitamin
  A deficiency 360
  B6 232
  D 83
Vitreous 376
Vitritis 375
Vogt–Koyanagi–Harada
  disease 375
Voiding symptoms, evaluation
  of 300
Volatile organic compounds 315
Vomiting 234
von Willebrand factor 295
Vulvovaginal candidiasis 329

## W

Weakness 69
Wegener granulomatosis 362
Weight gain
  insufficient 351
  restricting 96
Weight loss 24
Weight reduction 123
Weill–Marchesani
  syndrome 363
White dot syndromes 376
White-coat hypertension 274, 278
Widal test 335
Wilson's disease 184, 231, 241, 242, 245
Woman's body 383

Women empowerment 352
Women's health 387
  across nation 142
Women's ischemia syndrome
  evaluation 32
World Health Organization
  17-19, 130, 139, 163, 226, 408

## X

X chromosome inactivation 101

## Y

Yentl syndrome 33, 36

## Z

Zoledronic acid 256
Zonisamide 166, 167